HOW TO
SURVIVE
A PANDEMIC

Also by Michael Greger, MD, FACLM

How Not to Die

How Not to Die Cookbook

How Not to Diet

The How Not to Diet Cookbook
(December 2020)

HOW TO
SURVIVE
A PANDEMIC

MICHAEL GREGER,
MD, FACLM

AFTERWORD BY
KENNEDY SHORTRIDGE,
PH.D., DSC(HON), CBIOL, FIBIOL

bluebird
books for life

First published 2020 by Flatiron Books

First published in the UK 2020 Bluebird
an imprint of Pan Macmillan
The Smithson, 6 Briset Street, London, EC1M 5NR
Associated companies throughout the world
www.panmacmillan.com

ISBN 978-1-5290-5491-0

3 5 7 9 8 6 4

A CIP catalogue record for this book is available from the British Library.

Printed and bound by CPI Group (UK) Ltd, Croydon, CR0 4YY

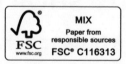

Visit **www.panmacmillan.com** to read more about all our books
and to buy them. You will also find features, author interviews and
news of any author events, and you can sign up for e-newsletters
so that you're always first to hear about our new releases.

In honor of Dr. Li Wenliang, 1986–2020

Contents

Preface

After I graduated from medical school, I went to work in a public health hospital. It housed a maximum-security prison unit, a homeless shelter, and one of the last few locked tuberculosis wards in the country. It was like practicing medicine on a Doctors Without Borders mission, only right in the Boston suburbs.

The hospital also had an entire floor dedicated to AIDS patients. This was before the revolution in HIV antiviral drugs, and victims were dying of all manner of bizarre, horrifying infections. With their immune systems ravaged, they fell prey to fungal pneumonias, parasitic brain diseases, and purulent tumors that looked like cauliflower when they erupted from their skin. Throughout my medical training, I had never seen anything more heart-wrenching. What was an infectious disease specialist's dream was a patient's nightmare.

I can still see their sunken eyes. Often, the best I could offer was just morphine and massage. When I was growing up, there was no such thing as HIV/AIDS. *Where did this virus come from?* The question echoed in my head as I tended to patient after patient. That question fueled my interest in emerging infectious disease.

Today I am largely known for my achievements in lifestyle medicine, but years before I launched NutritionFacts.org and shifted my focus to the study of chronic illness, it was my infectious disease work that formed the bulk of my scientific publications and afforded me the opportunities to testify before Congress, appear on *The Colbert Report,* and help defend Oprah Winfrey in that infamous meat defamation trial. Many are surprised to learn that *How Not to Die* was my fourth book, not my first, and the one immediately prior was on preventing and surviving pandemic disease.

The current coronavirus crisis provided the impetus—and time—to revisit that body of work. I was in the midst of a two-hundred-city speaking tour for *How Not to Diet,* my most recent book, when COVID-19 started spreading around the globe. I was sadly disappointed my lectures and travel had to be suspended, but it enabled me to seize this opportunity to once again dive deep into the literature on pandemic preparedness to bring you the latest science amid so much of the prevailing noise and nonsense.

The time is not for panic but for common-sense measures to protect your family and community both now and in the future against emergent outbreaks.

The current coronavirus pandemic may just be a dress rehearsal for the coming plague. Decades ago, a flu virus was discovered in chickens—H5N1—that would forever change our understanding of how bad pandemics could get. It was a flu virus that appeared capable of killing more than half the people it infected. Imagine if a virus like that started explosively spreading from human to human. Consider a pandemic a hundred times worse than COVID-19, one with a fatality rate not of one in two hundred but rather a coin flip of one in two. Thankfully, H5N1 has so far remained a virus mainly of poultry, not people, but H5N1 and other new and deadly animal viruses like it are still out there, still mutating, with an eye on the eight-billion-strong buffet of human hosts. With pandemics, it's never a matter of if, but when. A universal outbreak with more than a few percent mortality wouldn't just threaten financial markets but civilization itself as we know it.

This book contains what you need to know to protect yourself and your family from the current threat, but it also digs deeper into the roots of the problem and tackles the fundamental question: *How can we stop the emergence of pandemic viruses in the first place?* If there is one concept to draw from my work on preventing and reversing chronic disease, it's that we must—whenever possible—*treat the cause.*

Prologue

On December 30, 2019, Dr. Li Wenliang, an ophthalmologist at Wuhan Central Hospital in the Hubei province of China, messaged his fellow physicians, alerting them to the appearance of a concerning cluster of pneumonia cases. In response, he was summoned to the Public Security Bureau and reprimanded for "spreading rumors" and "making false statements that disturbed the public order." Thirty-nine days later, after becoming infected with the very virus he had tried to warn his colleagues about, he was dead at age thirty-three.[1] By that time, the disease had already spread to dozens of countries.[2]

His initial message read "7 SARS cases confirmed at Hua'nan Seafood Market."[3] SARS stands for *severe acute respiratory syndrome,* which, seventeen years earlier, had been the first deadly global outbreak known to be triggered by a coronavirus. (Sadly, the doctor who first alerted the world to that epidemic, Carlo Urbani, also succumbed to the disease.[4]) Coronaviruses are named for their crown-like appearance under an electron microscope—from the Latin *corona* for "crown," as in coronation—due to a fringe of protein spikes that radiate from the surface.[5] Before the outbreak of SARS in 2002, only two coronaviruses were known to cause disease in humans, and both caused little more than the common cold.[6] But the SARS coronavirus went on to kill about one in ten people it infected.[7]

A decade later, in 2012, another deadly coronavirus emerged: the Middle East respiratory syndrome coronavirus. Like SARS, MERS spread to infect thousands across dozens of countries, but this time, one in three died.[8] Imagine if a disease like that went viral and caused a pandemic. COVID-19 is the third deadly human coronavirus to emerge since the turn of the century.

Emerge from where? Where do new infectious diseases come from? All human viral infections are believed to originate in animals.[9]

The Emergence of MERS

Most human coronaviruses appear to have arisen originally in bats,[10] which make good viral hosts. Up to two hundred thousand can crowd together in dense roosting colonies, and they can fly more than a thousand miles, acquiring and spreading new viral strains.[11] Their unique navigational tool—echolocation—may even facilitate bat-to-bat transmission by spraying out respiratory secretions.[12] Bats are considered the primordial hosts, the "gene pool" from which genetic fragments of coronaviruses can mix and match,[13] but breaching the species barrier to infect people appears to have involved intermediate hosts in whom coronaviruses can adapt, amplify, and access human populations.[14] In the case of MERS, the intermediate hosts were found to be camels.[15]

A bat in Saudi Arabia was found carrying the MERS coronavirus,[16] but it is contact with the bodily fluids of infected camels—particularly their nasal secretions—that is considered the major risk factor for human infection. Once camels infect people, MERS can then be spread human-to-human.[17] Those in the camel business denied the link between MERS and camel exposure, responding to the government warnings that those in close camel contact "wear proper personal protective equipment at all times" with a social media campaign entitled Kiss Your Camel.[18]

But we domesticated camels three thousand years ago.[19] What happened to turn camel slobber into a potential kiss of death? Archived samples of camel blood show MERS had long been circulating in them for decades before spilling over into the human population.[20] Why now?

Camels used to be allowed to forage outdoors, but as more and more camels were being raised, desertification from overgrazing forced the industry to transition to thousands of camel farms using enclosed, high-density housing systems where they were confined indoors. The high-intensity contact between camels alongside their workers is thought to be what helped drive the spillover of the MERS coronavirus from camels to humans. By 2011, open grazing was completely banned in Qatar, the Middle Eastern country with the highest camel density. The next year, the first human cases of MERS were reported.[21]

The Emergence of SARS

Before MERS, there was SARS, the first new global disease outbreak of the twenty-first century.[22] Many of the first cases of SARS were tied to the same kind of place most of the first cases of COVID-19 appeared to come from: live animal "wet" markets in China.[23,24]

Freshly slaughtered animals are thought to be more nutritious by many regional consumers,[25] and some seek *ye wei,* the "wild taste," believing the consumption of exotic animals bestows benefits to health and social status.[26] This combination leads to a perfect storm for zoonotic—animal-to-human—disease transmission, where crowded cages in these markets are contaminated with the blood, urine, and feces of countless species mixed together in a potential cauldron of contagion.[27]

There was a vast expansion of the wildlife trade in the 1990s to supply the emerging urban middle-class demand in China.[28] Many of the wild animals, typically while still alive, entered China through Vietnam from Lao PDR (commonly known as Laos), where the wildlife meat trade rose to become the second-largest income source for rural families.[29] A study of a single Laotian market estimated the annual sale of eight to ten thousand of at least twenty-three different types of mammals, six to seven thousand of more than thirty-three types of birds, and three to four thousand reptiles, for a total weight exceeding thirty-six tons.[30]

As demand surpassed supply, the transboundary wildlife trade was supplemented with the creation of intensive, captive production farms where wild animals could be raised under poor sanitation in unnatural stocking densities[31] before being transported and caged at markets for sale. Six million people are involved in China's wildlife farming industry, which is valued at $18 billion.[32]

The genetic building blocks for the SARS virus have since been identified from eleven different strains of coronaviruses found in Chinese bats,[33] but there are bat-borne coronaviruses around the world. The reason China in particular has been ground zero for multiple jumps of deadly human coronavirus epidemics may be these wet markets.[34]

In the case of SARS, the intermediate host appeared to be the masked palm civet, a catlike animal prized for its meat, the purported aphrodisiac qualities of its penis,[35] and the taste imparted to coffee beans they are fed to confer a scent from their perianal glands.[36] Coronaviruses found in civets at wild animal markets were almost identical to the SARS virus.[37] While civets at wildlife farms supplying the live markets were found largely free of infection, up to 80 percent of sampled civets at the markets showed evidence of exposure.[38] This suggests that most infections happened at the market, perhaps due to a combination of crowded interspecies mixing and the immunosuppressive effect of stress.[39]

Live animal markets not only allow for cross-species transmission, human exposure, and viral amplification but viral modification, too. Apparently, civets are not just passive conduits for the virus; they appear to be incubators for human-adapting mutations in the virus itself.[40] The virus uses its corona of spikes like a key in a lock to latch onto host receptors and gain entry into its victims' cells. To switch from infecting one species to another, the genes that code for the spikes have to mutate to fit the spikes into the new host's receptors.[41] A new lock requires a new key. Both SARS-CoV, the virus that causes SARS, and SARS-CoV-2, the virus that causes COVID-19, attach to a specific enzyme coating the cells of our lungs.[42] By the time a mishmash of bat coronaviruses[43] made it into civets, the docking spikes of the virus were only two mutations away from locking in the configuration that bound to human receptors,[44] and the SARS epidemic was born.

After the initial SARS outbreak ended in July 2003, four new human cases were confirmed in China the following winter. Unlike most of the previous cases, the four individuals had not had close contact with infected persons, and they presented with mild symptoms. Viruses sampled from palm civets both kept at a local market and served at the restaurant where most of the new patients had previously eaten were found to be nearly identical to those discovered in the new, milder human cases. The new civet viruses shared one of the two civet-to-human spike mutations found in all the new human patients but none of the previous year's civet coronaviruses. These findings suggest that intermediate hosts can help transform coronaviruses from the primordial reservoir in bats into greater human infectivity.[45]

Yes, bats are trapped for meat in Asia, and most bat hunters report getting bitten.[46] Yes, the handling and consumption of undercooked bat meat is still practiced in China, Guam, and other parts of Asia,[47] with some markets reportedly selling five or six thousands bats a week.[48] But it appears intermediate hosts may be needed as a stepping-stone for bat coronaviruses to trigger a human outbreak, and it's hard to imagine a system that could be better designed to trip this kill switch than a live animal wet market.

In response to the SARS outbreak, the Chinese government implemented strict controls over the wildlife trade,[49] including a ban on the sale of civet cats. Though the permanent closure of live animal markets has been called the "strongest deterrent to another zoonotic disease outbreak,"[50] within months, the ban was lifted and trade resumed as before.[51] Had authorities in China learned their lesson from SARS and enacted a permanent ban on live animal markets, it's possible humanity would not now be suffering the worst pandemic in a century.

The Emergence of COVID-19

A review published in the December 2019 issue of the journal *Infectious Disease Clinics of North America* concluded: "The SARS epidemic demonstrated that novel highly pathogenic viruses crossing the animal-human barrier remain a major threat to global health security."[52] Little did the authors know that by the date of publication, just such a virus was brewing. "[I]t will not be surprising if new coronaviruses emerge in the near future," read a review a few months earlier.[53] Read another: "[I]t is highly likely that future SARS- or MERS-like coronavirus outbreaks will originate from bats, and there is an increased probability that this will occur in China."[54]

These warnings are not new. They date back well before I first started writing about the threat of emerging coronaviruses more than a decade ago, in 2006.[55] From a review published around that time: "The presence of a large reservoir of SARS-like coronaviruses in bats, together with the culture of eating exotic mammals in southern China, is a time bomb."[56] A time bomb that just went off.

We can now understand why Dr. Li's "7 SARS cases confirmed at Hua'nan Seafood Market" forewarning was so ominous. It wasn't SARS-CoV, though—it was a virus that would come to be known as SARS-CoV-2, the cause of COVID-19, short for *coronavirus disease 2019*.[57] Before it became known as SARS-CoV-2, however, it was known as the Wuhan seafood market pneumonia virus.[58]

According to the director of the Chinese Center for Disease Control and

Prevention, ground zero for the COVID-19 pandemic was the Hua'nan Market in Wuhan, China,[59] where most of the first human cases could be traced back.[60] Described as the largest wholesale seafood market in Central China,[61] the Hua'nan Market reportedly also sold seventy-five species of wild animals.[62] (To see photos of what the market looked like, visit bit.ly/HuananMarket.[63]) Although there are fish coronaviruses,[64] more than 90 percent of the samples that turned up positive for the virus were found in the section of the half-million-square-foot[65] seafood market that trafficked in exotic animals sold for food.[66]

The fact that the genetic sequences of the viruses obtained from some of the early human victims were 99.98 percent identical despite the rapid mutation rate of coronaviruses suggests the current pandemic originated within a very short period from a single source.[67] Although there have been documented reports of SARS-CoV escaping from laboratories,[68] the fact that the COVID-19 coronavirus, SARS-CoV-2, was optimized for binding to human cells in a novel way suggests that the new pandemic we now face is a product of natural selection. To achieve the necessary mutations, the "animal host would probably have to have a high population density,"[69] but which animal host might that have been?

The new coronavirus appears to share a common ancestor with the original SARS virus, with which it is about 80 percent identical, but it's more than 95 percent identical with a coronavirus found in a bat in 2013.[70] The current thinking is that the COVID-19 virus originated in bats but then jumped to humans only after passing through an intermediate host.[71] The pandemic emerged in winter, after all, when most bat species in Wuhan are hibernating, and no bats were reportedly found at the Hua'nan Market.[72] It's possible a bat virus might have escaped from labs located in proximity to the market,[73] but the virus was apparently found in environmental samples taken from the market itself.[74] Unfortunately, the market was closed and cleared before the animals were tested, complicating the forensic search for the source.[75] Scientists would have to use genetic fingerprinting techniques to identify the animal most likely to have played the role of intermediate host.

The leading suspect for the stepping-stone civet of the current outbreak is the pangolin.[76] Also known as scaly anteaters, pangolins look like a cross between a sloth and a pine cone. Between the demand for their meat as a delicacy and their scales for use in traditional medicines, pangolins are the most trafficked mammal in the world.[77] Pangolins are served in high-end restaurants in China. Once the order is placed, the animal may be hammered to death in front of the customers as a guarantee of the meat's freshness. The blood is drained and usually given to the customer to take home or used to make pangolin-blood fried rice.[78]

Although other potential intermediate hosts were investigated, including snakes[79] and turtles,[80] most attention has turned to pangolins, after a coronavirus found in diseased pangolins being smuggled from Malaysia into China was found to be about 90 percent identical with the COVID-19 virus.[81] Samples taken from pangolins earlier in the year in a different Chinese province revealed similar findings. What's more, the critical receptor binding region of the pangolin coronavirus spike protein is virtually identical to the human strain.[82]

Regardless of which animal it was, that one meal or medicine may end up costing humanity trillions of dollars and millions of lives.

China's Temporary Ban on Consuming Wildlife

Given the role exotic animal trafficking appears to have played in the current global health crisis, some in the international scientific community have called for a ban on the sale of wild animals[83] and a closure of live animal markets.[84] "[S]hut down those things right away," said Anthony Fauci, director of the National Institute of Allergy and Infectious Diseases.[85] Even infectious disease experts within Wuhan started calling for "completely eradicating wildlife trading."[86] On January 26, 2020, the Chinese government responded, announcing a total ban on the trade and sale of wild animal meat,[87] reportedly shutting down or quarantining almost twenty thousand wildlife farms across seven Chinese provinces.[88] The ban is only set to be temporary, however.[89] After the SARS outbreak in 2003, Chinese officials enacted a similar ban on the trade of civet cats, but within months, the ban was lifted and the animals were back on the menu.[90]

Much of the wildlife trade was already illegal in China in the first place,[91] with flaunted bans dating back more than a decade.[92] The Chinese pangolin, for example, is officially considered a critically endangered species.[93] That's part of the draw, though, as a serving of extra-rare meat may project wealth and prestige.[94] A thriving black market already exists, and it could be driven further underground by government action.[95] "The ultimate solution," wrote a group of scientists supported by the National Natural Science Foundation of China, "lies in changing people's minds about what is delicious, trendy, prestigious, or healthy to eat."[96] Having spent the bulk of my professional life trying to get people to eat more healthfully to prevent chronic diseases, I can certainly relate.

Even in the unlikely[97] event the current wildlife meat ban were to be made permanent and was enforced effectively, there remains a glaring loophole: The ban exempts the use of wild animals for traditional Chinese medicine. So, while it's currently illegal to eat pangolin meat, it's not illegal to eat other pangolin parts.[98] Pangolin blood is said to "promote . . . circulation."[99] How ironic that the pandemic appears to have arisen in a market selling remedies purported to promote immunity and longevity.[100]

For only about thirty dollars a pound, anyone can go online and buy Chinese bat feces (*Yè ming shǎ*) to "treat . . . eye disorders."[101] While the drying of excrement would presumably inactivate coronavirus, the handling and trade of live and recently killed bats for use in traditional remedies could infect people directly or introduce opportunities for cross infection with other susceptible hosts.[102] Even now the Chinese government has been pushing traditional animal-based remedies for the treatment of COVID-19.[103]

It's easy for xenophobic Westerners to condemn cultures consuming rhino horns, tiger bones, or pangolin scales,[104] or twenty-first-century manifestations such as *mukbangs,* livestreaming broadcasts of people eating bat soup and the like.[105] But, as I discuss in "Tracing the Flight Path," the last pandemic virus, the 2009 H1N1 swine flu, arose not from some backwater wet market in Asia but largely from industrial pig operations in the United States. So, for the emergence of SARS-CoV-3, we may need look no further than the food we put on our own plates.

Coronaviruses Infect Pigs Right Off the Bat

As we've seen, COVID-19 is only one of many coronavirus diseases to jump from bats in the twenty-first century to cause deadly outbreaks—not only SARS in 2002 and MERS in 2012 but SADS in 2016. A new disease killing up to 90 percent of young piglets, swine acute diarrhea syndrome devastated industrial pig farms in the same region in China where SARS had broken out. SADS-CoV was traced to a coronavirus discovered in a bat cave in the vicinity.[106] The combination of deforestation and intensive pork production,[107] with millions of pigs encroaching on bat habitat, may have facilitated the coronavirus spillover from bats to pigs.[108]

Porcine epidemic diarrhea virus is another presumed bat-to-pig coronavirus.[109] In 2010, a highly virulent strain emerged in China that caused massive outbreaks when it hit the United States three years later, killing millions of pigs, approximately 10 percent of the U.S. herd.[110] Porcine deltacoronavirus (PDCoV) is the third new pig coronavirus to emerge from China in the last decade,[111] rapidly spreading coast to coast once it reached U.S. shores in 2014.[112] This pattern of emergence and outbreaks of new coronaviruses appears to be accelerating, in part because "intensive farm-management practices result in thousands of animals being housed together in a closed environment."[113]

Although continued public health monitoring is considered necessary,[114] none of these emerging pig coronaviruses appears able to infect humans at this time. However, coronaviruses are known for their high rates of mutation and recombination, the process by which viruses swap parts of their genetic code to better adapt to their hosts or find new ones. The fact that many livestock coronaviruses cause persistent infections that can spread rapidly among thousands of intensively confined animals increases the likelihood that a coronavirus mutant could arise with an "extended host range,"[115] meaning the potential to invite humanity to the party.

To trigger a pandemic of respiratory disease, the virus would first have to spread to the lungs. Most coronaviruses in bats and livestock to date have been intestinal infections.[116] The exception is infectious bronchitis virus (IBV) in chickens, the first coronavirus ever discovered.[117] IBV is a major cause of respiratory infections in the nine billion chickens raised for meat in the United States every year, but it is prevalent in all countries with industrial poultry production, with infection rates often approaching 100 percent.[118] Currently, the only way IBV has been shown to cause disease in mammals, though, is by being directly injected into the brain.[119]

With so many different coronaviruses circulating among so many different species, it is considered likely a matter of when, not if, the next recombinant coronavirus will emerge and burst into the human population.[120] Already, the spikes of porcine deltacoronavirus attach to receptors found not only in pig intestines[121] but also in the respiratory tract of humans.[122] In a petri dish, PDCoV can infect both human and chicken cells,[123] and we know PDCoV can infect chickens[124] (just like a bovine coronavirus in calves can infect turkeys).[125]

PDCoV can then spread rapidly from chicken to chicken.[126] Given the susceptibility of human cells to infection, Ohio State University researchers in the February 2020 issue of the Centers for Disease Control and Prevention's *Emerging Infectious Diseases* journal concluded: "Research regarding how PDCoV is adapting and mutating in different species and whether it infects humans is critical to determining if PDCoV poses a pandemic health risk."[127]

SADS-CoV can also infect human cells in a petri dish and infect mice in a laboratory. Given the "ability of SADS-CoV to grow efficiently in human cell lines," a team of researchers recently concluded, "we should not underestimate the risk that this bat-origin CoV may 'jump' from pigs to humans."[128] Pigs, not only pangolins, may act as the mixing vessel of the generation of new coronaviruses with pandemic potential.[129]

Coronaviruses are increasingly emerging[130] and circulating among livestock populations around the world. The more novel coronaviruses we have mixing in more and more animals, the greater the likelihood that strains with pandemic potential may emerge.[131] While global pangolin populations are in drastic decline,[132] we produce and slaughter more than a billion pigs each year, nearly half in China alone,[133] raising the specter that the next pandemic may arise from domestic rather than wild animals, an event that may actually have already happened.

COVID-19 May Not Have Been the First Coronavirus Pandemic

Coronaviruses are the second-most common cause of the common cold.[134] So far, we've discovered four human cold coronaviruses, so that makes seven coronaviruses in all that can cause human disease. We suspect we got SARS from civets, MERS from camels, and COVID-19, perhaps, from pangolins. Where did we get the common cold coronaviruses?

The origin of two of the four mild coronaviruses remains a mystery, but one—HCoV-229E—has been traced back to camels[135] and the other—HCoV-OC43—to cattle or pigs.[136] Well, if the jump by the common cold from camels to humans foreshadowed the deadly MERS species jump that went on to kill one in three infected, might the mild coronavirus jump from livestock to humans portend a deadly human outbreak as well? Some speculate it may already have.

So-called molecular clock analyses dating the emergence of human coronavirus OC43 suggest that the bovine coronavirus now causing "shipping fever" disease jumped to humans around the year 1890. That's interesting timing. There was a pandemic in 1890. While the 1889–1890 pandemic has traditionally been presumed to be influenza, the timing of the emergence of HCoV-OC43 has led some to conjecture that instead, it may have been a COVID-19-like interspecies transmission of a coronavirus. This is bolstered by the fact that in the years leading up to the pandemic, there were massive culling operations to eradicate a deadly respiratory disease devastating cattle herds the world over.[137]

We may never know what caused the 1889–1890 outbreak, but we can take steps to prevent the next one. To understand COVID-19 and other deadly diseases, we have to understand their history and evolution. We have to take lessons from the past to protect ourselves in the future. That's the main subject of this book—pandemic prevention. The best way to survive a pandemic is not to have one in the first place.

Introduction

> *"It was 'the perfect storm'—a tempest that may happen only once in a century—a nor'easter created by so rare a combination of factors that it could not possibly have been worse. Creating waves 10 stories high and winds of 120 miles an hour, the storm whipped the sea to inconceivable levels few people on Earth have ever witnessed."*
>
> —SEBASTIAN JUNGER, *THE PERFECT STORM:*
> *A TRUE STORY OF MEN AGAINST THE SEA*

Millions around the world may die in the COVID-19 pandemic.[138] In the United States, a "best guess" estimate presented to the American Hospital Association was about a half a million American deaths.[139] With sufficient social distancing, however, that may be reduced to around a hundred thousand.[140] Even at half a million, it still, unbelievably, could be much, much worse.

With thousands already dead, millions projected to perish, billions in lockdown, and trillions lost as markets tumble, COVID-19 is still only shaping up to be a Category 2 pandemic.[141]

Fashioned after the Hurricane Severity Index to define the destructive capacity of a storm, the Pandemic Severity Index (figure 1) is the CDC's attempt at classifying the destructive capacity of pandemics.[142] It is based on case fatality rate, the percentage of those who fall ill who eventually succumb

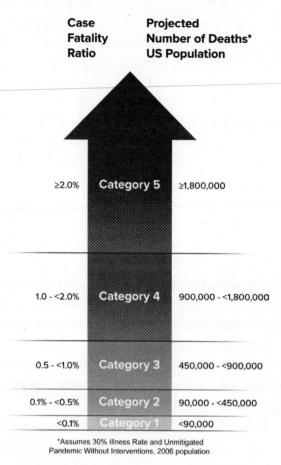

Figure 1. Pandemic Severity Index (Courtesy of the Centers for Disease Control and Prevention,[143] reformatted for print by Dustin Kirkpatrick)

to the infection. In the worst plague in history, the 1918 flu pandemic, nearly one in three fell ill and, of those, about 2 percent died.[144,145] That made the 1918 pandemic a Category 5 pandemic, analogous to a "super typhoon" with sustained winds exceeding 150 miles per hour.[146] The rate of those dying from COVID-19 is much lower, probably closer to 0.4 percent,[147] based both on where the most extensive testing has been done to date[148,149,150] and historical trends when trying to capture such estimates in real time.[151]

As you can see in the figure, a 2 percent case fatality rate like that of the 1918 pandemic is just where Category 5 starts. COVID-19 shows that SARS-like coronaviruses can escape our grasp and spark a full-blown pandemic. SARS was rapidly stamped out by fever-monitoring travelers, but by the time it was all over, there were 774 deaths out of 8,096 cases.[152] That's a case fatality ratio of about 10 percent. Thank heavens we're dealing with a SARS-CoV-2 pandemic and not a SARS-CoV pandemic. Even more lethal, MERS killed 858 out of 2,494.[153] That's 34 percent, a one in three chance of dying if you get it.

Since 2002 with SARS and then 2012 with MERS, we learned that coronaviruses could become extremely deadly. They're not just the common cold viruses we thought they were. Now, with COVID-19, we realize this family of viruses can also explode unfettered onto the global stage. So coronaviruses have already shown us they can do both. It's not hard to imagine a combination of transmissibility and lethality that makes the next coronavirus pandemic worse by an order of magnitude or more.

There's an even greater cautionary tale to be told, though, which is the primary subject of this book. We've long known about the pandemic potential of influenza, but the deadliest it ever appeared to get was the 2 percent fatality rate of the 1918 flu. Now, 2 percent was enough to kill up to a hundred million people, making it the single deadliest event in human history[154]—but in 1997, H5N1 was discovered, the flu virus in chickens, with an apparent fatality rate exceeding 50 percent.[155] What if a virus like that triggered a pandemic? What if instead of a 2 percent death rate, it was a flip of a coin?

The COVID-19 pandemic is devastating, but food is still being restocked in our grocery stores. The internet may be slow, but it's still up. The lights are still on, and safe drinking water is still flowing from the tap. Doctors and nurses are still showing up to work. If the predictions are correct and "only" a hundred thousand Americans die,[156] that's less than one in three thousand. In the pandemic of 1918, in which 2 percent of the cases succumbed, about one in a hundred and fifty Americans died.[157] Imagine if it were ten times as bad as 2 percent with one in fifteen dying. Or twenty-five times as bad, killing one in six of us.

Coronavirus or influenzavirus, the good news is that there is something we can do about it. And just as eliminating the exotic animal trade and live animal markets may go a long way toward preventing the next coronavirus pandemic, reforming the way we raise domesticated animals for food may help forestall the next killer flu.

I. Storm Gathering

1918

> *"Humanity has but three great enemies: fever, famine and war; of these by far the greatest, by far the most terrible, is fever."*
>
> —Sir William Osler[158]

Most of us know the flu—influenza—as a nuisance disease, an annual annoyance to be endured along with taxes, dentists, and visits with the in-laws. Why worry about influenza when there are so many more colorfully gruesome viruses out there like Ebola? Well, because influenza is scientists' top pick for humanity's next killer plague. Up to 60 million Americans come down with the flu every year. What if it suddenly turned deadly, like it did in 1918?

It started back then, harmlessly enough, with a cough drowned out by the raging world war. It was known as Spanish influenza only because censorship by the warring governments wouldn't allow reports of the spreading illness for fear it would damage morale.[159] However, Spain, being neutral, allowed its press to publicize what was happening. The first cable read, "A STRANGE FORM OF DISEASE OF EPIDEMIC CHARACTER HAS APPEARED IN MADRID." Because of the censors, even as millions were dying around the globe, the world press was apt to report little about the pandemic beyond what Spanish King Alfonso's temperature was that morning.[160] In Spain, they called it the French flu.[161]

"The year 1918 has gone," the editors of the *Journal of the American Medical*

Association wrote in the Christmas issue, "a year momentous as the termination of the most cruel war in the annals of the human race; a year which marked the end, at least for a time, of man's destruction of man; unfortunately a year in which developed a most fatal infectious disease."[162] That most fatal disease killed about ten times more Americans than did the war.[163] In fact, according to the World Health Organization (WHO), "The 1918 influenza pandemic killed more people in less time than any other disease before or since,"[164] the "most deadly disease event in the history of humanity."[165]

The word "epidemic" comes from the Greek *epi,* meaning "upon," and *demos,* meaning "people." The word "pandemic" comes from the Greek word *pandemos,* meaning "upon *all* the people."[166] Most outbreaks of disease are geographically confined, just like most disasters in general. Wars, famines, earthquakes, and acts of terror, for example, tend to be localized both in time and space. We look on in horror, but may not be affected ourselves. Pandemics are different. Pandemics are worldwide epidemics. They happen everywhere at once, coast to coast, and can drag on for more than a year.[167] "With Hurricane Katrina, people opened their homes, sent checks and people found safe havens," wrote a global economic strategist at a leading investment firm about one of the deadliest natural disasters in U.S. history, but with a pandemic "there is nowhere to turn, no safe place to evacuate."[168]

The word "influenza" derives from the Italian *influentia,* meaning "influence," reflecting a medieval belief that astrological forces were behind the annual flu season.[169] In 1918, though, the Germans called it *Blitzkatarrh.*[170] To the Siamese, it was *Kai Wat Yai,* The Great Cold Fever.[171] In Hungary, it was The Black Whip. In Cuba and the Philippines, it was *Trancazo,* meaning "a blow from a heavy stick." In the United States, it was the Spanish Lady, or, because of the way many died, the Purple Death.

Purple Death

What started for millions around the globe as muscle aches and a fever ended days later with many victims bleeding from their nostrils, ears, and eye sockets.[172] Some bled inside their eyes;[173] some bled around them.[174] They vomited blood and coughed it up.[175] Purple blood blisters appeared on their skin.[176]

Chief of Medical Services, Major Walter V. Brem, described the horror at the time in the *Journal of the American Medical Association,* writing that "often blood was seen to gush from a patient's nose and mouth."[177] In some cases, blood reportedly spurted with such force as to squirt several feet.[178] The patients were bleeding into their lungs.

As victims struggled to clear their airways of the bloody froth that poured from their lungs, their bodies started to turn blue from the lack of oxygen, a condition known as violaceous heliotrope cyanosis.[179] U.S. Army medics noted that this was "not the dusky pallid blueness that one is accustomed to in failing pneumonia, but rather [a] deep blueness . . . an indigo blue color."[180] The hue was so dark that one physician confessed that "it is hard to distinguish the colored men from the white."[181] "It is only a matter of a few hours then until death comes," recalled another physician, "and it is simply a struggle for air until they suffocate."[182] They drowned in their own bloody secretions.[183]

"It wasn't always that quick, either," one historian added. "And along the way, you had symptoms like fingers and genitals turning black, and people reporting being able to literally smell the body decaying before the patient died."[184] "When you're ill like that you don't care," recalled one flu survivor, at a hundred years old. "You don't care if you live or die."[185]

Major Brem described an autopsy: "Frothy, bloody serum poured from the nose and mouth when the body was moved, or the head lowered. . . . Pus streamed from the trachea when the lungs were removed."[186] Fellow autopsy surgeons discussed what they called a "pathological nightmare," with lungs up to six times their normal weight, looking "like melted red currant jelly."[187] An account published by the National Academies of Sciences describes the lungs taken from victims as "hideously transformed" from light, buoyant air-filled structures to dense sacks of bloody fluid.[188]

There was one autopsy finding physicians reported having never seen before. As people choked to death, violently coughing up as much as two pints of yellow-green pus per day,[189] their lungs would sometimes burst internally, forcing air under pressure up underneath their skin. In the *Proceedings of the Royal Society of Medicine,* a British physician noted "one thing that I have never seen before—namely the occurrence of subcutaneous emphysema"—pockets of air accumulating just beneath the skin—"beginning in the neck and spreading sometimes over the whole body."[190] These pockets of air leaking from ruptured lungs made patients crackle when they rolled onto their sides. In an unaired interview filmed for a PBS American Experience documentary on the 1918 pandemic, one Navy nurse compared the sound to a bowl of Rice Krispies. The memory of that sound—the sound of air bubbles moving under people's skin—remained so vivid that for the rest of her life she couldn't be in a room with anyone eating that popping cereal.[191]

> *"[A] dead man has no substance unless one has actually seen him dead; a hundred million corpses broadcast through history are no more than a puff of smoke in the imagination."*
>
> —ALBERT CAMUS, THE PLAGUE[192]

In 1918, it is estimated that half the world became infected.[193] Unlike the regular seasonal flu, which tends to kill only the elderly and infirm, the flu virus of 1918 killed those in the prime of life. Public health specialists at the time noted that most influenza victims were those who "had been in the best of physical condition and freest from previous disease."[194] Ninety-nine percent of excess deaths were among people under sixty-five years old.[195] Mortality peaked in the twenty- to thirty-four-year-old age group.[196] Women under thirty-five accounted for 70 percent of all female influenza deaths. In 1918, the average life expectancy in the United States dropped precipitously to only thirty-seven years.[197]

Calculations made in the 1920s estimated the global death toll in the vicinity of twenty million, a figure medical historians now consider "almost ludicrously low."[198] The number has been revised upward ever since, as more and more records are unearthed. The best estimate currently stands at fifty to a hundred million people dead.[199] In some communities, like in Alaska, 50 percent of the population perished.[200]

The 1918 influenza pandemic killed more people in a single year than the bubonic plague—the "black death"—in the Middle Ages killed in a century.[201] The 1918 virus also killed more people in twenty-five weeks than AIDS killed in twenty-five years.[202] According to one academic reviewer, this "single, brief epidemic generated more fatalities, more suffering, and more demographic change in the United States than all the wars of the Twentieth Century."[203]

> *"Has one ever seen anything like this, ever heard reports of a similar occurrence? In what annals has one ever read that the houses were empty, the cities deserted, the farms untended, the fields full of corpses, and that everywhere a horrible loneliness prevailed?"*
>
> —PETRARCH, *CIVILIZATION AND DISEASE*

In September 1918, according to the official published account of the American Medical Association, the deadliest wave of the pandemic spread over the world "like a tidal wave."[204] On September 11, Washington officials disclosed that it had reached U.S. shores.[205] September 11, 1918—the day Babe Ruth led the Boston Red Sox to victory in the World Series—three civilians dropped dead on the sidewalks of neighboring Quincy, Massachusetts.[206] It had begun.

When a "typical outbreak" struck Camp Funston in Kansas, the commander, a physician and former Army Chief of Staff, wrote the governor, "There are 1440 minutes in a day. When I tell you there were 1440 admissions in a day, you realize the strain put on our Nursing and Medical forces."[207] "Stated briefly," summarized an Army report, "the influenza . . . occurred as an explosion."[208]

October 1918 became the deadliest month in American history[209] and the last week of October was the deadliest week from any cause, at any time. More than twenty thousand Americans died in that week alone.[210] Numbers, though, cannot reflect the true horror of the time.

> *"They died in heaps and were buried in heaps."*
>
> —DANIEL DEFOE, 1665

One survivor remembers the children. "We had little caskets for the little babies that stretched for four and five blocks, eight high, ten high."[211] Soon, though, city after city ran out of caskets.[212] People were dying faster than carpenters could make them.[213] The dead lay in gutters.[214] One agonized official in the stricken East sent an urgent warning west: "Hunt up your wood-workers and set them to making coffins. Then take your street laborers and set them to digging graves."[215] When New York City ran out of gravediggers, they had to follow Philadelphia's example and use steam shovels to dig trenches for mass graves.[216] Even in timber-rich Sweden, the dead were interred in cardboard boxes or piled in mass graves because they simply ran out of nails.[217]

Another survivor recalls:

A neighbor boy about seven or eight died and they used to just pick you up and wrap you up in a sheet and put you in a patrol wagon. So the mother and father are screaming, "Let me get a macaroni box"—macaroni, any kind of pasta, used to come in this box, about 20 pounds of macaroni fit in it—"please, please let me put him in a macaroni box, don't take him away like that."[218]

One nurse describes bodies "stacked in the morgue from floor to ceiling like cordwood." At the peak of the epidemic she remembers toe-tagging and wrapping more than one still-living patient in winding sheets. In her nightmares, she wondered "what it would feel like to be that boy who was at the bottom of the cordwood in the morgue."[219]

They brought out their dead. Corpses were carted away in anything— wheelbarrows, even garbage trucks.[220] Often, though, the bodies were just pushed into corners and left to rot for days. People too sick to move were discovered lying next to corpses.[221]

All over the country, farms and factories shut down and schools and churches closed. Homeless children wandered the streets, their parents vanished.[222] The New York Health Commissioner estimated that in New York City alone, twenty-one thousand children lost both parents to the pandemic.[223]

Around the world, millions were left widowed and orphaned.[224] *The New York Times* described Christmas in Tahiti.[225] "It was impossible to bury the dead," a Tahitian government official noted. "Day and night trucks rumbled throughout the streets filled with bodies for the constantly burning pyres."[226] When firewood to burn the bodies ran out in India, the rivers became clogged with corpses.[227] In the remote community of Okak in northern Labrador, an eight-year-old girl reportedly survived for five weeks at 20 below zero—among the corpses of her family. She kept herself alive by melting snow for water with the last of her Christmas candles while she lay listening to the sound of dogs outside feasting off the dead.[228]

Colonel Victor Vaughan, acting Surgeon General of the Army and former head of the AMA, lived through the pandemic. "If the epidemic continues its mathematical rate of acceleration," Vaughan wrote in 1918, "civilization could easily disappear from the face of the earth."[229]

But the virus did stop. It ran out of human fuel; it ran out of accessible people to infect. Those who lived through it were immune to reinfection, so many populations were, for the most part, either immune or dead. "[I]t's like a firestorm," one expert explained. "[I]t sweeps through and it has so many victims and the survivors developed immunity."[230] Influenza is "transmitted so effectively," reads one virology textbook, "that it exhausts the supply of susceptible hosts."[231]

As soon as the dying stopped, the forgetting began. As Arno Karlen wrote in *Man and Microbes,* "Many Americans know more about mediaeval plague than about the greatest mass death in their grandparents' lives."[232] Commentators view the pandemic as so traumatic that it had to be forced out of our collective memory and history. "I think it's probably because it was so awful while it was happening, so frightening," one epidemiologist speculates, "that people just got rid of the memory."[233]

For many, however, the virus lived on. As if the pandemic weren't tragic enough, in the decade that followed, a million people came down with a serious Parkinson's-like disease termed "encephalitis lethargica," the subject of the book and movie *Awakenings.*[234] Some researchers now consider this epidemic of neurological disease to be "almost certainly" a direct consequence of viral damage to the brains of survivors.[235] The latest research goes a step further to suggest the pandemic had ripples throughout the century, showing that those in utero at the height of the pandemic in the most affected areas seemed to have stunted lifespans and lifelong physical disability.[236]

> *"This is a detective story. Here was a mass murderer that was around 80 years ago and who's never been brought to justice. And what we're trying to do is find the murderer."*
>
> —JEFFERY TAUBENBERGER, MOLECULAR PATHOLOGIST
> AND ARCHE-VIROLOGIST[237]

What caused the 1918 pandemic? Popular explanations at the time included a covert German biological weapon, the foul atmosphere conjured by the war's rotting corpses and mustard gas, or "spiritual malaise due to the sins of war and materialism."[238] This was before the influenza virus was discovered, we must remember, and is consistent with other familiar etymological examples—malaria was contracted from *mal* and *aria* ("bad air") or such quaintly preserved terms as catching "a cold" and being "under the weather."[239] The committee set up by the American Public Health Association to investigate the 1918 outbreak could only speak of a "disease of extreme communicability."[240] Though the "prevailing disease is generally known as influenza," they couldn't even be certain that this was the same disease that had been previously thought of as such.[241] As the *Journal of the American Medical Association* observed in October 1918, "The 'influence' in influenza is still veiled in mystery."[242]

In the decade following 1918, thousands of books and papers were written on influenza in a frenzied attempt to characterize the pathogen. One of the most famous medical papers of all time, Alexander Fleming's "On the Antibacterial Actions of Cultures of Penicillium," reported an attempt to isolate the bug that caused influenza. The full title was "On the Antibacterial Actions of Cultures of Penicillium, with Special Reference to Their Use in the Isolation of *B. Influenzae*." Fleming was hoping he could use penicillin to kill off all the contaminant bystander bacteria on the culture plate so he could isolate the bug that caused influenza. The possibility of treating humans with penicillin was mentioned only in passing at the end of the paper.[243]

The cause of human influenza was not found until 1933, when a British research team finally isolated and identified the viral culprit.[244] What they discovered, though, was a virus that caused the typical seasonal flu. Scientists still didn't understand where the flu virus of 1918 came from or why it was so deadly. It would be more than a half century before molecular biological techniques would be developed and refined enough to begin to answer these questions—but, by then, where would researchers find 1918 tissue samples to study the virus?

The U.S. Armed Forces Institute of Pathology originated more than 150 years ago. It came into being during the Civil War, created by an executive order from Abraham Lincoln to the Army Surgeon General to study diseases in the battlefield.[245] It houses literally tens of millions of pieces of preserved human tissue, the largest collection of its kind in the world.[246] This is where civilian pathologist Jeffery Taubenberger first went to look for tissue samples in the mid-1990s. If he could find enough fragments of the virus, he felt he might be able to decipher the genetic code and perhaps even resurrect the 1918 influenza for study, the viral equivalent of bringing dinosaurs back to life in "Jurassic Park."[247]

He found remnants of two soldiers who succumbed to the 1918 flu on the same day in September—a twenty-one-year-old private who died in South Carolina and a thirty-year-old private who died in upstate New York. Tiny cubes of lung tissue preserved in wax were all that remained. Taubenberger's team shaved off microscopic sections and started hunting for the virus using the latest advances in modern molecular biology that he himself had helped devise. They found the virus, but only in tiny bits and pieces.[248]

The influenza virus has eight gene segments, a genetic code less than fourteen thousand letters long. (The human genome, in contrast, has several billion.) The longest strands of RNA (the virus's genetic material) that Taubenberger could find in the soldiers' tissue were only about 130 letters long. He needed more tissue.[249]

The 1918 pandemic littered the Earth with millions of corpses. How hard could it be to find more samples? Unfortunately, refrigeration was essentially nonexistent in 1918, and common tissue preservatives like formaldehyde tended to destroy any trace of RNA.[250] He needed tissue samples frozen in time. Expeditions were sent north, searching for corpses frozen under the Arctic ice.

Scientists needed to find corpses buried below the permafrost layer, the permanently frozen layer of subsoil beneath the topsoil, which itself may thaw in the summer.[251] Many teams over the years tried and failed. U.S. Army researchers excavated a mass grave near Nome, Alaska, for example, only to find skeletons.[252] "Lots of those people are buried in permafrost," explained Professor John Oxford, co-author of two standard virology texts, "but many of them were eaten by the huskies after they died. Or," he said, "*before* they died."[253]

On a remote Norwegian Island, Kirsty Duncan, a medical geographer from Canada, led the highest profile expedition in 1998, dragging twelve tons of equipment and a blue-ribbon academic team to the gravesite of seven coal miners who had succumbed to the 1918 flu.[254] Years of planning and research combined with surveys using ground-penetrating radar had led the team to believe that the bodies of the seven miners had been buried deep in the eternal permafrost.[255] Hunched over the unearthed coffins in biosecure space suits, the team soon realized their search was in vain.[256] The miners' naked bodies, wrapped only in newspaper, lay in shallow graves above the permafrost. Subjected to thawing and refreezing over the decades, the tissue was useless.[257]

Nearly fifty years earlier, scientists from the University of Iowa, including a graduate student who had recently arrived from Sweden named Johan Hultin, had made a similar trek to Alaska with similarly disappointing results.[258] In the fall of 1918, a postal carrier delivered the mail—and the flu—via dogsled to a missionary station in Brevig, Alaska.[259] Within five days, seventy-two of the eighty or so missionaries lay dead.[260] With help from a nearby Army base, the remaining eight buried the dead in a mass grave.[261] Governor Thomas A. Riggs spent Alaska into bankruptcy caring for the orphaned children at Brevig and across the state. "I could not stand by and see our people dying like flies."[262]

Learning of Taubenberger's need for better tissue samples, Johan Hultin returned to Brevig in 1997, a few weeks before his seventy-third birthday.[263] Hultin has been described as "the Indiana Jones of the scientific set."[264] In contrast to Duncan's team, which spent six months just searching for the most experienced gravediggers, Hultin struck out alone.[265] Hultin was "there with a pickaxe," one colleague relates. "He dug a pit though solid ice in three days. This guy is unbelievable. It was just fantastic."[266]

Among the many skeletons from the missionary station lay a young woman whose obesity insulated her internal organs. "She was lying on her back, and on her left and right were skeletons, yet she was amazingly well preserved. I sat on an upside-down pail, amid the icy pond water and the muck and fragrance of the grave," Hultin told an interviewer, "and I thought, 'Here's where the virus will be found and shed light on the flu of 1918.'"[267] He named her Lucy. A few days later, Taubenberger received a plain brown box in the mail containing both of Lucy's lungs.[268] As Hultin had predicted, hidden inside was the key to unlock the mystery.

Many had assumed that the 1918 virus came from pigs. Although the human influenza virus wasn't even discovered until 1933, an inspector with the U.S. Bureau of Animal Industry had been publishing research as early as 1919 that suggested a role for farm animals in the pandemic. Inspector J. S. Koen of Fort Dodge, Iowa, wrote:

The similarity of the epidemic among people and the epidemic among pigs was so close, the reports so frequent, that an outbreak in the family would be followed immediately by an outbreak among the hogs, and vice versa, as to present a most striking coincidence if not suggesting a close relation between the two conditions. It looked like "flu," and until proven it was not "flu," I shall stand by that diagnosis.[269]

According to the editor of the medical journal *Virology,* Koen's views were decidedly unpopular, especially among pig farmers who feared that customers "would be put off from eating pork if such an association was made."[270] It was never clear, though, whether the pigs were the culprits or the victims. Did we infect the pigs or did they infect us?

With the entire genome of the 1918 virus in hand thanks to Hultin's expedition, Taubenberger was finally able to definitively answer the Holy Grail question posed by virologists the world over throughout the century: *Where did the 1918 virus come from?* The answer, published in October 2005,[271] is that humanity's greatest killer appeared to come from avian influenza—bird flu.[272]

Evidence now suggests that *all* pandemic influenza viruses—in fact all human and mammalian flu viruses in general—owe their origins to avian influenza.[273] Back in 1918, schoolchildren jumped rope to a morbid little rhyme:

I had a little bird,
Its name was Enza.
I opened the window,
And in-flu-enza.[274]

The children of 1918 may have been more prescient than anyone dared imagine.

Resurrection

Sequencing the 1918 virus is one thing; bringing it back to life is something else. Using a new technique called *reverse genetics,* Taubenberger teamed up with groups at Mount Sinai and the U.S. Centers for Disease Control and Prevention (CDC) and set out to raise it from the dead.[275] Using the genetic blueprint provided by Lucy's frozen lungs, they painstakingly recreated each of the genes of the virus, one letter at a time. Upon completion, they stitched each gene into a loop of genetically manipulated bacterial DNA and introduced the DNA loops into mammalian cells.[276] The 1918 virus was reborn.

Ten vials of virus were created, each containing ten million infectious virus particles.[277] First they tried infecting mice. All were dead in a matter of days. "The resurrected virus apparently hasn't lost any of its kick," Taubenberger noted. Compared to a typical non-lethal human flu strain, the 1918 virus generated thirty-nine thousand times more virus particles in the animals' lungs. "I didn't expect it to be as lethal as it was," one of the co-authors of the study said.[278]

The experiment was hailed as a "huge breakthrough,"[279] a "tour de force."[280] "I can't think of anything bigger that's happened in virology for many years," cheered one leading scientist.[281] Not knowing the true identity of the 1918 flu had been "like a dark angel hovering over us."[282]

Critics within the scientific community, however, wondered whether the box Taubenberger had received from Hultin might just as well have been addressed to Pandora. One scientist compared the research to "looking for a gas leak with a lighted match."[283] "They have constructed a virus," one biosecurity specialist asserted, "that is perhaps the most effective bioweapon known."[284] "This would be extremely dangerous should it escape, and there is a long history of things escaping," warned a member of the Federation of American Scientists' Working Group on Biological Weapons.[285] Taubenberger and his collaborators were criticized for using only an enhanced Biosafety Level 3 lab to resurrect the virus rather than the strictest height of security, Level 4. Critics cited three separate examples where deadly viruses had escaped accidentally from high-security labs.[286]

In 2004, for example, a strain of influenza that killed a million people in 1957 was accidentally sent to thousands of labs around the globe within a routine testing kit. Upon learning of the error, the World Health Organization called for the immediate destruction of all the kits. Miraculously, none of the virus managed to escape any of the labs. Klaus Stöhr, former head of the World Health Organization's global influenza program, admitted that it was fair to say that the laboratory accident with the unlabeled virus could have started a flu pandemic. Remarked Michael Osterholm, the director of the Center for Infectious Disease Research and Policy at the University of Minnesota, "Who needs terrorists or Mother Nature, when through our own stupidity, we do things like this?"[287]

Not only was the 1918 virus revived, risking an accidental release from the lab, but in the interest of promoting further scientific exploration, Taubenberger's group openly published the entire viral genome on the internet, letter for letter. This was intended to allow other scientists the opportunity to try to decipher the virus's darkest secrets. The public release of the genetic code, however, meant that rogue nations or bioterrorist groups had been afforded the same access. "In an age of terrorism, in a time when a lot of folks have malicious intent toward us, I am very nervous about the publication of accurate [gene] sequences for these pathogens and the techniques for making them," said a bioethicist at the University of Pennsylvania.[288] "Once the genetic sequence is publicly available," explained a virologist at the National Institute for Biological Standards and Control, "there's a theoretical risk that any molecular biologist with sufficient knowledge could recreate this virus."[289]

Even if the 1918 virus were to escape, there might be a graver threat waiting in the wings.

As devastating as the 1918 pandemic was, the mortality rate was less than 5 percent on average.[290] But the H5N1 strain of bird flu virus that first emerged in 1997 and spread to more than sixty countries[291] seems to kill about 50 percent of its known human victims,[292] on par with Ebola,[293] making it potentially ten times as deadly as the worst plague in human history.[294,295]

Leading public health authorities, from the CDC to the World Health Organization, feared that this bird flu virus was but mutations away from spreading efficiently though the human population, triggering the next pandemic. "The lethal capacity of this virus is very, very high; so it's a deadly virus that humans have not been exposed to before. That's a very bad combination," said Irwin Redlener, former director of the National Center for Disaster Preparedness at Columbia University.[296] Scientists speculate worst-case scenarios in which H5N1 could end up killing a billion[297] or more[298] people around the world. "The only thing I can think of that could take a larger human death toll would be thermonuclear war," said Council on Foreign Relations senior fellow Laurie Garrett.[299] H5N1 had the potential to become a virus as ferocious as Ebola and as contagious as the common cold.

MASTER OF METAMORPHOSIS

"The single biggest threat to man's continued dominance on the planet is a virus."

—JOSHUA LEDERBERG, NOBEL LAUREATE[300]

If, as Nobel laureate Peter Medawar has said, a virus "is a piece of bad news wrapped in a protein,"[301] the world may have had all the bad news it could handle with the emergence of the H5N1 virus.

For more than a century, scientists marveled at how a virus, one of the simplest, most marginal life forms, could present such a threat. "It's on the edge of life," explains a former director of the CDC's viral diseases division, "between living organism and pure chemical—but it seems alive to me."[302]

For a virus, less is more. Viruses are measured in millionths of a millimeter.[303] As one writer described them, "Like tiny terrorists, viruses travel light, switch identity easily and pursue their goals with deadly determination."[304]

Viruses are simply pieces of genetic material, DNA or RNA, enclosed in a protective coat. As such, they face three challenges. First, they have genes, but no way to reproduce, so they must take over a living cell and parasitically hijack its molecular machinery for reproduction and energy production. The second problem viruses face is how to spread from one host to another. If the virus is too passive, it may not spread during the host's natural lifespan and thus will be buried with its host. The virus must not be too virulent, though. If a virus comes on too strong, it may kill its host before it has a chance to infect others, in which case the virus will also perish. Finally, all viruses need to be able to evade the host's defenses. Different viruses have found different strategies to accomplish each of these tasks.[305]

"A hen is only an egg's way of making another egg."

—SAMUEL BUTLER

A virus is a set of instructions to make the proteins that allow it to spread and reproduce. Viruses have no legs, no wings, no way to move around. They even lack the whip-like appendages that many bacteria use for locomotion.

So viruses must trick the host into doing the spreading for them. One sees similar situations throughout nature. Plants can't walk from place to place, so many have evolved flowers with sweet nectar to attract bees who spread the plants' reproductive pollen for them. Cockleburs have barbs to hitch rides on furry animals; berries developed sweetness so that birds would eat them and excrete their seeds miles away. Viruses represent this evolutionary instinct boiled down to its essence.

The rabies virus, for example, is programmed to infect parts of the animal brain that induce uncontrollable rage, while at the same time replicating in the salivary glands to spread itself best through the provoked frenzy of biting.[306] Toxoplasma, though not a virus, uses a similar mechanism to spread. The parasite infects the intestines of cats, is excreted in the feces, and is then picked up by an intermediate host—like a rat or mouse—who is eaten by another cat to complete the cycle. To facilitate its spread, toxoplasma worms its way into the rodent's brain and actually alters the rodent's behavior, amazingly turning the animal's natural anti-predator aversion to cats into an imprudent attraction.[307]

Diseases like cholera and rotavirus spread through feces, so, of course, they cause explosive diarrhea. Ebola is spread by blood, so it makes you bleed. Blood-borne travel is not very efficient, though. Neither is dog or even mosquito saliva, at least not for a virus that sets its sights high. Viruses that "figure out" how to travel the respiratory route, or the venereal route, have the potential to infect millions. Of the two, though, it's easier to practice safe sex than it is to stop breathing.

Something in the Air

Viruses like influenza and coronavirus have only about a week to proliferate before the host kills them or, in extreme cases, they kill the host. During this contagious period, there may be a natural selection toward viruses of greater virulence to overwhelm host defenses.

Our bodies fight back with a triple firewall strategy to fend off viral attackers. The first is our set of barrier defenses. The outermost part of our skin is composed of fifteen or more layers of dead cells bonded together with a fatty cement.[308] A new layer forms every day as dead cells are sloughed off, so the entire layer is completely replaced about every two weeks.[309] Since viruses can only reproduce in live functional cells and the top layers of skin are dead, our intact skin represents a significant barrier to any viral infection.

But the respiratory tract has no such protection. Not only is our respiratory tract lined with living tissue, it represents a primary point of contact with the external world. We only have about two square yards of skin, but the surface area within the convoluted inner passageways of our lungs exceeds that of a tennis court.[310] And every day we inhale more than five thousand gallons of air.[311] For a virus, especially one not adapted to survive stomach acid, the lungs are the easy way in.

Our bodies are well aware of these vulnerabilities, however. It's not enough for a virus to be inhaled—it must be able to physically infect a live cell. This is where mucus comes in. Our airways are covered with a layer of mucus that keeps viruses at arm's length from our cells. And many of the cells themselves are equipped with tiny sweeping hairs that brush the contaminated mucus up to the throat to be coughed up or swallowed into the killing acid of the stomach. One of the reasons smokers are especially susceptible to respiratory infections in general is that the toxins in cigarette smoke paralyze and destroy these fragile little sweeper cells.[312]

Our respiratory tract produces a healthy half cup of snot every day,[313] but can significantly ramp up production in the event of infection. However, influenza viruses belong to the orthomyxovirus family, from the Greek *orthos-myxa-*, meaning "straight mucus." And these flu viruses have found a way to cut through this mucus barrier defense.

Unlike most viruses, which have a consistent shape, influenza viruses may exist as round balls, spaghetti-like filaments, or any shape in between.[314] One characteristic they all share, though, is the presence of hundreds of spikes protruding from all over the surface of the virus, much like pins in a pincushion.[315] There are two types of spikes. One is a triangular, rod-shaped enzyme called *hemagglutinin*.[316] The other is a square, mushroom-shaped enzyme called *neuraminidase*.

There have been multiple varieties of both enzymes described, so far eighteen hemagglutinin (H1 to H18) and eleven neuraminidase (N1 to N11). Influenza strains are identified by which two surface enzymes they display. The strain identified as "H5N1," for example, denotes that the virus is studded with the fifth hemagglutinin in the WHO-naming scheme, along with spikes of the first neuraminidase.[317]

There is a reason the flu virus has neuraminidase jutting from its surface. Described by virologists as having a shape resembling a "strikingly long-stalked mushroom,"[318] this enzyme has the ability to slash through mucus like a machete, dissolving through the mucus layer to attack the respiratory cells underneath,[319] before moving aside as the hemagglutinin spikes take over.

Like the spike proteins coating coronaviruses, hemagglutinin is the key the flu virus uses to get inside our cells. The cells of our body are sugar-coated. The external membrane that wraps each cell is studded with glycoproteins—complexes of sugars and proteins—that are used for a variety of functions, including cell-to-cell communication. The viral hemagglutinin binds to one such sugar called *sialic acid* (from the Greek *sialos* for "saliva") like Velcro. In fact, that's how hemagglutinin got its name. If you mix the influenza virus with a sample of blood, the hundreds of surface hemagglutinin spikes on each viral particle form crosslinks between multiple sialic acid–covered red blood cells, effectively clumping them together. It agglutinates (*glutinare* or "to glue") blood (*heme-*).[320]

The docking maneuver prompts the cell to engulf the virus. Like the classic *Saturday Night Live* "landshark" skit, the virus fools the cell into letting it inside. Once inside, it takes over, turning the cell into a virus-producing factory. The conquest starts with the virus chopping up our own cell's DNA and retooling the cell to switch over production to make more virus with a single-mindedness that eventually leads to the cell's death through the neglect of its own needs.[321] Why has the virus evolved to kill the cell, to burn down its own factory? Why bite the hand that feeds it? Why not just hijack half of the cell's protein-making capacity and keep the cell alive to make more virus? After all, the more cells that end up dying, the quicker the immune system is tipped off to the virus's presence.

The virus kills because killing is how the virus gets around.

Influenza transmission is legendary. The dying cells in the respiratory tract trigger an inflammatory response, which triggers the cough reflex. The virus thus uses the body's own defenses to infect other potential hosts. Each cough releases billions of newly made viruses from the body at an ejection velocity exceeding seventy-five miles an hour.[322] Sneezes can exceed one hundred miles per hour[323] and hurl germs as far away as forty feet.[324] That's why it's so important to cover your mouth when you cough or sneeze. Standing six feet apart may not protect you from an uncovered cough.[325]

Furthermore, the viral neuraminidase's ability to liquefy mucus promotes the formation of tiny aerosolized droplets,[326] which are so light they can hang in the air for minutes before settling to the ground.[327] Each cough produces about forty thousand such droplets[328] and each microdroplet can contain millions of viruses.[329] One can see how easily a virus like this could spread around the globe.

In terms of viral strategy, another advantage of the respiratory tract is its tennis court–sized surface area, which allows the virus to go on killing cell after cell, thereby making massive quantities of virus without killing the host too quickly. The virus essentially turns our lungs into flu virus factories. In contrast, viruses that attack other vital organs like the liver can only multiply so fast without taking the host down with them.[330]

Unlike some other viruses, like the herpes virus, which go out of their way *not* to kill cells so as not to incur our immune system's wrath, the influenza virus has no such option. It must kill to live, kill to spread. It must make us cough, and the more violently the better.

Makings of a Killer

Once our barrier defenses—the first line of our triple firewall against infection—are breached, we have to rely on an array of nonspecific defenses known as the "innate" arm of our immune system. These include Pacman-like roving cells called *macrophages* (literally from the Greek for "big eaters"), which roam the body chewing up any pathogens they can catch. In this way, any viruses caught outside our cells can get gobbled up. Once viruses invade our cells, however, they are effectively hidden from our roaming defenses. This is where our interferon system comes in, another piece of the innate immune system.

Interferon is one of the body's many cytokines, inflammatory messenger proteins produced by cells under attack that can warn neighboring cells of an impending viral assault.[331] Interferon acts as an early warning system, communicating the viral threat and activating a complex self-destruct mechanism in the cell should nearby cells find themselves infected. Interferon instructs cells to kill themselves at the first sign of infection and take the virus down with them. They should take one for the team and jump on a grenade to protect the rest of the body. This order is not taken lightly; false alarms could be devastating to the body. Interferon pulls the pin, but the cell doesn't drop the grenade unless it's absolutely sure it's infected.

This is how it works: When scientists sit down and try to create a new antibiotic (*anti-bios,* "against life") they must find some difference to exploit between our living cells and the pathogen in question. It's like trying to formulate chemotherapy to kill the cancer cells but leave normal cells alone. There is no doubt that bleach and formaldehyde are supremely effective at destroying bacteria and viruses, but the reason we don't chug them at the first sign of a cold is they are toxic to us as well.

Most antibiotics, like penicillin, target the bacterial cell wall. Since animal cells don't have cell walls, these drugs can wipe out bacteria and leave us still standing. Pathogenic fungi don't have bacterial cell walls, but they do have unique fatty compounds in their cell membranes that our antifungals can target and destroy. Viruses, however, have neither cell walls nor fungal compounds, and, therefore, these antibiotics and antifungals don't work against viruses. There's not much to a virus to single out and attack. There's the viral RNA or DNA, of course, but that's the same genetic material as in our cells.

Human DNA is double-stranded (the famous spiral "double helix"), whereas human RNA is predominantly single-stranded.[332] To copy its RNA genome to repackage into new viruses, the influenza virus carries along an enzyme that travels the length of the viral RNA to make a duplicate strand. For a split second, there are two intertwined RNA strands. That's the body's signal that something is awry. When a virus is detected, interferon tells neighboring cells to start making a suicide enzyme called *PKR* that can shut down all protein synthesis in the cell—stopping the virus, but also killing the cell in the process.[333] To start this deadly cascade, PKR must first be activated, but how? By double-stranded RNA.[334]

What interferon does is prime the cells of the body for viral attack. Cells preemptively build up PKR to be ready for the virus. An ever-vigilant sentry, PKR continuously scans cells for the presence of double-stranded RNA. As soon as PKR detects that characteristic signal of viral invasion, PKR kills the cell and hopes to take the virus down with it. Our cells die, but they go down fighting. This defense strategy is so effective in blunting a viral onslaught that biotech companies have long been trying to genetically engineer double-stranded RNA to be taken in pill form during a viral attack in hopes of accelerating this process.[335]

Cytokines like interferon have beneficial systemic actions as well. Interferon release leads to many of the other symptoms we associate with the flu, such as high fever, fatigue, and muscle aches.[336] The fever is valuable since viruses like influenza tend to replicate poorly at high temperatures. Some like it hot, but not the influenza virus. The achy malaise encourages us to rest so our bodies can shift energies to mounting a more effective immune response.[337] On a population level, these intentional side effects may also limit the spread of the virus by limiting the spread of the host, who may feel too lousy to go out and socialize. Cytokine side effects are our body's way of telling us to call in sick.

Normally when you pretreat cells in the lab with powerful antivirals like interferon, the cells are forewarned and forearmed and viral replication is effectively blocked.[338] Not so with H5N1. Viruses have evolved a blinding array of ways to counter our body's finest attempts at control. The smallpox virus, for example, actually produces what are called *decoy receptors* to bind up the body's cytokines so that less of them make it out to other cells.[339] "I am in awe of these minute creatures," declared a Stanford microbiologist. "They know more about the biology of the human cell than most cell biologists. They know how to tweak it and how to exploit it."[340]

So how exactly does H5N1 block interferon's interference? After all, the virus can't stop replicating its RNA. The H5N1 virus carries a trick up its sleeve called *NS1* (for "Non-Structural" protein). If interferon is the body's antiviral warhead, then the NS1 protein is H5N1's antiballistic missile.[341] NS1 itself binds to the virus's own double-stranded RNA, effectively hiding it from the cell's PKR cyanide pill, preventing activation of the self-destruct sequence. Interferon can pull the pin, but the cell can't let go of the grenade. NS1 essentially foils the body's attempt to protect itself by covering up the virus's tracks. Influenza viruses have been called a "showcase for viral cleverness."[342]

All influenza viruses have NS1 proteins, but H5N1 carries a mutant NS1 with enhanced interferon-blocking abilities. H5N1's viral countermove isn't perfect, but it doesn't have to be. The virus just needs to buy itself enough time to spew out new virus. After that, it doesn't care if the cell goes down in flames—in fact, the virus prefers that because the cell's death may trigger more coughing. "This is a really nasty trick that this virus has learnt: to bypass all the innate mechanisms that cells have for shutting down the virus," laments the chief researcher who first unearthed H5N1's deadly secret. "It is the first time this mechanism has shown up and we wonder if it was not a similar mechanism that made the 1918 influenza virus so enormously pathogenic."[343]

Once researchers actually had the 1918 virus in hand, the mechanism was one of the first things they tested in hopes of understanding why the apocalyptic pandemic was so extraordinarily deadly. They tested the virus in a tissue culture of human lung cells, and, indeed, the 1918 virus was using the same NS1 trick to undermine the interferon system.[344] As the University of Minnesota's Osterholm told Oprah Winfrey on her television program, H5N1 is a "kissing cousin of the 1918 virus."[345] Could H5N1 or a virus like it come to mean 1918 all over again?

"But what gave this pestilence particularly severe force was that whenever the diseased mixed with healthy people, like a fire through dry grass or oil, it would run upon the healthy."

—BOCCACCIO'S DESCRIPTION OF THE PLAGUE IN FLORENCE
IN HIS CLASSIC *DECAMERON*, PUBLISHED IN 1350 [346]

H5N1 shares another ominous trait with the virus of 1918: they both have a taste for the young. One of the greatest mysteries of the 1918 pandemic was, in the words of the Acting Surgeon General of the Army at the time, why "the infection, like war, kills the young vigorous robust adults."[347] As the American Public Health Association put it rather crudely: "The major portion of this mortality occurred between the ages of 20 and 40, when human life is of the highest economic importance."[348]

Seasonal influenza, on the other hand, tends to seriously harm only the very young or the very old. The death of the respiratory lining that triggers fits of coughing accounts for the sore throat and hoarseness that typically accompany the illness. The mucus-sweeping cells are also killed, which opens up the body for a superimposed bacterial infection on top of the viral infection. This bacterial pneumonia is typically how stricken infants and elderly may die during flu season every year. Their immature or declining immune systems are unable to fend off the infections in time.

The resurrection of the 1918 virus offered a chance to solve the great mystery. The reason the healthiest people were the most at risk, researchers discovered, was that the virus tricked the body into attacking itself. It used our own immune systems against us.

Those who suffer anaphylactic reactions to bee stings or food allergies know the power of the human immune system. In their case, exposure to certain foreign stimuli can trigger a massive overreaction of the body's immune system that, without treatment, could literally drop them dead within minutes. Our immune systems are equipped to explode at any moment, but there are layers of fail-safe mechanisms that protect most people from such an overreaction. The influenza virus has learned, though, how to flick off the safety.

Both the 1918 virus and the H5N1 threat seem to trigger a "cytokine storm," an overexuberant immune reaction to the virus. In laboratory cultures of human lung tissue, infection with the H5N1 virus led to the production of ten times the level of cytokines induced by regular seasonal flu viruses.[349] The chemical messengers trigger a massive inflammatory reaction in the lungs. "It's kind of like inviting in trucks full of dynamite," says the lead researcher who first discovered the phenomenon with H5N1.[350] A similar storm can rage in severe cases of COVID-19.[351]

While cytokines are vital to antiviral defense, the virus may trigger too much of a good thing.[352] The flood of cytokines overstimulates immune components like natural killer cells, which go on a killing spree, causing so much collateral damage that the lungs start filling up with fluid. "It actually turns your immune system on its head, and it causes that part to be the thing that kills you," explains Osterholm.[353] "All these cytokines get produced and [that] calls in every immune cell possible to attack yourself. It's how people die so quickly. In 24 to 36 hours, their lungs just become bloody rags."[354]

People between twenty and forty years of age tend to have the strongest immune systems. You spend the first twenty years of your life building up your immune system, and then, starting around age forty, the system's strength begins to wane. That is why this age range is particularly vulnerable to such viruses, because it's your own immune system that may kill you.[355] A new dog learning old tricks, H5N1 may already be following in the 1918 virus's footsteps.[356]

Quite simply, either we wipe out the virus within days or the virus wipes us out. The virus doesn't care either way. By the time the host wins or dies, the virus expects to have moved on to virgin territory. And, in a dying host, the cytokine storm may even produce a few final spasms of coughing, allowing the virus to jump the burning ship. As one biologist recounted, the body's desperate shotgun approach to defending against infection is "somewhat like trying to kill a mosquito with a machete—you may kill that mosquito, but most of the blood on the floor will be yours."[357]

| *"There is nothing permanent except change."*

—HERACLITUS

The final wall of defense, after barrier methods and the best attempts of the innate immune system have failed, is the "adaptive" (or "acquired") arm of the immune system: the ability to make antibodies. Antibodies are like laser-guided missiles specific for a particular foreign invader. They are made by immune cells called *B cells* that arise in our bone marrow. We make a billion of these cells every day of our lives, each recognizing a specific target. Once one of these B cells is activated, it can pump out thousands of antibodies a second.[358] And some of the B cells can remember prior activations and attacks.

So-called memory B cells retain a memory of past invaders and lie in wait for a repeat attack. If that same invader ever tried anything again, the body would be armed and ready to fight it off before it could gain a foothold. This is why once you get chicken pox, you tend never to get it again. Our adaptive immune system is the principle behind vaccination. People can get vaccinated against measles as infants, for example, setting in place a "memory" of the virus, and retain immunity for life.

Why can you get a few shots against something like mumps as a kid and forget about it, whereas there's a new flu vaccine out every year? Because the influenza virus, in the words of the World Health Organization, is a "Master of Metamorphosis."[359]

Influenza viruses are like Hannibal Lecter. Like the COVID-19 coronavirus, they bud from infected cells and cloak themselves in a stolen swatch of the cell's own membrane, wrapping itself in our cells' own skin as a disguise. The virus can't hide completely, though. Out of necessity, it must poke neuraminidase and hemagglutinin spikes through the membrane to clear through mucus and bind to new cells. These spikes are the primary targets, then, that our antibodies go after. So that it doesn't go the way of chicken pox, the influenza virus's only chance for reinfection is to stay one step ahead of our antibodies by presenting an ever-moving target.

The World Health Organization describes influenza viruses as "sloppy, capricious, and promiscuous."[360] Sloppy, because an RNA virus thrives on mutation. The human genetic code is billions of DNA letters long. Every time one of our cells divides, each of those letters has to be painstakingly copied to provide each progenitor cell with the identical genetic complement. This is a tightly controlled process to prevent the accumulation of mutations (errors) in our genetic code. RNA replication is different.

RNA viruses tend to have no spell-checker, no proofreading mechanism.[361] A virus like influenza is no perfectionist. When RNA viruses make copies of their genomes, they intentionally include mistakes, so odds are that each new virus is unique.[362] Once a cell is infected and its molecular machinery pirated, it starts spewing out millions of viral progeny, each a bit different from the next, a population of viruses known in the scientific world as a "mutant swarm."[363] Essentially, every virus is a mutant.[364]

Most of the new viruses are so mutated, so crippled, that they won't survive to reproduce, but thousands of the fittest will.[365] This represents millennia of evolution by the hour. This is how other RNA viruses like HIV and hepatitis C can exist for years within the same individual; they are constantly changing, constantly evading the immune system.[366] One of the reasons we haven't been able to come up with a vaccine against HIV is that it mutates so rapidly[367]—and the influenza virus mutates even faster.[368] This is why it's so hard for our immune system to get a handle on influenza. By the time we've mounted an effective antibody response, the virus has changed appearances ever so slightly, a process called *genetic drift*. Thus, influenza can come back year after year.

Professor Kennedy Shortridge, the virologist who first identified H5N1 in Hong Kong's chickens, describes influenza as being caused by an "unintelligent, unstable virus."[369] A fellow colleague put it bluntly: "Flu's not clever. Forget this idea that the virus is clever. The virus is *clumsy*. It makes lots of mistakes when it's copying itself, the ones that have an advantage get selected, and that's why it's successful."[370] No other human respiratory virus has this kind of mutation rate.[371] It's like the worst of all worlds: respiratory spread of a deadly virus with a high mutation rate. Scientists fear a virus like H5N1 could become like an airborne HIV—half the mortality rate of untreated HIV, but able to kill us within days.

Viral Sex

The few genes the influenza virus has are distributed among eight discrete strands of RNA within each virus. It must be a nightmare for the virus to package each new outgoing progenitor with the correct RNA octet. Why not just keep all its genes on a single strand? Because with separate strands, influenza viruses can have sex.[372]

Variability is the engine of evolution. Survival of the fittest only works if there are some more fit than others. That is how natural selection works, how, over time, species can adjust to unpredictable changes in their environment. If all progeny are identical, if all progeny are simply clones of the parent, then the species has less flexibility to adapt. This is thought to be why the birds and the bees (and many plants) evolved to combine genetic endowments with one another in order to reproduce. This genetic mixing greatly increases variation among the offspring.

Suppose two completely different types of influenza viruses take over the same cell. They each make millions of copies of their eight individual RNA strands. Then what happens? As each new progeny virus buds from the cell, it can mix and match genes from both "parents." This segmented nature of the genome allows different flu viruses to easily "mate" with each other, swapping segments of RNA to form totally new hybrid viruses.[373] This is one way pandemics can be made.

Only one strain of influenza has historically tended to dominate at any one time within the human population.[374] Since 1968, one such strain has been H3N2. Each year, the virus's protruding spikes drift subtly in appearance, but the virus is still H3N2, so antibodies we made against the virus in previous years still recognize it as somewhat familiar and confer us some protection. As such, year after year for decades now, H3N2 has been kept in check by our immune systems, thanks to our prior run-ins with the virus.

If the virus didn't change its appearance at all from year to year, our immunity could be absolute, and, as with chicken pox, we'd never get the flu again. But, because the appearance of the virus does drift a bit annually, every year some of us come down with the flu. For most of us, though, the illness only lasts a few days before our prior partial immunity can vanquish the familiar foe and we can get on with our lives.

Pandemics happen when a dramatically different virus arrives on the scene, a virus to which we have no prior immunity. This can happen when the virus undergoes an entire shift, acquiring a new H spike. And that is where gene swapping can come in.

The 1918 pandemic virus was H1N1. It came back in subsequent years, but by then it was old hat. Those who had survived the virus during the pandemic retained much of their immunity. The annual flu strain remained H1N1, infecting relatively few people every year for decades until 1957, when an H2N2 virus suddenly appeared as the "Asian flu" pandemic. Because the world's population had essentially only acquired immunity to H1 spikes, the virus raced around the globe, infecting a significant portion of the world's population. For example, half of U.S. schoolchildren fell ill.[375] Thankfully, it was not very virulent and only killed about a million people worldwide.[376] H2N2 held seasonal sway for eleven years. In 1968, the H3N2 "Hong Kong Flu" virus triggered another pandemic and has been with us every year since. It attacked even fewer people than the H2N2 flu—only about 40 percent of U.S. adolescents got sick—and killed fewer still. Experts suspect that partial immunity to at least the N2 spike afforded a baseline level of protection.[377] Since 95 percent of the surface spikes are hemagglutinin and only 5 percent are neuraminidase,[378] though, and because the hemagglutinin directly determines infectivity since it is what attaches to host receptors, it is the appearance of a new H spike that triggers a pandemic.[379]

If only a limited number of types of human virus dominate at one time, with which viruses can the dominant virus swap genes? Birds are the reservoir from which nearly all human and nonhuman animal influenza genes originate. Thus, pandemic viruses can arise when human influenza dips into the bird flu gene pool and pulls out some avian H or N combination that the present human generation has never seen before. The human virus has lots to choose from, since birds harbor sixteen different hemagglutinin spikes and nine different spikes of neuraminidase.[380] (Two new Hs and Ns have been recently discovered in bats.[381])

Researchers speculate that sometime shortly before February 1957, somewhere along the road between Kutsing and Kweiyang in southern China, an H2N2 bird flu virus may have infected either a pig or a person already suffering from the regular H1N1 seasonal human flu, and an unholy viral matrimony took place.[382] From one of those co-infected cells came a human-bird crossbreed virus containing five of the original human viral gene segments and three new segments from the bird virus, including the new H and new N spikes.[383] Then, in 1968, the virus swapped its H2 for an H3 from another bird flu strain. With each new avian addition, the virus became sufficiently alien to the human immune system and quickly blanketed the globe.

So there were three influenza pandemics in the twentieth century—in 1918, 1957, and 1968—but, as the director of the National Institute for Allergy and Infectious Diseases has said, "There are pandemics and then there are pandemics."[384] The half-and-half bird/human hybrid viruses of 1957 and 1968 evidently contained enough previously recognizable human structure that the human population's prior partial exposure dampened the pandemic's potential to do harm. In contrast, the pandemic strain of 1918 was wholly avian-like.[385] Instead of diluting its alien avian nature, the 1918 bird flu virus "likely jumped straight to humans and began killing them," noted Taubenberger, the man who helped resurrect it.[386] The same could be happening with the new spate of avian influenza viruses sporadically infecting people in more recent years, like H5N1. The human immune system had never been known to be exposed to an H5 virus before. As the WHO points out, "Population vulnerability to an H5N1-like pandemic virus would be universal."[387]

H5N1 developed a level of human lethality not thought possible for influenza. Half of those known to have come down with that flu so far have died.[388] H5N1 is good at killing, but not at spreading. To trigger a pandemic, the virus has to learn how to spread efficiently from person to person. Now that the genome of the 1918 virus has been completely sequenced, we understand that it may have taken only a few dozen mutations to turn a bird flu virus into humanity's greatest killer,[389] and we have seen some of those changes taking form in H5N1.[390] The further H5N1 spreads and the more people it infects, the greater the likelihood that it might lock in mutations that could allow for efficient human-to-human transmission. "And that's what keeps us up at night," said the chair of the Infectious Diseases Society of America's task force on pandemic influenza.[391]

Research funded by the National Institutes of Health (NIH) suggests that influenza viruses mutate even faster than previously thought.[392] Some scientists theorize the existence of a "mutator mutation" that makes replication even sloppier, predisposing the virus for the species jump.[393] As if its sloppiness and segmentation don't create enough novelty for our immune system, influenza viruses have devised a third way to mutate. The process of swapping genes between two viruses has been named "reassortment," like reshuffling two decks of cards—one human deck and one bird deck with eight cards each. A process now known as *recombination* allows influenza viruses to swap mere pieces of individual RNA strands with each other. It's as if the virus not only reshuffles both decks together, but also cuts each card in half and then randomly tapes the halves back together.[394] Masters of metamorphosis indeed.

All influenza viruses are capable of high rates of mutation, but never had the scientific world seen a virus like H5N1. Very few human pathogens even approach 50 percent mortality. The director of the Center for Biosecurity of the University of Pittsburgh noted this at a congressional briefing: "Death rates approaching this order of magnitude are unprecedented for any epidemic disease." University of Minnesota's Osterholm described the specter of a deadly superflu as "the beast lurking in the midnight of every epidemiologist's soul"—the "Ace of Spades in the influenza deck."[395]

It's hard to believe a flu virus could be that deadly, though. The 50 percent fatality figure is calculated by taking the number of people who have died and dividing it by the total number of cases, but what if we don't have an accurate count? What if there are people who got infected but were overlooked because they showed little or no symptoms? In that case, the 50 percent mortality could be a gross overestimate.

The results of an investigation to help answer this question were published by the CDC.[396] In the Cambodian province of Kampot, dozens of chicken flocks were dying from H5N1, but there was only one reported human case, a young farmer who subsequently died. This was the signal for researchers to swoop in and take blood from every family in the area to determine the actual human infection rate. How many cases were we missing? How many infected people had been overlooked? They analyzed bloodwork from 351 area villagers. Not a single person showed evidence of present or past infection.[397]

There are two conclusions we can draw from this study. First, at present, H5N1 remains almost exclusively a bird virus. In the decades since it was discovered, less than a thousand people seem to have gotten infected, even though it has led to the deaths of hundreds of millions of birds. The concern, of course, is that the virus will mutate into a human form that is easily transmissible from one person to the next, thereby triggering the next pandemic. This leads us to conclusion number two: If this study is an accurate reflection of what's happening on the ground, then the human case mortality rate may really be on the order of 50 percent. Based on that study, we don't seem to be missing many cases.

A total of twenty-nine other such similar surveys in Bangladesh,[398] Cameroon,[399] China,[400] Germany,[401] Indonesia,[402] Nigeria,[403] South Korea,[404] Thailand,[405] Turkey,[406] and Vietnam[407] have found no evidence of significant numbers of asymptomatic or clinically mild cases even among those with frequent high-risk exposures, suggesting that the high case fatality ratio may accurately reflect the severity of infection.[408] And if a flip-of-a-coin death rate isn't bad enough, experimental data suggest that a pandemic H5N1 pathogen could initiate neurodegenerative disorders such as Parkinson's and Alzheimer's diseases in the survivors.[409]

Even if H5N1 does indeed have Ebola-like human lethality at this time, for it to be able to mutate into an easily transmissible human form, many assume the virus would necessarily have to ratchet down its ferocity. A panel of experts convened by the World Health Organization, however, brought that assumption into question, positing that it could retain its extreme lethality.[410] Pandemic influenza has the potential to infect billions of people. If H5N1 is able to preserve its ability to kill a significant proportion of its victims, "it could be more lethal than anything we've ever seen in history," said one WHO scientist.[411] Or as another flu expert remarked, "All bets would be off."[412]

Robert Webster, chair of the Virology Division of St. Jude Children's Research Hospital in Tennessee, is arguably the world's top bird flu expert. He is often referred to as the "pope" of influenza researchers.[413] In characteristically unpapal language, Webster puts it bluntly. H5N1, he said, is "the one that scares us shitless."[414]

H5N1

Hong Kong, 1997

It seems to have started with a three-year-old boy in Hong Kong who had a sore throat and tummy ache.[415] On May 14, 1997, Lam Hoi-ka was admitted to Queen Elizabeth Hospital with a fever; a week later he was dead. The causes of death listed were acute respiratory failure, acute liver failure, acute kidney failure, and "disseminated intravascular coagulopathy." Basically, on top of the multiple organ failure, his blood had curdled.[416]

The top specialist of the government virus unit was called in.[417] Samples were taken from the boy's throat. As far as anyone knew at the time, human beings were susceptible to getting sick only from H1, H2, and H3 viruses. When the samples came back positive for influenza, but negative for all known human strains, Hong Kong's chief virologist forwarded the mystery samples to the world's top labs in London, Holland, and Atlanta, to the CDC.[418]

The Dutch were the first to make the discovery. Virologist Jan de Jong, now a senior investigator at Rotterdam's Erasmus University, received the sample. He found that the boy had been killed by an H5 virus, H5N1.[419] The scientific world was stunned.

"We thought we knew the rules," recalled the director of the Center for Public Health Preparedness at Columbia University, "and one of those rules was that H1, H2 and H3 cause flu in humans, not H5. This is like the clock striking 13."[420] H5 was supposed to cause disease only in birds, not in people.

Within two days, de Jong was on a plane to Hong Kong. "We had to act very, very quickly," he remembers. "We realized this could be a pandemic situation."[421] Keiji Fukuda, chief of epidemiology in the CDC's influenza branch, followed shortly behind. It had been a hard death. The child had had to have a breathing tube inserted and reportedly had been in great pain. Fukuda at the time was the father of two young children. "It drove home for me how much suffering there might be if this bug took off."[422]

If H5N1 had spread from Hong Kong in 1997, Lam Hoi-ka would have been patient zero for a new global pandemic.[423] Keiji Fukuda was asked in an interview years later what his first thought had been upon hearing the news that an H5 virus had killed a child. He said that he distinctly remembered hanging up the phone and thinking, "This is how it begins."[424]

What this first death showed, according to the director of Holland's National Influenza Center, "was what everyone until then had thought impossible—that the virus could leap directly from birds to humans."[425] "This had never happened before in history," agreed the head of the University of Hong Kong's Emerging Pathogens Group. "It was terrifying." These statements, however, were taken before the 1918 virus was resurrected in 2005.[426]

In fact, it *had* happened before in history, many scientists now believe, in 1918—and that makes it all the more terrifying.

Fowl Plague

More than a century ago, researchers confirmed the first outbreak of a particularly lethal form of avian influenza that they called "fowl plague."[427] Plague comes from the Greek word meaning "blow" or "strike."[428] Later, the name "fowl plague" was abandoned and replaced by "highly pathogenic avian influenza" or HPAI.[429]

Domesticated poultry can also become infected with a low-grade influenza, so-called low pathogenic avian influenza, or LPAI, which may cause a few ruffled feathers and a drop in egg production.[430] Influenza viruses with H5 or H7 spikes, however, are able to mutate into the high-grade variety that can cause devastating illness among the birds. Webster's term for H5 and H7 strains of flu says it all: "the nasty bastards."[431] And you don't get nastier than H5.

Webster is credited as being the one who first discovered the part avian influenza plays in triggering all known flu pandemics. *The Washington Post* described him as "arguably the world's most important eye on animal influenza viruses."[432] Webster had more reason than most to be especially concerned about the death in Hong Kong. He had seen H5 before; he knew what it could do.

In 1983, an H5N2 virus struck commercial chicken operations in Pennsylvania and seventeen million chickens died or had to be killed. It quickly became the world's largest outbreak of avian influenza and the most costly animal disease control operation in U.S. history[433]—until an even bigger H5N2 chicken epidemic struck in 2015 that wiped out fifty million birds, that is.[434] As striking as the numbers of deaths are, it is the *way* the chickens died that continues to haunt scientists. In the veterinary textbooks, the deaths are described as "a variety of congestive hemorrhagic, transudative and necrobiotic changes."[435] One researcher described it in lay terms: The chickens were essentially reduced to "bloody Jell-O."[436]

In the spring of 1997, two months before Lam Hoi-ka fell ill, the same thing started happening in Hong Kong. Thousands of chickens were dying from H5N1. "Their bodies began shaking," one farmer described, "as if they were suffocating and thick saliva starting coming out of their mouths . . . The faces then went dark green and black, and then they died."[437] Some of the birds were asphyxiating on large blood clots lodged in their windpipes.[438] "One minute they were flapping their wings," another reported, "the next they were dead."[439] Others had given birth to eggs without shells.[440] In the lab, the virus was shown to be a thousandfold more infectious than typical human strains.[441] The virus, one Hong Kong scientist remarked, "was like an alien."[442]

Kennedy Shortridge, then chair of the University of Hong Kong's Department of Microbiology, went personally to investigate. Growing up in Australia, Shortridge was shaken by his mother's haunting stories of the 1918 pandemic and decided to dedicate his life to trying to understand the origins of influenza pandemics.[443] He had already been working for twenty-five years on this question in Hong Kong before H5N1 hit. He found "chickens literally dying before our eyes."[444] "One moment, birds happily pecked their grain," he recalled, "the next, they fell sideways in slow motion, gasping for breath with blood slowly oozing from their guts."[445] On necropsy, pathologists found that the virus had reduced the birds' internal organs to a bloody pulp. "We were looking at a chicken Ebola," Shortridge recalled.[446] "It was an unbelievable situation, totally frightening. My mind just raced," he remembered. "I thought, 'My God. What if this virus were to get out of this market and spread elsewhere?'"[447]

Close Call

The second human to die in Hong Kong was a thirteen-year-old girl with a headache. She soon started coughing blood as her lungs began hemorrhaging. The internal bleeding spread to her intestinal tract, and then her kidneys shut down.[448] She fought for weeks on a ventilator before she died. "To me," remarked Webster, "the startling thing about the second case is that there is a second case." The experts still couldn't believe that a virus supposed to be "strictly for the birds" was directly attacking human children.[449]

These initial cases started with typical flu symptoms—fever, headache, malaise, muscle aches, sore throat, cough, and a runny nose. They weren't dying of a superimposed bacterial pneumonia as one tends to see in seasonal influenza deaths of the elderly and infirm. H5N1 seemed to have gotten the immune system to do the dirty work.

Autopsies were performed on two of the first six victims, the thirteen-year-old girl in Hong Kong and a twenty-five-year-old Filipino woman. Both died of multiple organ failure. Their lungs were filled with blood, their livers and kidneys clogged with dead tissue, and their brains swollen with fluid.[450]

In both cases, cytokine levels were found elevated as expected. The virus evidently had tricked the body into unleashing massive cytokine storms, burning their livers, kidneys, and lungs in their immune systems' not-so-friendly fire. Interestingly, viral cultures taken at autopsy from all their organs came up negative. It seems that in their bodies' brutal counter-attack, their immune systems were able to triumph in a way and kill off the virus. Of course, in burning down the village in order to save it, the patients were killed off as well.[451]

Most of the 1997 victims had either bought chickens (or, in one case, chicken feet) or had shopped next door to a chicken merchant.[452] Lam Hoi-ka may have been infected by baby birds in his preschool's "feathered pet cor-ner."[453] The strongest risk factor to shake out of the subsequent investigations was "either direct or indirect contact with commercial poultry."[454]

Human-to-human transmission remained very limited. An infected banker, for example, didn't pass the virus on to coworkers, but when a two-year-old boy had "played with and been hugged and kissed by his symptom-atic 5-year old female cousin," he joined her in the hospital three days later.[455] Thankfully, they both recovered. The virus only seemed to be spread by close, rather than casual, contact. One of Lam Hoi-ka's doctors came up positive for the virus, for example, but it is believed she had come in contact with his tears.[456] The virus was still learning, but the scientific community was bent on putting an end to its education.

Realizing the disease was coming from chickens, leading scientists called for every chicken in the entire territory to be killed at once to stop any and all new human cases. "The infection was obviously tearing away at the inside of the birds," Shortridge realized. "My reaction was: 'This virus must not es-cape from Hong Kong.'"[457] Biologically the plan made sense, but politically it was a tough sell. "It was absolutely terrifying," Shortridge remembered. "You could feel the weight of the world pressing down on you."[458]

The weight of world opinion may indeed have been what finally led to the government's concession. Hong Kong had just been reunified with China and with eyes focused on the fledgling power, it could not afford to be perceived as endangering the rest of the world.[459] Amid mounting panic, Margaret F. C. Chan, who would go on to lead the investigation into SARS and become the World Health Organization's influenza chief, ordered the death sentence for more than a million birds.[460]

For four days, hundreds of Hong Kong's government workers—many of them desk workers—engaged in the slaughter.[461] Scuffles broke out with chicken vendors. Buddhist monks held a seven-day prayer chant for the souls of the birds.[462]

Overnight, new human infections ceased. The last human case in the 1997 Hong Kong outbreak was recognized the day before the slaughter commenced.[463] In all, only eighteen people got sick and only six people died.

"Next to a battle lost, the greatest misery is a battle gained."

—DUKE OF WELLINGTON

Books have been written about the 1997 outbreak. Noted journalist Pete Davies was with Webster eight months after the mass slaughter, perched on an Arctic mountainside within miles of the North Pole. He asked Webster if they had done the right thing killing all those chickens in Hong Kong. "It was a killer—like 1918 on its way."[464] If the chickens hadn't been killed, Webster replied, "I would predict that you and I would not be sitting here talking now. Because one of us would be dead."[465]

Other experts agree. "Imagine if that virus obtained a little additional capacity to be freely transmitted in humans," said Klaus Stöhr, head of the World Health Organization's influenza program, "a large proportion of the population of the world would presumably have died."[466] Fukuda explained: "When you look at the people who died . . . [most] were basically healthy young adults. These are not the kinds of people you normally see dying from influenza . . . and most of them died from illnesses generally consistent with viral pneumonia—so it's *very* similar to the picture we saw in 1918. It's disturbingly similar—and that's what gave this added sick feeling in all our stomachs."[467]

The Hong Kong government took heat from the poultry industry for its decision to kill more than a million birds, but was vindicated by a 1998 joint proclamation signed by nineteen of the world's experts on influenza, including the World Health Organization's chief authority, expressing gratitude for Hong Kong's decision. The proclamation concluded: "We may owe our very lives to their actions."[468]

Only years later did intensive research on the H5N1 virus reveal how close the world had truly come to facing a pandemic. There was evidence that during the Hong Kong crisis the virus was rapidly adapting to the new human host, acquiring mutations that increased its ability to replicate in human tissue. Shortridge, who first identified H5N1 in Hong Kong's chickens, wrote in 2000, "It is probably fair to say that a pandemic had been averted."[469]

The Hong Kong Medical Association's infectious disease expert, however, warned that this may not have been the end to H5N1. "And as long as we have the circumstances which can favour the spread of H5N1," he said, "it can occur again."[470] The CDC's Keiji Fukuda was asked in an interview whether the prospect of H5N1's return robbed him of any sleep. "More nights than I like," he admitted.[471]

Closely studying the Hong Kong H5N1 virus, Webster estimated that it may have taken only months for it "to acquire whatever mutations are needed for transmitting between people—but it would have done it," he said. "And if it had got away, my God. . . . I am convinced that this virus was probably like 1918. It was wholly avian, yes—but it had human aspects that we've never seen before."[472] We now suspect the 1918 virus was wholly avian as well, a "human adapted variant of a pathogenic avian strain."[473]

Mike Ryan, founding member of the Global Outbreak Alert and Response Network at the World Health Organization, described H5N1 in birds as "a disease of biblical proportion."[474]

In a textbook published by Oxford University, Webster wrote this about the Pennsylvania H5 outbreak in 1983:

How do we cope with such an epidemic? The Agriculture Department used the standard methods of eradication, killing the infected chickens and exposed neighboring birds and burying the carcasses. But we can't help asking ourselves what we would have done if this virus had occurred in humans. We can't dig holes and bury all the people in the world.[475]

What Happens to a Pandemic Deferred?

The killing of all the chickens in Hong Kong in 1997 stopped H5N1, but not for long. The same underlying conditions that originally led to its emergence were still in place; it was just a matter of time.

Experts think human influenza started about 4,500 years ago with the domestication of waterfowl like ducks, the original source of all influenza viruses.[476] According to Professor Shortridge, this "brought influenza viruses into the 'farmyard,' leading to the emergence of epidemics and pandemics."[477] Before 2500 B.C.E., it's likely that nobody ever got the flu.

Duck farming dramatically spread and intensified over the last five hundred years, beginning during the Ching Dynasty in China in A.D. 1644.[478] Farmers moved ducks from the rivers and tributaries onto flooded rice fields to be used as an adjunct to rice farming. This led to a permanent year-round gene pool of avian influenza viruses in East Asia in close proximity to humans.[479] The domestic duck of southern China has been considered the principal host of all influenza viruses with pandemic potential.[480]

This is probably why two of the last three flu pandemics started in China.[481] According to the United Nations' Food and Agriculture Organization (FAO), China is the largest producer of chicken, duck, and goose meat for human consumption.[482] It accounts for 70 percent of the world's tonnage of duck meat and more than 90 percent of global goose meat.[483] China has more than two dozen species of waterfowl.[484] As Osterholm has said, "China represents the most incredible reassortment laboratory for influenza viruses that anyone could ever imagine."[485]

Extensive sampling of Asian waterfowl in the years following the Hong Kong outbreak seems to have tracked H5N1 to a farmed goose outbreak in 1996, the year the number of waterfowl raised in China exceeded two billion birds.[486] The virus seemed to have been playing a game of Duck, Duck, Goose . . . then Chicken.

In 2001, the virus arose again from the primordial reservoir of waterfowl to make a comeback among chickens in Hong Kong.[487] Once again, all the chickens were destroyed—this time before anyone fell ill.[488] Sporadic outbreaks continued through 2002, but people didn't start dying again in Hong Kong until 2003.[489] By the end of that year, the virus would escape China and start its rampage across the continent.

As revelers got ready to ring in 2004, the FAO and other international organizations began to hear rumors of widespread outbreaks of a virulent disease obliterating chicken flocks across the region.[490] Reports were coming from so many directions at the same time that authorities didn't know which to believe. Within a month, though, they were all confirmed. H5N1 had burst forth from China, erupting across eight countries nearly simultaneously. It quickly became the greatest outbreak of avian influenza in history.[491]

Given the pattern and timing of outbreaks, trade in live birds was blamed for the spread throughout Southeast Asia.[492] For example, chickens made nearly a thousand-mile trek from the Ganzu province in China to Tibet via truck.[493] The Vietnamese Prime Minister quickly imposed a ban on all transport of chickens,[494] but the widespread smuggling of birds is thought to have continued the viral spread throughout the region.[495] It would be another year before the virus would learn how to hitch rides on migratory waterfowl to wing its way westward,[496] although the poultry trade may also have played a role in the spread of H5N1 to the Middle East, Europe, and Africa.[497] Even in the United States, a shipment of chicken parts marked "jellyfish" was allegedly smuggled in from Thailand and distributed to ten states before it was confiscated.[498] At a single port in California, customs agents intercepted illegal shipments of nearly seventy-five tons of poultry smuggled in from Asia and about a hundred thousand eggs within a three-month period in 2005.[499] One biologist remarked that the reason why the focus has remained on the birds in the poultry trade is that "[c]orporations pay more taxes than migratory birds do."[500]

Within a few months, more than a hundred million birds across Asia were killed by the disease or culled.[501] Birds were buried alive by the millions in Thailand and burned alive in China.[502] Birds were stomped to death in Taiwan and beaten to death in Vietnam.[503] The French media reported: "Soldiers stripped to the waist pound terrified ducks with bloody sticks; farmers dressed in grubby clothes grab chickens squawking from their cages to wring their necks, and twitching bags stuffed with live birds are tossed into a ditch and covered in dirt."[504] Lest Westerners judge, the U.S. egg industry has thrown live hens with waning egg productivity into wood chippers[505] and continues to drop living male baby chicks of egg-laying breeds into high-speed grinders.[506] Humane considerations aside, the World Health Organization is concerned that the methods of culling and disposal could increase the risk of human exposure. "If [the killing of birds] is done in such a way that exposes more people [to the virus]," said one WHO spokesperson, "then this . . . could be increasing the risk of developing a strain that you would not want to see."[507]

Despite the culling, the virus came back strong in the fall of 2004, first spreading its wings throughout Southeast Asia[508] and then the Middle East, Africa, and Europe.[509] As 2004 came to an end, former U.S. Secretary of Health and Human Services Tommy G. Thompson told reporters in his farewell news conference that H5N1 was his greatest fear, eclipsing bioterrorism. Bird flu, he said, was a "really huge bomb."[510]

Year of the Rooster

The year 2005, the Chinese zodiac's Year of the Rooster, saw a resurgence of human deaths. By June, more than a hundred laboratory-confirmed cases were reported to the WHO, with more than fifty deaths.[511] The year also saw the continuation of an alarming trend in the growth of H5N1's learning curve.

The WHO's Klaus Stöhr explained in an editorial in *The New England Journal of Medicine*: "Recent laboratory and epidemiologic studies have yielded disturbing evidence that the H5N1 virus has become progressively more pathogenic in poultry, has increased environmental resistance, and is expanding its mammalian host range."[512] By 2003, H5N1 had undergone more than a dozen reassortments with other influenza viruses since its re-emergence among domestic poultry in 2001, trading genes like baseball cards and forming a powerhouse H5N1 mutant known to scientists as type *Z*. The virus was shuffling between more than a dozen decks, picking all the best cards. The adaptations that allowed *Z* to survive in the ambient environment augmented the virus's ability to infect, spread, and mutate even further. Within a year, the mutant *Z+* was born.[513]

Z+ led to the explosion of cases across Asia in 2004. H5N1 had slowly but surely mastered the ability to spread among chickens with supreme efficiency, flooding across poultry-raising nations. It had also gotten better at killing.

University of Wisconsin virologists were the first to show that the virus's lethality was not limited to birds. Influenza viruses don't typically kill mammals like mice, but in the lab, *Z+* killed 100 percent of the test population, practically dissolving their lungs.[514] "This is the most pathogenic virus that we know of," declared the lead investigator. "One infectious particle— one single infectious virion—kills mice. Amazing virus."[515] Crystallography studies showed that on a molecular level the virus had begun structurally to look more like the virus of 1918.[516]

H5N1 began taking more species under its wing. Reports came from China that pigs were infected,[517] raising a concern that these animals could act as additional gene "swap meets." Since pigs can be infected with both hu- man and avian flu, they are thought to act as "mixing vessels" for influenza viruses.[518]

Pet cats began to die.[519] This was the first time on record that cats had *ever* come down with the flu. Cats had always been considered resistant to getting the disease.[520] "If avian influenza has one predictable property, it is that it is not predictable," lamented an Ohio State University biologist. "It has made a fool of us more than once."[521]

Tigers and leopards in zoos who were fed chickens from the local slaughterhouse fell ill and died.[522] In Thailand's largest tiger zoo, more than a hundred big cats were killed. There was suggestive evidence that the virus was able to spread from tiger to tiger,[523] and experimental studies seem to have confirmed the suspicion.[524] Webster's lab discovered that ferrets could also be infected with the virus, leading to rapid paralysis and death. "The outbreaks indicate that the virus has become highly pathogenic to more and more species," reported Shigeru Omi, former WHO regional director for the Western Pacific region. "The virus remains unstable, unpredictable and very versatile. Anything could happen. Judging from the way the virus has behaved it may have new and unpleasant surprises in store for us."[525]

The feline outbreaks had researchers very concerned. The virus was be- coming better adapted to kill mammals. "Every species leap [by H5N1] rep- resents a new virus mutation, increasing the chance that one will become highly infectious to humans," explained one WHO epidemiologist.[526] Not only was the virus getting a better feel for mammalian biology, it was begin- ning to learn how to spread mammal to mammal.

Because cats, unlike pigs, are resistant to human influenza, they would presumably not be able to act as mixing vessels in which viral gene shuffling could potentially form bird/human hybrid viruses like those that triggered the pandemics of 1957 and 1968. But what the cat could drag in is a facili- tation of the stepwise adaptation of the avian virus towards direct human infection and transmission, as presumably occurred in the pandemic of 1918. These home and zoo outbreaks also suggest viral infection in the meat.

PLAYING CHICKEN

"Where chicken soup used to cure the flu, now it gives you the flu."

—JAY LENO[527]

To avoid contracting bird flu, an influenza expert at the UK Health Protection Agency warned, "[a]void being in touching distance [of birds who could be affected]. Don't kiss chickens."[528] Kissing aside, what is the risk of putting our lips on them in other ways?

Investigators suspect that at least five people living near Hanoi contracted H5N1 after dining on congealed duck blood pudding, a traditional Vietnamese dish called *tiet canh vit* prepared from a duck's blood, stomach, and intestines.[529] This led the FAO to advise, "People should not eat raw blood."[530] But what about the skeletal muscle tissue we know as meat?

In 2001, the virus was found and confirmed in frozen Pekin duck meat exported from mainland China. The investigators concluded, "The isolation of an H5N1 influenza virus from duck meat and the presence of infectious virus in muscle tissue of experimentally infected ducks raises concern that meat produced by this species may serve as a vehicle for the transmission of H5N1 virus to humans."[531]

Inexplicably, after meeting with the Chinese president in April 2006, then President George W. Bush agreed to allow the resumption of poultry imports from China starting in May. Although the meat would be cooked before export, which should kill the virus, members of the U.S. House and Senate agriculture committees expressed concern about quality control in Chinese processing plants.[532] Some critics suspect that this concession was made in return for China's promise to drop the mad cow disease–related ban on U.S. beef imports.[533]

The finding of H5N1-contaminated poultry meat triggered a more extensive survey. Investigators randomly sampled duck meat from China and found that thirteen of fourteen imported lots all contained up to a thousand infectious doses of virus. The researchers concluded that "the isolation of H5N1 viruses from duck meat reveals a previously unrecognized source for human exposure to potential highly pathogenic viruses."[534]

Top flu researchers at the U.S. Department of Agriculture (USDA) looked into chicken. Chickens who inhaled H5N1 became infected even more systemically than did ducks.[535] The virus spread through the internal organs, into the muscle tissue, and even out into the skin. Virus was found in both white and dark meat.[536]

There is a precedent for bird-borne virus-infected meat.[537] Unlike bacteria, viruses can remain infective for prolonged periods even in processed foods. Some methods of preservation, like refrigeration, freezing, or salting, may even extend the persistence of viruses in food.[538] On the other hand, since viruses cannot replicate without living tissue, improper storage of food is less problematic.[539]

When someone gets hepatitis from eating strawberries, it didn't come from the strawberries—the fruits don't have livers. The virus came from human or nonhuman fecal material, the cause of nearly all foodborne illness. For the same reason that people are likelier to get mad cow disease than Dutch elm disease or never seem to come down with a really bad case of aphids, food products of animal origin are the source of most cases of food poisoning,[540] with chicken the most common culprit.[541] Poultry and eggs seem to cause more food poisoning cases than red meat, seafood, and dairy products combined.[542]

Due to viral contamination of meat in general, those who handle fresh meat for a living can come down with unpleasant conditions with names like contagious pustular dermatitis. Fresh meat is so laden with viruses that there is a well-defined medical condition colloquially known as "butcher's warts," affecting the hands of those who handle fresh poultry,[543] fish,[544] and other meat.[545] Even wives of butchers seem to be at higher risk of cervical cancer,[546] a cancer definitively associated with wart virus exposure.[547] Concerns about viral infection even led to recommendations that pregnant women and people with AIDS not work the slaughter lines.[548] Proper cooking of the meat, though, utterly kills all known viruses.

Isolated viruses like influenza can be killed by exposure to 158 degrees Fahrenheit for less than a minute in a laboratory setting.[549] In the kitchen, however, it's a little more complicated. While some authorities feel that one can just cook until the meat is no longer pink and the juices run clear, USDA bird flu guidelines insist on the use of a meat thermometer. USDA recommends cooking whole birds to 180°F as measured in the thigh, while an individual breast need only reach an internal 170°F. Drumsticks, thighs and wings cooked separately should reach 180°F inside, but ground turkey and chicken need only be cooked to 165°F, though the minimum oven temperature to use when cooking poultry should never drop below 325°F.[550]

Because proper cooking methods kill the virus[551] no matter how deadly it is, the standard government and industry line remains: "There is no risk of getting avian influenza from properly cooked poultry and eggs."[552] But that's what they say about all foodborne illnesses. The CDC estimates that forty-eight million Americans come down with food poisoning every year. Annually, an estimated three thousand Americans die as a result of foodborne illness.[553] And every single one of those millions of infections, every single one of those thousands of deaths, was caused by a virus or bacteria that should have been utterly destroyed by "proper" cooking. So why are tens of millions of Americans still falling ill?

Cooking the Crap Out of It

Cross-contamination—the infection of kitchen implements, surfaces, or food during preparation *before* cooking—may be considered the predominant cause of food poisoning.[554] "It does not require much imagination," reads a public health textbook, "to appreciate the ease with which a few hundred bacteria can be transferred from, say, a fresh broiler [chicken] covered in a million bacteria to a nearby bit of salad or piece of bread."[555]

Knowing that poultry is the most common cause of food poisoning in the home, microbiologists had fifty people take chicken straight from a supermarket and prepare a meal with it as they normally would in their own kitchen. The researchers then took samples from such kitchen staples as sponges, dishcloths, and hand towels, and tested them for the presence of disease-causing bacteria like *Campylobacter* and *Salmonella*. They found multiple contaminated samples. "Antibacterial" dishwashing liquid did not seem to offer any protection. They concluded, "Pathogenic bacteria can be recovered relatively frequently from the kitchen environment."[556] Some animal parts are so contaminated that the CDC recommends that during preparation the household meat handler find caretakers to supervise his or her children so as not to infect them.[557]

The World Health Organization describes where most bird flu infections have originated: "[D]irect touching of poultry or poultry feces contaminated surfaces, eating uncooked poultry products (e.g., blood) or preparing poultry have been considered the probable routes of exposure leading to infection in most older children and adults."[558] Unfortunately, the "poultry feces contaminated surfaces" may be our countertops.

Medical researchers at the University of Minnesota took more than a thousand food samples from multiple retail markets and found evidence of fecal contamination in 69 percent of the pork and beef and *92 percent* of the poultry samples, as evidenced by contamination with the intestinal bug *E. coli.*[559] This confirms USDA baseline data stating, astonishingly, that "greater than 99% of broiler carcasses had detectable *E. coli.*"[560] "If chicken were tap water," journalist Nicols Fox wrote in her widely acclaimed book *Spoiled,* "the supply would be cut off."[561]

Most Americans don't realize that our poultry supply is contaminated with fecal matter. Delmer Jones, past president of the U.S. Meat Inspection Union, described USDA labels as misleading to the public. He suggested, "The label should declare that the product has been contaminated with fecal material."[562] Eric Schlosser in *Fast Food Nation* proposed a more straightforward approach: "There is shit in the meat."[563]

How did it get there? After chickens are shackled, stunned, have their necks cut, and bleed to death, they are scalded, defeathered, and have their heads and feet removed. The next step is evisceration. Birds are typically gutted by a machine that uses a metal hook to pull out the guts.[564] The intestines are often ripped in the process, spilling the contaminated contents over the carcass. If even a single bird is infected, the machinery is then contaminated and can pass infection down the line. In one study, when one chicken was inoculated with tracer bacteria, the next forty-two birds subsequently processed were found to be cross-infected. Sporadic contamination occurred up to the 150th bird.[565] The World Health Organization concludes that large, centralized, and mechanized slaughter plants may "create hazards for the human food chain."[566]

Millions of chickens miss the killing blade and are drowned in the scalding tanks every year[567] because the USDA does not include poultry under the protections of the federal Humane Methods of Slaughter Act.[568] The birds, still conscious, may defecate in the tanks and inhale water polluted by fecal leakage into their lungs,[569] which can lead to further contamination of the carcass down the line.[570] Controlled atmosphere killing, which uses inert gases to essentially put the birds to sleep, is a more hygienic method of slaughter.[571]

According to former USDA microbiologist Gerald Kuester, "there are about 50 points during processing where cross-contamination can occur. At the end of the line, the birds are no cleaner than if they had been dipped in a toilet."[572] The toilet, in this case, is the chill water bath at the end of the line in which the birds' remains may soak for an hour to increase profitability by adding water weight to the carcass. At this point, the bath water is more of a chilled fecal soup. This collective soak has been shown to increase contamination levels by almost a quarter. "That extra 24% of contamination the chill water adds," writes Nicols Fox, "can be credited to pure greed."[573]

As Fox points out in *Spoiled,* the microbiologist's assertion that the "final product is no different than if you stuck it in the toilet and ate it" is not gross hyperbole. (Gross, perhaps, but not hyperbole.) In fact, the toilet might actually be safer than your sink. Researchers at the University of Arizona found more fecal bacteria in the kitchen—on sponges, dish towels, the sink drain, and countertops—than they found swabbing the rim of the toilet.[574] Comparing surfaces in bathrooms and kitchens in the same household, the investigators note, "consistently, kitchens come up dirtier."[575] The excess fecal contamination is presumed to come from raw animal products brought into the home. As Fox points out, "The bathroom is cleaner because people are not washing their chickens in the toilet."[576]

Handle with Care

Animal manure is the source of more than a hundred pathogens, including bacteria, parasites, and viruses that could be transmitted from animals to humans, such as influenza.[577] According to the WHO's International Food Safety Authorities Network, when it comes to bird flu viruses like H5N1, "handling of frozen or thawed raw poultry meat before cooking can be hazardous if good hygiene practices are not observed."[578] According to the USDA, this includes washing hands, cutting boards, knives, utensils, and all countertops and surfaces with hot, soapy water after cutting raw meats. All meats and their "juices" need to be quarantined away from all other foods. Further, cutting boards need to be sanitized with a chlorine bleach solution

(1 teaspoon bleach in 1 quart of water) and food thermometers should be used without exception.[579]

One state epidemiologist describes what she does to avoid foodborne illness risks in general: "I assume that poultry is contaminated, and that any package of hamburger I buy is grossly contaminated too. When I'm preparing a turkey or hamburger, I have everything out and ready, the pan on the counter, right where my meat is, so that I don't have to go in the cupboard to get it. Then I've got the soap handy, of course. After I handle the meat, I use my wrists to turn on the faucet so I'm not touching it with my dirty hands. I wash my hands thoroughly for at least thirty seconds."[580]

This is why the official U.S. poultry industry's slogan "Avian Influenza: It's not in your food"[581] may be so misleading. That's like saying *Salmonella* is not in your food. Or *Campylobacter* is not in your food. Tell that to the millions of Americans who fall ill every year from these poultry pathogens.[582] Would we go to the store and pick up a package of meat that might be contaminated with HIV or hepatitis, even if there was a certainty that the virus was killed by cooking? We presumably wouldn't want to risk bringing any potentially deadly viruses into our home.

A WHO spokesperson added the critical caveat: "The chicken is safe to eat if it is well cooked, provided that the people preparing the chicken have not contaminated themselves from somewhere."[583] Thai government officials reportedly confirmed that a forty-eight-year-old man died of bird flu after cooking and eating a neighbor's infected chickens.[584] Maybe he didn't properly Clorox his cutting board or he accidentally used his hand to turn on the kitchen faucet. Maybe he didn't sterilize his meat thermometer every time he checked to see if the fecal viruses had been killed. "To me," writes Nicols Fox, "it is really asking the consumer to operate a kind of biohazard lab."[585]

Consider the CDC's recommended disposal methods for carcasses known to be infected with bird flu:

* Disposable gloves made of lightweight nitrile or vinyl or heavy duty rubber work gloves that can be disinfected should be worn. . . . Gloves should be changed if torn or otherwise damaged. Remove gloves promptly after use, before touching non-contaminated items and environmental surfaces.

- Protective clothing, preferably disposable outer garments or coveralls, an impermeable apron or surgical gowns with long cuffed sleeves, plus an impermeable apron should be worn.
- Disposable protective shoe covers or rubber or polyurethane boots that can be cleaned and disinfected should be worn.
- Safety goggles should be worn to protect the mucous membranes of eyes.
- Disposable particulate respirators (e.g., N-95, N-99, or N-100) are the minimum level of respiratory protection that should be worn. . . . Workers must be fit-tested to the respirator model that they will wear and also know how to check the face-piece to face seal. Workers who cannot wear a disposable particulate respirator because of facial hair or other fit limitations should wear a loose-fitting (i.e., helmeted or hooded) powered air purifying respirator equipped with high-efficiency filters.[586]

This should give pause to those of us who might unknowingly dispose of infected carcasses through consumption.

Bird flu viruses like H5N1 can survive in feces as long as thirty-five days at low temperatures.[587] We can't just wash it off? Poultry companies have actually been revising labeling to steer consumers away from the age-old practice of washing a fresh bird inside and out.[588] In fact, federal dietary guidelines have specifically recommended that "meat and poultry should not be washed or rinsed." The USDA is concerned that this practice could cause viral or bacterial splatter from "raw meat and poultry juices." Animals, of course, are not fruit; they don't really have "juice," per se. "Chicken juice" is the fecal broth absorbed in the chill bath.

The *Tufts University Health and Nutrition Letter* explains: "Your own hands, where they grasped the meat while washing it, could become just as bacteria-laden as the surface of the food . . . The best bet is to leave meat or poultry untouched until you start cooking it."[589] What are we supposed to do, *levitate* it into the oven? Research suggests we could infect ourselves before even leaving the grocery store.

Researchers published a study in the *Journal of Food Protection* in which they swabbed the plastic-wrapped surface of prepackaged raw meat in grocery stores for fecal contamination. Even though most of the packages looked clean on the outside, the researchers found *Salmonella, Campylobacter,* and multidrug-resistant *E. coli* on the outer surface of the packages, suggesting that just picking up a package of meat in the store could put one at risk. Poultry beat the competition for the most contamination. A single swab picked up more than ten thousand live *E. coli* bacteria. The researchers concluded, "The external packaging of raw meats is a vehicle for potential cross-contamination by *Campylobacter, Salmonella,* and *E. coli* in retail premises and consumers' homes."[590]

Realizing this level of contamination, bird flu experts at a CDC symposium reminded consumers not to touch our mucous membranes—rub our eyes or noses—while handling any raw poultry products.[591] Vegetarian? Risk applies to non-meat-eaters as well: Any fecal-fluid drippings of bird droppings trailing down the checkout counter conveyer belt could easily contaminate fresh produce.

A cooked fly in one's soup poses no danger. Fecal matter, once properly shaked and baked, may be perfectly safe, but we may still not want to feed it to our family. "After all," as *Consumer Reports* put it, "sterilized poop is still poop."[592] What would we do if we found out there was a small chance that, in the back of the grocery store, some malicious prankster had smeared our dinner with bird droppings? Would we still buy it? What if the chance of contamination was greater than 90 percent?

There are a number of toxins that can make one ill that are denatured (destroyed) by cooking, such as botulinum toxin, the cause of botulism. Even if such a toxin was rendered utterly and completely harmless by cooking, would we still consider bringing contaminated products into our homes, putting them onto the kitchen counter, and feeding them to our kids, knowing that one accident on our part, one little spill, one little drip, could potentially land our loved ones in the hospital?

Some suggest keeping birds out of the kitchen altogether. During an interview recorded by the Government Accountability Project, a USDA meat inspector stated:

> *I will not buy inspected product—only what I raise. I do not eat out, and I don't allow my children to eat at school. We didn't use to have to put warning labels on product for "safe handling" but we do now. This is just a politically correct way of saying "cook good, this product may contain fecal matter and other poor sanitary handling bacterias." I was told by a supervisor some time back that if you cook a piece of [feces] to 170 degrees you can eat it and it*

won't hurt you. But I don't really think the consumer is aware of the [feces]
they are being fed.[593]

Soft-Boiled Truth

What about eggs? "Be careful with eggs," the World Health Organization has warned.[594] "Eggs from infected poultry could also be contaminated with the [H5N1] virus and therefore care should be taken in handling shell eggs or raw egg products."[595] This includes first washing eggs with soapy water and then afterward washing our hands and all surfaces and utensils thoroughly with soap and water.[596] Given that pigs fed eggs from an infected flock fell ill, researchers maintain that the "survival time of the viruses . . . on surfaces such as eggs is sufficient to allow wide dissemination."[597] According to the European Centre for Disease Prevention and Control, the biggest risk from eggs is that the shells may harbor traces of excrement containing the virus.[598]

The comic strip *One Big Happy* by Rick Detorie once explained the layers of infection. A father and daughter are in the grocery store. "That's a cow's tongue?!" the girl exclaims, face contorted in disgust. "EEEEww . . . I would never eat anything that was in a cow's mouth!" "Me neither," replies the father, not looking up from his shopping list. "Let's see, where are the eggs?" The daughter stops, eyes wide in realization: "Wait a minute!" Eggs do, after all, come out of a chicken's rear (vagina and rectum combine into the cloaca).

Like *Salmonella,* bird flu viruses can infect the chickens' ovaries, so the virus can come prepackaged within the egg as well.[599] During the 1983 Pennsylvania outbreak, the virus was found festering within both the egg white and the yolk, making proper cooking essential.[600] To reduce the risk of contracting bird flu from eggs, the Mayo Clinic warns about mayo: "Avoid eating raw or undercooked eggs or any products containing them, including mayonnaise, hollandaise sauce and homemade ice cream."[601] Other potential sources of raw or undercooked eggs include mousse, Caesar salad, homemade eggnog, lemon meringue pie, tiramisu, raw cookie dough, and eggs that are soft boiled, lightly poached, or cooked sunny side up or "over easy" with a runny yolk. The latest CDC[602] and WHO[603] recommendations are adamant on this point—whether it's to avoid bird flu or *Salmonella,* egg yolks should not be runny or liquid. Researchers concluded in the *Journal of the American Medical Association* that "no duration of frying 'sunnyside' (not turned) eggs was sufficient to kill all the *Salmonella*."[604]

But haven't people been cooking eggs that way for a hundred years? Diseases like bird flu and *Salmonella* were practically unknown a handful of decades ago. Our grandparents could drink eggnog with wild abandon while their grandkids could eat raw cookie dough without fear of joining the more than a thousand Americans who may die every year from *Salmonella* poisoning. There was a time when medium-rare hamburgers, raw milk, and steak tartare were less dangerous, a time when Rocky Balboa could more safely drink his raw-egg smoothies. Blaming customers for mishandling or improper cooking is only possible when all of this is forgotten.

Said USDA microbiologist Nelson Cox, "Raw meats are not idiot-proof. They can be mishandled and when they are, it's like handling a hand grenade. If you pull the pin, somebody's going to get hurt." While some may question the wisdom of selling hand grenades in the supermarket, Cox disagrees: "I think the consumer has the most responsibility but refuses to accept it."[605] Patricia Griffin, director of Epidemiological Research at the Centers for Disease Control, responded famously to this kind of blame-the-victim attitude. "Is it reasonable," she asked, "that if a consumer undercooks a hamburger . . . their three-year-old dies?"[606]

Pre-processed foods, however, are undeniably industry's responsibility. Eggs used in processed food products are pasteurized first to ensure safety. Because the use of eggs is so widespread in the processed food industry (about one-third of the eggs Americans consume are eaten in products),[607] USDA researchers studied standard industry pasteurization protocols to make certain that no bird flu virus was left alive. Although they found that pasteurization did kill the virus in liquid eggs (used in products like Egg Beaters®), the standard method used to pasteurize dried egg products—which are ubiquitously used as ingredients by the processed food and baking industries—was not effective in eliminating the deadliest bird flu viruses. The USDA researchers showed that while the industry standard "low temperature pasteurization protocol"—one week at 130 degrees Fahrenheit—killed the low-grade bird flu viruses naturally adapted to wintering in ice-cold Canadian lakes, the high-grade bird flu viruses like H5N1 adapted to land-based domestic poultry survived more than two weeks at that temperature. The length of time required to kill the virus, about fifteen days, was considered inconsistent with "commercial application."[608]

Tastes Like Chicken

Government reactions to egg and poultry food safety recommendations in light of bird flu were mixed. In Indonesia and Pakistan,[609] health ministers called upon people to stop consuming chicken and eggs for the time being,[610] whereas the Prime Minister of Thailand promised 3 million baht ($76,000) to relatives of anyone dying from cooked eggs or chicken.[611] The international airport in Rome promised the "destruction by incineration of any poultry-based food found in the luggage of passengers traveling from risk areas."[612] A European Food Safety Authority advisory panel advised Europeans to cook all eggs and chicken carefully in light of the disease spreading from Asia.[613] They also cautioned that down and feathers originating from affected areas "may be infective due to contamination with infective faeces or other body fluids" and noted that processing methods for these materials "vary widely as regards virus reduction."[614]

U.S. officials appeared less concerned. During a 2002 outbreak of low-grade avian influenza across Virginia, West Virginia, and North Carolina, most of the millions of infected and potentially infected carcasses were disposed of in landfills at a cost of up to $140 per ton of carcasses. (Incineration is more expensive, costing producers $500 per carcass ton.[615]) USDA's chief flu researcher David Swayne recommended producers try to recoup the costs of culling by selling sick birds for human consumption. They argued that since only high-grade viruses have been found in skeletal muscle meat, it was okay for producers to market birds infected with low-grade viruses for food as a cheap "method of elimination."[616]

Remarkably, Swayne has since disclosed that a scientist in his own lab demonstrated in the early 1990s that even low-grade bird flu viruses infect the birds' abdominal air sacs that extend up into the breastbone and the humerus on the wing. "[S]o there would be obviously a potential for air sac contamination of the associated meat products if they contained bone," Swayne admitted.[617]

Still, Swayne suggests that even birds infected with high-grade bird flu viruses could be used as meat as long as they were sent for further processing and turned into precooked products.[618] The Food and Agriculture Organization of the United Nations disagrees. "Poultry from infected flocks should be disposed of by environmentally sound methods and should not be processed for animal and human food consumption."[619] The FAO evidently frowns on the disposing of infected carcasses by putting them on our dinner plates. Even suspect birds not yet showing signs of infection, according to the FAO, should be destroyed and disposed of, should "not be allowed to enter the human food chain or be fed directly or indirectly to other animals including zoo animals."[620]

During the 2002 outbreak, even the rendering industry—which turns slaughterhouse waste, roadkill, and euthanized pets into farm animal feed and pet food[621]—was reluctant to accept birds from an avian influenza outbreak because of the stigma attached to the disease.[622] Too tainted for pets, but not for kids?

WORSE THAN 1918?

Higher Human Learning

The Z+ strain of H5N1 not only got better at killing other mammals like mice, pigs, and cats, but it learned how to burrow deep into human lungs. The scientist who discovered the SARS virus explains how H5N1 has mutated to better effect our death: "Unlike the normal human flu, where the virus is predominantly in the upper respiratory tract so you get a runny nose, sore throat, the H5N1 virus seems to go directly deep into the lungs so it goes down into the lung tissue and causes severe pneumonia."[623] Then director of Oxford University's Clinical Research Unit in Ho Chi Minh City describes how shocked he was by what he was seeing. "I've never experienced anything like it in terms of its destructive power."[624]

H5N1 and the virus of 1918 share a proclivity for the lungs, but H5N1 doesn't always stop there. It may dig deeper, invading the bloodstream to ravage other internal organs. What starts as a respiratory infection may become a whole-body infection. Researchers were surprised to find that the 1918 virus, with all its fury, had not mutated to destroy other organs. This is thought to be why H5N1 may be more than ten times more lethal than the virus that sparked the greatest medical tragedy in human history.[625]

As human contagious diseases go, only Ebola and untreated HIV infection are deadlier.[626] But H5N1 could go airborne. In a tone one rarely finds in scholarly medical journals, *Lancet,* perhaps the most prestigious medical journal in the world, editorialized, "In view of the mortality of human influenza associated with this strain, the prospect of a worldwide pandemic is massively frightening."[627]

One of the organs H5N1 can devastate, the medical world swiftly realized, is the human brain. The first case report in *The New England Journal of Medicine* started with the line: "In southern Vietnam, a four-year-old boy presented with severe diarrhea, followed by seizures, coma, and death." His nine-year-old sister had died similarly two weeks earlier. She was fine one day and dead five days later. Her brother lasted a week. The bird flu virus seemed to attack their central nervous systems, plunging them into rapidly progressing fatal comas. The Oxford investigators concluded, "These reports suggest that avian influenza A (H5N1) virus is progressively adapting to mammals and becoming more neurologically virulent."[628]

Researchers weren't sure how the virus got to the brain. They assumed it traveled there through the bloodstream where live virus has been found,[629] but experimental studies showed a possible alternate route. Once inhaled, the virus may creep up the olfactory nerves used for our sense of smell, leading to direct brain invasion though the nose.[630] H5N1 is like no flu virus anyone has ever seen. "Just when you start to think that you've understood what it can do then it pulls another one out of the bag," St. Jude's Robert G. Webster said. "It's one of the most crafty of all infectious disease agents. It's got such a repertoire of tricks."[631] But H5N1 is still having trouble, to date, learning how to pull off its greatest trick of all—efficient human-to-human spread.

Mano-a-Mano

First, her chickens died. Then, her niece died, coughing blood as she expired in her mother's arms.[632] In 2005, *The New England Journal of Medicine* reported the first documented case of deadly human-to-human transmission of H5N1. Until that point, nearly all the human deaths had "involved people who lived or worked with poultry, poultry meat or eggs in Southeast Asia."[633] While the eleven-year-old girl was exposed to sick chickens while living in a village with her aunt, her mother arrived from the Bangkok suburbs to care for her and had no known exposure to chickens, sick or otherwise. The day after the funeral, the mother started to feel sick, too, and after severe illness, died.

The aunt also fell sick, but recovered.[634] Both she and her sister tested positive for the same virus that had killed the child.[635]

The report sent shivers down the spine of the scientific and medical community.[636] In the week following the report, the European science publication *New Scientist* ran an editorial titled "Bird Flu Outbreak Could Kill 1.5 Billion People."[637] The director of the U.S. Centers for Disease Control described it as the number-one health threat in the world and called it a "very ominous situation for the globe."[638] The head of the World Health Organization in Asia held a press conference and said, "We at WHO believe that the world is now in the gravest possible danger of a pandemic."[639]

The case compelled Thailand to launch a massive search for other cases of human spread, involving as many as one million volunteers going door-to-door. Thankfully, no further clusters of cases were found.[640] The virus still had some learning to do. Currently infection requires more than just a sneeze, a handshake, or a breath. So far, all officially suspected human-to-human transmissions have involved "close physical contact that included hugging, kissing, or cuddling the infected individuals to whom they were exposed."[641]

H5N1 has shown itself to be a gifted learner. Grasping the mutant swarm concept is critical to understanding how the virus got from strain *A* to *Z+*, and how it may get from *Z+* to the pandemic strain. One individual may theoretically only be infected by a single virus particle, but one infected cell can start sloppily churning out millions of mutant progeny. H5N1 has a large graduating class. This dynamic mutant swarm breaks out and tries to reinfect other cells. The ones that are best at infecting other human cells are naturally selected to live long and prosper, passing on their genes. Only the strong survive; it's a mammoth campaign of trial and error.

Out of millions of competing viruses, the ones whose N spikes best worm their way through human mucus, the ones whose H spikes are best at unlocking human cells, the ones with NS1 proteins that best block human interferon—those are the ones that may best survive to make millions more in the next cell. By death, their hosts' lungs are saturated with more than a billion infectious viral doses per ounce of tissue.[642] "The clock keeps ticking," Robert Webster fretted. "Every time this virus replicates, it makes mistakes. Sooner or later it will make the mistakes that will allow it to go human-to-human."[643]

Former Senate Majority Leader Bill Frist, M.D., compared H5N1 to a gambler. From the floor of the Senate, Frist explained: "Billions of mutations of the virus are occurring every day. With each mutation, the virus multiplies its odds of becoming transmissible from human to human. It's like pulling the lever on a Vegas slot machine over and over again. If you pull enough times, the reels will align and hit the jackpot."[644]

In the end, the virus that wins, the virus that succeeds in making the most copies of itself, is the virus that outperforms the others, passaging through thousands of individual cells to learn how best to infect the human species. It is that virus that gets breathed into the next person's lungs and the process starts all over so the virus can get even smarter.

Within a single individual, a virus evolves, adapts, learns. It hits dead ends and tries something new, slowly notching up mutations that may lock into place the ability to effectively survive in, and transmit between, people. Every single person who gets infected presents a risk of spawning *the* pandemic virus. Describes one virologist, "You're playing Russian roulette every time you have a human infection."[645] Experts fear that as more and more people become infected, a virus will finally figure out the combination—the right combination of mutations to spread not just in one elevator or building, but in every building, everywhere, around the globe. Then it won't just be peasant farmers in Vietnam dying after handling dead birds or raw poultry—it will be New Yorkers, Parisians, Londoners, and people in every city, township, and village in the world dying after shaking someone's hand, touching a doorknob, or simply inhaling in the wrong place at the wrong time. It's happened before, and it may soon happen again.

No Shot

Experts fear a modern pandemic could "eclipse 1918,"[646] but how could that be? We live in the age of modern medicine. We have vaccines and ventilators, antibiotics and antivirals, and the latest in medical technology. In 1918, they essentially didn't know what a virus was. One former president of the American Medical Association pointed out that the doctors of 1918 "knew no more about the flu than fourteenth-century Florentines had known about Black Death."[647] Essentially all doctors could do was advise people to get on waiting lists for caskets.[648] Sadly, though, we're not in much better shape today.

Osterholm explains why twenty-first century medical advances are not expected to make a significant dent in the coming pandemic:

We really have no armamentarium today that is any different on a [sic] whole than what we had 100 years ago, at least in terms of what's available to the world's population. We have vaccines, we have some antivirals, but they will be in such insufficient quantities as to be what we like to say filling Lake Superior with a garden hose in overall impact.[649]

Vaccines are the cornerstone in our fight against viral disease. By introducing a killed or weakened version of the target virus, we can prime our adaptive immune systems to recognize the attacker in the future and mobilize a more rapid response. Unfortunately, influenza viruses in general, and H5N1 in particular, mutate so rapidly that it is impossible to present the body with a perfect match. With H5N1, for example, we could try making vaccines out of the Z type or any of the ten different H5 bird flu lineages that have since been spawned,[650] but any strain that would eventually "go human" and trigger a pandemic may appear so differently to the body as to render the vaccine ineffective. Therefore "adequate supplies of vaccine will not be available at the start of a pandemic in any country," concludes the World Health Organization.[651] From the moment a pandemic strain is recognized, mass production of a workable flu vaccine is expected to take six to eight months. In other words, please wait six to eight months for delivery. Webster asks: "How many people are going to die in the meantime?"[652]

It may take a full year to produce enough for the United States,[653] and, by then, the pandemic may be over. With today's limited production capacity, we would not expect to be able to vaccinate more than about 14 percent of the world's population within a year of a pandemic striking.[654] The greatest problem then, according to the WHO, is production capacity.[655]

The tenuousness of modern vaccine manufacture—even for seasonal influenza[656]—became clear in 2004, when half of the expected flu vaccine for the United States had to be tossed due to sterility concerns.[657] A former director of the Center for Bioethics at the University of Pennsylvania suggested this precedent should cast doubt upon reassurances from politicians that vaccines could be distributed effectively during a pandemic. "Rhetoric about the orderly and carefully thought-out rationing of a scarce life-saving resource—flu vaccine—turned [in 2004] into a cacophony of cheating, hoarding, lying and selfishness."[658]

One of the main problems is the outdated method of vaccine production. According to the National Academy of Medicine, the basic technology for the production of influenza vaccine hasn't changed in well over fifty years,[659] dating back to when slide rules were the state of the art for mathematical calculation.[660] This archaic method involves growing the virus for vaccine production in live fertile chicken eggs, a problem if you're trying to grow a bird flu virus that may be 100 percent lethal to chickens and their eggs. Researchers have since surmounted this hurdle by using cell-based technologies, but there is no guarantee that an emerging pandemic strain could be cultivated fast enough.[661] The prospects for developing a safe, effective vaccine for COVID-19 in a timely manner are even less certain.[662] "We have to get the message out loud and clear that vaccine will not save us," emphasizes Osterholm. "We will have very little of it, and it will get here too late."[663]

Bitter Pill

Antibiotics may be even less help. We live in a global, just-in-time economy, which allows manufacturers worldwide to streamline their production to precisely meet demand, thereby reducing inventory warehousing costs and waste. The problem is that a single glitch in the supply chain can almost instantly dry up supply. During a crisis in which we shut down our borders, globalized supply chains will be shattered and vital goods like pharmaceuticals in general will be in short supply or unavailable.[664]

Antibiotics only work against bacteria. Although they can be effective in treating secondary bacterial infections, they are useless against viral pneumonia. Antibiotics were useful during the 1957 and 1968 pandemics because these were essentially just bad flu seasons when more people than expected came down with the flu due to the novelty of the bird/human hybrid viruses. The influenza of 1918 was different because many people were killed by their own immune systems in the cytokine firestorm sparked by the virus.[665] Antibiotics may not have been much help in 1918,[666] and it is feared we may face the same situation with a virus like H5N1.[667]

In the 1960s, though, a breakthrough was made. A new class of drugs—

anti*viral* drugs—hit the market, drugs that could actually block influenza viruses from entering cells.[668] The medical community breathed a collective sigh of relief. The CDC's report of the 1997 Hong Kong outbreak confidently declared, "Two antiviral drugs, amantadine and rimantadine, inhibit replication of virtually all naturally occurring human and animal strains of influenza type A [meaning influenza strains with pandemic potential] and therefore can be useful for prophylaxis and treatment of influenza A infections."[669]

The devastating news broke in June 2005. For years, Chinese chicken farmers had been slipping the drugs into the chickens' water supply to prevent economic losses from bird flu. Because of this practice, the emerging H5N1 became totally resistant to these potentially life-saving drugs. "Bird Flu Drug Rendered Useless," headlined *The Washington Post*'s exposé.[670] The scientific community's fears had been realized.[671] "In essence," one expert wrote, "this finding means that a whole class of antiviral drugs has been lost as treatment for this virus."[672]

China learned this trick from us. The use of amantadine in the water supply of commercial poultry as prophylaxis against avian influenza was pioneered in the United States after the 1983 outbreak in Pennsylvania.[673] Even then it was shown that drug-resistant mutants arose within nine days of application.[674] Although Europe has banned the use of antibiotics of human importance in farm animals for non-treatment purposes since 1998, producers in the United States continue to legally spike farm animal feed with more than a dozen antibiotics. In fact, the Union of Concerned Scientists estimated that fully 70 percent of antibiotics used in the United States have been fed to farm animals for nontherapeutic purposes. U.S. poultry eat nearly two million pounds of antibiotics important to human medicine.[675] With few, if any, new classes of antibiotics in clinical development,[676] an expert on antibiotic resistance at the Institute for Agriculture and Trade Policy warned that "we're sacrificing a future where antibiotics will work for treating sick people by squandering them today for animals that are not sick at all."[677]

In 1999, a new class of antivirals came onto the market, notably oseltamivir (brand name Tamiflu®).[678] Based on a 2003 review of ten manufacturer-funded trials that showed Tamiflu supposedly reduced flu hospitalizations and complications,[679] governments spent billions stockpiling the drug. As the world scrambled during the 2009 pandemic, a Japanese pediatrician named Keiji Hayashi pointed out that data from eight of the original ten trials were never published. Roche, the drug company that made Tamiflu and ran the trials, refused to release the data.[680] Now we know why. In 2013, when the full clinical data were finally obtained, no such benefits were found.[681] The "Tamiflu fiasco" was over, but not before Roche had raked in $18 billion in sales.[682]

The Chinese poultry industry's actions created, as one world's authority on bird flu put it, a "very, very dangerous" situation.[683] Even if Tamiflu worked as advertised, it's a relatively unstable compound, expiring after just a few years, which makes it difficult to stockpile. Amantadine, on the other hand, is adamantine; it's sticking around. Researchers had taken amantadine that had already been sitting on the shelf for literally decades, then boiled it for a few hours. It still retained full antiviral activity.[684] "Thus," the researchers had concluded, "amantadine and rimantadine could be synthesized in large quantities and stored for at least one generation without loss of activity in preparation for the next influenza A pandemic in humans."[685] Not anymore, though, thanks to global poultry industry practices.[686] Amantadine was no panacea—it had rare but serious side effects, and resistance may well have developed with human use as well[687]—but it may have been our best bet,[688] a bet we gambled away.

Profit Motive

What about advances in medical technology? With a virus such as H5N1 and in severe cases of COVID-19, the immune system's attack on the lungs can cause a condition called *acute respiratory distress syndrome,* a devastating, often lethal, inflammatory form of severe lung failure seen in other conditions such as extensive chemically seared lung burns.[689] Treatment involves paralyzing the patients, producing a drug-induced coma, and mechanically ventilating them with a tube down the windpipe connected to a ventilator—that is, hooking them up to a breathing machine. This allows doctors to increase the flow of oxygen while suctioning fluid from the lungs, a treatment unavailable in 1918.

The mortality rates coming out of Asia, though, were not a function of outmoded medical facilities. Osterholm toured the facilities and was amazed at the care patients received. He said at the time: "Many of those patients get as good care as you are going to get at most medical centers in this country. But they still crash and burn—the point being, the cytokine storm, even under the best of conditions, is extremely difficult. I don't care if you're in the intensive care unit at Johns Hopkins or the Mayo Clinic or in Hanoi. It's a very difficult clinical condition to manage."[690] "In general terms," Osterholm continued, "we are not much better able to handle acute respiratory distress syndrome, in any number of cases today, than we were in 1918." "So," he told a reporter, "do not go back and say, well, it is different today, it is not 1918. Unfortunately, folks, it is 1918 all over again, even from a clinical response standpoint."[691] If it happens again, Osterholm concluded, "modern medicine has little in its arsenal to fight it."[692]

A former director of the National Institutes of Health described how the scene is likely to look: "Hospital wards will be choked with thousands of victims young and old. They will be hooked up to respirators, lying in comas, and dying as their heart and blood vessels fail massively. Others will be waiting in the corridors."[693] Indeed, even with COVID-19, many of our hospitals are overwhelmed, and it may be on the order of a hundred times less deadly than a pandemic could be with a virus like H5N1.

Fifty percent of those falling sick from H5N1 are dying despite our best treatments, and in the event of a pandemic, even those therapies won't be sufficiently available. There are fewer than a hundred thousand full-feature ventilators in all of America's hospitals,[694] and most are already in use at any given time for everyday medical care year round.[695] Experts like Irwin Redlener, then director of Columbia University's National Center for Disaster Preparedness, saw the ventilator shortage as being emblematic of the country's overall lack of preparedness. "This is a life-or-death issue, and it reflects everything else that's wrong about our pandemic planning," Redlener said.[696]

Within days of a pandemic, ventilators will be just one of many pieces of medical equipment that would be in short supply with the collapse of global supply chains. "Throughout the crisis," Osterholm wrote in the public policy journal *Foreign Affairs,* "many of these necessities would simply be unavailable for most health-care institutions."[697] With COVID-19, we're seeing a desperate lack of even basic protective gear for health-care workers, such as masks and gowns.

Redlener described insufficient hospital capacity as our "biggest weak link."[698] Unlike most other health-care systems in the world, health care in the United States is largely profit driven. The reconstruction of the U.S. medical system around managed care led to the closure of hundreds of hospitals across the country,[699] leaving many cities with little surge capacity to deal with an abnormal influx of patients.[700] HMO corporate stock profiles can ill afford to provide extra beds and ventilators for some indeterminate future surge of patients.[701]

A 2016 report by the American College of Emergency Physicians (ACEP), for example, found that 90 percent of the country's emergency departments were already understaffed and overcrowded.[702] The founder of the ACEP disaster medicine section described emergency care in the United States as being "like a house of cards waiting for a big wind to collapse it."[703] Just as visits to the nation's emergency rooms are reaching an all-time high,[704] the number of emergency departments in the nation has been decreasing.[705] "We [would] be caring for people in gymnasiums and community centers," said Osterholm, "just like in 1918."[706]

Then CDC's top flu expert, Keiji Fukuda, elaborated in a *New York Times* interview: "The United States medical system has been moving toward fewer hospital beds, less unused capacity. This makes sense from a business

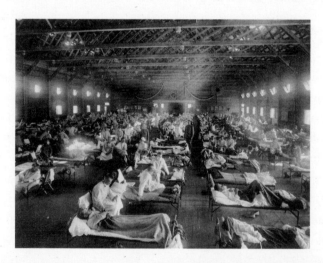

Emergency hospital during the 1918 pandemic (Courtesy of the National Museum of Health and Medicine, Armed Forces Institute of Pathology, Washington, D.C. [NCP 1603])

standpoint." His voice then reportedly dropped to a softer, sadder register. "I come from a generation of doctors who didn't think of what we do as first and foremost a business. But I suppose we're dinosaurs. We have to operate in the real world where medicine is run on a cost-benefit basis."[707]

According to a survey in the *Economist,* the United States was ranked 55th in the world in terms of acute care beds per capita,[708] comparable more to the developing world than to Europe, which has about twice the number of population-adjusted beds.[709] Over the past generation, wrote the editor of *Lancet,* "the U.S. public health system has been slowly and quietly falling apart."[710]

There is also concern about severe staff shortages.[711] Clarified one system director of emergency and continuity management for a large hospital chain, "The question becomes not how many beds you have but how many beds you can staff."[712] During the SARS crisis in Toronto, many health-care workers didn't turn up for work for fear of taking the infection home to their families. Indeed, almost half of the cases in the outbreak were health-care workers, and two nurses and one doctor died.[713] A Johns Hopkins survey of public health employees in Maryland found that "nearly half of the local health department workers are likely not to report to duty during a pandemic."[714]

For more than a century, the American Medical Association code of ethics included a noble obligation that mirrored the Canadian Medical Association's: "When pestilence prevails, it is their (physicians') duty to face the danger, and to continue their labours for the alleviation of suffering, even at the jeopardy of their own lives." The AMA duty-to-care clause has since been removed.[715] According to the journal of the American Bar Association, though, thirty-two state governments have considered legislation that would effectively force health-care workers to show up for work in a medical crisis by threatening to yank their licensure.[716]

Population Bust

A Category 5 pandemic today could be many times worse than the pandemic of 1918, the world's greatest medical catastrophe. In 1918 we were, as a nation and as a people, much more self-sufficient.[717] Now, with the corporate triumph of free trade, just-in-time inventory management and global supply chains characterize all major economies and business sectors.[718] Economic analysts predict a pandemic would cause a global economic collapse unprecedented in modern history.[719] With the world's population at an historical high, this could lead to unprecedented human suffering, something the global community is getting a taste of due to the COVID-19 pandemic.

A short one hundred thousand years ago, all members of the human race lived in eastern Africa.[720] The 7.8 billion people alive today represent roughly one out of every fourteen people who have ever inhabited the Earth.[721] In 1918, cities like London were smaller, with just over one million residents. Today there are twenty-six megacities in the world, each with more than ten million people.[722] With this kind of tinder, experts like the WHO's Klaus Stöhr have predicted a pandemic will "explosively" hit world populations "like a flash flood."[723]

"The rapidity of the spread of influenza throughout a country is only limited by the rapidity of the means of transportation," explained the 1918 New York State Health Commissioner.[724] Back then, the fastest way to cross the world was by steamship.[725] In the past, a trip around the world took a year; today we and our viruses can circle the globe in twenty-four hours.[726] The number of human globe-trotters now exceeds one billion people a year.[727] HIV left Africa on an aircraft, and the fear was that H5N1 may leave Asia the same way COVID-19 escaped, only a plane ride away.

Between record population levels and the unprecedented current speed, volume, and reach of global air travel, any pandemic virus could wreak unparalleled havoc.[728] H5N1, though, promised to be more than just any pandemic virus. At a congressional briefing, Gregory A. Poland of the Mayo Clinic and the Infectious Diseases Society of America tried to get members of Congress to imagine the unimaginable—an H5N1 pandemic. "I want to emphasize the certainty that a pandemic will occur," he began. "When this happens, time will be described, for those left living, as before and after the pandemic."[729] The top virologist in Russia attempted to tally the worst-case scenario potential human death count: "Up to one billion people could die around the whole world in six months . . . We are half a step away from a worldwide pandemic catastrophe."[730]

| *"Get rid of the 'if.' This is going to occur."*
—ANTHONY FAUCI, DIRECTOR OF THE NATIONAL INSTITUTE OF ALLERGY AND INFECTIOUS DISEASES[731]

In a talk in 2005 at his alma mater, Harvard Medical School, former Senate Majority Leader Frist described the horrors of 1918—at least fifty million dead from an "avianlike" virus.[732] Frist asked:

> *How would a nation so greatly moved and touched by the 3,000 dead of September 11th react to half a million dead? In 1918–1919 the mortality rate was between 2.5% and 5%, which seems merciful in comparison to the 55% mortality rate of the current avian flu. In just 18 months, this avian flu has killed or forced the culling of more than 100 million animals. And now that it has jumped from birds to infect humans in 10 Asian nations, how many human lives will it or another virus like it take? How, then, would a nation greatly moved and touched by 3,000 dead, react to 5 or 50 million dead?[733]*

Other public health authorities expressed similar sentiments on a global scale. Former World Health Organization executive director David Nabarro was appointed the bird flu czar of the United Nations. At a press conference at UN headquarters in New York, Nabarro tried to impress upon journalists that "we're dealing here with world survival issues—or the survival of the world as we know it."[734]

Similar fears reportedly kept former U.S. Secretary of Health and Human Services Mike Leavitt awake at night. "It's a world-changing event when it occurs," Leavitt said in an interview. "It reaches beyond health. It affects economies, cultures, politics and prosperity—not to mention human life, counted by the millions."[735] Yes, but what are the odds of it actually happening with a virus like H5N1?

What are the odds that a killer flu virus will spread around the world like a tidal wave, killing millions? "The burning question is, will there be a human influenza pandemic," Secretary Leavitt told reporters. "On behalf of the WHO, I can tell you that there will be. The only question is the virulence and rapidity of transmission from human to human."[736] "The world just has no idea what it's going to see if this thing comes," then head of the

CDC's International Emerging Infections Program in Thailand said, but then stopped. "When, really. It's when. I don't think we can afford the luxury of the word 'if' anymore. We are past 'if's.'"[737]

The chief medical officer of Great Britain,[738] the director-general of Health of Germany,[739] the director of the U.S. Centers for Disease Control,[740] the senior United Nations coordinator for avian and human influenza,[741] and the director of the U.S. National Security Health Policy Center[742] all agreed that another influenza pandemic is only a matter of time. As then director of Trust for America's Health put it, "This is not a drill. This is not a planning exercise. This is for real."[743]

WHEN, NOT IF

"It is coming."

—LEE JONG-WOOK, THE LATE DIRECTOR-GENERAL
OF THE WORLD HEALTH ORGANIZATION[744]

The National Academy of Medicine described a pandemic as "not only inevitable, but overdue."[745] This was based in part on the understanding that there have been twelve pandemics recorded since global travelers embarked approximately three centuries ago.[746] Pandemics have averaged every twenty-seven and a half years,[747] with forty-one years presented as the longest known interval between pandemics.[748]

Said a WHO spokesperson about a virus like H5N1, "All the indications are that we are living on borrowed time."[749] A senior associate at the Center for Biosecurity listed the indications: "The lethality of the virus is unprecedented for influenza, the scope of the bird outbreak is completely unprecedented and the change that needs to happen to create a pandemic is such a small change—it could literally happen any day."[750]

Never before H5N1 had bird flu spread so far, so fast,[751] and the longer the virus circulates in poultry production systems the higher the likelihood of additional human exposure.[752] Virology professor John Oxford explained:

The problem is one chicken can contain hundreds of thousands of strains of H5N1. Let's say there are a billion chickens in Asia and 10% are infected—

that's a vast population of viruses, more than the entire human population of the planet. Now let's further suppose some of these strains have mutated so they can latch not only onto a chicken but onto you or me, but they cannot do it very efficiently. That's the position we appear to be in. If a child catches the virus from a chicken they may transmit it to their mother, but the mother won't be able to go out and infect the grocer. At the moment it's a slow greyhound of a virus. It's when it develops into a normal greyhound that we're in for it.[753]

In 1968, the year of the H3N2 pandemic, there were thirteen million chickens in China. Now, there are billions. And since the time from hatching to slaughter is only a matter of weeks or months, depending on whether the chicken is raised for meat or eggs, there are multiple cycles of these billions passing through the system in the course of the year. Back in the 1960s, there were five million pigs in China; now there are nearly five *hundred* million.[754] "High concentrations of animals," concluded the International Food Policy Research Institute, "can become breeding grounds for disease."[755]

H5N1 may be here to stay. "This virus cannot now be eradicated from the planet," said Center for Biosecurity director O'Toole. "It is in too many birds in too many places."[756] The virus seemed to be getting more entrenched. "If you described it as a war, we've been losing more battles than we've won," a WHO spokesman told *The Financial Times*. "From a public health point of view, and an animal health point of view, this virus is just getting a stronger and stronger grip on the region."[757]

In a tone uncharacteristic of international policy institutions, the FAO wrote: "Over this bleak landscape sits a black cloud of fear that the virus might become adapted to enable human-to-human transmission and then spread around the globe."[758] The urgency and alarm among those tracking H5N1's building momentum was palpable.[759] "It's like watching a volcano getting ready to erupt," described a spokesperson of the World Organization for Animal Health (known as OIE, for Office Internationale des Epizooties).[760] "We're all holding our breath," said Julie Gerberding, former head of the CDC.[761]

Two Minutes to Midnight

When would the H5N1 pandemic strike? The experts were vague on that point, and "probably sooner rather than later,"[762] "any time now,"[763] "this year or next"[764] were common refrains. Some wondered why it hadn't happened already.[765] "It's tough to make predictions," said Yogi Berra, "especially about the future."

Some attempted to take comfort in the fact that the virus had been in existence for almost ten years and hadn't sparked a pandemic yet.[766] Evidence suggests, though, that the 1918 virus was "smouldering" for at least eleven years before it went pandemic.[767]

Even if greater numbers of people started falling ill, the virus may still need to fine-tune its human appetite. Historians have found evidence of suspicious outbreaks of severe respiratory illness in the year preceding the pandemic of 1918. "We think these outbreaks in these army camps started in 1917," concluded one expert, "then it took another year of an extra few mutations before it really exploded into the great wide world."[768] Gerberding told a meeting of the American Association for the Advancement of Science that H5N1 represented the "most important threat" the world is currently facing. She said, "I think we can all recognize a similar pattern probably occurred prior to 1918."[769]

Unlike annual seasonal influenza, which tends to strike the northern hemisphere in winter,[770] pandemics have been known to occur at any time of the year.[771] Although there does not seem to be a concrete seasonal pattern, based on an analysis of a dozen past pandemics, appearance in the summer was more common than the winter,[772] which may coincide with the placing of ducks onto China's flooded rice fields.[773] The increased poultry sales and mass travel in the days leading up to the Tet Lunar New Year festival (which starts February 9) may also be a high-risk time.[774] The emergence of COVID-19 coincided with the Lunar New Year, the most celebrated holiday in China, for which billions of trips are made by individuals traveling back and forth to their hometowns.[775] Experts admit that they really don't know.

"It would be irresponsible to say we are absolutely going to get there this year or next year because we just don't understand virus evolution enough," said one Harvard epidemiologist. "It is, I think, correct to say that we are in a period where the risk is growing and where it's higher than we've ever known it to be."[776] What most scientists do agree on is that each day brings us one day closer to the pandemic, though they admit it is unknown which virus will ultimately trigger the pandemic or how severe the next one will be. The current coronavirus pandemic—the first of its kind—is certainly testament to that.

"With the advent of AIDS, avian flu, Ebola and SARS," a Tulane researcher noted, "the question of what launches new epidemics and pandemics is extremely important. The somewhat shocking answer is that we actually know nothing about the factors that launch animal viruses into epidemics or pandemics."[777] A few scientists have toyed with the idea of trying to find out.

By mixing H5N1 and human influenza viruses together in a lab, one might be able to estimate how much time we might have left by identifying how many mutations H5N1 may be away from creating a pandemic strain. The World Health Organization was cautious about this approach and called for a formal scientific consensus, believing that global decisions that entail global risks require global review. For any one country to undertake the project on its own, WHO's former principal flu scientist Klaus Stöhr said, "is like a decision to start testing nuclear weapons unilaterally."[778] Proponents argued that any pandemic H5N1 virus they created would be sequenced, but then promptly destroyed. With a genetic description of the virus, though, and the easy availability of its progenitors, it could be recreated. "You can destroy this virus," one critic remarked, "but it will never really be gone."[779] The Dutch scientist who proposed the original idea admitted, "You could create a monster. But it's a monster that nature could produce as well."[780]

Flu Year's Eve

Once a pandemic hits, scientists disagree on how fast it will spread around the world. The WHO expects it could hit every country on Earth in a matter of weeks.[781] Others imagine it may take weeks just to break out of its presumed Asian country of origin.[782] Once it does get moving, though, some authorities suspect it will hit Western shores within one week (if it indeed originates in Asia).[783] Others argue one day.[784] Or twelve hours.[785] Once in a country like the United States, supercomputer simulations at the Los Alamos weapons lab show the virus blanketing the country "with remarkable speed and efficiency."[786]

In 1918, the entire Earth was engulfed within weeks—and that was before commercial airline travel.[787] In an attempt to model the spread of the 1997 Hong Kong outbreak (had it gone pandemic), scientists calculated how many travelers had passed through Hong Kong's Kai Tak Airport. During the two-month outbreak in Hong Kong in 1997, more than four million people left that one airport.[788] Viruses now travel at jet speed. Within months, COVID-19 had spread to more than two hundred countries and territories on six continents.[789]

The next pandemic is expected to come in multiple waves. Based on prior pandemics, two or three waves of infection have been predicted, spaced several months apart, with each global surge of infection expected to last perhaps six to eight weeks.[790] The second wave may be deadlier than the first as the virus fine-tunes its killing power.[791]

Imagine this scenario: "A gentleman checks into a four star Hong Kong hotel to attend a wedding. He seems to have a bad cold—coughing and sneezing—but actually has something much worse. The wedding ends. Guests depart. The virus coughed by one man spreads to five countries within 24 hours."[792]

This is actually the true story of SARS, which brought the world to the brink of a pandemic influenza-like scenario in 2002–2003.[793] Within months, the virus had spread to thirty countries on six continents.[794] The WHO Global Outbreak Alert and Response team later marveled, "A global outbreak was thus seeded from a single person on a single day on a single floor of a Hong Kong hotel."[795]

The transmission rate of SARS pales in comparison to influenza.[796] "The world was lucky with SARS," a top expert explained. "It turned out to be a dachshund of a virus akin to smallpox, and not a sprinting greyhound like . . . influenza."[797] Little did we know then that a SARS-like coronavirus was able to trigger a pandemic after all.

Catching the Flu

According to the former WHO's director of Communicable Diseases Surveillance and Response, "History has told us that no one can stop a pandemic."[798] But this is the twenty-first century. With enough advance warning, couldn't a smoldering pandemic be stamped out, or at least controlled?

In 2005, then President George W. Bush issued an executive order authorizing the use of quarantines inside the United States.[799] The man in charge of preparing America for a pandemic was then Secretary of Health and Human Services, Michael Leavitt. "We would do all we could to quarantine," said Secretary Leavitt. "It's not a happy thought. It's something that keeps the president of the United States awake. It keeps me awake."[800] But experts fear that not only would quarantines be wholly impractical and ineffective, they may make matters worse.

The World Health Organization recommends against such measures in part given the impracticality of enforcement.[801] "It shows a fundamental lack of understanding of public health emergencies," says a Federation of American Scientists spokesperson. "I would be fascinated to see whether the president has a plan to quarantine a city like Washington, D.C., New York or Boston with so many roads in or out."[802] President Trump's proposal to enact an "enforceable" quarantine in regions of New York, New Jersey, and Connecticut for COVID-19 was quickly withdrawn.[803]

Following the 1916 polio epidemic in New York City, the head of the Health Department wrote that given the "countless instances of inconvenience, hardship, yes, real brutal inhumanity which resulted from the application of the general quarantine,"[804] it was no wonder that so many people "developed a most perverse ingenuity in discovering automobile detours."[805] The Federation of American Scientists spokesperson could not imagine how the quarantine could be enforced in this day and age. "Is he going to send in tanks and armed men?" he asked.[806] Perhaps. President Bush asked Congress to give him authority to call in the military to contain an outbreak.[807]

That had some commentators worried. An op-ed in *The Houston Chronicle* asked, "If a health worker, drug addict or teenager attempted to break the quarantine, what would soldiers do? Shoot on sight?" Teenagers and health workers were found to be the prime violators of quarantine rules in Toronto during the SARS outbreak in 2003.[808] Stating the obvious in regard to the difference between stopping the 1997 Hong Kong outbreak among chickens and stopping a human outbreak, experts have written, "Slaughter and quarantine of people is not an option."[809]

"Even if it was possible to cordon off a city," noted then Center for Biosecurity's O'Toole, "that is not going to contain influenza."[810] Based on failed historical attempts along with contemporary statistical models,[811] influenza experts are confident that efforts at quarantine "simply will not work."[812] Experts consider quarantine efforts "doomed to fail"[813] because of the extreme contagiousness of influenza,[814] which is a function of its incubation period and mode of transmission.

SARS, in retrospect, was an easy virus to contain because people essentially became symptomatic *before* they became infectious.[815] People showed signs of the disease before they could efficiently spread it, so tools like thermal image scanners at airports to detect fever or screening those with a cough could potentially stem the spread of the disease.[816]

The influenza virus, however, gets a head start. The incubation period for influenza, the time between when you get infected and when you actually start showing the first symptoms of disease, can be up to four days.[817] During this time, we are both infected and infectious. Just as those with HIV can spread the virus though they may appear perfectly healthy, at least twenty-four hours before any flu symptoms arise, we may be exhaling virus with every breath.[818] As many as half of those infected may never show symptoms at all, but may still shed virus to others.[819]

Some respiratory diseases seem only to be spread by droplets of mucus and therefore are not airborne in the truest sense. These aerosolized globs of mucus—though tiny—eventually settle to the floor and are not spread very far. Bird flu, on the other hand, can truly take wing. Influenza viruses in general, though predominantly spread by larger droplets, may also travel on microscopic residual specks of evaporated droplets less than a few millionths of a meter in diameter. These "droplet nuclei" can float suspended in air like particles of perfume[820] and hence may spread through ventilation systems.[821] Some investigators have even issued the dubious speculation that airborne viral transmission of influenza can occur over thousands of miles on intercontinental wind currents driven by low pressure weather fronts.[822]

Boots on the Ground

The threat of quarantine can sometimes make things worse in a pandemic. The detainment, isolation, and stigma associated with quarantine tend to dissuade communities from the timely reporting of outbreaks. Sending soldiers to quarantine large numbers of people may even create panic and cause people to flee, further spreading the disease. During the SARS epidemic, for example, rumors that Beijing would be quarantined led to a quarter of a million people pouring out of the city that night.[823] Throughout history, according to the National Academy of Medicine, "for the most part quarantine policies did more harm than good."[824]

Irwin Redlener, former director of the National Center for Disaster Preparedness, called the president's suggestion to use the military to cordon off communities stricken by disease an "extraordinarily draconian measure." "The translation of this," Redlener told *The Washington Post,* "is martial law in the United States."[825]

The president's proposal drew rancor from both ends of the political spectrum. The conservative Cato Institute joined George Mason University's Mercatus Center[826] in warning that Bush risked undermining "a fundamental principle of American law."[827] The Posse Comitatus Act of 1878 has effectively barred the military from playing a policing role on U.S. soil. "That reflects America's traditional distrust of using standing armies to enforce order at home, a distrust that's well justified," the Institute's website read. Since soldiers are not trained as police officers, the Cato Institute feared that putting them in charge of civilian law enforcement could "result in serious collateral damage to American life and liberty."[828]

After the September 11 attacks, FEMA—the Federal Emergency Management Agency—was folded into the Department of Homeland Security. According to an emergency management expert at the Institute for Crisis, Disaster and Risk Management at George Washington University, this move "downgraded" FEMA from being a well-functioning, small, independent agency in the 1990s to being "buried in a couple of layers of bureaucracy." One former FEMA director testified before Congress in 2004:

> *I am extremely concerned that the ability of our nation to prepare for and respond to disasters has been sharply eroded. I hear from emergency managers, local and state leaders, and first responders nearly every day that the FEMA they knew and worked well with has now disappeared. In fact one state emergency manager told me, "It is like a stake has been driven into the heart of emergency management."[829]*

His fears were realized a year later with the response to Katrina, which, read one *USA Today* editorial, "was nearly as disastrous as the hurricane itself."[830] Bush went on to hand authority for coordinating pandemic response to the same agency that handled Katrina, the Department of Homeland Security.

Business Week's bird flu cover story "Hot Zone in the Heartland" featured Osterholm contrasting Katrina with the prospect of a pandemic. "The difference between this and a hurricane is that all 50 states will be affected at the same time," said Osterholm. "And this crisis will last a year or more. It will utterly change the world."[831] Even those sympathetic to the administration have cast doubt on its abilities to manage the crisis. Colonel Lawrence Wilkerson, for example, who was Colin Powell's right-hand man at the State Department, said, "If something comes along that is truly serious . . . like a major pandemic, you are going to see the ineptitude of this government in a way that will take you back to the Declaration of Independence."[832]

II. When Animal Viruses Attack

THE THIRD AGE

Emerging Infectious Disease

In 1948, the U.S. Secretary of State pronounced that the conquest of all infectious diseases was imminent.[833] Twenty years later, victory was declared by the U.S. Surgeon General: "The war against diseases has been won." But, as the chair of Medical Microbiology at the University of Edinburgh wrote in retrospect, "He was spectacularly wrong."[834]

The National Academy of Medicine called the post-WWII period the "era of complacency."[835] The overconfidence of the time was understandable. We had conquered polio, nearly eradicated smallpox, developed childhood vaccinations, and assembled an arsenal of more than twenty-five thousand different "miracle drug" antibiotic preparations.[836] Even Nobel Laureates were seduced into the heady optimism. To write about infectious disease, one Nobel-winning virologist wrote in the 1962 text *Natural History of Infectious Disease,* "is almost to write of something that has passed into history." "[T]he most likely forecast about the future of infectious disease," he pronounced, "is that it will be very dull."[837]

The year smallpox was declared history, human immunodeficiency virus began its colonization of Africa and the world with HIV/AIDS.[838] In some countries, the prevalence of HIV exceeded 25 percent of the adult population.[839] The global efforts sparked by the WHO decision to "eliminate all malaria on the planet"[840] succeeded, as another Nobel Laureate put it, "in eradicating malariologists, but not malaria." The malaria parasites are now antibiotic-resistant and the mosquitoes carrying them are insecticide-resistant as well.[841] "Even the diseases once thought subdued," the WHO finally had to concede, "are fighting back with renewed ferocity."[842] Infectious disease remains the number-one killer of children worldwide.[843]

It's getting worse.[844] "We claimed victory too soon," said the co-chair of Yale University's committee on emerging infections. "The danger posed by infectious diseases has not gone away. It's worsening."[845] After decades of declining infectious disease mortality in the United States, the trend reversed[846] and the number of Americans dying from infectious diseases started going back up.[847] A bitter pill of a joke circulates among infectious disease specialists: "The 19th century was followed by the 20th century, which was followed by the . . . 19th century."[848]

A vice chair of the U.S. National Foundation for Infectious Diseases was once asked, "Are we having more plagues?" "The answer is an unequivocal yes," he replied. "These plagues are coming back with greater fury and in much greater profusion because they're killing more people than they did in centuries gone by."[849]

The concept of "emerging infectious diseases" has changed from a mere curiosity in the field of medicine to an entire discipline.[850] As recorded in the database of the U.S. National Library of Medicine, more scientific journal articles have been written on emerging infectious diseases in the last eight years than in the previous century.[851] Emerging diseases have been moving to center stage in human medicine.[852]

Since about 1975,[853] previously unknown diseases have surfaced at a pace unheard of in the annals of medicine[854]—more than thirty new diseases in thirty years, most of them newly discovered viruses.[855] *What's going on? Why is it getting worse? Where are these emerging diseases emerging from?* An increasingly broad consensus of infectious disease specialists has concluded that "nearly all" of the emergent disease episodes in the United States and around the world in recent years have come to us from the animal world.[856]

Their Bugs Are Worse Than Their Bite

Almost by definition, "novel" viruses tend to come from other species.[857] In 1959, the World Health Organization defined the term "zoonosis" to describe this phenomenon,[858] from the Greek *zoion* for "animal" and *nosos* for "disease." Most emerging infections are RNA viruses such as Ebola, HIV, or influenza[859]—not surprising, given their ability to mutate rapidly, evolve, and adapt to new hosts.[860] Although many doctors learned in their medical school textbooks that viruses were species-specific and therefore couldn't jump from animals to people,[861] we now know that viruses are, as the Mayo Clinic describes, "masters of interspecies navigation."[862]

The exact proportion of emerging human diseases that have arisen from animals is unknown. In 2004, the director of the CDC noted that "11 of the last 12 emerging infectious diseases that we're aware of in the world, that have had human health consequences, have probably arisen from animal sources."[863] An editorial in *Lancet* published the same year insisted that "[a]ll human diseases to emerge in the past 20 years have had an animal source."[864] In any case, experts agree that it's a sizeable majority.[865] Eleven out of the top twelve most dangerous bioterrorism agents were noted to be zoonotic pathogens as well.[866] The National Academy of Medicine published a report on the factors implicated in the emergence of disease in the United States. "The significance of zoonoses in the emergence of human infections," it concluded, "cannot be overstated."[867]

According to the World Health Organization, the increasing numbers of animal viruses jumping to humans is expected to continue.[868] The zoonotic virus pool is by no means exhausted.[869] "If you look at the animal kingdom—from goats, sheep, camels, poultry, all fish, just about any animal you can name—they [each] have probably 30 or 40 major diseases," noted the WHO expert who led the fight against SARS. "So the possibility for exposure is huge."[870] Estimates as to the number of zoonotic diseases run into the thousands.[871] "For every virus that we know about, there are hundreds that we don't know anything about," said one professor of tropical medicine at Tulane studying emerging viruses in Africa. "Most of them," he said, "we probably don't even know that they're out there."[872]

As I've discussed, transmissions of disease from animal to person are not new.[873] Most of the human infectious diseases that exist today originally came from animals.[874] Many of humanity's greatest scourges—including influenza—can be traced back ten thousand years to the domestication of animals.[875]

> *"Most and probably all of the distinctive infectious diseases of civilization have been transferred to human populations from animal herds."*
>
> —WILLIAM H. MCNEILL,
> *PLAGUES AND PEOPLES*[876]

Humanity's biblical "dominion over the fish of the sea and over the birds of heaven; and every living thing that moved upon the earth" has unleashed a veritable Pandora's ark full of humankind's greatest killers.[877] Some diseases, such as herpes and shingles, seem to have always been with us, passed down the evolutionary chain, but most modern human infectious diseases were unknown to our hunter and gatherer ancestors.[878] Early humans may have suffered sporadic cases of animal-borne diseases such as anthrax from wild sheep or tularemia ("rabbit skinner's disease") from wild rabbits,[879] but the domestication of animals triggered what a director of Harvard's Center for Health and the Global Environment called the mass "spillover" of animal disease into human populations.[880]

Archeological evidence suggests that small, nomadic groups hardly suffered from contagious disease. With the advent of agriculture, though, communities settled and grew in relatively fixed locations, increasing their close exposure to their own waste and reservoirs of disease. Populations that domesticated only plants became more exposed to the few diseases they already harbored, but it was the domestication of animals that brought people in contact with a whole new array of pathogenic germs.[881]

Epidemic diseases tend to be harbored only by those animal species that herd or flock together in large numbers. This concentration allows for the evolution and maintenance of contagious pathogens capable of rapidly spreading through entire populations. Unfortunately, this same quality—the herd instinct—is what makes these animals particularly desirable for domestication, and it is domestication that brought these animals once appreciated mainly from afar (along with their diseases) into close proximity and density with human settlements. As a Johns Hopkins research team concluded, "The spread of microbes from animals to humans was then inevitable."[882]

Tuberculosis, "the captain of all these men of death,"[883] is thought to have been acquired through the domestication of goats.[884] In the twentieth century, tuberculosis killed approximately a hundred million people.[885] Today, tuberculosis continues to kill more than a million people a year.[886] The World Health Organization declared tuberculosis a global health emergency in 1993 and estimated that nearly one billion people may be newly infected from the year 2000 to 2020. What started out in goats went on to infect one-third of humanity.[887]

Domesticated goats seemed to have beaten domesticated cattle to the punch. Between 1850 and 1950, *bovine* tuberculosis, acquired mostly by children drinking unpasteurized milk, was responsible for more than eight hundred thousand human deaths in Great Britain alone.[888] Interestingly, it can go both ways. *The British Journal of Biomedical Science* recounted that dozens of cases of bovine TB were traced back to a "curious farm-worker practice of urinating on the hay, perhaps on the folklore premise that the salts in urine are beneficial to the cattle." Of course, when it turns out the workers have genitourinary tuberculosis infections, it's not so beneficial.[889]

Bovine tuberculosis continues to infect milk-drinkers to this day.[890] In a study published in the journal of the American Academy of Pediatrics in 2000, doctors tested children with tuberculosis in San Diego and found that one third of the tuberculosis wasn't human. One in three of the children was actually suffering from tuberculosis caught not from someone coughing on them, but, the researchers suspect, from drinking inadequately pasteurized milk from an infected cow. The investigators concluded, "These data demonstrate the dramatic impact of this underappreciated cause of zoonotic TB on U.S. children."[891]

Measles is thought to have come from domesticated sheep and goats, a mutant of the rinderpest virus.[892] The measles virus has so successfully adapted to humans that livestock can't get measles and we can't get rinderpest. Only with the prolonged intimate contact of domestication was the rinderpest virus able to mutate enough to make the jump.[893] Though now considered a relatively benign disease, in roughly the last 150 years, measles has been estimated to have killed about 200 million people worldwide.[894] These deaths can be traced to the taming of the first sheep or goats a few hundred generations ago.[895]

Smallpox may have resulted from camel domestication.[896] We domesticated pigs and got whooping cough, domesticated chickens and got typhoid fever,[897] and domesticated ducks and got influenza.[898] The list goes on.[899] Leprosy came from water buffalo,[900] the cold virus from cattle[901] or horses.[902] How often did wild horses have opportunity to sneeze into humanity's face before they were broken and bridled? Before then, the common cold was presumably common only to them.

New zoonotic infections from domesticated farm animals continue to be discovered. The 2005 Nobel Prize in Medicine was awarded to the scientists who discovered in 1982 that bacteria living in the human stomach, which they called *Helicobacter pylori,* caused stomach cancer and the vast majority of peptic ulcers worldwide.[903] Roughly half of the world's population is infected.[904] These ulcer-causing bacteria are thought to have originated in sheep's milk but are now spread person to person via oral secretions—saliva or vomit—or perhaps, like cholera, the fecal-oral route due to poor handwashing following defecation. What has become probably the most common chronic infection afflicting humanity,[905] according to the CDC, came about because humanity started to drink the milk of another species thousands of years ago.[906]

A recent addition to the list of infectious farm animal bacteria is a cousin of *H. pylori,* known as *Heliobacter pullorum* (from the Latin *pullus* for "chicken"),[907] infecting a large proportion of chicken meat. *H. pullorum* is thought to cause a diarrheal illness in people who contract it through the consumption of improperly cooked chicken fecal matter.[908]

Yet another fecal pathogen, hepatitis E, is one of the more recent additions to the family of hepatitis viruses. It can cause fulminating liver infection in pregnant women, especially during the third trimester, with a mortality rate of up to 20 percent. Scientists began to suspect that this virus was zoonotic when they found it rampant in North American commercial pork operations.[909] A recent sampling from more than five thousand pigs at twenty-five slaughterhouses in ten U.S. states found 6 percent were actively infected with the virus in their blood at the time of slaughter.[910] Direct evidence of cross-species transmission was obtained in 2003.[911] Unlike a disease like trichinosis, which humans only get by eating improperly cooked pork, once a disease like hepatitis E crosses the species line, it can then be spread person to person. Between 1 and 2 percent of blood donors in the United States have been found to have been exposed to this virus.[912]

"Wherever the European has trod, death seems to pursue the aboriginal."

—CHARLES DARWIN, 1836[913]

UCLA professor Jared Diamond explored how pivotal the domestication of farm animals was in the course of human history and medicine in his Pulitzer Prize–winning book *Guns, Germs, and Steel.* In the chapter "Lethal Gift of Livestock," he argued convincingly that the diseases we contracted through the domestication of animals may have been critical for the European conquest of the Americas in which as many as 95 percent of the indigenous peoples were decimated by plagues the Europeans brought with them. Natives had no prior exposure or immunity to diseases like tuberculosis, smallpox, and measles. Parallels were seen throughout the world with single missionaries unintentionally exterminating the entire target of their religious zeal with one of livestock's "lethal gifts."[914]

Why didn't the reverse happen? Why didn't Native American diseases wipe out the landing Europeans? Because there essentially weren't any epidemic diseases. Medical historians have long conjectured that the reason there were so many plagues in Eurasia was that "crowd" diseases required large, densely-populated cities, unlike the presumed small tribal bands of the Americas—but that presumption turned out to be wrong. New World cities like Tenochtitlan were among the most populous in the world.[915]

The reason the plagues had never touched the Americas is that there were far fewer domesticated herd animals. There were buffalo, but no domesticated buffalo, so there was presumably no opportunity for measles to arise. No pigs, so no pertussis; no chickens, so no Typhoid Marys. While people died by the millions of killer scourges like tuberculosis in Europe, none were dying in the "new world" because no animals like goats existed to domesticate. The last ice age killed off most of the easily domesticated species in the western hemisphere, such as American camels and horses, leaving the indigenous population only animals like llamas and guinea pigs to raise for slaughter, neither of which seem to carry much potential for epidemic human disease.[916]

The Plague Years

According to the Smithsonian, there have been three great epidemiological transitions in human history. Epidemiology is the study of the distribution of epidemic disease. The first era of human disease began with the acquisition of diseases from domesticated animals, such as measles and smallpox. Entire ancient civilizations fell prey to diseases birthed in the barnyard.[917]

The second era came with the Industrial Revolution of the eighteenth and nineteenth centuries, resulting in an epidemic of the so-called diseases of civilization, including cancer, heart disease, stroke, and diabetes.[918] Chronic diseases now account for seven out of ten deaths in the United States[919] and the majority of deaths worldwide.[920] Thankfully, these diseases are considered "largely preventable" through changes in diet and lifestyle.[921]

We have now entered into the third age of human disease, which started around forty years ago—the emergence (or re-emergence) of zoonotic diseases.[922] Medical historians describe these last decades as the age of "the emerging plagues."[923] Never in medical history have so many new diseases appeared in so short a time, and the trend is continuing. We may soon be facing, according to the National Academy of Medicine, a "catastrophic storm of microbial threats."[924]

We know that most of these new diseases are coming from animals, but animals were domesticated ten thousand years ago. Why now? What is responsible for this recent fury of new and re-emerging zoonotic disease?

Starting in the last quarter of the twentieth century, medicine has been examining emerging disease within an increasingly ecological framework. According to then director of Australia's National Centre for Epidemiology and Population Health, we shouldn't be surprised by the recent explosion in zoonotic disease given recent environmental changes. "We need to think ecologically," he said. "These viruses are trying to evolve."[925] Just as plants and animals in the wild try to adapt to new environments to spread their species, viruses also expand to exploit any newly exposed niches. "Show me almost any new infectious disease," said the executive director of the Consortium of Conservation Medicine, "and I'll show you an environmental change brought about by humans that either caused or exacerbated it."[926] To quote the comic-strip character Pogo, "We have met the enemy and he is us."[927]

Two centuries ago, Edward Jenner, the founder of modern vaccines, proposed that the "deviation of man from the state in which he was originally placed by nature seems to have proved him a prolific source of diseases."[928] This observation dates back to the second century, when Plutarch argued that new classes of diseases followed profound changes in the way we live.[929] The same can be said for animals. "Something is not right," reflected Professor Shortridge. "Human population has exploded, we are impinging on the realms of the animals more and more, taking their habitats for ourselves, forcing animals into ever more artificial environments and existences."[930]

According to the World Health Organization's coordinator for zoonoses control, "The chief risk factor for emerging zoonotic diseases is environmental degradation by humans."[931] This includes degradation wrought by global climate change, deforestation, and, as described by the WHO, "industrialization and intensification of the animal production sector."[932] That may be a particularly important factor. A 2019 review on emerging human infectious diseases concluded that most new animal-to-human diseases have been a result of how we now raise animals for our food.[933] Along with human culpability, though, comes hope. If changes in human behavior can cause new plagues, changes in human behavior may prevent them in the future.[934]

MAN-MADE

AIDS: A Clear-Cut Disaster

In 1933, Aldo Leopold, the "founding father of wildlife ecology,"[935] declared, "The real determinants of disease mortality are the environment and the population," both of which he said were being "doctored daily, for better or for worse, by gun and axe, and by fire and plow."[936] Since Leopold wrote those lines, more than half of the Earth's tropical forests have been cleared.[937] According to the UN Food and Agriculture Organization, expanding livestock production is one of the main drivers of tropical rainforest destruction, particularly in Central and South America.[938] This "hamburgerization" of the rainforests sets the stage for disease emergence and transmission in a number of ways.

Many disease-carrying mosquitoes prefer to breed out in the open along partially cleared forest fringes, rather than deep in the forest.[939] Clear-cutting trees can also create a windfall for disease-bearing rodents. When livestock are grazed on the cleared land, the animals serve as warm-blooded meals for disease vectors like mosquitoes and biting flies, which may become so numerous they seek out blood meals from humans.[940] One mosquito-borne disease, Rift Valley Fever, probably wouldn't have even occurred in humans without the necessary amplification in agricultural animals.[941]

In India, what was initially thought to be a severe outbreak of yellow fever was in fact a novel disease caused by a tick-borne monkey virus that was then named after the recently deforested Kyasanur forest.[942] The cleared land was used for the grazing of cattle, a major host for the tick species, carrying the virus out from its primate reservoir to subsequently cause as many as a thousand human cases in a single year.[943]

With leading cattle-producing nations at war during WWII, Argentina took advantage of this situation by dramatically expanding its beef industry at the expense of its forests. The ensuing explosion in field mouse populations led to the surfacing of the deadly Junin virus, the cause of Argentine hemorrhagic fever,[944] a disease characterized in up to one-third of those infected by extensive bleeding, shock, seizures, and death.[945] On cleared cropland, unprotected agriculture workers are on the front line, as harvesting machinery produces clouds of potentially infectious dust and aerosols of blood from animals crushed in the combines.[946]

This scenario was repeated as humankind intruded into other remote virgin forests. In Bolivia, we discovered the Machupo virus, or, rather, the Machupo virus discovered us. In Brazil we uncovered the Sabia virus. The Guanarito virus resulted in Venezuelan hemorrhagic fever.

Inroads into Africa's rainforests exposed other hemorrhagic fever viruses—the Lassa virus, Rift Valley Fever, and Ebola. According to the WHO, all dozen or so[947] hemorrhagic fever viruses so far unearthed have been zoonotic, jumping to us from other animals.[948] "These zoonotic viruses seem to adhere to the philosophy that says, 'I won't bother you if you don't bother me,'" explained a former *Nature* editor.[949] But then, she said, as people began "pushing back forests, or engaging in agricultural practices that are ecologically congenial to viruses, the viruses could make their way into the human population and multiply and spread."[950]

Radical alterations of forest ecosystems can be hazardous in the Amazon Basin or the woods of Connecticut, where Lyme disease was first recognized in 1975. Since then, the disease has spread across all fifty states[951] and affected an estimated one hundred thousand Americans.[952] Lyme disease is spread by bacteria-infested ticks that live on deer and mice, animals with whom people have always shared wooded areas. What happened recently was suburbia. Developers chopped America's woods into subdivisions, scaring away the foxes and bobcats who had previously kept mouse populations in check. Animal ecologists have recovered some seven times more infected ticks from one- and two-acre woodlots than lots of ten to fifteen acres.[953]

The forests of Africa were not, however, cut down to make golf courses. The inroads into Africa's rainforests were logging roads, built by transnational timber corporations hacking deep into the most remote regions of the continent. This triggered a mass human migration into the rainforests to set up concessions to support the commercial logging operations. One of the main sources of food for these migrant workers is bushmeat—wild animals killed for human consumption.[954] This includes upward of twenty-six different species of primates,[955] including thousands of endangered great apes—gorillas and chimpanzees—who are shot, butchered, smoked, and sold as food.[956] To support the logging industry infrastructure,[957] a veritable army of commercial bushmeat hunters are bringing the great apes to the brink of extinction.[958] "These logging companies have been promoting the bushmeat trade themselves," claimed one expert. "It is easier to hand out shotgun shells than to truck in beef."[959]

The reason french fries can be eaten with abandon without fear of coming down with potato blight is that pathogens adapted to infect plants don't infect people. The evolutionary span is too wide. Eating animals can certainly give us animal diseases, but near-universal taboos against cannibalism have well served the human race by keeping more closely adapted viruses off our forks.[960] Having finally sequenced the genome of the chimpanzee, though, scientists realize we may share more than 95 percent of our DNA with our fellow great apes.[961] "Darwin wasn't just provocative in saying that we descend from the apes—he didn't go far enough," one primatologist said. "We are apes in every way."[962] By cannibalizing our fellow primates, we are exposing ourselves to pathogens particularly fine-tuned to human physiology. Human outbreaks of Ebola, for example, have been traced to exposure to the dead bodies of infected great apes hunted for food.[963] Ebola, one of humanity's deadliest infections, is not efficiently spread, though, compared to a virus like HIV.

The year 1981 brought us Ronald Reagan taking the oath, MTV's first broadcast, Pacman-mania, *Raiders of the Lost Ark,* and the release of IBM's first personal computer. In June, the Centers for Disease Control issued a bulletin of nine brief paragraphs. Five gay men in Los Angeles had died with a strange cluster of symptoms.[964] From humble beginnings, AIDS has killed millions.[965]

The relaxation of sexual mores, blood banking, and injection drug use aided the spread of the AIDS virus, but where did this virus come from? The leading theory is "direct exposure to animal blood and secretions as a result of hunting, butchering, or other activities (such as consumption of uncooked contaminated meat)."[966] Experts believe the most likely scenario is that HIV arose from humans sawing their way into the forests of west equatorial Africa on logging expeditions, butchering chimpanzees for their flesh along the way.[967]

In Botswana, 39 percent of the country's adults were infected with HIV. There are countries in which 15 percent or more of the nation's children have been orphaned by AIDS killing both parents. To this day, a person dies from AIDS every minute. Although there has been tremendous progress in the treatment of AIDS, attempts at a vaccine have been undermined by the uncontrollable mutation rate of HIV. Someone butchered a chimp a few decades ago and now thirty million people are dead.[968]

The bushmeat industry may already be cooking up a new AIDS-like epidemic. Samples of blood were taken from rural villagers in Cameroon, known for their frequent exposure to wild primate body fluids from hunting. Ten were found to be infected with foreign ape viruses.[969] "Our study is the first to demonstrate that these retroviruses are actively crossing into people," the chief investigator said.[970] Their article published in *Lancet* ends, "Our results show simian retroviral zoonosis in people who have direct contact with fresh non-human primate bushmeat, and suggest that such zoonoses are more frequent, widespread, and contemporary than previously appreciated."[971] In the accompanying *Lancet* editorial, we are reminded that zoonotic cross-species infections are "among the most important public health threats facing humanity."[972]

While zoonotic diseases like rabies kill about fifty thousand people globally a year,[973] humans generally end up as the dead-end host for the virus. In terms of global public health implications, the greatest fear surrounds viruses that can not only jump from animals to humans, but then spread person to person. Only a few people eat chimpanzees, but many people in the world have sex.

Aggressive Symbiosis

Richard Preston wrote in *The Hot Zone*: "In a sense, the earth is mounting an immune response against the human species."[974] His fanciful "revenge of the rainforest" theme makes for good reading but lacks a grounding in science. There is an emerging evolutionary theory, however, that may help provide a biological basis for the lethality of emerging infectious disease.

Viruses have long been thought of as the ultimate parasite, "feeding" off the host organism while contributing nothing of value in return. This view may be changing. Frank Ryan, a British physician-researcher, has introduced the concept of "aggressive symbiosis." As opposed to parasitism, where one organism exclusively exploits the other, symbiotic relationships in biology can be characterized by both species benefiting in some way. *Symbiosis* is Greek for "companionship," whereas parasite is from the Greek *parasitos,* meaning "person who eats at someone else's table."[975] The classic symbiotic relationship is of the sea anemone and the clown fish. The clown fish is afforded protection among the stinging tentacles of the anemone. This is mutually beneficial for the sea anemone, which refrains from stinging the clown fish in return for help luring other prey into its grasp. Not all symbiotic relationships are as tender, though.

In Borneo, a species of rattan cane has developed a symbiotic relationship with a species of ants. The ants construct a nest around the cane and drink at its sugary sap. When an herbivore approaches to nibble its sweet leaves, the ants rush out and attack to defend their sugar daddy.[976] Ryan draws an analogy between this kind of behavior—which he terms "aggressive symbiosis"—and that of new zoonotic agents of disease. He argues that when it comes to emerging animal viruses, animals are the cane and ants are the virus.

For example, a herpes virus, *Herpesvirus saimiri,* has seemingly developed a symbiosis with the squirrel monkey, passing harmlessly from mother to baby. If a rival species like a marmoset monkey invades their territory, the virus jumps species and wipes out the challenger, inducing fulminant cancers in the invaders. In this way, the virus protects the squirrel monkeys' habitat from invading primates. It is in the squirrel monkeys' evolutionary best interest *not* to try to purge the virus from their systems, and so the virus is able to replicate free of immune interference. Another similar virus, *Herpesvirus ateles,* protects spider monkeys in South American jungles in much the same way, killing virtually 100 percent of encroaching monkeys lacking immunity. The spider monkeys pass both the virus and immunity to the virus from mother to child, benefiting all. This "jungle immune system" protects the inhabitants from invading primate species, even when that invading species is us.[777]

This may explain why Ebola is so virulent—*too* virulent, in fact. The disease evoked by the Ebola virus is so fierce that victims don't make it very far to infect others, which would seem to make the virus an evolutionary failure. Under the aggressive symbiosis hypothesis, however, the virus may be fulfilling its evolutionary purpose after all, protecting a host species we simply haven't identified.[978] Interestingly, it works both ways. The herpes virus that causes nothing more serious in humans than cold sores at the corner of one's mouth can pose a risk of lethal infection to monkeys in Central and South America.[979]

Simian (from the Latin *simia* for "ape"[980]) immunodeficiency virus is considered the precursor to the human AIDS virus, HIV.[981] Chimpanzees have SIV, but never get AIDS.[982] SIV is harmless in the African green monkey but can cause acute disease in the yellow baboon.[983] Hanta viruses are likewise harmless to their natural rodent hosts.[984] Aggressive symbiosis is an argument for keeping viruses confined to their natural niches.

Wild Tastes

In central Africa, consumers eat an estimated five hundred million wild mammals every year, totaling billions of pounds of meat. But the trade in bushmeat is not limited to Africa. In the Amazon basin, another few hundred million pounds of wild animal meat may be consumed, including six to sixteen million individual mammals.[985] "All considered," wrote two chief wildlife veterinarians in the Council on Foreign Relations journal *Foreign Affairs,* "at least a billion direct and indirect contacts among wildlife, humans, and domestic animals result from the handling of wildlife and the wildlife trade annually."[986]

The intensive commercial bushmeat trade started in the live animal markets of Asia,[987] particularly in Guangdong, the southern province surrounding Hong Kong from which H5N1 arose.[988] Literature from the Southern

Song Dynasty (1127–1279) describes the residents of Guangdong eating "whatever food, be it birds, animals, worms, or snakes."[989] Today, live animal "wet" markets cater to the unique tastes of the people of Guangdong, where shoppers can savor "Dragon-Tiger-Phoenix Soup," a brew made up of snake, cat, and chicken,[990] or delicacies like *san jiao,* "three screams." The wriggling baby rat is said to scream first when hefted with chopsticks, a second time as it is dipped into vinegar, and a third time as it is bitten.[991]

In China, animals are eaten for enjoyment, sustenance, and their purported medicinal qualities. There have been reports of dogs being "savagely beaten before death to increase their aphrodisiac properties."[992] Cats may be killed and boiled down into "cat juice," used to treat arthritis. Many of the cats are captured ferals in ill health, so "consuming such diseased cats is a time bomb waiting to explode," claimed the chief veterinarian of the Australian RSPCA.

As I mentioned in the prologue, the catlike masked palm civet has been a popular commodity in Chinese animal markets.[993] In addition to being raised for their flesh, civet cat penis is soaked in rice wine for use as an aphrodisiac.[994] These animals also produce the most expensive coffee in the world.[995] So-called fox-dung coffee is produced by feeding coffee beans to captive civets and then recovering the partially digested beans from the feces.[996] A musk-like substance of buttery consistency secreted by the anal glands gives the coffee its characteristic flavor and smell.[997] One might say this unique drink is good to the last dropping.

The masked palm civet has been blamed for the SARS epidemic.[998] "A culinary choice in south China," one commentator summed up in *Lancet,* "led to a fatal infection in Hong Kong, and subsequently to 8,000 cases of severe acute respiratory syndrome (SARS), and nearly 1,000 deaths in 30 countries on six continents."[999] Ironically, one reason civets are eaten is for protection from respiratory infections.[1000] As noted in *The China Daily,* "We kill them. We eat them. And, then, we blame them."[1001]

Wildlife have been hunted for more than a hundred thousand years[1002]— why the payback now? Growing populations and increasing demand for wildlife meat exceed local supplies of these animals.[1003] This has resulted in an enormous (and largely illegal) transboundary trade of wildlife and the setting up of intensive captive production farms in which wild animals are raised under poor sanitation in unnatural stocking densities. These animals are then packed together into markets for sale. These factors favor the spread and emergence of mutant strains of pathogens capable of infecting hunters, farmers, and shoppers.[1004] "You have a bird pooping on a turtle that poops on a civet," said the head of the Research Institute of Wildlife Ecology. "For getting new viruses to emerge, you couldn't do it much better even if you tried."[1005]

Following the SARS outbreak, the Chinese government reportedly confiscated more than eight hundred thousand wild animals from the markets of Guangdong.[1006] Animals sold live guarantee freshness in the minds of consumers, but in all their "freshness," the animals cough and defecate over one another, spewing potential pathogens throughout the market wet with blood and urine.[1007] These viral swap meets are blamed for the transformation of coronaviruses, previously known for causing the common cold, into a killer.[1008] If hindsight were twenty-twenty and the wet markets had been closed permanently, maybe we wouldn't be suffering a pandemic in 2020.

Shipping Fever

The bushmeat trade is not the viruses' only ticket around the world. More than fifty million live farm animals—cattle, sheep, and pigs—are traded across state lines in the United States alone every year, along with untold numbers of live birds on their way to slaughter.[1009] A pound of meat can travel a thousand miles "on the hoof" in the United States before reaching dinner tables.[1010] Live farm animal long-distance transport not only spreads disease geographically, but can also make animals both more infectious and more vulnerable to infection.

According to the FAO, "Transport of livestock is undoubtedly the most stressful and injurious stage in the chain of operations between farm and slaughterhouse," leading to significant "loss of production."[1011] This stress impairs immune function, increasing the animals' susceptibility to any diseases they might experience on their prolonged, often overcrowded journeys.[1012] Some pathogens that would not lead to disease under normal conditions, for example, become activated during transport due to stress-induced immunosuppression, triggering a wide variety of diarrheal and respiratory diseases. So-called shipping fever, the bovine version of which has cost U.S. producers more than $500 million a year, is often caused by latent pathogens—including a coronavirus[1013]—which may become active when shipping live cattle long distances.[1014] Given the increased disease risk, the European Commission's Scientific Committee on Animal Health and Animal Welfare recommended that "[j]ourneys should be as short as possible."[1015]

Once an animal is infected, the stress of transport can lead to increased shedding of the pathogen.[1016] In one study at Texas Tech University, for example, the average prevalence of *Salmonella* within feces and on the hides of cattle was 18 percent and 6 percent, respectively, before transport. But cram animals onto a vehicle and truck them just thirty to forty minutes, and the levels of *Salmonella* found in feces jumped from 18 percent to 46 percent and the number of animals covered with *Salmonella* jumped from 6 percent to 89 percent upon arrival at the slaughter plant, where fecal contamination on the hide or within the intestines can end up in the meat.[1017] Similar results were found in pigs.[1018] The physiological stress of transport thus increases a healthy animal's susceptibility to disease,[1019] while at the same time enhancing a sick animal's ability to spread contagion.[1020]

No surprise, then, that the FAO has blamed "[t]ransport of animals over long distances as one cause of the growing threat of livestock epidemics."[1021] Dozens of outbreaks of foot and mouth disease, for example, have been tied to livestock movements[1022] or contaminated transport vehicles.[1023]

The FAO has described live animal transport as "ideally suited for spreading disease" given that animals may originate from different herds or flocks and are "confined together for long periods in a poorly ventilated stressful environment."[1024] Given the associated "serious animal and public health problems," the Federation of Veterinarians of Europe have called for the replacement of the long-distance transportation of animals for slaughter as much as possible to a "carcass-only trade."[1025] I detail the role long-distance live animal transport played in the last pandemic in "Tracing the Flight Path."

America's Soft Underbelly

According to the Government Accountability Office, long-distance live animal transport not only places countries at risk for catastrophic disease outbreaks,[1026] but it makes them vulnerable to bioterrorism as well.[1027] U.S. animal agriculture has been described as a particularly easy target,[1028] not only as "one of the probable threats for an economic attack on this country,"[1029] according to former U.S. Deputy Secretary of Agriculture, but also as a direct attack on our citizenry.

In 2004, the RAND Corporation prepared a report on agroterrorism for the Office of the Secretary of Defense titled *Hitting America's Soft Underbelly.* They blamed America's vulnerability in part on the "concentrated and intensive nature of contemporary U.S. farming practices."[1030] According to the last USDA census, the top 1 percent of the nation's feedlots produced about half of the cattle[1031] and 1 percent of U.S. egg farms confine more than 90 percent of the nation's egg-laying hens.[1032] Given that "highly crowded" animals are reared in "extreme proximity" in the United States, one infected animal could quickly expose thousands of others.[1033]

The RAND corporation points out that individual animals raised by U.S. agriculture have become progressively more prone to disease as a result of increasingly routine invasive procedures:

> *Herds that have been subjected to such modifications—which have included everything from sterilization programs to dehorning, branding, and hormone injections—have typically suffered higher stress levels that have lowered the animals' natural tolerance to disease from contagious organisms and increased the viral and bacterial "volumes" that they normally shed in the event of an infection.[1034]*

Long-distance live transport could then ferry the spreading infection, according to USDA models, to as many as twenty-five states within five days.[1035] Curtailing the long-distance live transport of animals, as well as the concentration and intensification of the food animal industry, could thus potentially be a matter of national security.

Pet Peeves

"It's corny and it's a cliché," said one veterinary virologist, "but Mother Nature is the world's worst bioterrorist."[1036] Her viruses can escape the rainforests in animals living or dead, as pets or as meat. The international trade in exotic pets is a multibillion-dollar industry, and exotic pets can harbor exotic germs.[1037] Wildlife trafficking, the illegal trade in wildlife and wildlife parts, is a soaring black market worth as much as $10 billion a year in the United States alone.[1038] Before, the only wings with which viruses could typically fly were those of the mosquito. Now they also have jumbo jets. The U.S. imports an unbelievable 350,000 different species of live animals. According to testimony by then deputy director of the U.S. Fish and Wildlife Service before a Senate committee in 2003, the United States imports more than 200 million fish, 49 million amphibians, 2 million reptiles, 365,000 birds, and 38,000 mammals in a single year. With fewer than a hundred U.S. inspectors monitoring traffic nationwide, even if they worked 24-7, this would allow less than one second to inspect each incoming animal.[1039]

Whether for exotic pets or exotic cuisine, imported animals transported together under cramped conditions end up in holding areas in dealer warehouses, where they and their viruses can mingle further.[1040] The 2003 monkeypox outbreak across half a dozen states in the Midwest was traced to monkeypox-infected Gambian giant rats shipped to a Texas animal distributor along with eight hundred other small mammals snared from the African rainforest. The rodents were co-housed with prairie dogs who contracted the disease and made their way into pet stores and swap meets via an Illinois distributor. One week the virus is in a rodent in the dense jungles of Ghana, along the Gold Coast of West Africa; a few weeks later, that same virus finds itself in a three-year-old Wisconsin girl whose mom bought her a cute little prairie dog at a 4-H swap meet. "Basically you factored out an ocean and half a continent by moving these animals around and ultimately juxtaposing them in a warehouse or a garage somewhere," said Wisconsin's chief epidemiologist.[1041] Nobody ended up getting infected directly from the African rodents; they caught the monkeypox from secondary and tertiary contacts inherent to the trade.[1042]

The international pet trade in exotics has been described as a "major chink in the USA public health armor."[1043] As one expert quipped, "It was probably easier for a Gambian rat to get into the United States than a Gambian."[1044] Previously, monkeypox was typically known only to infect bushmeat hunters living in certain areas of Africa who ate a specific species of monkey.[1045] "Nothing happens on this planet that doesn't impact us," noted the chair of medicine at the Medical College of Wisconsin. "Could there be a more poignant example than this [monkeypox outbreak] happening in Wisconsin? People in Wisconsin don't even know where Gambia is."[1046]

Monkeypox is caused by a virus closely related to human smallpox, but currently has only a fraction of the lethality.[1047] Human-to-human transmission has been known to occur, however, and there is concern that monkeypox could evolve into a more "successful human pathogen."[1048] The CDC editorialized that the U.S. monkeypox outbreak "highlights the public health threat posed by importation, for commercial purposes, of exotic pets into the United States."[1049] "As long as humans are going to associate in a close way with exotic animals," said the dean of the University of Texas Medical Branch in Galveston, "they're going to be at risk."[1050]

Pigs Barking Blood

As H5N1 was emerging in Hong Kong in 1997, more than ten million acres of virgin forest were burning in Borneo and Sumatra. The resulting haze is thought to have caused a mass migration of fruit bats searching for food. Forced out of the forests and into areas of human cultivation, some of these "flying foxes" nested in mango trees overlying huge Malaysian pig farms. The fruit bats dribbled urine and half-eaten fruit slobbered with saliva into the pig pens.[1051] The bat urine and saliva were both later found to contain a virus[1052]—named the Nipah virus, after the village with the first human fatality. That virus was harmless to the fruit bats, but far from harmless to everyone else.[1053]

The pigs developed an explosive cough that became known as the "one-mile cough," because the violent hacking could be heard from far away. The disease was called *barking pig syndrome* after the unusual, loud barking cough.[1054] Pigs started coughing blood[1055] and developing neurological symptoms. Sows pressed their heads against the walls, started twitching, became paralyzed, or seized into spasms. Many died within twenty-four hours.[1056]

Using pigs as its conduit, the virus turned its attention to others. Almost every animal in the vicinity started falling ill—other farm animals like goats and sheep, companion animals like dogs, cats, and horses, and wild animals like deer fell into fatal respiratory distress.[1057] Human animals were no exception. People broke out in high fevers and headaches as their brains began to swell. Many started to convulse. Those who went into a coma never woke up.[1058] On autopsy, their brains and lungs were swollen with fluid.[1059]

The disease erupted in the northern part of the Malaysian peninsula, but ultimately swept nationwide on a seven-month rampage, thanks to long-distance animal transport.[1060] "A hundred years ago, the Nipah virus would have simply emerged and died out," the Thai Minister of Public Health explained; "instead it was transmitted to pigs and amplified. With modern agriculture, the pigs are transported long distances to slaughter. And the virus goes with them."[1061] A one-mile cough is still only a one-mile cough in a country that is almost five thousand miles around.[1062]

The Nipah virus was finally stamped out by stamping out much of the Malaysian pig population.[1063] Pig farmers started the cull, beating the animals to death with batons, but the Malaysian army needed to come in to finish the job, killing more than one million pigs.[1064]

The Nipah virus turned out to be one of the deadliest of human pathogens, killing 40 percent of those infected, a toll that propelled it onto the U.S. list of potential bioterrorism agents.[1065] Nipah is also noted for its "intriguing ability" to cause relapsing brain infections in some survivors[1066] many months after initial exposure.[1067] Even more concerning, a 2004 resurgence of Nipah virus in Bangladesh showed a case fatality rate on par with Ebola—75 percent—and showed evidence of human-to-human transmission.[1068]

The surfacing of the Nipah virus demonstrates how slash-and-burn deforestation may contribute to disease emergence in unexpected ways. Remote rainforest intrusions can bring humans into contact with viruses they had never before been in contact with, or, as in the case of Nipah, it can bring the new viruses out to us. One zoologist described the outbreak: "Nipah appears to be a case of the bats getting some payback."[1069] This may not have been possible without collusion from the pig industry.

It is likely no coincidence that the Nipah outbreak began on one of the largest pig farms in the country.[1070] Raising pigs was not new in Malaysia, but intensive industrial production was. The Leong Seng Nam farm, where the epidemic broke out, confined more than thirty thousand pigs. The Nipah virus, like all contagious respiratory diseases, is a density-dependent pathogen,[1071] requiring a certain threshold density of susceptible individuals to spread, persist, and erupt from within a population.[1072] Scientists suspect it may have taken more than a year of circulating in this unnaturally massive herd before it learned to fully adapt and mutate into a strain that explodes into other mammals.[1073] "Without these large, intensively managed pig farms in Malaysia," the director of the Consortium for Conservation Medicine said, "it would have been extremely difficult for the virus to emerge."[1074]

China is the world's largest producer of pork.[1075] Much of the pig production is concentrated in the Sichuan province, which in 2005 suffered an unprecedented outbreak in scope and lethality of *Streptococcus suis,* a newly emerging zoonotic pig pathogen.[1076] *Strep. suis* is a common cause of meningitis in intensively farmed pigs worldwide[1077] and presents most often as meningitis in people as well,[1078] particularly those who butcher infected pigs or later handle infected pork products.[1079] Due to involvement of the auditory nerves connecting the inner ears to the brain, half of the human survivors become deaf.[1080]

The World Health Organization reported that it had never seen so virulent a strain[1081] and blamed intensive confinement conditions as a predisposing factor in its sudden emergence, given the stress-induced suppression of the pigs' immune systems.[1082] The USDA explains that these bacteria can exist as a harmless component of a pig's normal bacterial flora, but stress due to factors like crowding and poor ventilation can drop the animal's defenses long enough for the bacteria to become invasive and cause disease.[1083] China's Assistant Minister of Commerce admitted at the time that the disease was "found to have direct links with the foul environment for raising pigs."[1084] The disease can spread through respiratory droplets or directly via contact with contaminated blood on improperly sterilized castration scalpels, tooth-cutting pliers, or tail-docking knives.[1085] China boasts more than ten thousand confined animal feeding operations (CAFOs),[1086] colloquially known as factory farms, which, as I've discussed, tend to have stocking densities conducive to the emergence and spread of disease.[1087]

The United States is the world's second-largest pork producer,[1088] and *Strep. suis* infection has also been an emerging pathogen in North America pig production, especially in intensive confinement settings.[1089] According to the *Journal of Swine Health and Production,* human cases of meningitis in North America are likely underdiagnosed and mis-identified[1090] due to the lack of adequate surveillance.[1091] The WHO encourages careful pork preparation,[1092] and North American agriculture officials urge *Strep. suis* disease awareness for people "who work in pig barns, processing plants, as well as in the home kitchen."[1093]

The first human case of *Strep. suis* was not in Asia or in the United States, however, but in Europe. The Dutch pig belt, extending into parts of neighboring Belgium and Germany, has the densest population of pigs in the world, more than twenty thousand per square mile. This region has been hit with major epidemics within recent years of hog cholera and foot and mouth disease, leading to the destruction of millions of animals. "With more and more pigs being raised intensively to satisfy Europe's lust for cheap pork, epidemics are inevitable," wrote *New Scientist*'s Europe Correspondent. "And the hogs may not be the only ones to get sick."[1094]

Even industry groups, like the American Association of Swine Veterinarians, have blamed "[e]merging livestock production systems, particularly where they involve increased intensification" as a main reason why zoonotic diseases are of increasing concern. These intensive systems, in addition to their high population density, "may also generate pathogen build-ups or impair the capacity of animals to withstand infectious agents."[1095] Increasing consumer demand for animal products worldwide over the past few decades has led to a global explosion in massive animal agriculture operations which have come to play a key role in the Third Age of emerging human disease.[1096]

LIVESTOCK REVOLUTION

Breeding Grounds

In response to the torrent of emerging and re-emerging zoonotic diseases jumping from animals to people, the world's three leading authorities—the Food and Agriculture Organization of the United Nations, the World Health Organization, and the World Organization for Animal Health (OIE)—held a joint consultation in 2004 to determine the key underlying causes. Four main risk factors for the emergence and spread of these diseases were identified. Bulleted first: "Increasing demand for animal protein."[1097] This has led to what the CDC refers to as "the intensification of food-animal production," the factor blamed in part for the increasing threat.[1098]

The way we kept animals when we first domesticated them ten thousand years ago is a far cry from how they are reared today. Chickens used to run around the barnyard on small farms. Now, "broiler" chickens—those raised for meat—are typically warehoused in long sheds confining an average of twenty thousand to twenty-five thousand birds.[1099] A single corporation, Tyson, can churn out more than twenty million pounds of chicken meat a

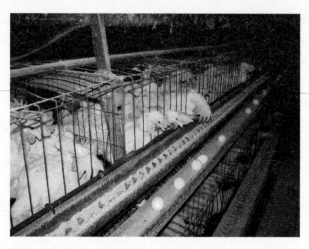

Battery cages[1100]

day.[1101] Worldwide, an estimated 70 to 80 percent of egg-laying chickens are intensively confined in battery cages,[1102] small barren wire enclosures stacked several tiers high and extending down long rows in windowless sheds.[1103] The cages are stocked at such densities that each hen is typically allotted less floor space than a standard letter-sized piece of paper.[1104] It is not uncommon for egg producers to keep hundreds of thousands—or even a million—hens confined on a single farm.[1105] Half the world's pig population—now approaching one billion—is also crowded into industrial confinement operations.[1106] This represents the most profound alteration of the animal-human relationship in ten thousand years.[1107]

Driven by the population explosion, urbanization, and increasing incomes,[1108] the per capita consumption of meat, eggs, and dairy products has skyrocketed in the developing world,[1109] leading to a veritable Livestock Revolution beginning in the 1970s, akin to the 1960s Green Revolution in cereal grain production.[1110] World meat production has risen more than 500 percent over the past decades.[1111]

To evaluate the global risks of infectious animal diseases, the Iowa-based, industry-funded[1112] Council for Agricultural Science and Technology created a task force that included public health experts from the WHO, veterinary experts from the OIE, agriculture experts from the USDA, and industry experts from the likes of the National Pork Board. Its report was released in 2005 and traced the history of livestock production from family-based farms to industrial confinement. It found that traditional systems are being replaced by intensive systems at a rate of more than 4 percent a year, particularly in Asia, Africa, and South America. "A major impact of modern intensive production systems," the report reads, "is that they allow the rapid selection and amplification of pathogens that arise from a virulent ancestor (frequently by subtle mutation), thus there is increasing risk for disease entrance and/or dissemination." Modern animal agriculture provides "significant efficiency in terms of economy of scale," but the "cost of increased efficiency" is increased disease risk. "Stated simply," the report concluded, "because of the Livestock Revolution, global risks of disease are increasing."[1113]

In the United States, the average numbers of animals on chicken, pig, and cattle operations approximately doubled between 1978 and 1992.[1114] This increasing population density seems to be playing a key role in triggering emerging epidemics. In terms of disease control, according to the FAO, "[t]he critical issue is the keeping [of] more and more animals in smaller and smaller spaces."[1115] The unnaturally high concentration of animals confined indoors in a limited airspace producing enormous quantities of manure provides, from a microbiologist's perspective, "ideal conditions for infectious diseases."[1116]

Back to the Dark Ages

Before the Sanitary Revolution of the nineteenth century established sewage collection and treatment, cities were centers of filth and pestilence. "Thousands of tons of midden filth filled the receptacles, scores of tons lay strewn about where the receptacles would receive no more," observed an English medical officer in Leeds in 1866. "Hundreds of people, long unable to use the privy because of the rising heap, were depositing on the floors."[1117] Fecal diseases from squalor and overcrowding, like cholera and typhoid fever, were rampant. Animals are increasingly raised for food today in conditions straight out of the Middle Ages.[1118]

Award-winning science journalist and author Madeline Drexler compared modern meat production facilities to a "walled medieval city, where waste is tossed out the window, sewage runs down the street, and feed and drinking water are routinely contaminated by fecal material."[1119] In the United States, farm animals produce more than one billion tons of manure each year—the weight of ten thousand Nimitz-class aircraft carriers.[1120] That is one huge load of crap. Each steer can produce seventy-five pounds of manure a day, turning feedlots into wading pools of waste.[1121] "Animals are living in medieval conditions and we're living in the 21st century," the chief of the CDC's foodborne and diarrheal diseases branch pointed out. "Consumers have to be aware that even though they bought their food from a lovely modern deli bar or salad bar, it started out in the 1600s."[1122]

The slum conditions on factory farms are breeding grounds for disease.[1123] The British Agriculture Ministry walks us through the microbiological hazards of modern pig production:

> Treatment may be given to sows for metritis, mastitis, and for diseases such as erysipelas and leptospirosis. In most indoor herds antibiotic treatment starts soon after birth. Piglets will receive drugs for enteritis and for respiratory disease. From weaning (usually three weeks) all piglets are gathered, mixed and then reared to finishing weights. Weaners usually develop post-weaning diarrhea caused by E. coli which occurs on day 3 post-weaning. . . . Post-weaning diarrhea is quickly followed by a range of other diseases. Glasser's Disease (Haemophilus parasuis) occurs at 4 weeks, pleuropneumonia at 6–8 weeks, proliferative enteropathy from 6 weeks and spirochaetal diarrhea and colitis at any time from 6 weeks onward. . . . At 8 weeks the pigs are termed growers and moved to another house. Here they will develop enzootic pneumonia, streptococcal meningitis (Streptococcus suis), and, possibly, swine dysentery. Respiratory disease may cause problems until slaughter.[1124]

According to animal scientists at Purdue and the University of Georgia, the late nineteenth and early twentieth centuries ironically "might well have been the golden age for domesticated livestock in terms of welfare and disease control."[1125]

High-density production allows for disease to spread faster to greater numbers of animals.[1126] Because intensive operations are vulnerable to catastrophic losses from disease,[1127] the USDA considers animal disease "the single greatest hindrance to efficient livestock and poultry production on a global basis."[1128] Industrial animal factories lead not only to more animal-to-animal contact, but also to more animal-to-human contact, particularly when production facilities border urban areas.[1129]

Due to land constraints around the world, massive livestock operations have been moving closer to major urban areas in countries like Bangladesh.

This is bringing together the worst of both worlds[1130]—the congested inner cities of the developing world, combined with the congested environment on industrial farms.[1131] The United Nation's FAO considers this a dangerous nexus, providing "flash points" for the source of new diseases.[1132]

There are other systemic factors that inherently increase the susceptibility of these animals to disease. The USDA cites a loss of genetic diversity in herds and flocks.[1133] A former chief of the Special Pathogens Branch of the CDC explains: "Intensive agricultural methods often mean that a single, genetically homogeneous species is raised in a limited area, creating a perfect target for emerging diseases, which proliferate happily among a large number of like animals in close proximity."[1134]

The stress associated with the routine mutilations farm animals are subjected to without anesthesia[1135]—including castration, branding, dehorning, detoeing, teeth clipping, beak trimming, and tail docking[1136]—coupled with the metabolic demands of intensive production, such as artificially augmented reproduction, lactation, early weaning, and accelerated growth rates, leave animals, according to one review, "extremely prone to disease."[1137] Never before have microbes had it so good. In the twenty years between 1975 (around the time when the dean of Yale's School of Medicine famously told students that there were "no new diseases to be discovered"[1138]) and 1995, seventeen foodborne pathogens emerged, almost one every year.[1139] With billions of feathered and curly-tailed test-tubes for viruses to incubate and mutate within, a WHO official described the last few decades as "the most ambitious short-term experiment in evolution in the history of the world."[1140]

Stomaching Emerging Disease

Most of the animal manure produced in the United States every year (five tons for every man, woman, and child in the country)[1141] goes unclaimed, but some of it ends up in our food and water. Excess manure nitrates can cause a condition called *methemoglobinemia,* or "blue-baby syndrome," a rare but under-recognized cause of illness and death among U.S. infants, as well as asphyxiating aquatic ecosystems with algae blooms.[1142] In the 1990s, this latter ecological problem bloomed into a public health issue as well with the emergence of the carnivorous algae *Pfiesteria piscicida* (Latin for "fish killer").[1143]

Likened to grass feeding on sheep, this tiny plankton releases a toxin that skins fish alive to feed on their flesh. More than one billion fish have been killed,[1144] and fish are not the only ones affected. Fishers, recreational boaters, and swimmers along the eastern seaboard of the United States started developing skin lesions and neurological deficits, such as memory loss, disorientation, and speech impediments. One *Pfiesteria* researcher was sent to the hospital[1145] and was still experiencing neurological symptoms years later.[1146] Experts blamed poultry manure runoff for the emergence of this "cell from hell,"[1147] which led to tighter poultry industry regulation.[1148]

In our kitchens, animal excrement leads to food poisoning. The risks associated with this "plate waste" have intensified along with the industry that created it. In its landmark 1992 report, *Emerging Infections: Microbial Threats to Health in the United States,* the National Academy of Medicine stated that "the introduction of feedlots and large-scale poultry rearing and processing facilities has been implicated in the increasing incidence of human pathogens, such as *Salmonella,* in domestic animals over the past 30 years."[1149] As microbiologist John Avens said at a poultry meeting, "*Salmonella* infection of animals will occur more frequently and affect more individual animals as concentration of confinement increases."[1150]

The World Health Organization sets the number killed worldwide from foodborne microbial diseases at twenty million a year, with animal products topping the list of causes.[1151] The WHO attributes the global rise in foodborne illness not only to the "greater consumption of foods of animal origin," but also the "methods of intensive production" required to supply such a demand.[1152] About half of all known foodborne pathogens have been discovered within just the past few decades.[1153]

In industrialized countries, the incidence of reported infectious food- and waterborne illnesses has more than doubled since the 1970s.[1154] According to the best estimate of the CDC, an astonishing 48 million Americans come down with foodborne illness annually. That's nearly one in seven of us every single year. Remember that "twenty-four-hour flu" you or a family member may have had last year? There's no such thing as a twenty-four-hour flu. It may very well have been food poisoning.[1155] In the food safety lottery, each year, Americans may have approximately a 1 in 2,500 chance of being hospitalized, and about a 1 in 100,000 chance of dying, simply from eating.[1156]

It may be from *E. coli* O157:H7 in hamburgers, *Salmonella* in eggs, *Listeria* in hot dogs, "flesh-eating" bacteria in oysters,[1157] or *Campylobacter* in Thanksgiving turkeys. According to an executive editor of *Meat Processing* magazine,

"Nearly every food consumers buy in supermarkets and order in restaurants can be eaten with certainty for its safety—except for meat and poultry products."[1158]

The latest comprehensive analysis of sources for foodborne illness outbreaks found that chickens were the primary cause overall. In fact, poultry and eggs caused more cases than red meat, seafood, and dairy products combined.[1159] A British analysis showed that fruits and vegetables carried the lowest disease and hospitalization risk, and poultry carried the highest. The researchers concluded, "Reducing the impact of indigenous foodborne disease is mainly dependent on controlling the contamination of chicken."[1160] Good luck. In the United States, the overwhelming majority of the nine billion chickens raised each year are stocked in densities between ten[1161] and twenty[1162] birds per square yard, unable even to fully stretch their wings.[1163] Under the avian carpet is a fecal carpet of filth most of the birds spend their lives upon.[1164]

Chicken of the Sea® is an ironic brand name for canned tuna. The only animal industry with greater stocking density than poultry production is fish farming, where tanks routinely squeeze up to a ton of animals into a dozen cubic yards of water (9 m^3).[1165] Floating cages have been known to hold up to four times more.[1166] The water can become so saturated with feed and feces that these fish-in-a-barrel operations may be more aptly dubbed fish-in-a-toilet. As the chief of the CDC's Special Pathogens branch once pointed out, whether in a human megacity, a broiler chicken shed, or an aquaculture tank, any time one crowds a monoculture of a single species together, one is asking for trouble.[1167] Combined with the stress associated with overcrowding and poor water quality, it is not hard to imagine how the factory farming methods associated with the so-called Blue Revolution expansion of fish farming in the 1980s[1168] resulted in the emergence of another zoonotic disease.[1169]

Discovered first in an Amazon dolphin in the 1970s from which it got its name, *Streptococcus iniae* (*inia* is the Guarayo Indian word for "dolphin"[1170]) started wiping out fish stocks on intensive fish farms around the world with epidemics of acute meningitis.[1171] By the 1990s, the dolphin wasn't the only mammal discovered to be infected. In 1995, the first confirmed spread to humans who handled fish in their kitchens was published in *The New England Journal of Medicine*. Most of the human reports involved just skin infections, but in a few cases, the bacteria became invasive, spread through victims' bloodstreams, seeding infection in their joints, heart, or even brain. Thankfully, no one has died yet from this emerging disease.[1172]

"The demonstration of another new pathogen linked to the food industry is not surprising," concluded the investigators, "considering that changes in the production, storage, distribution, and preparation of food, as well as environmental changes, provide increased opportunity for humans to be exposed to new organisms that may be pathogenic."[1173] Other pathogens emerging on aquaculture farms include a class that threatens immunocompromised persons in particular,[1174] as well as wildlife pathogens escaping from hatcheries and threatening the survival of wild rainbow trout, for example, in many streams in the western United States.[1175]

A recent foodborne pathogen linked to poultry is ExPEC. Urinary tract infections (UTIs) are the most common bacterial infections in women of all ages,[1176] affecting millions every year in the United States. From a physician's perspective, they are getting harder and harder to treat as antibiotic resistance among the chief pathogen, E. coli, becomes more and more common.[1177]

When most people think of E. coli, they think about E. coli O157:H7, the strain best known for the 1993 Jack-in-the-Box outbreak that infected more than five hundred kids and adults when burgers contaminated with infectious fecal matter were distributed to ninety-three restaurants.[1178] Infection starts as hemorrhagic colitis (profuse bloody diarrhea) and can progress to kidney failure, seizures, coma, and death. While E. coli O157:H7 remains a leading cause of acute kidney failure in U.S. children,[1179] fewer than a hundred thousand Americans get infected every year, and fewer than a hundred die.[1180] But millions get "extraintestinal" E. coli infections—urinary tract infections that can invade the bloodstream and cause an estimated thirty-six thousand deaths annually in the United States.[1181] That's more than five hundred times as many deaths as E. coli O157:H7. We know where E. coli O157:H7 comes from—fecal contamination from the meat, dairy, and egg industries[1182]— but where do these other E. coli come from?

Medical researchers at the University of Minnesota published a clue to the mystery in the April 2005 issue of The Journal of Infectious Disease. Taking more than a thousand food samples from multiple retail markets, they found evidence of fecal contamination in 69 percent of the pork and beef and 92 percent of the poultry samples, as evidenced by E. coli contamination. More surprising was that more than 80 percent of the E. coli they recovered from beef, pork, and poultry were resistant to one or more antibiotics, and greater than half of the samples of poultry bacteria "were resistant to >5 drugs!" (One rarely finds exclamation points in the medical literature.) What was most surprising was that half of the poultry samples were contaminated with the extraintestinal pathogenic *E. coli* bacteria, abbreviated ExPEC. UTI-type *E. coli* may be foodborne pathogens as well.[1183]

Scientists suspect that by eating chicken and other meat, women infect their lower intestinal tract with these antibiotic-resistant bacteria, which can then creep up into their bladder.[1184] Commonsense hygiene measures to prevent UTIs have included wiping from front to back after bowel movements and urinating after intercourse to flush out any infiltrators. Commenting on this body of research, *Science News* suggested meat avoidance as an option to "chicken out" of urinary tract infections.[1185]

Even if we avoided meat, though, we would still not be able to escape exposure to pathogens found in animal wastes. Apple cider freshly squeezed from apples collected in an orchard where an infected calf grazed caused an outbreak of cryptosporidiosis, a parasitic disease.[1186] This was the same disease that caused a record 420,000 cases of severe gastroenteritis in the Milwaukee area in 1993, when cattle excreted upstream of a major source of the metropolitan water supply.[1187]

The alfalfa sprouts lining the whole-grain avocado sandwiches of the California health conscious led to a *Salmonella* outbreak in 2001.[1188] Since the first reported sprout outbreak in 1973, there have been at least two dozen more in the United States,[1189] including both *Salmonella* and *E. coli* O157:H7, infecting thousands of people.[1190] How did bacteria from chickens and cattle get onto sprouts? The bacteria were in manure used as fertilizer.[1191] As the level of infection in herd and flock feces has risen with intensification, so has the contamination of produce crops it has fertilized.[1192]

Even though spout producers may soak sprout seeds in a solution of bleach, pathogens seem to be able to hide inside microscopic crevices in the seeds. One outbreak in California led both the CDC and FDA to reiterate their recommendations that everyone cook their sprouts before eating them.[1193] Of course, while sprouts have been associated with about one hundred infections annually in the United States, eating eggs is estimated to sicken seventy-nine thousand.[1194]

Tragically, food poisoning can be the gift that keeps on giving. Although thousands die from food poisoning every year in the United States, the vast majority suffer only acute self-limited episodes. Up to 15 percent of those who contract *Salmonella,* however, go on to develop serious joint inflammation that can last for years. An estimated one hundred thousand to two hundred thousand Americans suffer from arthritis arising directly from foodborne infections every year.[1195] One of the most feared long-term complications of food poisoning is Guillain-Barré syndrome, in which infection with *Campylobacter,* a bacteria contaminating about a quarter of retail chicken meat in the United States,[1196] can lead to being paralyzed for months on a ventilator.[1197] With the virtual elimination of polio, poultry products are now the most common cause of acute flaccid paralysis in the developed world.[1198]

Campylobacter is a spiral-shaped poultry bacteria[1199] that corkscrews its way into the lining of the intestine "with a speed that cannot be matched by other bacteria."[1200] Just as *H. pylori* bacteria has been linked to stomach cancer, *Campylobacter* may trigger cancer as well, a rare lymphoma of the intestines.[1201] *Campylobacter,* not even proven to cause human illness until the 1970s,[1202] is now the suspected cause of up to 25 percent of cases of irritable bowel syndrome[1203] and is currently the number-one bacterial cause of food poisoning, sickening millions of Americans every year.[1204] The bacteria in a single drop of chicken "juice" are enough to make one sick[1205] and can persist on a cutting board for hours.[1206]

The U.S. meat inspection system—HACCP (Hazard Analysis Critical Control Point system)—was originally designed by NASA and represented a welcome scientific departure from the century-old "poke and sniff" method.[1207] Unfortunately, its implementation was handed over to the industry guarding its own henhouses, leaving some USDA inspectors to deride HACCP as more of a "Have A Cup of Coffee and Pray" system.[1208] "As an analogy," said the president of the U.S. Meat Inspection Union, "imagine that as a driver you must write yourself a ticket every time you exceed the speed limit because you're breaking the law. Some [chicken packing] plants cheat; others won't cheat until they're forced to in a competitive environment."[1209]

Few public health issues are more public than food safety, yet not only do the state and federal governments continue to lack the power to order mandatory recalls of contaminated meat, the meat and poultry industry don't even have to divulge where the infected meat went. Federal agencies have more power to recall defective toys than meat. When the industry is left to do it voluntarily, less than half of the tainted meat is recovered. Following one of the largest meat recalls in U.S. history—"ready to eat" chicken and turkey products harboring *Listeria* bacteria[1210]—the Government Accountability Office, the watchdog arm of Congress, called for an overhaul of the process in 2004, including granting the federal government mandatory meat recall authority.[1211]

The U.S. poultry industry, instead of cleaning up its own act—by reducing the overcrowding of birds, relieving production stresses, and improving hygiene to lower infection rates—has tended to push for more cost-effective alternatives, such as irradiation to kill off bacteria and viruses in the fecal material remaining on carcasses before they hit the store. One former USDA meat inspection administrator claimed, "All irradiation will do is add partially decontaminated fecal matter to the American diet . . . The solution to the food safety problem is to produce safe food."[1212]

One novel solution that "holds great promise" is the application of bacteria-destroying viruses to chicken meat, although the industry expressed concern over initial reports revealing "consumer resistance" to the idea.[1213] For a similar reason, the industry prefers the term "cold pasteurization" to irradiation.[1214]

The industry has even considered "gluing shut the rectal cavities of turkeys and chicken broilers" in the slaughter plants before they hit the scalding tanks to cover up its dirty secret of fecal contamination.[1215] There are concerns, though, about glue residues contaminating the final product. Other ideas for sealing up the birds' rectums include some type of mechanical plug or stapling technology.[1216] The name of the poultry superglue product is "Rectite®."[1217]

Offal Truth

Global public health experts have identified "dubious practices used in modern animal husbandry" beyond the inherent overstocking, stress, and filth that have directly or indirectly launched deadly new diseases.[1218] One such "misguided" brave new farm practice is the continued feeding of livestock slaughterhouse waste, blood, and excrement to animals to save on feed costs.[1219]

Feed expenditures remain the single largest industry expense.[1220] The livestock industry has experimented with feeding newspaper, cardboard, cement dust, and sewer sludge to farm animals.[1221] A *U.S. News and World Report* article summarized the gambit: "Cattle feed now contains things like manure and dead cats."[1222] The Animal Industry Association defends these practices, arguing that the average U.S. farm animal "eats better than the average U.S. citizen."[1223] Forcing natural herbivores like cows and sheep to be carnivores and cannibals turned out to have serious public health implications.

A leading theory on the origin of mad cow disease is that cows got it by eating diseased sheep.[1224] In modern corporate agribusiness, protein concentrates (or "meat and bone meal," euphemistic descriptions of "trimmings that originate on the killing floor, inedible parts and organs, cleaned entrails, fetuses"[1225]) are fed to dairy cows to increase milk production,[1226] as well as to most other livestock.[1227] According to the World Health Organization, nearly ten million metric tons of slaughterhouse waste is fed to livestock every year.[1228] The recycling of the remains of infected cattle into cattle feed was probably what led to the British mad cow epidemic's explosive spread[1229] to nearly two dozen countries around the world in the subsequent twenty years.[1230] Dairy producers may use corn or soybeans as a protein feed supplement, but slaughterhouse by-products can be cheaper.[1231]

An editorial in the *British Medical Journal* described mad cow disease as resulting "from an accidental experiment on the dietary transmissibility of prion disease between sheep and cows."[1232] A subsequent "accidental experiment"—with humans—started in the late 1980s as meat contaminated with mad cow disease entered the food supply.[1233] Prions—infectious proteins—are the unconventional pathogens that cause mad cow-like diseases. Unlike other foodborne pathogens that can be treated with antibiotics and killed by proper cooking, prions are practically indestructible, surviving incineration[1234] at temperatures hot enough to melt lead.[1235]

More than two hundred people have been killed in this experiment by the human form of mad cow disease, called *variant Creutzfeldt-Jakob disease (vCJD)*,[1236] whose standard clinical picture can involve weekly deterioration[1237] into blindness and epilepsy[1238] while the brain becomes riddled with holes.[1239] vCJD produces a relentlessly progressive[1240] and invariably fatal dementia.[1241] "vCJD always results in death, and the disease process is highly dreaded—mute, blind, incontinent, immobile/paralyzed/bedridden."[1242] It may take decades between the act of eating infected meat and coming down with the initial symptoms of a vCJD death sentence.[1243] To this day, as many as one in two thousand of those living in the UK carry the infection[1244] and may yet succumb with what Britain's Secretary of Health called the "worst form of death" imaginable.[1245]

Decades ago, the World Health Organization called for the exclusion of the riskiest bovine tissues—cattle brains, eyes, spinal cord, and intestine—from the human food supply and from all animal feed.[1246] Unfortunately, the United States still feeds some of these potentially risky tissues to people, pigs, pets, poultry, and fish.[1247] Then, pig remains can be fed back to cattle.[1248] Cattle remains are still fed to chickens, and the poultry litter (the mixture of excrement, spilled feed, dirt, feathers, and other debris that is scooped from the floors of bird sheds[1249]) is fed back to cows.[1250] In these ways, prions may continue to be cycled back into cattle feed and complete the cow "cannibalism" circuit.

Ecologists assert that animal fecal wastes pose public health risks "similar to those of human wastes and should be treated accordingly,"[1251] yet in animal agriculture today, fecal wastes are fed to other animals. Although excrement from other species is fed to livestock in the United States, chicken droppings are considered more nutritious for cows than pig feces or cattle dung.[1252] Because poultry litter can be as much as eight times cheaper than foodstuffs like alfalfa,[1253] the U.S. cattle industry feeds poultry litter to cattle.[1254] A thousand chickens can make enough waste to feed a growing calf year round.[1255]

A single cow can eat as much as three tons of poultry waste a year,[1256] yet the manure does not seem to affect the taste of the subsequent milk or meat.[1257] Taste panels have found little difference in the tenderness, juiciness, and flavor of beef made from steers fed up to 50 percent poultry litter. Beef from animals fed bird droppings may in fact even be juicier and more tender.[1258] Cows are typically not given feed containing more than 80 percent poultry litter, though, since it's not as palatable[1259] and may not fully meet protein and energy needs.[1260]

The industry realizes that the practice of feeding poultry manure to cattle might not stand up to public scrutiny. It understands that the custom carries "certain stigmas,"[1261] "presents special consumer issues,"[1262] and poses "potential public relations problems."[1263] It seems puzzled as to why the public so "readily accepts organically grown vegetables" grown with composted manure, while there is "apparent reluctance on the part of the public" to accept the feeding of poultry litter to cattle.[1264] "We hope," says one industry executive, "common sense will prevail."[1265]

The editor of *Beef* magazine commented, "The public sees it as 'manure.' We can call it what we want and argue its safety, feed value, environmental attributes, etc., but outsiders still see it simply as 'chicken manure.' And, the most valid and convincing scientific argument isn't going to counteract a gag reflex."[1266] The industry's reaction, then, has been to silence the issue. According to *Beef,* public relations experts within the National Cattlemen's Beef Association warned beef producers that discussing the issue publicly would only "bring out more adverse publicity."[1267] When the Kansas Livestock Association dared to shine the spotlight on the issue by passing a resolution urging the discontinuation of the practice, irate producers in neighboring states threatened a boycott of Kansas feed-yards.[1268]

In compliance with World Health Organization guidelines, Europe has forbidden the feeding of all slaughterhouse and animal waste to livestock.[1269] The American Feed Industry Association called such a ban "a radical proposition."[1270] The American Meat Institute agreed, stating, "[N]o good is accomplished by . . . prejudicing segments of society against the meat industry."[1271] As far back as 1993, Gary Weber, director of Beef Safety and Cattle Health for the National Cattlemen's Beef Association, admitted that the industry could find economically feasible alternatives to feeding rendered animal protein to other animals, but that the Cattlemen's Association did not want to set a precedent of being ruled by "activists."[1272]

Gary Weber was the beef industry spokesperson who appeared on the infamous episode of the Oprah Winfrey show in 1996. An internal U.S. government PR crisis management document showed that the government knew such feeding practices would be "vulnerable to media scrutiny."[1273] Indeed, alarmed and disturbed that cows in the United States are fed the remains of other cattle, Oprah swore she would never eat another burger.[1274] After Oprah tried to remind the audience that cows were supposed to be herbivores, Weber defended the practice by stating, "Now keep in mind, before you—you view the ruminant animal, the cow, as simply a vegetarian—remember that they drink milk."[1275] The absurdity of the statement aside, it's not even accurate. In modern agribusiness, humans drink the milk. Calves typically get milk "replacer."

Like all mammals, cows can only produce milk after they've had a baby. Most newborn calves in the United States are separated from their mothers within twelve hours—many immediately after birth—so the mother's milk can be marketed for human consumption.[1276] Though some dairy farmers still wean calves on whole milk, the majority of producers use milk replacer,[1277] which too often contains spray-dried cattle blood as a cheap source of protein.[1278] The chief disadvantage of blood-based milk replacer, according to the vice president of product development for the Animal Protein Corporation, is simply its "different color." Milk replacer containing blood concentrate typically has a "chocolate brown" color which can leave a dark residue on the bottles, buckets, and utensils used to feed the liquid.[1279] "For some producers," the company official remarked, "the difference is difficult to accept at first, since the product does not look 'like milk.'" But the "[c]alves don't care," he was quick to add.[1280]

The calves may not care, but Stanley Prusiner does. Prusiner won the Nobel Prize in Medicine for his discovery of prions. He was quoted in *The New York Times* as calling the practice of feeding cattle blood to young calves "a really stupid idea."[1281] The European Commission also condemned the practice of "intraspecies recycling of ruminant blood and blood products"— the practice of suckling calves on cows' blood protein.[1282] Even excluding the fact that brain emboli may pass into the trough that collects the blood once an animal's throat is slit,[1283] the report concludes, "As far as ruminant blood is concerned, it is considered that the best approach to protect public health at present is to assume that it could contain low levels of infectivity."[1284] Calves in the United States may still be drinking up to three cups of "red blood cell protein" concentrate every day.[1285]

The American Protein Corporation boasts it's the largest spray-dryer of blood in the world[1286] and advertises blood products that can even be fed "through the drinking water" to calves and pigs.[1287] The majority of pigs in the United States are evidently raised in part on spray-dried blood meal.[1288] According to the National Renderers Association, although young pigs may find spray-dried blood meal initially unpalatable, they eventually get used to it.[1289]

Dateline NBC quoted D. Carleton Gajdusek, the first to be awarded a Nobel Prize in Medicine for his work on prion diseases,[1290] as saying, "[I]t's got to be in the pigs as well as the cattle. It's got to be passing through the chickens."[1291] Paul Brown, medical director for the U.S. Public Health Service, also believed that pigs and poultry could be harboring mad cow disease and passing it on to humans, adding that pigs are especially sensitive to the disease. "It's speculation," he says, "but I am perfectly serious."[1292]

Since 1996, the World Health Organization has recommended that all countries stop feeding remains of cows to cows, yet the U.S. government still allows dairy farmers to feed calves gallons of a mixture of concentrated cow blood and fat collected at the slaughterhouse.[1293] Industry representatives continue to actively support this practice.[1294] "It was the farmers' fault," one young victim whispered to her mother from the bed where she waged and lost a painful, prolonged battle against vCJD.[1295]

Since 1996, the World Health Organization has recommended that all countries test their downed cattle—those animals too sick or crippled even to walk—for mad cow disease, yet the U.S. government tests but a fraction of this high-risk population. The beef industry calls U.S. surveillance "aggressive"[1296] and doesn't think more testing is necessary.[1297] Stanley Prusiner, the world's authority on these diseases, called the level of surveillance "appalling."[1298]

Since 1996, the World Health Organization has recommended that all countries stop feeding risky cattle organs (like brains) to all livestock. The Food and Agriculture Organization of the United Nations agrees with this no-brainer.[1299] The U.S. government continues to violate the guidelines. The American Meat Institute and fourteen other industry groups vocally opposed the ban.[1300] The British government's Official Inquiry into mad cow disease (also known as bovine spongiform encephalopathy, or BSE) concluded: "BSE developed into an epidemic as a consequence of an intensive farming practice—the recycling of animal protein in ruminant feed. This practice, unchallenged over decades, proved a recipe for disaster."[1301]

The meat industry has long known that cannibalistic feeding practices could be harmful, as *Salmonella* epidemics in poultry linked to the recycling of animal remains back into animal feed had been described well before the mad cow disease epidemic.[1302] Even if the meat industry didn't realize the scope of the potential human hazard then, it certainly should now. Yet it remains opposed to a total ban on the feeding of slaughterhouse waste, blood, and excrement to farm animals.[1303]

Veterinarian, author, and journalism professor Mark Jerome Walters returned to the scene of mad cow disease's birth in rural England. The farmer who harbored the first discovered case confessed:

> In retrospect, I'm appalled at what I didn't know about my own cows. I didn't know they were being fed other cows and sheep that had been ground into a powder. We've forced these hoofed grazers into cannibalism. On some farms they're fed growth promotants, and that's probably causing other problems. In many places in the world, livestock are kept in deplorable conditions, all

for convenience and profit. We've put cows on an assembly line and we take them off at the other end and butcher them. Did we really think we could just rearrange the world in any way we pleased? Nobody could have wished for or foreseen this awful thing called BSE. But should we be all that surprised? [1304]

Big Mac Attack

Unnatural feeding practices have also been blamed for the emergence of *E. coli* O157:H7, the strain I mentioned earlier that caused the 1993 Jack-in-the-Box outbreak.[1305] McDonald's, however, was ground zero for the first *E. coli* O157:H7 outbreak the decade before.[1306] A mother offers an eyewitness account of what the bug did to her eight-year-old daughter, Brianne:

The pain during the first 80 hours was horrific, with intense abdominal cramping every 10 to 12 minutes. Her intestines swelled to three times their normal size and she was placed on a ventilator. Emergency surgery became essential and her colon was removed. After further surgery, doctors decided to leave the incision open, from sternum to pubis, to allow Brianne's swollen organs room to expand and prevent them from ripping her skin. Her heart was so swollen it was like a sponge and bled from every pore. Her liver and pancreas shut down and she was gripped by thousands of convulsions, which caused blood clots in her eyes. We were told she was brain dead. [1307]

Brianne did survive, though suffering permanent kidney, liver, and brain damage.[1308] Alexander Thomas Donley, age six, did not. He stopped screaming only after *E. coli* toxins destroyed his brain before his death. "I was so horrified and so shocked and so angered by what happened to him," said his mother, Nancy, who became president of Safe Tables Our Priority, a Chicago-based advocacy organization. She continued:

I had no idea that there was any problem in our food supply. I loved my child more than anything in this world. And then to find out that he died because there were contaminated cattle feces in a hamburger. And to find out that had been recognized as a problem for a while. Why hadn't it been fixed?

Steve Bjerklie, as editor of the U.S. trade journal *Meat and Poultry*, described the industry's mantra: "It's spoken by dozens of industry leaders and government regulators, even intoned by fact-finding academicians who should know better," he wrote. "Over and over, at convention after convention, meeting after meeting, one hears the words droned by industry speaker after industry speaker, as if the existence of the words as sound waves in the air confirmed their truth: 'We have the safest meat and poultry supply in the world.'"[1309] Unfortunately, he admits, the facts don't support the claim.

Most European nations don't allow profitable but risky practices like the chilling baths that add water weight—and bacteria—to poultry in the United States. Sweden's poultry is virtually *Salmonella*-free. In Sweden, it's not just a good idea, it's the law—and it has been since 1968 after a *Salmonella* outbreak caused nine thousand illnesses.[1310] In the United States, eggs continue to infect more than seventy-nine thousand Americans annually.[1311] The U.S. industry trade group United Egg Producers has openly bragged about obstructing public health measures, crowing in its "Washington Report" that it added language to the USDA inspection budget that effectively killed the *Salmonella* testing program.[1312] According to Marion Nestle, former director of Nutrition Policy at the U.S. Department of Health and Human Services and longtime chair of the nutrition department at New York University, "major food industries oppose pathogen-control measures by every means at their disposal."[1313]

In the United States, *Salmonella* continues to infect about one in sixteen chickens sampled.[1314] The chair of the department of epidemiology at the University of Maryland School of Medicine and former official in the Agriculture Department's Food Safety and Inspection Service told *The New York Times* that when it comes to poultry products, "[i]t continues to be buyer beware."[1315]

The Netherlands' *E. coli* O157:H7 testing program, according to Bjerklie, "makes USDA's look like quality control at the 'Laverne and Shirley' brewery." This may be because their meat inspection program falls under the Netherlands' Ministry of Health, not the Ministry of Agriculture.[1316] As far back as 1979, the National Research Council,[1317] the Government Accountability Office,[1318] the National Academy of Medicine[1319]—and even the conservative Food Marketing Institute[1320]—have called for the formation of an independent food safety authority similar to what exists in Europe, but to no avail.[1321]

In 2002, ConAgra recalled nineteen million pounds of *E. coli* O157:H7-contaminated ground beef in one of the biggest meat recalls in U.S. history,[1322] yet it raised little public alarm. Where was the beef? "If nineteen million pounds of meat distributed to half of this country had been contaminated with a deadly strain of *E. coli* bacteria by terrorists," wrote one columnist, "we'd go nuts. But when it's done by a Fortune 100 corporation, we continue to buy it and feed it to our kids."[1323]

Given the alleged collusion between industry and government,[1324] parents are forced to take responsibility. One public health official put it bluntly:

> *Somebody had to come right out and say, because it wasn't getting said because people were tiptoeing around the issue, "Parents, if you've got a child in a hospital laying there with [organ failure] . . . and you're the one who served them red hamburger, you're as responsible for the illness as if you had put them in the front seat of a car without a seat belt or a car seat and drove 90 miles an hour through red lights."[1325]*

This sentiment is typical of the industry's blame-the-victim attitude. A more appropriate analogy might be sitting one's child in a pre-1970s car with no seatbelts before the consumer movement forced auto makers to include them.

E. coli O157:H7 means children can now die from going to a petting zoo.[1326] Since 1990, the CDC has reported more than two dozen separate outbreaks in children linked to petting zoos.[1327] There is no reason for anyone's children to get *E. coli* poisoning from this or any other source. *E. coli* O157:H7, like many of these other diseases, is thought to be a byproduct of our new intensive confinement system of animal agribusiness.

The changes in the digestive tracts of cattle fattened in feedlots with energy-dense grain to marble the flesh with saturated fat (instead of natural cattle foodstuffs like hay) has been blamed for the emergence of *E. coli* O157:H7. Grain-fed beef may be more tender, but grass-fed beef may be safer.[1328] In a familiar refrain, instead of altering feeding practices or eliminating the crowded feedlots that lead to manure-encrusted hides, the industry has decided it's more cost-effective to invest in chemical carcass dehairing technologies to lessen fecal contamination.[1329] Cost-effective, perhaps, as long as children's lives are not figured into the bottom line.

Animal Bugs Forced to Join the Resistance

At the American Chemical Society annual meeting in Philadelphia in 1950, the business of raising animals for slaughter changed overnight. Scientists announced the discovery that antibiotics make chickens grow faster.[1330] By 1951, the FDA approved the addition of penicillin and tetracycline to chicken feed as growth promotants, encouraging pharmaceutical companies to mass-produce antibiotics for animal agriculture. Antibiotics became cheap growth enhancers for the meat industry.[1331]

Healthy animals raised in hygienic conditions do not respond in the same way. If healthy animals housed in a clean environment are fed antibiotics, their growth rates don't change. Factory farms are considered such breeding grounds for disease that much of the animals' metabolic energy is spent just staying alive under such filthy, crowded, stressful conditions;[1332] normal physiological processes like growth are put on the back burner.[1333] Reduced growth rates in such hostile conditions cut into profits, but so would reducing the overcrowding. Antibiotics, then, became another crutch the industry can use to cut corners and cheat nature.[1334] Mother Nature, however, does not stay cheated for long.

The poultry industry, with its extreme size and intensification, continues to swallow the largest share of antibiotics. By the 1970s, 100 percent of all commercial poultry in the United States were being fed antibiotics. By the late 1990s, poultry producers were using more than ten million pounds of antibiotics a year.[1335] So many antibiotics have been fed to poultry that there have been reports of chickens dying from antibiotic overdoses.[1336] These thousands of tons of antibiotics were not going to treat sick animals; more than 90 percent of the antibiotics were used just to promote weight gain.[1337] The majority of the antibiotics produced in the world go not to human medicine but to prophylactic usage on the farm.[1338] This may generate antibiotic resistance.

When one saturates an entire shed-full of broiler chickens with antibiotics, this kills off all but the most resistant bugs, which can then spread and multiply. When Chinese chicken farmers put amantadine into their flocks' water supply, there was a tremendous environmental pressure on the virus to mutate resistance to the antiviral. Say there's a one in a billion chance of an influenza virus developing resistance to amantadine. Odds are, any virus we would come in contact with would be sensitive to the drug. But each infected bird poops out more than a billion viruses every day.[1339] The rest of their viral colleagues may be killed by the amantadine, but that one resistant strain of virus will be selected to spread and burst forth from the chicken farm, leading to widespread viral resistance and emptying our arsenal against bird flu. The same principles apply to the feeding of other antimicrobials.[1340]

According to the CDC, at least seventeen classes of antimicrobials are approved for farm animal growth promotion in the United States,[1341] including many families of antibiotics, such as penicillin, tetracycline, and erythromycin, that are critical for treating human disease.[1342] Each year, twenty million pounds of medically important antibiotics are laced into the feed and water of farm animals in the United States.[1343] As the bugs become more resistant to the antibiotics fed to healthy chickens, they may get more resistant to the antibiotics needed to treat sick people. According to the latest national survey, half of the *Salmonella* in retail meat sampled in the United States— chicken, turkey, beef, and pork—is resistant to tetracycline. About a quarter of the bugs are now resistant to three or more entire classes of antibiotics, including some resistant to ceftriaxone,[1344] which is a critically important drug we use to treat severe *Salmonella* infections, especially in children.[1345] Though the industry continues to deny culpability,[1346] the link between antibiotic use in farm animals and antibiotic resistance in humans is considered unequivocal and an urgent threat to human health.[1347]

Tragically, things are getting worse, not better. U.S. animal agriculture is using more antibiotics now than ever before,[1348] and it's not just that we're raising more animals. Antibiotic sales for meat production in the United States are outpacing meat production itself.[1349] Quite simply, we may be on the path to untreatable infections by using even some of our last-resort antibiotics, like carbapenems, just to shave a few cents off a pound of meat.[1350]

The European science magazine *New Scientist* editorialized that the use of antibiotics to make animals grow faster "should be abolished altogether." That was in 1968.[1351] Pleas for caution in the overuse of antibiotics can be traced back farther to Sir Alexander Fleming, the inventor of penicillin, who told *The New York Times* in 1945 that inappropriate use of antibiotics could lead to the selection of "mutant forms" resistant to the drugs.[1352] While Europe banned the use of many medically important antibiotics as farm animal growth promoters years ago,[1353] no such comprehensive step has yet taken place in the United States. The combined might of Big Ag and Big Pharma, who profit from all the drugs, have fought bitterly against efforts by the World Health

Organization,[1354] the American Medical Association,[1355] and the American Public Health Association[1356] to enact a similar ban in the United States.[1357]

The U.S. Government Accountability Office has acknowledged that "[m]any studies have found that the use of antibiotics in animals poses significant risks for human health," but, notably, has not recommended banning the practice,[1358] as a ban on the use of antibiotics as growth promoters could in part result in a "reduction of profits" for the industry. Even a partial ban would "increase costs to producers, decrease production, and increase retail prices to consumers." By how much? The National Academy of Sciences once estimated that a total ban on the widespread feeding of antibiotics to farm animals would raise the price of poultry anywhere from one to two cents per pound and the price of pork or beef around three to six cents a pound, costing the average meat-eating American consumer up to $9.72 a year.[1359] Meanwhile, antibiotic-resistant infections in the United States cost an estimated $30 billion every year[1360] and kill ninety thousand people.[1361]

When the FDA first considered revoking the license for the use of antibiotics strictly as livestock growth promoters, the drug industry went hog wild. The late Thomas H. Jukes, a drug industry official formerly involved with one of the first commercial producers of antibiotics for livestock, blamed the FDA's consideration on a "cult of food quackery whose high priests have moved into the intellectual vacuum caused by the rejection of established values." Jukes was so enamored with the growth benefits he saw on industrial farms that he advocated for antibiotics to be added to the human food supply. "I hoped that what chlortetracycline did for farm animals it might do for children." We should especially feed antibiotics to children in the Third World, he argued, to compensate for their unhygienic overcrowding, which he paralleled to the conditions "under which chickens and pigs are reared intensively."[1362] "Children grow far more slowly than farm animals," he wrote. "Nevertheless, there is still a good opportunity to use low-level feeding with antibiotics . . . among children in an impoverished condition."[1363]

The poultry industry blames the dramatic rise in antibiotic-resistant bacteria on the overprescription of antibiotics by doctors.[1364] While doctors undoubtedly play a role, according to the CDC, more and more evidence is accumulating that livestock overuse is particularly worrisome.[1365] Take, for example, the September 2005 FDA victory against the Bayer Corporation.[1366]

Typically, *Campylobacter* causes only a self-limited diarrheal illness ("stomach flu") which doesn't require antibiotics. If the gastroenteritis is particularly severe, though, or if doctors suspect that the bug may be working its way from the gut into the bloodstream, the initial drug of choice is typically a quinolone antibiotic like Cipro. Quinolone antibiotics have been used in human medicine since the 1980s, but widespread antibiotic-resistant *Campylobacter* didn't arise until after quinolones were licensed for use in animal feed as growth promoters in the early 1990s. In countries like Australia, which reserved quinolones for human use only, resistant bacteria are practically unknown.[1367]

The FDA concluded that the use of Cipro-like antibiotics in chickens compromised the treatment of nearly ten thousand Americans a year, meaning that thousands infected with *Campylobacter* who sought medical treatment were initially treated with an antibiotic to which the bacteria was resistant, forcing the doctors to switch to more powerful drugs.[1368] Studies involving thousands of patients with *Campylobacter* infections showed that this kind of delay in effective treatment led to up to ten times more complications— infections of the brain, the heart, and, the most frequent serious complication they noted, death.[1369]

When the FDA announced that it was intending to join other countries and ban quinolone antibiotic use on U.S. poultry farms, the drug manufacturer Bayer threatened to sue. Despite successfully hamstringing the process for five years while continuing to corner the estimated $15 million a year market,[1370] Bayer eventually did back down and ended its game of chicken with America's health.[1371]

Meanwhile, poultry factories continue to spike the water and feed supply with other antibiotics critical to human medicine. Retail chicken samples from factories that used antibiotics are more than 450 times likelier to carry antibiotic-resistant bugs. Even companies like Tyson and Perdue, which supposedly stopped using antibiotics years ago, are still churning out antibiotic-resistant bacteria-infected chicken. Scientists think bacteria that became resistant years before are still hiding within the often dirt floors of the massive broiler sheds or within the water supply pipes. Another possibility is that the carcasses of the chickens raised under so-called "Antibiotic Free" conditions are contaminated with resistant bacteria from slaughterhouse equipment that can process more than two hundred thousand birds in a single hour.[1372]

Relying on the poultry industry to police itself may not be prudent. This is the same industry that pioneered the use of the synthetic growth hormone diethylstilbestrol (DES) to fatten birds—and producers' wallets—despite the fact that it was a known carcinogen. Although some women were prescribed DES during pregnancy—a drug advertised by manufacturers to produce "bigger and stronger babies"[1373]—the chief exposure for the American people to DES was through residues in meat. Even after it was proven that women who were exposed to DES gave birth to daughters who developed high rates of vaginal cancer, the meat industry was able to stonewall a ban on DES in chicken feed for years.[1374] According to a Stanford University health policy analyst, only after a study found DES residues in marketed poultry meat at 342,000 times the levels found to be carcinogenic did the FDA finally ban it as a growth promotant in poultry in 1979.[1375]

The industry defends its antibiotic-feeding practices. Before Bayer's antibiotic was banned, a National Chicken Council spokesperson told a reporter, "It improves the gut health of the bird and its conversion of feed, what we call the feed efficiency ratio . . . And if we are what we eat, we're healthier if they're healthier."[1376] Chickens in modern commercial production are profoundly *un*healthy. Due to growth-promoting drugs and selective breeding for rapid growth, many birds are crippled by painful leg and joint deformities.[1377] The industry journal *Feedstuffs* reported that "broilers now grow so rapidly that the heart and lungs are not developed well enough to support the remainder of the body, resulting in congestive heart failure and tremendous death losses."[1378]

The reality is that these birds exist under such grossly unsanitary conditions, cramped together in their own waste, that the industry may feel forced to lace their water supply with antibiotics. "Present production is concentrated in high-volume, crowded, stressful environments, made possible in part by the routine use of antibacterials in feed," the congressional Office of Technology Assessment wrote as far back as 1979. "Thus the current dependency on low-level use of antibacterials to increase or maintain production, while of immediate benefit, also could be the Achilles' heel of present production methods."[1379]

In 2005, the CDC released data showing that antibiotic-resistant *Salmonella* has led to serious complications.[1380] Foodborne *Salmonella* emerged in the Northeast in the late 1970s and has spread throughout North America. One theory holds that multidrug-resistant *Salmonella* was disseminated worldwide in the 1980s via contaminated feed made out of farmed fish fed routine antibiotics,[1381] a practice condemned by the CDC.[1382] Eggs are currently the primary vehicle for the spread of *Salmonella* bacteria to humans, causing an estimated 80 percent of outbreaks. The CDC is especially concerned about the rapid emergence of a strain resistant to nine separate antibiotics, including the primary one used in children.[1383] *Salmonella* kills hundreds of Americans every year, hospitalizes thousands,[1384] and sickens more than a million.[1385]

The director-general of the World Health Organization feared that this global rise in antibiotic-resistant "superbugs" is threatening to "send the world back to a pre-antibiotic age."[1386] As resistant bacteria sweep aside second- and third-line drugs, the CDC's antibiotic-resistance expert said that "we're skating just along the edge."[1387] The bacteria seem to be evolving resistance faster than our ability to create new antibiotics. "It takes us 17 years to develop an antibiotic," explained a CDC medical historian. "But a bacterium can develop resistance virtually in minutes. It's as if we're putting our best players on the field, but the bench is getting empty, while their side has an endless supply of new players."[1388] Remarked one microbiologist, "Never underestimate an adversary that has a 3.5 billion-year head start."[1389]

For critics of the poultry industry, the solution is simple. "It doesn't take rocket science," said the director of the Union of Concerned Scientists food division, "to create the healthy, non-stressful conditions that make it possible to avoid the use of antibiotics."[1390] The trade-off is between immediate economic benefit for the corporations and longer-term risks shared by us all, a theme that extends to the control of avian influenza.[1391]

In 2004, the Worldwatch Institute published an article, "Meat: Now, it's not personal!"[1392] They were alluding to intensive methods of production that have placed all of us at risk, regardless of what we eat. In the age of antibiotic resistance, a simple scrape can turn into a mortal wound and a simple surgical procedure can be anything but simple. But at least these "superbugs" are not effectively spread from person to person. Given the propensity of factory farms to churn out novel lethal pathogens, though, what if they produced a virus capable of a global pandemic?

The Last Great Plague

A National Academy of Sciences report investigating the rising tide of new diseases spoke of myriad factors creating the microbial equivalent of a "perfect storm." "However, unlike a major climactic event where various meteorologic forces converge to produce a tempest," they wrote, "this microbial perfect storm will not subside. There will be no calm after the epidemic; rather the forces combining to create the perfect storm will continue to collide and the storm itself will be a recurring event."[1393] And there is no storm like influenza.

The dozens of emerging zoonotic disease threats that have characterized this third era of human disease must be put into context. SARS infected thousands of human beings and killed hundreds. Nipah only infected hundreds and killed scores. *Strep. suis* infected scores and only killed dozens. Influenza infects billions and can kill millions.

Influenza, the "last great plague of man,"[1394] is the only known pathogen capable of truly global catastrophe.[1395] Unlike other devastating infections like malaria, which is confined equatorially, or HIV, which is only fluid-borne, influenza was considered by the CDC's Keiji Fukuda to be the only pathogen carrying the potential to "infect a huge percentage of the world's population inside the space of a year."[1396] Now we know coronaviruses may be capable of the same feat.

Because of its extreme mutation rate, influenza is a perpetually emerging disease. Dr. Fauci called it "the mother of all emerging infections."[1397] In its 4,500 years infecting humans since the first domestication of wild birds, influenza has always been one of the most contagious pathogens.[1398] Only since 1997 has it also emerged as one of the deadliest. If influenza is the "lion king" of all emerging infections,[1399] a virus like H5N1 is feared to become the king of kings. H5N1 seems to be a full order of magnitude more lethal than every known human influenza virus on record, completely off the charts. To reduce the risk of future escalating pandemics, we must trace its origin in greater detail to understand how a monster like H5N1 could be hatched.

TRACING THE FLIGHT PATH

Pandora's Pond

Prior to Graeme Laver and Robert Webster's landmark experimental work proving the avian origin of human influenza—Webster's self-described "barnyard theory"[1400]—any links between bird flu and human flu were scoffed at, Laver remembers, as "scornful remarks about 'Webster and his obsession with chicken influenza.'"[1401] No one is scoffing anymore. Analyzing the genome of H5N1, scientists now suspect that the 1997 outbreak arose when an H5 goose virus combined with an N1 duck virus with quail acting as the mixing vessel (another species "raised under battery conditions"[1402] like egg-laying hens). The virus then jumped from quail to chickens and then from chickens to humans.[1403]

In 2001, in what seems to be a separate emergence, that same H5 goose virus combined with an N1 duck virus in a duck, then jumped to chickens directly, bypassing the quail.[1404] In both cases, the H5 virus first isolated from a farmed domestic goose population in Guangdong province was found,[1405] surprisingly, to be already partially adapted to mammals.[1406] Scientists speculate that this could have been a result of the virus acclimating to a pig—especially, perhaps, given Asia's unique fish-farming technique.[1407]

Pig-hen-fish aquaculture involves perching battery cages of chickens directly over feeding troughs in pig pens, which in turn are positioned above fish ponds. The pigs eat the bird droppings and then defecate into the ponds. Depending on the species of fish, the pig excrement is then eaten directly by the fish[1408] or acts as fertilizer for aquatic plant fish food.[1409] The pond water can then be piped back up for pig and chicken drinking water.[1410] The efficiency of integrated aquaculture in terms of reduced feed and waste disposal costs is considered key to the economics of chicken farming in some areas in Asia,[1411] and, as such, led to increasing support from international aid agencies.[1412] "The result," wrote experts from the German Institute for Virology in the science journal *Nature,* "may well be creation of a considerable potential human health hazard."[1413]

In parts of Asia, human feces may also be added to the ponds for additional enrichment.[1414] For pathogens spread via a fecal-oral route, this aquaculture system is a dream come true. These fully integrated systems are blamed for the high incidence of an emerging strain[1415] of cholera in shrimp farmed in the Calcutta region of India.[1416] According to aquaculture experts, rampant disease on Asian aquaculture farms is considered the primary constraint to the industry's growth. Even back in 2005, they wrote that "the aquaculture industry has been overwhelmed with its share of diseases and problems caused by viruses, bacteria, fungi, parasites, and other undiagnosed and emerging pathogens."[1417] Concluded another review, "Although the recycling of excrements in integrated agriculture–aquaculture farming systems offers many advantages, the spread of diseases to man via aquatic organisms multiplying in excreta-laden water needs special attention."[1418] Much of that attention has focused on influenza.[1419]

"The ducks, the ducks, the ducks are the key to the whole damned thing," Webster once exclaimed to a *Newsday* reporter.[1420] Due to the growing industrialization and pollution of migratory aquatic flyways, wild ducks are landing in increasing numbers on these farmed fish ponds.[1421] The influenza virus found naturally and harmlessly in the ducks' intestines are excreted in the water. The chickens may drink the virus-laden water. The pigs then eat the virus-laden chicken feces. The ducks then drink the pond water contaminated by the virus-laden pig excrement, and the cycle can continue. The pond water ends up a "complete soup" of viruses, admitted the head of the Hong Kong environmental think tank Civic Exchange.[1422] Dead ducks or chickens may also be fed to pigs, providing another potential route of infection. This risky practice is not limited to Asia. In an H5N2 outbreak in the United States in the 1980s, pigs raised under chicken houses in Pennsylvania and fed dead birds came down with the infection as well.[1423]

Integrating pigs and aquaculture affords this waterborne duck virus a rather unique opportunity to cycle through a mammalian species, accumulating mutations that may better enable it to adapt to mammalian physiology. Migratory ducks could then theoretically fly the mutant virus thousands of miles to distribute it into other ponds, pigs, and ducks across the continent. Although there is concern that the virus could infiltrate the abdominal fluid or even the muscle meat of the farmed fish,[1424] the aquatic animals are largely thought to be innocent bystanders.[1425] Without the Trojan duck vectors, fish farming wouldn't pose a pandemic threat. Likewise, without the pigs, the fish farms would be no riskier than the thousands of Canadian lakes where ducks congregate and discharge virus into the water every summer. Any spoonful of lake water from this "veritable witches' brew of avian influenza," as Webster put it, may contain virus, but as long as it stays between ducks, as it has for millions of years up until domestication, it poses no pandemic threat.[1426]

The aquaculture industry disagrees that its practices are potentially hazardous.[1427] Fish farming advocates argue that integrated aquaculture is "uncommon."[1428] One aquaculture professor estimated that at most, only 20 percent of pigs in China may be involved in aquaculture production.[1429] However, 20 percent is tens of millions of pigs, plenty of fodder for viruses to potentially extract adaptive pearls from swine.[1430] An industry insider admitted that aquaculturists have too often adopted a "bury-your-head-in-the-sand" attitude when it comes to human disease threats.[1431] While fish farmers continue to downplay the risks, medical historians speculate that integrated aquaculture may have played a role in the increasing threat of pandemic influenza.[1432] "As these agricultural practices increase," wrote one commentator in the journal *Science,* "so does the likelihood that new potentially lethal influenza viruses will increase at the same time."[1433]

Hog Ties

Before the 1997 outbreak of H5N1 and the realization that the 1918 virus was also likely purely avian in origin, pigs, as I've mentioned, were thought to be the prime vessels in which human and avian influenza viruses could potentially mix and match their genes to create strains capable of infecting people. All influenza viruses use cellular sialic acid receptors to dock onto cells and infect them. The sialic acid receptors lining the intestines of ducks have what are called *alpha-2,3 linkages,* whereas human lungs have sialic acid receptors with *alpha-2,6 linkages.* Influenza strains tend only to bind effectively with one type of receptor or the other. This difference in receptor compatibility helps form a species barrier, keeping the bird strains in the birds and the human strains in the humans.[1434] How then, could a hybrid bird-human virus ever arise?

Researchers discovered that the respiratory tracts of pigs have both types of molecular linkages. Since pigs display both bird-type and human-type virus receptors, pigs could potentially be simultaneously infected with bird flu and human flu. With both viruses slobbering throughout the pigs' respiratory systems, the strains might re-assort to create a hybrid virus that could recognize human-type receptors but retain enough avian novelty to escape pre-existing human immunity. This could theoretically trigger mild pandemics as were seen in 1957 and 1968,[1435] thought to be mild because humans retained at least some immune memory to the human fraction of the hybrid virus.

There is building evidence that this scenario may be more than just speculation; pigs may indeed play some role in avian influenza's adaptation to people. During the 1918 pandemic, millions of pigs fell ill. Did they give it to us, or did we give it to them?[1436]

Our current understanding is that the 1918 pandemic was triggered when an H1N1 bird virus in its entirety—all eight gene segments—jumped into human beings with or without adaptation in an intermediate host.[1437] We then apparently passed it along to pigs, sickening millions of them as well. After the 1918 pandemic passed, a reassortment of the 1918 virus turned into the regular seasonal flu, and in pigs, a reassortment turned into what we call classic swine flu,[1438] one of the most common causes of respiratory disease on North American pig farms.[1439] Before 1918, there weren't reports of pigs ever getting the flu at all.[1440]

So, throughout the Roaring Twenties, every year, people got the regular flu and pigs got swine flu. Same with the Thirties and same with the Forties. In 1957, though, an H2N2 bird virus combined with the seasonal flu. It swapped in three genes, triggered the relatively mild 1957 pandemic, and then turned into a seasonal flu.[1441] Nothing happened to swine flu, though, which remained completely stable.

In 1968, an H3 bird virus combined with the seasonal flu. This time, it swapped in two genes and triggered the mild 1968 pandemic before turning into the seasonal flu we've had ever since.[1442] Still nothing happened with swine flu, which continued to remain stable and unchanging through the Seventies and the Eighties in North America. But then, by 1999, everything changed. A never-before-described triple species flu virus arose.[1443]

The classic swine flu virus, after being stable for eighty consecutive years, picked up three gene segments from the circulating human flu virus and two gene segments from a bird flu virus to create the first triple-animal reassortment virus ever described. Our first discovered human-pig hybrid viral mutant was uncovered in August 1998[1444] in Newton Grove, North Carolina, at an industrial pig production operation owned by a massive pork conglomerate called Hog Slat.[1445] Within months of the discovery, the triple hybrid virus had shown up in Texas, Minnesota, and Iowa.[1446] Within a year, it had spread across the United States.[1447] That was the virus that went on to seed our last pandemic in 2009.

The rapid dissemination of this virus across the country has been blamed on long-distance live animal transport.[1448] In the United States, livestock may travel an average of one thousand miles[1449] and pigs can travel from coast to coast. They can be bred in North Carolina, fattened in the corn belt of Iowa, and slaughtered in California.[1450] It's cheaper to bring the pigs to the corn than the corn to the pigs. While this may reduce short-term costs for the pork industry,[1451] the highly contagious nature of diseases like influenza (perhaps made further infectious by the stresses of transport,[1452] as I've discussed) needs to be considered when calculating the true cost of long-distance live animal transport. This factor alone confirms the link between industrial pork production and the last pandemic.[1453] How *else* could a virus get to Minnesota, Mexico,[1454] and Malaysia?[1455] The answer is *when pigs fly*. And indeed they now do fly, thanks to the market globalization.[1456] Maybe this little piggy should have stayed home.

After eight decades of stability, what led to the unprecedented emergence and spread of this unique, never-before-seen triple reassortment hybrid swine flu virus? Scientists postulate that a human flu virus may have started circulating in U.S. pig farms as early as 1995, but "through mutation or simply by obtaining a critical density, caused disease in pigs and began to spread rapidly through swine herds in North America."[1457] It is therefore likely no coincidence that the first hybrid virus emerged in North Carolina, the home of the nation's largest pig production operation. What's more, North Carolina has the densest pig population in North America and reportedly boasts more than twice as many corporate pig mega-factories as any other state.[1458]

The year of emergence, 1998, was the year North Carolina's pig population hit ten million, up from two million just six years earlier.[1459] Concurrently, the number of pig farms was decreasing, from 15,000 in 1986 to 3,600 in 2000. How can five times as many animals be raised on nearly five times fewer farms? By crowding about twenty-five times as many pigs into each operation. In the 1980s, more than 85 percent of all North Carolina pig farms had fewer than a hundred animals. By the end of the 1990s, operations confining more than a thousand animals controlled about 99 percent of the state's pig population.[1460]

In the influenza pandemic of 1918, a U.S. Army regiment whose barracks allowed only approximately 4.2 square meters (45 square feet) per soldier reportedly had a flu incidence more than ten times that of a regiment afforded about 7.25 square meters (78 square feet) per person.[1461] In pigs, respiratory diseases,[1462] such as chronic pleuritis and pneumonia, have reportedly been strongly correlated to increased crowding of pigs per pen[1463] and per building.[1464] Similar studies on influenza in commercial pig operations have come to the same conclusion: An increased density of pigs per pen, pigs per operation, and pigs per municipality all have been shown to be associated with increased risk of swine flu infection.[1465] Swine flu went from a seasonal infection to one raging year-round.[1466] A professor of Medical Microbiology at the University of Edinburgh concluded that "overcrowded farms are a hot-bed of genetic mixing for flu viruses."[1467]

Whether talking about pigs in a shed or sniffly kids in a preschool, the greater the number of contacts, the greater the risk of spread. A systematic review and meta-analysis of risk factors for swine flu infection of pig herds found the two most important factors were pig density and the sheer number of pigs on each farm.[1468] One study found that the likelihood of swine flu infection was twenty-five times higher for operations confining more than a thousand pigs,[1469] and each additional thousand pigs may quadruple the odds of infection.[1470] Researchers blame the increased risk in part on diminished air volume per animal, increasing the concentration of infectious particles and thereby facilitating aerosol spread.[1471] A study in Brazil found evidence of swine flu exposure in about a quarter of the pigs in confinement operations, but not a single case at any of the fifty-six open-air farms they sampled.[1472]

Starting in the early 1990s, the U.S. pig industry restructured itself after Tyson's profitable chicken model of massive industrial-sized units.[1473] As a headline in the trade journal *National Hog Farmer* announced, "Overcrowding Pigs Pays—If It's Managed Properly."[1474] The majority of U.S. pig farms now confine more than five thousand animals each.[1475] Imagine five thousand people crammed into an elevator—and someone sneezes. China reportedly possesses some of the largest industrial pig units in the world, confining as many as 250,000 pigs in a single, six-story, concrete building.[1476] A review on the role these immense numbers play in disease risk concluded that because of the greater "gross margin per pig sold," producers are "unlikely to reduce herd size voluntarily."[1477]

Europe has faced a similar situation.[1478] Virginia-based Smithfield, the largest pork producer in the world, raked in more than $10 billion in annual revenue and posted record profits in 2005, in part because of its expansion of factory-sized pig farms in Europe.[1479] The trend has raised a stink among both environmentalists[1480] and public health officials.[1481]

By 1993, a bird flu virus had adapted to pigs, grabbed a few human flu virus genes, and infected two young Dutch children, even displaying evidence of limited human-to-human transmission.[1482] Denmark happens to be the North Carolina of Europe. In 1970, the number of pig farms with more than five hundred animals was zero. Between 1980 and 1994, 70 percent of the pig farms went out of business at the same time the pig population climbed to more than ten million.[1483] This tiny country is one of the largest exporters of pork in the world.[1484] Past bans on Asian poultry because of bird flu and U.S. beef because of mad cow disease, according to the chairman of Denmark's Bacon and Meat Council, began to "favourably affect demand."[1485]

"Influenza [in pigs] is closely correlated with pig density," said a European Commission–funded researcher studying the situation in Europe.[1486] As such, Europe's rapidly intensifying pig industry has been described in *Science* as "a recipe for disaster."[1487] Some researchers have speculated that the next pandemic could arise out of "Europe's crowded pig barns."[1488] The European Commission's agricultural directorate warns that the "concentration of production is giving rise to an increasing risk of disease epidemics."[1489] Concern over epidemic disease is so great that Danish laws capped the number of pigs per farm and put a ceiling on the total number of pigs allowed to be raised in the country.[1490] No such limit exists in the United States.

Complicating the U.S. picture, the swine viruses appear to be crossing back to commercial poultry, as reported in the CDC journal *Emerging Infectious Diseases*. The investigators warned: "Repeated introductions of swine influenza viruses to turkeys, which may be co-infected with avian influenza viruses, provide opportunities for the emergence of novel reassortments with genes adapted for replication in pigs or even humans."[1491] Dr. Robert Webster, one of the world's leading experts on flu virus evolution, decried as "unsound" the "recently evolving intensive farming practice in the USA, of raising pigs and poultry in adjacent sheds with the same staff."[1492] North Carolina isn't only packed with pigs. It's also one of the nation's largest poultry producers, slaughtering nearly three-quarters of a *billion* chickens each year[1493] and confining enough hens to produce three billion eggs.[1494] Exhaust fans can then potentially blow infectious particles from one operation to the next.[1495]

Before a swine flu virus killed upward of a half-million people in 2009,[1496] there were only a handful of documented human deaths from swine flu.[1497] These included a young pregnant woman in the United States in 1988. On day 1, the woman visited a county fair in Wisconsin. On day 4, she started exhibiting signs of the flu. On day 11, she was hospitalized and intubated on a ventilator for respiratory failure. On day 14, labor was induced and she gave birth to a healthy baby. On day 18, she died. CDC laboratory analysis showed she was killed by a swine flu virus that she presumably contracted at the agriculture fair.[1498] H5N1 and the virus of 1918 help argue, however, that pigs may not be needed to produce killer viruses with pandemic potential.[1499]

It turns out that the human respiratory tract, like the pig respiratory tract, has bird flu-type receptors after all, eliminating the need for an inter-mediate porcine host.[1500] Human beings can be directly infected with bird flu. As I've discussed, once sufficiently adapted for efficient human-to-human transmission, a wholly avian virus could potentially infect billions since there may be no prior immunity in humans. In this way, H5N1 has been said to be following in the 1918 virus's footsteps,[1501] though, in actuality, the footprints, so to speak, have been weathered away.[1502] Instead of reassorting to form hy-brids in some sort of transitional species mixing vessel such as pigs, H5N1 has been directly attacking the human species, as the 1918 virus is presumed to have done, via an "adaptation of a smoldering avian progenitor."[1503] The head of the American Public Health Association conjectured, "This organism is following the historical [pandemic] playbook step by step."[1504]

That avian progenitor may have acquired some mammalian adaptive traits cycling through pigs on aquaculture farms or wallowing though flooded rice fields awash with domestic ducks,[1505] but there is still a vast gulf between a harmless waterborne intestinal duck virus—which is how all flu viruses start out—and a killer airborne respiratory human virus. The influenza virus has the mutation machinery to bridge that gap, but it needs a lot of test tubes.

Although pork is the most popular meat in the world,[1506] the bigger pig-geries may only contain tens of thousands of animals.[1507] The bigger egg farms, on the other hand, may confine more than a million.[1508] It may take six months for a piglet to reach slaughter weight, but much of the global broiler chicken population is hatched and killed in as few as six weeks, dra-matically multiplying the annual number of new viral hosts. More than forty-five billion chickens pass through the world every year, compared to only about one billion pigs. Spread wing to wing, the number of chickens killed every *day* would wrap more than twice around the world's equator.[1509] Never before has the influenza virus had such an opportunity. Did the first-ever triple-animal reassortment virus jump at the chance? The harbinger of the subsequent pandemic came not with feathers, but a curly tail.

Hog Wild: The 2009 H1N1 Swine Flu Pandemic

Blood samples taken from 4,382 pigs across twenty-three states found that 20.5 percent tested positive for exposure to the triple hybrid swine flu virus by early 1999, including 100 percent of herds tested in Illinois and Iowa, and

90 percent in Kansas and Oklahoma.[1510] It soon spread into Canada,[1511] and, by 2003, the majority of animals tested in industrial pig operations in Mexico also showed evidence of exposure to our triple hybrid strain.[1512] We then exported it to Asia,[1513] and then the favor was apparently returned. After reshuffling with classic swine flu, our made-in-the-USA triple reassortment virus picked up two gene segments from a Eurasian swine flu line to create the flu pandemic of 2009.[1514]

Indeed, the primary progenitor of the 2009 pandemic virus was the same triple hybrid mutant that had emerged and had been spreading throughout factory farms in the United States for more than a decade.[1515] Researchers tried reproducing the 2009 pandemic virus by co-inoculating nine pigs with the two precursor viruses. It didn't work, suggesting that locking in the right reassortment was a "rare event."[1516] But packing thousands of pigs snout-to-snout in close confinement allows for the large viral loads considered necessary for the emergence of rare flu mutants that can rapidly transfer from animal to animal.[1517] Similarly, the explosion in diversity of swine flu viruses over the last decade[1518] has been attributed to "increased intensive farming practices,"[1519] rather than anything special about the genetics of the triple hybrid mutant. As Johns Hopkins Bloomberg School of Public Health professor Ellen Silbergeld put it: "Instead of a virus only having one spin of the roulette wheel, it has thousands and thousands of spins, for no extra cost. It drives the evolution of new diseases."[1520]

The stress of overcrowded confinement may also weaken immune function and predispose pigs to infection.[1521] The operation in North Carolina where the first hybrid swine flu virus was found was a breeding facility in which thousands of sows were confined in gestation crates, barren metal cages about two feet wide. These highly intelligent, social animals are basically kept isolated and locked in a box—week after week, month after month, for nearly their entire lives. If someone did this to a dog, they could get thrown in jail. Not only can these pregnant pigs not turn around, but they can barely move at all.

The rise in stress hormone levels in crated sows is thought to be the result of interference with the expression of natural maternal behaviors, like nest building, and this frustration may result in impaired immunity.[1522] Breeding sows restricted to narrow stalls, as is common during gestation and farrowing in intensive production, produce lower levels of antibodies in response to an experimental challenge.[1523]

Measures as simple as providing straw bedding may decrease morbidity and mortality in sows, compared to those confined on concrete slatted floors, presumably by eliminating the immunosuppressive stress of lying on bare concrete their whole lives, which may also lead to an increased infection risk.[1524] This minimal act—providing straw—has been shown to decrease the risk of swine flu,[1525] yet the sows are often denied even that modicum of mercy, to their detriment and, potentially, ours as well.

If overcrowding pigs so intensively increases the risk of the emergence and spread of new viruses, why does the industry do it? Evidently, pork producers can maximize their profits by confining each pig to a six-square-foot space. This basically means cramming a two-hundred-pound animal into an area equivalent to about two feet by three feet. An article in *National Hog Farmer* acknowledged that overcrowding presents problems, including inadequate ventilation and increased health risks, but concluded that sometimes, "crowding pigs a little tighter will make you more money."[1526] Though it makes sense for the pork industry's bottom line, we are only beginning to understand the true costs of this approach—the externalized costs to society.

Robert F. Kennedy Jr. described North Carolina's hog farms in greater detail:

> *Stadium-size warehouses shoehorn 100,000 sows into claustrophobic cages that hold them in one position for a lifetime over metal-grate floors. Below, aluminum culverts collect and channel their putrefying waste into 10-acre, open-air pits three stories deep from which miasmal vapors choke surrounding communities and tens of millions of gallons of hog feces ooze into North Carolina's rivers.*[1527]

Swine flu isn't only found in up to 100 percent of air samples tested inside pig operations but also more than a mile away downwind.[1528] This same long-distance airborne spread[1529] was implicated in the H5N2 outbreak of avian influenza in the United States in 2015 that affected more than fifty million chickens and turkeys, costing the poultry industry billions of dollars.[1530] Huge tunnel ventilation fans can suck up aerosolized pathogens and spew large volumes of infectious particles out into the countryside, which helps illustrate how loosely a term like *biosecurity* could ever really be applied to industrial animal agriculture.[1531] In this way, factory farms, also known as

CAFOs (for *confined animal feeding operations*), can act as amplifiers of influenza,[1532] not only infecting workers[1533] but potentially spreading contagion to surrounding communities.[1534]

The virus can also spread via the millions of gallons of excrement expelled into open-air cesspits, of which I have quite vivid childhood memories, having grown up near the largest pig production facility west of the Mississippi. Swine flu viruses have been shown experimentally to multiply in a pig's digestive tract and be released in feces,[1535] and they can survive in this slurry of urine and excrement for weeks.[1536] Ammonia released from decomposing waste may also burn the pigs' respiratory tracts and predispose them to respiratory infection in the first place.[1537] The spread of this untreated waste on nearby land as fertilizer may then further introduce the virus out into the environment—and into other herds directly[1538]—or be carried miles away by infestations of flies.[1539] Pig factory employees can dip their boots in antiseptic footbaths all they want, but you can't keep a fly out of a hog CAFO.

LIPSTICK ON A PIG

In response to the H1N1 outbreak, the pork industry, instead of changing its practices, concentrated on changing the pandemic's name. "Considerable energy has been expended trying to keep people from calling the virus swine flu," read an editorial in the prestigious journal *Nature*. "This focus on commerce can lead to conflicts of interest as well as policy positions that border on denial." Now designated as (H1N1)pdm09,[1540] the CDC quite accurately originally called it swine-origin influenza H1N1,[1541] but "[t]hat's not helpful to pork producers," argued the U.S. Agriculture Secretary, "that's not helpful to people who eat pork . . . So we're discussing, is there a better to way to describe this that would not lead to inappropriate actions on people's part."

On the one hand, it's true that it doesn't matter what you eat. Once a pandemic flu virus has jumped from livestock, the risk shifts from eating to breathing. On the other hand, in some ways, protecting ourselves against pandemics is all about what we eat. Yes, we should

probably stop eating scaly anteaters, but it's easier to blame practices that may be culturally foreign, such as wet markets and bushmeat, than it is to look at our own plates in the mirror.[1542]

Even the term *swine-origin influenza* doesn't tell the whole story.
People have been raising pigs and chickens in their backyards for
thousands of years before the triple hybrid mutant emerged and
spread through U.S. pig CAFOs. *Factory farm flu* might be more accurate.

Put all these factors together and what you get is the perfect cauldron for
the emergence and spread of dangerous strains of the flu. What can we do
to prevent this chain of events from occurring in the first place? We need to
give these animals more breathing room. They're the ones who could use
some social distancing. To lower our risk of generating increasingly dangerous farmed animal flu viruses, the global meat and egg industries must reverse course away from greater intensification. But how? As suggested in the
Annals of the New York Academy of Sciences, by "replacing large industrial units
with smaller [farms] with lower stocking densities,"[1543] potentially resulting
in less stress, less disease susceptibility, less intense infectious contact, and
smaller infectious loads.

Before we had factory farms, we had family farms. There were fewer animals, less crowding of farms, and less crowding of animals, who were actually able to move around. The pigs could go outside, where influenza viruses
get dehydrated to death in the breeze and zapped by sunshine. Manure was
composted and actually fertilized the earth, rather than contaminating it and
attracting swarms of flies. We didn't feed the animals drugs, and, even if a
new virus did arise, where would it go? The pigs ended up in a local butcher
shop, not halfway around the world.

Influenza isn't the only public health threat created in the crucible
of factory farming. In 2005, China experienced the world's largest and
deadliest outbreak of the emerging pig pathogen *Strep. suis* that I discussed earlier, causing meningitis and deafness in people handling infected
pork products.[1544] The USDA blamed "[s]tress due to poor housing conditions [of the pigs], such as crowding and inadequate ventilation,"[1545] and the
World Health Organization similarly blamed "'intensive' conditions that can
cause stress and subsequent immune suppression."[1546] Pig factories in Ma-

laysia birthed the Nipah virus, one of the deadliest of human pathogens, a contagious respiratory disease causing relapsing brain infections and killing 40 percent of people infected.[1547] The pork industry in the United States feeds pigs millions of pounds of human antibiotics every year just to promote growth and prevent disease in such a stressful, unhygienic environment, and now there are multi-drug-resistant bacteria and we physicians are running out of effective antibiotic options. As the UK's chief medical officer once put it, "[E]very inappropriate or unnecessary use [of antibiotics] in animals or agriculture is potentially a death warrant for a future patient."[1548]

The public health community has been shouting from the rooftops for years about the risks posed by factory farms. In 2008, the Pew Commission on Industrial Farm Animal Production concluded that industrialized animal agriculture posed "unacceptable" public health risks: "Due to the large numbers of animals housed in close quarters in typical [industrial farm animal production] facilities there are many opportunities for animals to be infected by several strains of pathogens, leading to increased chance for a strain to emerge that can infect and spread in humans."[1549]

Specific to the veal crate–like metal stalls that confine breeding pigs like those on the North Carolina factory farm from which the first hybrid swine flu virus was discovered in North America, the Pew Commission asserted that "[p]ractices that restrict natural motion, such as sow gestation crates, induce high levels of stress in the animals and threaten their health, which in turn may threaten human health."[1550] Unfortunately, we don't tend to "shore up the levees" until after the disaster, but now that we know swine flu viruses can evolve to efficiently transmit human-to-human, we need to follow the advice of the American Public Health Association and declare a national moratorium on factory farms[1551] and, in the very least, take the Pew Commission's recommendations to follow Europe's lead and phase out extreme confinement practices like gestation crates across the country, as has already been accomplished in ten states despite Big Ag's best attempts at stonewalling.[1552,1553,1554,1555,1556,1557,1558,1559,1560,1561]

With massive concentrations of farm animals within whom to mutate, these new swine flu viruses in North America seem to be on an evolutionary fast track, jumping and reassorting between species at an unprecedented rate.[1562] This reassorting, Webster's team concludes, makes the sixty-five-million-strong U.S. pig population an "increasingly important reservoir of viruses with human pandemic potential."[1563] Pigs may then act as stepping-stones to better adapt avian flu viruses to human infection.[1564] Research shows that serially passing an engineered flu virus through pigs only nine times readily induced dramatic adaptive mutations, increasing its pandemic potential by making it both more virulent and transmissible.[1565] Such "dual use" research is controversial since bioterrorists could apply the same techniques.[1566] However, such "experiments" are inadvertently being performed in industrial pig farms the world over every day. As the former executive director of the Pew Commission on Industrial Farm Animal Production described, "Industrial farms are super-incubators for viruses."[1567]

Influenza experts had warned about this triple hybrid mutant for years, describing it as a "mammalian-adapted virus that is extremely promiscuous." Given the appearance of the triple hybrid mutant in North America, one virologist was quoted in *Science* as saying that now "we need to look in our own backyard for where the next pandemic may appear."[1568] Six years after those prophetic words were spoken, that virus seeded the first pandemic of the twenty-first century.

There had been sporadic human cases of swine flu infection going back decades,[1569] like the swine flu scare at Fort Dix in New Jersey in 1976.[1570] What changed in 2009 was the realization that flu viruses can jump straight from pigs to pandemic, infecting a sizable chunk of humanity, including more than a hundred million Americans.[1571] Thankfully it was only a Category 1 pandemic,[1572] resulting in "only" about a half million deaths.[1573] Next time, we might not be so lucky.

Viral Swap Meets

We saw what happens when swine flu acquired easy human-to-human transmission, but what about avian influenza? Just as the swine flu exploded in, through, and out of pig factory farms, would the bird flu follow course? To take advantage of this feathered bounty, the H5N1 virus would first have to find a way out from the guts of waterfowl. How did the Guangdong goose H5 ever find the duck N1 in quail? How did the goose-duck H5N1 hybrid find its way from quail to Hong Kong chickens? And how did the virus spread from farm to farm? Although some have proposed live poultry delivery trucks improperly cleaned between separate hauls of different bird species as the culprit, the likelier explanation may be cross-contamination at live bird markets.[1574]

Professor Kennedy Shortridge, the virologist who first characterized H5N1 in Asia, may have predicted its site of emergence years before its appearance. In 1992, he urged surveillance in "Hong Kong, as the place with the most extensive contact with China and a possible place of exit of an emerging pandemic virus."[1575] What is it about China that makes it such a hotbed of influenza virus activity? Shortridge blames the "great diversity of influenza viruses in the duck population in this region"—a function, in large part, of "the mass production of ducks for human consumption."[1576]

For centuries, Guangdong province has had the largest concentration of poultry, pigs, and people in the world.[1577] The "Asian flu" of 1957 and the "Hong Kong flu" of 1968 are just two examples of pandemics arising in the region. Historical records dating back centuries link emerging influenza epidemics and pandemics to this area of the world, although the first pandemic for which we have cogent data was the one that preceded 1918, in 1889.[1578]

Guangdong surrounds and feeds Hong Kong, one of the most heavily populated areas in the world: The city's seven million people[1579] are packed into densities exceeding fifty thousand people per square mile in some areas.[1580] A survey of nearly a thousand Hong Kong households[1581] found that 78 percent prefer "warm" meat.[1582] One hundred thousand chickens stream into Hong Kong every day from Guangdong[1583] to be sold alive in more than a thousand retail markets, stalls, and shops.[1584] As one influenza expert quipped, "Hong Kong is one big bird market."[1585]

This preference for just-killed poultry provides what Shortridge calls an "avian influenza virus melting pot."[1586] Chickens, ducks, geese, and quail are crammed into small plastic cages stacked as many as five high in these live animal "wet" markets. Distressed birds defecate on those below them.[1587] Feathers and feces are everywhere,[1588] as are blood and intestines.[1589] According to the World Health Organization, the birds are often slaughtered on the spot, "normally with very little regard for hygiene."[1590] "The activities of humans have affected the evolution of influenza," reads a Cambridge University Press textbook on pathogen evolution, "but not to our advantage. Close confinement of various strains of fowl in live poultry markets provide conditions ripe for the formation of new reassortment viruses and their transmission to humans."[1591] If live animal markets effectively turned a cold virus into a killer in the case of SARS and COVID-19, it may help turn a flu virus into a mass killer.

According to the Hong Kong survey, householders buy an estimated thirty-eight million live chickens every year, generating millions of human-chicken contacts.[1592] According to the University of Hong Kong School of Public Health, vendors and consumers are inevitably contaminated with fecal dust at these markets.[1593] Bird flu viruses may literally be floating around. Just as you can sample swine flu viruses right out of the air at live animal markets in Minnesota,[1594] bird flu viruses have been found circulating in the air at a live poultry market in China.[1595] Animals in a lab who are simply *exposed* to the airspace in which H5N1-infected birds are being slaughtered fall sick and die.[1596] Scientists were not surprised, then, that H5N1 surfaced first in Hong Kong.[1597]

Birds who remain unsold at the end of the day may go back to the farms of Guangdong, taking whatever new viruses they picked up with them.[1598] Webster and colleague Diane Hulse wrote, "Highly concentrated poultry and pig farming, in conjunction with traditional live animal or 'wet' markets, provide optimal conditions for increased mutation, reassortment and recombination of influenza viruses."[1599] Once the cycle has been sufficiently repeated, a virus can then use Hong Kong to escape. As the travel and commercial hub of Pacific Asia, Hong Kong represents a viral portal between the intensive farms of rural China and the human populations of the world.[1600]

In response to the emergence of H5N1, the government of Hong Kong tried separating different species and ordered that all duck and goose intestines must be packed when being sold in live chicken stalls to reduce cross-contamination. Over the long term, the UN Food and Agriculture Organization asked Hong Kong to move toward centralized slaughter facilities, a touchy subject with political as well as economic implications.[1601]

However, even if all Hong Kong live markets were closed, argued Webster, this would be unlikely to reduce the overall pandemic risk unless live markets could be closed throughout China and elsewhere.[1602] According to estimates from the China Wildlife Conservation Association, within Guangdong province itself, several thousands of tons of wild birds may be consumed in special stores each year and may mix with farmed birds before they are slaughtered for food.[1603] Bird markets outside of Hong Kong may be subject to even less regulation and are likely accompanied by less intensive surveillance for disease.[1604] China set the precedent, however, of attempting[1605] to ban all live bird markets in Shanghai, its largest city, as well as the capital city of Beijing.[1606] Hong Kong also finally decided to phase them out.[1607] "Until the traditional practice of selling poultry in the live market changes," concluded Webster's team, "we will have to accept that live markets are breeding grounds for influenza viruses."[1608]

These breeding grounds are not limited to Asia.[1609] We must not forget that before H5N1, the biggest outbreak of bird flu in history wasn't in China—it was in Pennsylvania. In the 1980s, the United States suffered the most costly and extensive disease eradication it ever had, the outbreak of H5N2 that led to the deaths of seventeen million chickens at a cost to taxpayers and consumers exceeding $400 million.[1610] The outbreak may have been linked to live bird markets in the northeastern United States.[1611] Before then, highly pathogenic bird flu had struck in the 1920s and later occurred in Texas in 2004. Both of these other high-grade bird flu incidents,[1612,1613] as well as most of the latest U.S. discoveries of low-grade viruses, have also been tentatively linked to U.S. live poultry markets.[1614]

According to estimates from the USDA, more than twenty million birds of different species may pass through 150 known storefront live bird markets in northeast metropolitan areas every year.[1615] Unlike Hong Kong, which learned its lesson and now segregates waterfowl from terrestrial species, U.S. ducks and chickens are still crammed on top of one another.[1616] As in Hong Kong markets, cages are generally stacked four to five tiers high, ensuring plenty of fecal splatter from distressed birds.[1617] "If you have seen these markets, you know that the birds are under stressful conditions," said a veterinarian with New York's Department of Agriculture. "And birds under stress are much more prone to disease."[1618]

Though suspected to play a pivotal role in the spread of bird flu in the United States,[1619] the problem seems to be worsening. In New York City, for example, the number of live bird markets almost doubled from forty-four in 1994 to more than eighty in 2002.[1620] Given the risk, many in the U.S. commercial poultry industry are "absolutely determined" to have live markets eliminated, according to a Louisiana State University poultry scientist.[1621] Briefly but incisively, the president of the USA Poultry and Egg Export Council commented, "We can't jeopardize the entire U.S. [poultry] industry."[1622]

The USDA agrees that live bird markets have been shown to present a "major risk" to the nation's poultry industry.[1623] USDA scientists wrote, "The live bird markets of the Northeast remain the biggest concern for the presence of avian influenza in the United States."[1624] If both the industry and the USDA agree (as they tend to do), why have live bird markets persisted and indeed been allowed to flourish? Some industry officials fear that closing bird markets would drive the entire trade underground, making it even more difficult to regulate.[1625] After SARS, for example, customer demand in Asia drove up the cost of civet cats to $200, making it likely that such animals could be obtained regardless of legality.[1626] The USDA has therefore chosen to "manage or mitigate the risk rather than to outlaw it."[1627]

By its own admission, the USDA is doing a poor job of risk management. Speaking at the Fifth International Symposium on Avian Influenza in 2002, USDA poultry researchers said, "Considerable efforts are continuing on the part of industry and state and federal governments to control influenza in the LBM [live bird market] system, but currently the efforts have been unsuccessful."[1628] "Despite educational efforts, surveillance, and increased state regulatory efforts," the USDA admitted the following year that "the number of [bird flu] positive markets has persisted and increased."[1629] Live bird markets seem inherently risky. In response to virus isolations from New Jersey's markets, the State Veterinarian said, "They can be doing everything right and still have a market that tests positive."[1630]

Even if a segment of the live bird trade were forced underground, it might not get much worse. Record-keeping in live poultry markets is already sparse or nonexistent even as to the birds' country of origin.[1631] Currently, the purchase and sale of live birds is a cash business in which market owners are "disinclined to keep accurate records that would be costly if subjected to IRS scrutiny."[1632] One survey of handling practices at live bird markets found that fewer than 2 percent of suppliers followed the recommended biosecurity practices to prevent the spread of the disease, for example.[1633] USDA Science Hall of Famer[1634] Charles Beard expressed concern that U.S. live bird markets could be the portal by which H5N1 enters commercial poultry flocks in the United States.[1635]

Live bird markets continue to exist in the United States only because local health authorities continue to license them. They are exempt from federal meat inspection laws because they slaughter fewer than twenty thousand birds a year,[1636] an exemption that doesn't apply for other animals.[1637] Poultry specialists predict that if live bird markets had to be held to the same federal standards of inspection, cleanliness, and pathogen control as the commercial poultry industry or small producers of other animals, "authorities could virtually eliminate LBMs."[1638]

The University of Hong Kong School of Public Health laid out the pros and cons: "The trade-off between the preference for eating the flesh of freshly slaughtered chicken and the risk to local, regional, and global population health from avian influenza should be addressed directly, and in terms of a precautionary public health approach aimed at providing the greatest benefit to the maximum possible number of people."[1639]

Avian influenza authority Robert Webster concluded a landmark article on the emergence of pandemic strains of influenza with these words: "An immediate practical approach is to close all live poultry markets." He went on to note that with refrigeration systems widely available—even through much of the developing world—it is no longer necessary to sell live birds. "The reality is that traditions change very slowly," he said, but "a new pandemic could accelerate this process."[1640]

Gambling with Our Lives?

The explosion of H5N1 in early 2004, which led to the deaths of more than a hundred million chickens across eight countries in Southeast Asia, was traced to the trade in live birds.[1641] The timing and pattern were inconsistent with known migratory bird routes.[1642] The disease's initial spread seems to have been via the railways[1643] and highways, not the flyways.[1644]

The riskiest segment of trade may be in fighting cocks, transported within and beyond their own country's borders to be unwilling participants in the high-stakes gambling blood "sport."[1645] In cockfighting pits, roosters are set upon one another, often pumped full of steroids and stimulants, with sharpened razors strapped to their legs. The sprays of bloody droplets help ensure that any virus present travels back home across borders after the fights in newly infected birds—or people. A number of cockfighting enthusiasts and the children of cockfighters[1646] have died from H5N1.[1647]

The Thai Department of Disease Control described a case of a young man who had "very close contact to . . . fighting cocks by carrying and helping to clear up the mucus secretion from the throat of the cock during the fighting game by using his mouth." As one leading epidemiologist at the CDC commented dryly, "That was a risk factor for avian flu we hadn't really considered before."[1648]

The movement of gaming cocks was directly implicated in the rapid spread of H5N1. Malaysian government officials blamed cockfighters as the main "culprits" for bringing the disease into their country by taking birds to cockfighting competitions in Thailand and bringing them back infected.[1649] Thailand, with an estimated fifteen million fighting cocks,[1650] was eventually forced to pass a nationwide interim ban on cockfighting.[1651] The director of Animal Movement Control and Quarantine within the Thai Department of Livestock Development explained what led to the ban: "When one province that banned cockfights didn't have a second wave outbreak of bird flu and an adjacent province did, it reinforced the belief that the cocks spread disease."[1652] A study of Thailand published in 2006 concluded, "We found significant associations at the national level between HPAI [H5N1] and the overall number of cocks used in cock fights."[1653]

According to the FAO, cockfighting may have also played a role in making the disease so difficult to control.[1654] During mass culls in Thailand, bird owners receive around 50 baht, about $1.25, in compensation for each chicken killed—less than the bird's market value for meat.[1655] Some prized fighting cocks fetch $1,000, providing a disincentive for owners to report sick birds.[1656]

Fighting cocks were reportedly hidden from authorities and illegally smuggled across provincial lines and country borders. This not only complicated the attempt at eradicating H5N1, but potentially facilitated its spread,[1657] causing some officials to throw up their hands. "Controlling the epidemic in the capital is now beyond the ministry's competence," Thailand's Deputy Agriculture Minister told the *Bangkok Post,* "due to strong opposition from owners of fighting cocks, who keep hiding their birds away from livestock officials."[1658] The *Los Angeles Times* likened asking Thais to give up cockfighting to "asking Americans to abandon baseball."[1659]

A different poultry virus, the cause of exotic Newcastle disease, did hit a home run in California, thanks to U.S. cockfighters. Cockfighting is illegal in all fifty states in the United States, carrying felony charges in most of them.[1660] Cockfighting rings have found relative refuge, however, in some states like California that retained only misdemeanor penalties.[1661] In 2002, an outbreak of Newcastle disease in California caused the destruction of nearly four million chickens at a cost to taxpayers of upward of $200 million[1662] and led to a multinational boycott of U.S. poultry products.[1663]

Fighting roosters smuggled in from Mexico were blamed for its emergence,[1664] and, according to the State Veterinarian and the director of Animal Health and Food Services in California at the time, the high mobility of the gamecocks—meetings, training, breeding, and fighting activities—played a major role in the spread of the disease.[1665] Although agriculture inspectors could not pinpoint the exact route by which the disease then jumped to Las Vegas and into Arizona, law enforcement had an idea. "We'll raid a fight in Merced County and find people from Nevada, New Mexico, Mexico, Arizona, and Southern California," said a detective with the Merced County Sheriff's office. "They bring birds to fight and take the survivors home."[1666]

Cockfighting also played a role in the previous exotic Newcastle disease outbreak in California, which led to the deaths of twelve million chickens.[1667] Although Newcastle can be fatal to nearly all species of birds, it does not represent a significant health risk to humans.[1668] "Fighting cocks were responsible for the spread of Newcastle disease in USA," warned a company veterinarian of the world's leading poultry breeding corporation,[1669] "but equally the virus could have been Avian Influenza."[1670] An article in *The Gamecock* openly encourages U.S. breeders of fighting cocks to hide birds from health inspection authorities should bird flu arrive in the States.[1671]

"Don't be surprised," said U.S. Representative and senior member of the Permanent Select Committee on Intelligence Elton Gallegly, "if the deadly avian flu enters the United States in the blood of a rooster smuggled into the country for the barbaric sport of cockfighting."[1672] During the course of containment following the 2002 outbreak, agriculture officials were staggered by the number of illegal cockfighting operations they stumbled upon—up to fifty thousand gamecock operations in southern California alone, according to some estimates.[1673] Despite being illegal for more than a century[1674] and despite hundreds of arrests,[1675] state law enforcement officials have said that cockfighting continues to grow in popularity.[1676]

According to the cockfighters' trade association, the American Animal Husbandry Coalition, there are thousands of operations that raise fighting cocks across the country.[1677] In states where raising birds for blood sports is illegal, breeders claim the cocks are being raised as pets[1678] or for show.[1679] With American roosters participating in competitions in Asia,[1680] it's clear that birds are being shipped illegally around the world.[1681] All it may take is one contraband avian Typhoid Mary smuggled out of Asia and into some clandestine U.S. cockfight to potentially spread bird flu throughout the United States. Strengthening penalties and improving enforcement on interstate transport of fighting cocks in America may help protect the health of America's flocks and America's people.[1682]

The National Chicken Council, the trade association for the U.S. commercial poultry industry, agrees. The NCC damns cockfighting as not only "inhumane," but as posing a "serious and constant threat of disease transmission to the commercial industry."[1683] A spokesperson for the United Gamefowl Breeders Association cries foul at the notion that cockfighting is inhumane, arguing that birds don't feel pain.[1684]

When the president of the National Chicken Council wrote to the chair of the House Agriculture Committee saying, "We are concerned that the nationwide traffic in game birds creates a continuing hazard for the dissemination of animal diseases," the president of the United Gamefowl Breeders Association responded, "You blatantly attack our industry . . . [but] it is the commercial poultry industry that has threatened the livelihood of other birds by transporting poultry that can release airborne pathogens (e.g. feathers being released) through the open-side transportation methods used on U.S. highways."[1685] He's got a point.

The Food and Agriculture Organization of the United Nations blames the transport of live birds raised for human consumption as a primary culprit in the rapid spread of avian influenza throughout Asia.[1686] Poultry destined for southern China's live animal markets can be transported thousands of miles.[1687] One senior Thai public health officer told a *New Yorker* reporter, "Chickens used to live in our backyards. They didn't travel much. Now, throughout the world, farms have become factories. Millions of chickens are shipped huge distances every day. We can't stop every chicken or duck or pig. And they offer millions of opportunities for pathogens to find a niche."[1688]

Trucking live poultry has also been implicated in the spread of the disease in Europe.[1689] An FAO consultancy report on the genesis and spread of H5N1 concluded that a "longer term prevention measure would be to reduce local and international supply-demand discrepancies such as to reduce the local and long-distance trade."[1690] In the United States, live birds are even shipped in boxes via the U.S. Postal Service.[1691]

In 2005, the North Carolina Department of Agriculture Food and Drug Safety administrator told a gathering of federal and state officials that current U.S. Postal Service regulations "are inadequate and present great potential for contamination of the poultry industry."[1692] He estimated that thousands of fighting cocks and other birds lacking health certificates enter North Carolina each year, potentially placing the state's massive[1693] poultry industry at risk.[1694]

"Chickens find transport a fearful, stressful, injurious and even fatal procedure," one group of researchers concluded.[1695] This high level of stress has been shown to make birds—whether raised for fighting, food, or any other use—more susceptible to spreading disease.[1696] And the legal and illegal international trade in fighting cocks makes the blood sport no safe bet—in fact, the stakes may be higher than anyone imagined.

Stopping Traffic

Fighting cocks are not the only birds smuggled internationally. Wild birds are sold by the millions as part of the global pet trade. Before H5N1, a single market in Indonesia sold up to 1.5 million wild birds every year.[1697] With the development of electronic payment methods over the internet, the international trafficking of wild animals has surged.[1698] The U.S. Fish and Wildlife Service has estimated that Americans have imported more than 350,000 birds a year.[1699] Although imports of all birds from countries with documented H5N1 poultry outbreaks have been banned jointly by the CDC and the USDA,[1700] the combination of a thriving black market,[1701] lax laws in Southeast Asia,[1702] and the rapid spread of the disease to new countries[1703] threatens to turn the legal U.S. trade in pet birds into a cover for the laundering of smuggled Asian birds into the United States.

"It's big business," said a spokesperson for the U.S. Fish and Wildlife Service about the illegal smuggling of exotic birds, ranking it just behind drug smuggling as border control's chief law enforcement concern.[1704] According to U.S. State Department estimates, the illegal exotic animal trade may be a $10 billion industry.[1705] Many birds are illicitly imported from Asian countries battling bird flu.[1706] "We are genuinely concerned," said an administrator of USDA's animal health inspection service about the risk of smuggled birds bringing H5N1 to U.S. shores.[1707]

The risk is not theoretical. In late 2004, a man from Thailand was stopped for a routine random drug check in a Belgian airport. Authorities found a pair of rare crested hawk eagles stuffed into plastic tubes in his luggage.[1708] Both of the birds were found to be harboring H5N1.[1709] The report of the incident in the CDC's Emerging Infectious Diseases journal concluded: "[I]nternational air travel and smuggling represent major threats for introducing and disseminating H5N1 virus worldwide."[1710] "We were very, very lucky," said the chief influenza expert at Belgium's Scientific Institute of Public Health. "It could have been a bomb for Europe."[1711]

The West Nile Virus may actually have been brought to the Western Hemisphere by bird smuggling.[1712] West Nile hit New York in 1999 and has since spread across forty-eight states and Canada,[1713] infecting an estimated seven million Americans.[1714] Its continued expansion suggests that the virus has become permanently established in the United States, all, perhaps, because of a single illegally imported pet bird.[1715]

The FAO describes even the legal trade in wild birds as a "serious potential opportunity for new [bird flu] disease transmission."[1716] Wild birds come from jungles around the world, trapped by nets or glue smeared on branches. Traumatized by long hours confined in trucks and planes, as many as 75 percent may die between capture and sale. Those who do live through the ordeal do so with compromised immune systems crammed into cages with multiple species in holding centers.[1717] One former CDC lab director stated:

> People who have seen the animal holding facilities at London-Heathrow,
> New York-Kennedy, and Amsterdam-Schiphol [airports] describe ware-
> houses in which every type of bird and other exotic animals are kept cheek
> by jowl in conditions resembling those in Guangdong food markets, awaiting
> trans-shipment. There, poultry can come into close contact with wild-caught
> birds.[1718]

The USDA coordinated with U.S. Customs and Border Control to increase vigilance for any movement of cargo or passengers coming from countries where there has been avian influenza H5N1.[1719] Vigilance directed at imports from specific countries may provide a false sense of security, however, as traders have been successful in the past in concealing countries of origin by laundering the birds for export through unaffected countries. The case of the British parrot is a perfect example.

In October 2005, the British government announced that H5N1 had been discovered in a parrot imported from South America. What is a South American bird doing with H5N1? The working hypothesis is that the bird contracted the virus while housed in a quarantine facility with birds from Taiwan who were also found to be infected.[1720] But Taiwan, like South America, is supposedly free of bird flu. What happened? That same month, a freighter was caught trying to smuggle more than a thousand birds, some of whom were infected with H5N1, from China into Taiwan.[1721] Perhaps infected birds were smuggled from China into Taiwan for global export, infecting the Taiwanese birds, who were then legally imported to the UK to mix with and infect the South American parrot.[1722] The same thing could have happened in the United States, which imports as many as fifty thousand birds from Taiwan annually.[1723]

The president of the U.S. National Chicken Council claimed that the American ban on imports from affected countries effectively "locked, bolted and barred the door against anything that could conceivably be carrying the virus."[1724] Allowing the import of birds from *any* country, though, risks the introduction of birds smuggled into that country from a third, contaminated country. Similarly, waiting until H5N1 had been detected in a country to ban its imports may pose unnecessary risks. A complete ban on importation of birds for the pet trade, regardless of the supposed country of origin, would address this problem. This is the precautionary approach Europe took, passing an immediate interim ban on captive birds from all countries.[1725] Such a measure would not be without precedent in the United States.

After the 2003 Midwest monkeypox outbreak, the CDC and the FDA issued a joint emergency executive order prohibiting the importation of all African rodents into the United States.[1726] This action was taken less than a month after the first confirmed case.[1727] Given the much greater threat bird flu represents, suggestions to broaden the bird importation ban seem reasonable. Both the National Association of State Public Health Veterinarians and the Council of State and Territorial Epidemiologists have called for the federal ban to be expanded to outlaw the import and transport of *all* exotic wildlife to protect both human and animal health in America.[1728]

U.S. law requires that all birds imported from overseas undergo a thirty-day quarantine,[1729] a measure shown successful in catching a bird flu virus in Peking robins imported from China years ago.[1730] Birds smuggled illegally into the United States, however, bypass this firewall. The legal trade in pet birds provides a cover for the illicit trade by providing market opportunities for smugglers to sell their birds. In addition to banning the importation of captive birds, closing down poorly regulated markets where birds are sold—flea market–like bird swaps and fairs—may further reduce the risk.[1731] Asked about the possibility of smuggled birds transporting H5N1 into America, the USDA's chief influenza scientist warned, "We should be more worried than we are."[1732]

More than two hundred non-governmental organizations representing millions of members joined to urge a permanent ban on the importation of wild birds into the European Union.[1733] The United States has yet to enact even a precautionary temporary ban. The pet bird industry claims that such a ban would have the opposite of the desired effect by driving trade underground and thereby increasing public health risk.[1734] Not true, according to an agriculture minister who testified before Parliament that the current EU ban on bird imports is having the desired effect and there is no evidence to suggest an increase in smuggling.[1735] Historical evidence shows the same.[1736]

In 1992, the U.S. Wild Bird Conservation Act was passed to ban the importation of certain wild-caught birds in an attempt to save endangered species of birds from extinction. The pet industry made the same claims back then that illegal trade would increase, but the law worked as intended.[1737] Scientists studying bird populations collectively reported that poaching of birds dropped significantly after passage of the law, and U.S. Customs testified that the number of birds smuggled over the border had dropped as well.

Following the U.S. monkeypox outbreak, the infectious diseases edition of *Lancet* carried an editorial titled, "Trade in Animals: A Disaster Ignored," which stressed the links between the trade in wild animals and disease. The editorial concluded:

> *The practice of taking animals from the wild for the pet trade also should swiftly be brought to an end. There will be fierce opposition to any such moves, and some of the trade will move underground, but if we can abolish such entrenched cultural traditions as burning at the stake and slavery, we can abolish the clear danger to human health of the wildlife trade.[1738]*

Global restrictions on the cockfighting and wild bird trades may play important roles in slowing the proliferation of H5N1 and other viruses. But since H5N1 has already infected migratory bird species, it may not need our help to spread.[1739] The overlap of Asian and North American migratory bird paths in Alaska provide a flight risk for the virus to enter the western hemisphere as well—outside of any cargo hold.[1740] With the possibility of viruses with pandemic potential literally coming out of the blue, closing gaping slats in our picket-fence trade firewall may be merely stopgap measures. It wouldn't matter how many species a bird flu virus infected in global live animal markets, or how widely the virus traveled by plane, truck, or duck, as long as it remained harmless as it had for millions of years.[1741] What turned bird flu into a killer in the first place?

ONE FLU OVER THE CHICKEN'S NEST

Acute Life Strategy

Understanding the ecology of the virus in its so-called benign reservoir is imperative if we hope to develop strategies to prevent future catastrophic outbreaks.[1742] As I've discussed, the primordial source of all influenza viruses—avian and mammalian—is aquatic birds.[1743]

All bird flu viruses seem to start out harmless to both birds and people. In its natural state, the influenza virus has existed for millions of years as an innocuous, intestinal, waterborne infection of aquatic birds such as ducks.[1744] Some have blamed free-ranging flocks and wild birds for the emergence of H5N1, for example, but people have kept chickens in their backyards for thousands of years, and birds have been migrating for millions. What happened in recent years to trigger the unprecedented evolution-in-fast-forward changes we're now seeing with the virus?

The influenza gene pool is really more of a gene pond. Every year, untold numbers of wild ducks congregate on the world's lakes to mate, raise families, and spread the influenza virus to each other. The virus silently multiplies in the ducks' intestinal lining and is then excreted into the pond water to lie in wait for other ducks to touch down for a drink. The ducks gobble down the virus, and the cycle continues. The duck doesn't get sick because the virus doesn't need to make the duck sick to spread. In fact, it may be in the virus's best interest for the duck *not* to get sick so as to spread farther. Dead ducks don't fly. This had been going on for perhaps a hundred million years before the first person came down with the flu.[1745]

Most ducks are infected as ducklings. Studies of ducks on Canadian lakes show that up to 30 percent of juvenile birds are actively shedding the virus.[1746] The ducks excrete such massive titers of virus[1747] that researchers have been able to culture it straight out of a spoonful of lake water.[1748] Under the right conditions, the virus is estimated to be able to persist for years in cold water.[1749] With such high concentrations of virus, with such highly efficient transmission,[1750] and with such environmental stability, scientists estimate that virtually all of the millions of ducks in the world become infected sometime within their lives.[1751]

The ducks aren't infected for long, though.[1752] Most only shed virus for a few days, but the fecal-oral route of infection for aquatic birds is so efficient that this is thought to be enough to keep the virus spreading throughout the millennia.[1753] Millions of years of evolution have so tailored the parasite to its host, a so-called optimally adapted system, that the virus seems completely innocuous to the ducks.[1754] The virus exists in an "evolutionary stasis" in waterfowl,[1755] remaining unchanged despite its furious mutation rate.[1756]

Influenza viruses don't tend to retain any new mutations in ducks because they found their perfect niche. Sharks, for example, have remained basically unchanged for a hundred million years, even while other species evolved around them. Why? Presumably because sharks had already evolved to be such perfected killing machines.[1757] Similarly, evolution doesn't seem to be able to much improve influenza. The virus continues to churn out millions of mutants in wild ducks in an attempt to spread faster and farther, but since the virus-duck relationship seems so flawlessly fine-tuned, any deviant viral progeny are less successful and die out. The virus has achieved peak efficiency and is found ubiquitously throughout aquatic bird species around the world.[1758]

Because the influenza virus in its natural state is so finely attuned to its aquatic host, it not only doesn't harm the carrier duck, but it also seems unable to cause serious disease in people. There are only two reports of human infection from wild bird viruses in the medical literature. One case involved a woman who kept ducks and got a piece of straw caught in her eye while cleaning out her duck house,[1759] and the second was a laboratory field worker whose eye was sneezed into by a bird-infected seal.[1760] Despite direct inoculations of virus, the worst the influenza seemed able to do was cause a mild self-limited case of conjunctivitis, commonly known as pinkeye.[1761] Duck flu viruses don't seem to grow well in humans (or other primates), and human flu viruses don't seem to grow well in ducks.[1762]

Scientists have even attempted to directly infect human volunteers with waterfowl viruses, but to little avail. Test subjects snorted massive doses of virus—enough to infect up to a billion birds—yet most of the time the virus wouldn't take hold at all. And, when it did have an effect, it typically produced nothing more than a transitory local reaction.[1763] It's because the evolutionary gulf between duck gut and human lung is so broad that an intermediate host is thought to be needed to act as a stepping-stone for the virus.[1764] "And poultry," said a spokesperson for the Department of Homeland Security's National Center for Foreign Animal and Zoonotic Disease Defense, "are likely to be that host."[1765]

Bird flu viruses only "heat up," in the words of Dutch virologist Albert Osterhaus, "when they pass from wild birds to poultry."[1766] Drs. E. Fuller Torrey, director of the Stanley Medical Research Institute, and Robert H. Yolken, a neurovirologist at Johns Hopkins University School of Medicine, concluded in their book *Beasts of the Earth: Animals, Humans, and Disease,* "If ducks had not been domesticated, we might not even be aware of the existence of influenza."[1767]

Although for a brief period of the year remote Canadian lakes can swarm with virus,[1768] a greater danger for humans may lie in the raising of domesticated ducks year-round on southern China rice paddies, leading to what Shortridge calls a "virus soup" of stagnant water and duck feces.[1769] According to Iowa State University's Center for Food Security and Public Health, "Humans have altered the natural ecosystems of birds through captivity, domestication, industrial agriculture, and nontraditional raising practices. This has created new niches for AI [avian influenza] viruses."[1770] The combination of what may be the greatest concentration of virus in the world with densely domesticated poultry and pigs to act as stepping-stones may have been what enabled influenza to take on the human species.[1771]

For a virus so perfectly adapted to the gut of wild waterfowl, the human lung is a long way from home. What is influenza, an intestinal waterborne duck virus, doing in a human cough? Imagine an infected duck transported to a live poultry market. The duck is crammed into a cage stacked high enough to splatter virus-laden droppings everywhere. Even if the vendor or customer were hit directly by the infected feces, humans might be too alien for the unmutated duck virus to take hold. But what if the virus reached land-based birds like quail or chickens? Terrestrial birds are not natural hosts for influenza,[1772] but they are recognizable enough by the virus to infect them. The virus then faces a problem, and the solution may be hazardous to human health.

All viruses must spread or perish. Like a fish out of water, when the influenza virus finds itself in the gut of a chicken, it no longer has the luxury of easy aquatic spread. It can no longer remain a strictly waterborne virus. Although the virus can still spread through feces when chickens peck at each other's droppings, in the open air, it must, for example, resist dehydration better.[1773] It also presumably must adapt to the novel body temperature and pH of its new environment.[1774]

In aquatic birds, the virus is and has been in total evolutionary stasis.[1775] But, when thrown into a new environment, it quickly starts accumulating mutations to try to adapt to the new host.[1776] The virus must mutate or die.[1777] Thankfully for the virus, mutating is what influenza does best.[1778] And, given enough time and enough hosts within which to mutate, some bird flu viruses can learn how to invade other organs in search of a new mode of travel. Sometimes, it finds the lungs.

In ducks, the virus keeps itself in check. The virus relies on a healthy host to fly it from lake to lake. To protect its natural host, the virus seemed to evolve a built-in, fail-safe mechanism that allows it to replicate only in the intestine, so as not to infect other tissues and potentially hurt the duck. To prevent itself from replicating outside the digestive tract, millions of years of evolution seem to have engendered an activation step.

Before the virus can become infectious, its hemagglutinin spike first has to be cleaved in half to activate it. This cleavage is done by specific host enzymes found only in certain tissues, like the intestinal tract. In its natural state, the influenza virus essentially gets permission from the host before tissue infection. The limited bodily distribution of the specific cleavage enzyme restricts the virus to safe areas like the gut. It would not be able to replicate in the brain or other vital organs that lack the specific cleavage enzyme required for activation. This is a restriction the virus has seemingly imposed upon itself, evolving harmlessness to best pass on and spread its genes.[1779] But once it finds itself in unfamiliar species, all bets are off. Researchers have shown that H5N1 seemed to enter chicken populations as an intestinal virus but left as more of a respiratory virus.[1780] Avian influenza goes into chickens as an aquatic virus, but may come out as airborne flu.

Landing in foreign territory, it's advantageous for the virus to find new ways to spread, but even more than that, it faces a hostile immune response and finds itself fighting for its life. It's either you or me, it "reasons," so in certain cases, the virus is able to eliminate the fail-safe mechanism that restricts it to the gut. The hemagglutinin spike of H5 and H7 viruses can mutate over time to be activated by enzymes in *any* organ in the body, allowing the virus to go on a rampage and essentially liquefy the bird from the inside—the "flubola" phenomenon of highly pathogenic avian influenza.[1781]

Of course, viruses don't reason. This is an example of high-speed natural selection. Even in ducks, influenza viruses exist as a swarm of mutants, each subtly different from the others. Since time immemorial, though, the same perfected, harmless mutant has won out over all the others time and time again. Deadly mutants find themselves grounded by the shore in a dying bird never to propagate to other locales. Harmful viruses are dead ducks.

Like other parasites, viruses tend to evolve toward a common agenda over time. Only when backed into a corner in new hostile territory might it be beneficial for the parasite to kill its host. The virus can be forced into what evolutionary biologists call an "acute life strategy" in which its only choice may be to rapidly overwhelm the host to gain a foothold.[1782]

Syphilis, for example, emerged more than five hundred years ago as an acute, severe, debilitating disease, but has evolved into the milder chronic form. Known in Renaissance Europe as the Great Pox, it had the ability to ulcerate faces off victims like leprosy and form great abscesses of pus. "Boils are exploding in groins like shells," read one contemporary description, "and purulent jets of clap vie with the fountains in the Piazza Navona."[1783] For a sexually transmitted disease, however, virulence may not be conducive to transmissibility. Overt manifestations—like losing one's nose—may tip off (and turn off) potential sexual partners, reducing the selective advantage of aggressive strains of the disease.[1784]

The best studied example of this phenomenon is the intentional introduction of the rabbitpox virus into Australia. In the 1950s, rabbits were introduced for hunting purposes, but lacking natural predators, they rapidly populated the continent.[1785] To kill off the rabbits, scientists introduced a rabbitpox virus isolated from a Brazilian rabbit species to which the virus had co-evolved an aggressive symbiosis.[1786] Within a year, the virus had spread a thousand miles in every direction, killing millions of rabbits with a 99.8 percent mortality rate.[1787] To the bane of the farmers (but the benefit of the bunnies), by the second year, the mortality rate was down to 90 percent and eventually dropped to only 25 percent, frustrating attempts to eradicate the cotton-tailed menace.[1788]

The rabbitpox virus was faced with a trade-off. On the level of a single individual host, it was presumably in the virus's best interest to attain maximal virulence, replicating and destroying at full bore to overwhelm the rabbit's immune defenses in hopes of spreading outward to other rabbits. If the immune system got the upper hand first, there was little chance the virus could pass on its genes. This tendency toward maximum virulence, though, was counterbalanced by the need for effective transmission on a population level. By rapidly overcoming the host, the virus may have won the battle but lost the war.[1789]

If a virus kills the host too quickly, there is less opportunity to spread, both in time and space. Just as dead ducks don't fly, dead rabbits don't hop. Unless farmers could cram rabbits by the thousands into some kind of bunny barn, viral mutants with diminished lethality may have an overall advantage since the host may stay alive longer and have more occasion to pass on the virus. This is a risky strategy for the virus; if it becomes too weak, the hosts' defenses may quash it completely. Natural selection mediates this evolutionary process, choosing over time the virus with the perfect balance of lethality and contagion.[1790]

This doesn't always mean a transition toward lesser virulence. "If predator-like variants of a pathogen population out-produce and out-transmit benign pathogens," wrote one evolutionary medicine pioneer, "then peaceful coexistence and long-term stability may be precluded much as it is often precluded in predator-prey systems."[1791] H5N1, in this case, seemed the model predator.

The tendency of the influenza virus when finding itself locked in a host as unfamiliar as a chicken may be to become as virulent as possible to overpower the bird's defenses.[1792] The deadlier the better, perhaps. Don't the same constraints apply, though? If the virus kills the chicken too quickly, how can it then infect others? Enter intensive poultry production. When the next beak is inches away, there may be fewer limits to how nasty influenza can get.

> *"In our efforts to streamline farming practices to produce more meat for more people, we have inadvertently created conditions by which a harmless parasite of wild ducks can be converted into a lethal killer of humans."*
>
> —JOHNS HOPKINS NEUROVIROLOGIST ROBERT H. YOLKEN AND
> STANLEY MEDICAL RESEARCH INSTITUTE DIRECTOR
> E. FULLER TORREY[1793]

As I've discussed, all bird flu viruses seem to start out harmless, arising out of the perpetual, benign, stable reservoir of innocuous waterfowl influenza.

They begin as mild, low-grade, low-pathogenicity avian influenza, or LPAI viruses. But, H5 and H7 viruses, if you'll recall, have the potential to mutate into virulent high-grade "fowl plague" viruses—highly pathogenic avian influenza, or HPAI.

HPAI viruses aren't born; they're made. The World Health Organization explains in its 2005 assessment of the pandemic threat:

> *Highly pathogenic viruses have no natural reservoir. Instead, they emerge by mutation when a virus, carried in its mild form by a wild bird, is introduced to poultry. Once in poultry, the previously stable virus begins to evolve rapidly, and can mutate, over an unpredictable period of time, into a highly lethal version of the same initially mild strain.*[1794]

Scientists have demonstrated this transformation in a laboratory setting. A collaboration of U.S. and Japanese researchers started with a harmless virus isolated from waterfowl, H5N3 from a whistling swan in this case, and proceeded to do serial passages through baby chickens. First, the researchers took day-old chicks and squirted a million infectious doses into their lungs. Over the next few days, the virus would presumably start to adapt to the chicks' respiratory tracts, with the viral mutant that learned best, through trial and error, to undermine the hatchlings' defenses selected to predominate. After three days, they killed the chicks, ground up their lungs, and squirted the viral lung slurry down the throats of other chicks. They allowed a few days for the virus to adapt further before repeating the cycle two dozen times.

When they killed the last set of chicks, the researchers ground up their brains instead of their lungs and infected five additional rounds of healthy chicks with the brain pulp. With every passage, the virus grew more adept at overwhelming and outwitting the fledging birds' immune systems to best survive and thrive in its new environment. The final infected brain sample, after two dozen cycles though lungs and five cycles through brain, was squirted into the nostrils of healthy adult chickens. Nothing happens to the healthy adult chickens if you squirt the original swan virus into their nostrils—but influenza is a fast learner. By the eighteenth passage into the lungs of chicks, the virus was able to kill half of the chickens exposed. After the final five brain passages, the virus was capable of rapidly killing every single one. The researchers concluded: "These findings demonstrate that the avirulent [harmless] avian influenza viruses can become pathogenic during repeated passaging in chickens."[1795]

If mad scientists wanted to create a bird flu virus of unprecedented ferocity, they could try to continually keep cycling the virus through chickens. Imagine if the serial passaging was done not two dozen times, but twenty thousand times. What kind of virus would come out the other end?

The World Organization for Animal Health and the Food and Agriculture Organization of the United Nations agree that it has been "prove[n]"[1796] that once LPAI viruses gain access to poultry facilities, they "progressively gain pathogenicity in domestic birds through a series of infection cycles until they become HPAI."[1797] However, deadly bird flu viruses don't tend to arise in just any poultry operation. According to USDA researchers, it is the "high density confinement rearing methods" that give bird flu "a unique chance to adapt to the new species."[1798] That is, today's intensive farming practices may remove the natural obstacles to transmission that prevent the virus from becoming too dangerous.

David Swayne, the USDA's leading bird flu researcher and director of the USDA's chief poultry research laboratory, has authored more than two hundred scientific publications on avian influenza.[1799] According to him, there has never been a recorded emergence of an HPAI virus in any backyard flock or free-range poultry operation. This is not surprising.

Imagine an outdoor setting. A duck flying overhead dive-bombs a dropping laden with relatively innocuous virus into a grassy field in which a flock of hens is pecking. The hens may be exposed to the virus, but coming straight from waterfowl, the virus is so finely tuned to duck physiology that it may not gain a foothold in the hen before being wiped out by a healthy chicken's immune system. That's why in the lab, researchers *injected* infected lung tissue from one bird to another to facilitate transmission. "The conditions under which we generated highly virulent viruses from an avirulent strain are generally not duplicated in nature," the research team admitted. "However, viruses with low pathogenicity can cause viremia in physically compromised chickens."[1800] Viremia means successful invasion of the bloodstream by the virus, an incursion they deem likelier to occur in compromised hosts.

If an outdoor flock does manage to get infected, the virus still has to keep spreading to remain in existence. Influenza virus is rapidly killed by sunlight and tends to be dehydrated to death in the breeze. Its ability to spread efficiently from one chicken to the next outside in the open air is relatively limited. In a sparsely populated outdoor setting, there may simply be too few susceptible hosts nearby to passage between in order to build up enough adaptive mutations to do more than ruffle a few feathers. There was a deadly outbreak among wild sea-birds in South Africa in 1961[1801] and a 2004 outbreak on two outdoor ostrich farms,[1802] and rare sporadic outbreaks of highly pathogenic bird flu viruses date back more than a century,[1803] but these seem to be exceptions to the rule.[1804] According to bird flu expert Dennis Alexander of the UK's Central Veterinary Laboratory, with the possible exception of the ostriches, highly pathogenic influenza viruses have "never known to arise in an outdoor flock."[1805]

Now imagine the mad scientist scenario. Tens of thousands of chickens crammed into a filthy, football field–sized broiler shed, living beak-to-beak in their own waste. The air is choked with moist fecal dust and ammonia, which irritates the birds' respiratory passages, further increasing susceptibility in chickens already compromised by the stress of confinement. Since the birds are standing in their own excrement, the virus need not even develop true airborne transmission via nasal or respiratory secretions. Rather, the virus has an opportunity to be excreted in the feces and then inhaled or swallowed by the thousands of other birds confined in the shed, allowing the virus to rapidly and repeatedly circulate. With so many birds in which to readily mutate, low-virulence strains can sometimes turn into deadly ones. The dose of virus transmitted from one bird to another might also play a crucial role.

Earl Brown specializes in influenza evolution. He studies how the virus acquires virulence and adapts to new species. In a landmark study published in the *Proceedings of the National Academy of Sciences of the United States of America,* he showed "that a group of 11 mutations can convert an avirulent virus to a virulent variant that can kill at a minimal dose." Instead of studying waterfowl viruses in chickens, he studied human viruses in a similarly unnatural host—mice. Mice can be experimentally infected with human flu strains, but they don't get sick. The virus is adapted to taking over and killing human cells, not mouse cells. Human viruses tend to replicate so poorly within a mouse that the mouse's immune system wipes it out before the virus can cause so much as the sniffles. If the human virus is dripped directly into a mouse's nostrils, though, and then you grind up the mouse's lungs and drip the viral infected lung tissue into another mouse's nose and the cycle is repeated, in as few as a dozen cycles, the virus—despite having started out totally harmless—comes out the other end causing fatal pneumonia in the mice.[1806]

Investigators have found that the key to this ramping up of virulence may be the size of the infectious dose that gets transferred from one animal to another. In the swarm of viral mutants in every infected mouse's lungs, odds are that there are a few capable of "heightened exploitation of the host,"[1807] but if these mutants never find their way into another mouse, they will be wiped out along with the others. So, even if an infected mouse were to rub noses with another mouse and transfer some small level of infection, chances are slim that the few virulent mutants would happen to find their way into the next mouse. In fact, since influenza is so sloppy at replicating, the majority of mutants may be relatively dysfunctional, so a small transferred dose may actually cause the virus to lose potency.[1808] In this way, it's not just the number of animals that doses of virus get transferred between—size matters. The greater the number of viruses transferred or "passaged" from one animal to the other, the greater the pool natural selection has to select from.

Professor Brown described it to me like trying to win the lottery. If you only buy a few tickets at a time, the chance of winning the jackpot is slim. But what if you bought *all* the tickets? The evolution of *hyper*virulence, as seen in viruses like H5N1, may require an enormous viral load seen only in rather unique circumstances—artificial inoculation in a laboratory or animals intensively confined in their own waste, where there is high dose transmission through thousands of hosts—what Brown calls the "nub and the crux" of the development of extreme viral virulence.[1809] Highly pathogenic bird flu viruses are primarily the products of factory farming.[1810]

Chicken Surprise

The mad scientist scenario of intensive poultry production has been replicated around the globe. Viral transformations from harmless to deadly have been documented in the outbreaks in Pennsylvania in the 1980s; Mexico,[1811] Australia, Pakistan,[1812] and Italy in the 1990s; and in Chile, the Netherlands, and Canada since 2002.[1813] Some of the farms in which this transformation took place were massive—six hundred thousand broiler breeders on the farm in the Chilean outbreak,[1814] for example, and seven hundred thousand caged laying hens at the index farm in Pakistan.[1815] These outbreaks have collectively led to the deaths of millions upon millions of chickens, but are highly pathogenic bird flu viruses more dangerous to *humans*? The CDC thinks that is likely the case.[1816]

Adaptation to land-based birds involves alterations of the virus in ways that may present increased human risk.[1817] Any modification that enhances airborne transmission, for example, such as improved resistance to desiccation, could amplify risk to people. Certainly the mutation that allows the virus to rage throughout all organ systems may contribute to the ability of viruses like H5N1 to cross the species barrier into humans[1818] and present a greater threat.[1819] In order to create a human pandemic, though, the virus has to be able to bind effectively to human receptors.[1820] That's why we've been so concerned about pigs. As I've mentioned, ducks have the 2,3 linkages, humans have the 2,6 linkages, and pigs have both. So, in a pig, the duck virus could theoretically accustom itself to our receptors and burst throughout the human population.[1821] Unfortunately for humanity, researchers recently discovered that *chickens* have human 2,6 receptors in their lungs, too.[1822]

A pandemic virus faces a paradoxical twin challenge: it must be new to the human immune system, so there's no pre-existing immunity, while, at the same time, be supremely well adapted to infect us.[1823] Mikhail N. Matrosovich at the Russian Academy of Sciences in Moscow discovered what may be a critical piece of the pandemic puzzle by demonstrating that, unlike ducks, chickens can tightly bind human influenza viruses and vice versa. This, Matrosovich wrote, could lead to the emergence of bird flu viruses with "enhanced propensity for transmission to humans."[1824]

In addition to the presence of human-like 2,6 linkages in the respiratory tracts of chickens, there's evidence of a second sialic acid binding site on the virus, the significance of which is unknown. This second binding site is highly conserved in the aquatic bird reservoir, but lost in both chickens and humans—another similarity on a molecular level between the lungs of chickens and humans that may make viral adaptations to one applicable to the other.[1825]

A third line of molecular evidence that implicates chickens as the pale Trojan horse of the apocalypse has to do with the length of ganglioside sugar chains. Gangliosides are complex fatty molecules jutting out of our cell membranes that display chains of sugars. It is not enough for the influenza virus to hook onto the sialic acid receptors on one of our cells; the virus must then fuse with the cell and spill its nefarious contents inside to take over. The virus must not only dock, but pry open the bay doors. This may be where these ganglioside sugar chains come into play, facilitating the virus's fusion and entry process.[1826]

The exact role gangliosides play remains speculative, but we do know that influenza viruses from different species have distinct binding preferences as to the length of these sugary chains. Duck viruses have an affinity for the short chains that are abundant in duck intestines, whereas human viruses have an affinity for the longer chains found in primate lung tissue. Part of the duck-human species barrier, then, may be that duck viruses prefer short chains, yet human cells exhibit more long chains. Chickens are in the middle.

As a duck virus circulates among chickens, there may be a selection pressure on the virus to attach to longer—and therefore more human-like—chains to better adapt and spread within and between chickens. Think about H5N1. As a waterfowl virus, it presumably preferred short chains, but it has mutated in favor of an affinity for longer chicken chains, on a potential trajectory toward more efficient human infection. In fact, chicken flu viruses bind tighter to human cells than they do to duck cells. As a result of some strange twist of evolutionary fate, from the standpoint of the influenza virus, chickens may look more like people than they do like ducks. When waterfowl viruses that are essentially harmless infect chickens, they may start accumulating mutations that make them more dangerous to chickens and humans alike.[1827] Evidence continues to build to support this hypothesis.[1828] In developing a taste for chicken, these viruses may acquire a taste for us.

Analysis of the 1918 virus protein sequences suggests that the transformation into a pandemic virus may be easier than previously thought. As I've discussed, just a single point mutation may change a virus that binds duck 2,3 receptors to a virus that binds human 2,6 receptors.[1829] The researchers who resurrected the 1918 virus found that the receptor binding site on the virus differed from the binding site of its presumed avian precursor by just one or two tiny amino acid substitutions, presumably all it needed to go human. Many experts expected H5N1 to similarly strike gold, line up the cherries, and cash in at our expense.

Adaptation to a human host requires more than just viral access into human cells. The internal viral machinery still has to evolve to best take over our cells, but viral entry is the first step. This surreptitious similarity between chicken and human receptors may better enable bird flu viruses like H5N1 to transition from infecting billions of chickens to infecting billions of humans. This may be thought of as an example of exaptation, a concept in evolutionary biology by which an adaptation in one context coincidentally predisposes success in an unrelated context. Legionnaire's disease is the classic example.[1830]

Legionnaire's is caused by bacteria whose primary evolutionary niche is the scum lining the rocks of natural hot springs. As they evolved to thrive within this warm, moist environment, the bacteria happened to be evolving to thrive within the warm, moist environment of the human lung as well. Of course, the bacteria had little occasion to find themselves within our lungs, since we're good about keeping water out of our windpipes (lest we drown). But then machines like air conditioners were invented, which have the capacity to mist water into the air, as evidenced by the infamous Philadelphia outbreak in 1976 at an American Legion convention in which the hotel ventilation system conditioned the air with bacteria now known as *Legionella*.[1831] In the environment of the human respiratory tract, *Legionella*'s prior adaptations proved lethal. In the case of influenza viruses that may have pandemic potential, like H5N1, chickens may be thought of as acting as both hot springs and air conditioner, providing the media by which the virus can adapt and propagate to the populace.

The evolutionary distance from duck to human seems too far for a direct jump by influenza, but with chickens sharing binding characteristics of each, they may act as stepping-stones to bridge the huge species gap.[1832] There is evidence that other land-based domesticated fowl, such as quail and pheasant, can also act as intermediaries and may play a minor role,[1833] but we don't tend to raise them like we do chickens. Although there was an outbreak of H5N2 on a farm raising more than a hundred thousand quail in Oregon in the 1980s, operations that size for birds other than chickens are typically the exception.[1834] Indeed, chickens would seem the most threatening possible species to be exhibiting human virus binding attributes, as they are the one animal in the world we raise by the tens of billions every year. In nature, as a waterborne virus, influenza has been known to infect aquatic mammals like whales and seals,[1835] but how many whales can you fit in a broiler shed or a battery cage?

Out of the Trenches

In 1918, chickens were still pecking around the barnyard. Industrial chicken factories didn't take off until after the *second* World War. How then could a pandemic virus of such ferocity have arisen? Nobody knows for certain, but evolutionary theory allows us to speculate. The development of extreme virulence is thought to require an overcrowding of susceptible hosts who cannot escape from one another. Otherwise, the virus needs to restrain itself. As I've said, if a bird flu virus gets too vicious, if the bird gets too ill, too fast, the virus is less likely to infect others—unless the next beak is just inches away. That wasn't the case in 1918. There were no reports of mass bird dieoffs, nor would one expect any since the 1918 virus was H1, and only H5 and H7 viruses are thought capable of mutating into highly pathogenic forms in chickens. In 1918, there were no stress-compromised chickens teeming with virus and crammed into enclosed spaces en masse. In 1918, the virus didn't learn how to kill humans crowded in filthy chicken sheds. Instead, it may have gotten that education in the trenches of World War I. In 1918, the soldiers may have been the chickens.

Military medical historian Carol Byerly argues in her 2005 book *Fever of War: The Influenza Epidemic in the U.S. Army During World War I* that the 1918 virus built up its virulence in the transport ships, trains, and trenches of the Great War.[1836] Millions of young men were forced together in close quarters where there was no escaping a sick comrade. Instead of battery cages of egg-laying chickens, battery units of infantry dug themselves into festering trenches. Instead of ammonia to irritate the respiratory tracts of chickens and predispose them to infection, residues of poison gases like chlorine saturated the Western Front.[1837] The unspeakable conditions, the theory goes, led to the perfect breeding ground for influenza superstrains: a population of "physically compromised" individuals under intense confinement undergoing mass troop movements, not unlike live animal transports. In both cases, fodder for slaughter.[1838] Boxcars were labeled "8 horses or 40 men."[1839] Evolutionary biologist Paul Ewald agrees that the crowded, stressful, unhygienic WWI conditions could have favored the evolution of a "predator-like virus" that otherwise may have killed too quickly to spread with peak efficiency under normal conditions.[1840]

If this controversial theory is correct, how might the virus have gotten into the trenches in the first place? There are a number of competing theories as to the true origin of the virus, all of them contentious.[1841] University of Hong Kong's Shortridge thinks it may have originated in Asia, conveyed to the front by Chinese laborers brought in to dig trenches for the Allies.[1842] Contemporary accounts have the workers speaking the Cantonese dialect of Guangdong Province (then Canton), the region harboring domesticated ducks for centuries alongside the highest concentration of people, pigs, and poultry in the world.[1843] The 1918 U.S. Surgeon General's report on the Spanish flu indeed alluded to an Asian origin.[1844] An avian virus may have smoldered in the Chinese population before serendipitously finding itself in the trenches, like a duck virus in a broiler chicken shed.[1845]

Royal London Hospital's John Oxford, on the other hand, points to declassified military medical records showing excessive numbers of deaths from respiratory infection in French military camps *before* the Chinese laborers arrived.[1846] The "heliotrope cyanosis" (bluish-purple skin discoloration) described in these reports does share a resemblance to the millions of cases that were soon to come.[1847] He suggests that the virus arose in the battlefield.

"Wounded survivors of gas contaminated battlefields gather in the Great City British Army Camp of Etaples in northern France," Oxford explains, "in close proximity with each other, with geese and poultry markets of the area and even pig farms installed right into the army camp itself."[1848] On any one day, the army base crowded a hundred thousand soldiers into tents and temporary barracks, a ripe setting for a respiratory virus. Survivors from the trenches crossed paths with more than a million men from England on their way to the Western Front in the Etaples camp alone. Combine the population density with the geese, chickens, and pigs raised for slaughter in the camps, Oxford notes, and "[t]hose conditions mimic what naturally occurs in Asia."[1849] In the absence of air travel, the virus may have simmered for

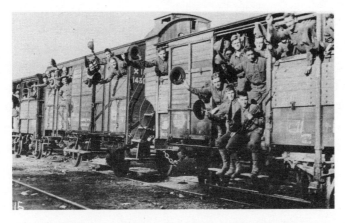

WWI troop transport in France (Courtesy of the
U.S. Army Military History Institute)

months or years in such a camp, relying on the demobilization in the fall of 1918 for rapid global dispersal.[1850]

Others think the pandemic 1918 virus was made in the United States. The American Medical Association sponsored what many consider to be the most comprehensive of several international investigations into the pandemic. Written by the editor of *The Journal of Infectious Disease,* the AMA report was published in 1927. The intervening years were spent reviewing evidence from around the world. The AMA concluded that the most likely site of origin of the 1918 virus was Haskell County, Kansas.[1851]

The first wave of the pandemic in the spring of 1918 was so mild that it did not merit special mention in the medical journals of the time.[1852] The virus still had a lot to learn. The AMA was able to track the spread of this mild spring wave from the first recorded case on March 4, 1918,[1853] at Camp Funston (now Fort Riley) in Kansas. Patient zero was a soldier recorded as cleaning pig pens prior to his infection.[1854] Maybe a Canada goose flew the virus to Kansas and infected a pig who infected a man. We will probably never know. From the Midwest, the flu virus spread along the rail lines from Army camp to Army camp,[1855] then into the cities, and finally traveled with the troops to Europe.[1856] The virus found itself not in Kansas anymore.

An equally authoritative multivolume British analysis of the pandemic agreed with the AMA: "The disease was probably carried from the United States to Europe."[1857] A Nobel Laureate who spent most of his research career studying influenza also concluded that the available evidence was "strongly suggestive" that the virus started in the United States and spread with "the arrival of American troops in France."[1858]

Over the summer of 1918, the virus mutated into a killer.[1859] Just as low-grade influenza viruses may infect free-range fowl, so too may they infect free-range Frenchmen. The highly unnatural wartime conditions may have allowed the virus to achieve its full lethal potential. The critical component, Ewald argues, "is something that chicken farms have in common with the Western Front: large numbers of hosts packed so closely that even immobilized hosts can transmit the virus to susceptibles."[1860] Once the ability of the virus to spread no longer depends on the host feeling well enough to move around in order to infect others, there may be little Darwinian limit to how fierce the virus can get.[1861]

In the wild, if a bird gets too sick, too fast, the virus isn't going anywhere. Stick a sick chicken in a broiler shed, though, or a sick soldier in a

troop transport, and the uninfected can no longer escape their sick companion. The key to the evolution of virulence may be the packing together of
the infected with the uninfected, beak-to-beak or shoulder-to-shoulder.[1862]
Ewald is uncompromising on this point:

> [W]e will continue to get severe influenza epidemics in chicken farms so
> long as the conditions in chicken farms, like the conditions at the Western
> Front, allow transmission from immobile chickens. This prediction has been
> confirmed by the lethal outbreaks of H5N1 in Asia and H5N2 in Mexico.
> Anyone who dismisses this analysis as speculation does not understand how
> the scientific process works or what scientific theory actually is, at least with
> regard to evolutionary biology.[1863]

The author of *Fever of War* emphasized the uniqueness of the conditions
that led to the pandemic. "The 1918 flu epidemic most likely will not happen
again," she said, "because we won't construct the Western Front again."[1864]
She failed to take into account that the same stress, filth, and crowding
of trench warfare exists in nearly every industrial egg farm and chicken
facility the world over. When you have a situation where the healthy cannot
escape the diseased and dying, when the virus can knock you flat and still
transmit from one to another just because you're so crowded, then there may
be no stopping rapidly mutating viruses from becoming truly ferocious.

Even Ewald, though convinced that the overcrowding of intensive poultry production made H5N1 into the killer it is today,[1865] seemingly failed to
recognize the genetic similarities between chickens and humans that make
viral evolution in the egg farm and the broiler house a sobering concern for
us all.[1866] The idiosyncratic likeness between the viral binding capacity to
both chicken and human respiratory linings may allow chickens to stand in as
our surrogates for the evolution of human lethality. Though millions fought
along the Western Front, we keep birds in the trenches by the billions.

A Chicken in Every Pot

America invented industrial poultry production, yet a century ago in the
United States, chickens were more prized as showpieces than dinner table
centerpieces. Chickens, like many fancy pigeon breeds of today, were bred

more for exhibition than consumption. Only around 1910 did raising these birds for eggs supersede raising them for show.[1867] When Herbert Hoover promised "a chicken in every pot" in 1928, America's entire annual per capita consumption could fit in a pot—Americans were eating an average of only a half-pound of chicken a year.[1868] By 1945, the figure stood at five pounds per year. The sea change happened after World War II.[1869] Current chicken consumption is around a hundred pounds a year,[1870] over half a bird a week.[1871] Chicken used to be more expensive than steak or lobster in the United States; poultry may now be cheaper than the potatoes with which it's served.[1872]

In past CEO Don Tyson's words, corporations "control the center of the plate for the American people"[1873] by turning a holiday or Sunday dinner into everyday fare through "least cost production,"[1874] an intense pressure to keep live production costs as low as possible.[1875] The first hurdle was to keep birds captive indoors in order to produce year-round.[1876] Without enough exercise and natural sunlight exposure, though, flocks raised in warehouses suffered from rickets and other developmental disorders. The discovery of the "sunshine" vitamin D in 1922[1877] finally allowed for total confinement,[1878] enabling producers to use near-continuous artificial light to increase feed-to-flesh conversion.[1879] As in the case of antibiotic growth promotants, such technological fixes have allowed the poultry industry to profit in the short term by undermining natural safeguards, but at what long-term cost?

Intensive confinement, while "more economical," according to USDA researchers, has the "unfortunate consequence that disease outbreaks occur more frequently and with greater severity."[1880] Many of the early indoor broiler chicken operations of the 1920s and 1930s were wiped out by contagious disease fostered by the crowded conditions,[1881] making it impossible to maintain large flocks economically.[1882] Overcrowding took over the egg industry, too. In 1945, the typical henhouse held five hundred egg-laying birds; today there are avian megalopolises, caging a hundred thousand or more hens in a single shed on a single egg farm.[1883] This was made possible in part by the antibiotic revolution. As one farmer admitted, "The more intensive farming gets, the more props you need. You crowd the animals to save every cent you can on space; then you have to give them more antibiotics to keep 'em healthy."[1884]

The history of the poultry industry is a history of disease. As soon as one epidemic was subdued, another one soon seemed to emerge.[1885] Bacterial diseases like fowl typhoid and tuberculosis gradually gave way over the century to viral scourges.[1886] In the 1960s, a hypervirulent form of Marek's disease was discovered, a destructive cancer virus that led to the condemnation of as many as one-fifth of U.S. broiler chicken flocks.[1887] In the 1970s, the exotic Newcastle disease, a viral invasion of the nervous system, caused the deaths of twelve million chickens.[1888] In the 1980s, H5N2 struck Pennsylvania and destroyed seventeen million chickens. It remained our worst bird flu outbreak in the United States[1889] until another series of H5 bird flu viruses struck again just a few years ago and laid waste to fifty million chickens and turkeys.[1890] In the 1990s, parasitic diseases like blackhead disease—once considered under control—re-emerged,[1891] and some bacteria reincarnated as antibiotic-resistant superbugs.[1892] In a review of the unrelenting global outbreaks of epidemic disease, a North Carolina veterinary poultry specialist wrote in *World Poultry,* "The intensification of the poultry industry seems to be paying its toll."[1893]

GRAIN, a respected agricultural research organization, pointed out a parallel between Newcastle disease and avian influenza in its briefing *Fowl Play: The Poultry Industry's Central Role in the Bird Flu Crisis.*[1894] Newcastle is another avian virus that can mutate into a highly pathogenic form if it finds its way into an intensive confinement environment. The GRAIN report pointed to the example of a sudden Australian outbreak of Newcastle in 1998 that led to the destruction of a hundred thousand chickens. Though the virus was originally assumed to have been brought into the country from overseas, virologists at the Australian Animal Health Laboratory concluded that a benign local strain had mutated into a highly virulent form.[1895] Vaccinations were mandated for all chickens on any farm with more than a thousand birds. The government explained why small farms and backyard flocks were exempt: "All the available evidence indicates that, for such a mutation to occur, it needs a large number of birds in a small area to 'generate' the virus mutation process. In simple terms, a small number of birds cannot generate enough virus for the mutation process to occur."[1896]

Even with total control over the animals' lives and movements, and an arsenal of vaccines, antimicrobials, and deworming agents, intensive farm animal industries remain plagued with disease epidemics.[1897] In intensive pig production, certain internal parasites have been eliminated, but respiratory diseases like influenza have intensified.[1898] In the poultry industry, according to an avian virology textbook, "confined, indoor, high-density" facilities "create an ideal environment for the transmission of viruses, particularly those that are shed from the respiratory or gastrointestinal tract."[1899] The flu virus can be shed from both.

> *"You have to say that high intensity chicken rearing is a perfect environment for generating virulent avian flu virus."*
>
> —UNIVERSITY OF OTTAWA VIROLOGIST EARL BROWN[1900]

Given the existence of diseases like bird flu with potentially disastrous human health consequences, the propensity of large-scale poultry production to generate disease—"industrial ecology created by intensive confinement"—has, as an academic technology journal described, "ramifications far beyond the chicken house."[1901] In the end, chickens may not be the only ones to fall sick.

Modern corporate chicken sheds cluster tens or hundreds of thousands of chickens into what are essentially giant slums.[1902] These animals spend their entire short lives eating, sleeping, and defecating in the same cramped quarters, breathing in particles of their neighbors' waste and the stinging ammonia of decomposing feces. Their first breath of fresh air is on the truck to the slaughter plant. In this kind of environment, mass disease outbreaks may be inevitable.[1903]

"The primary driver has been economics—short-term gain," said the director of the Toronto General Hospital's Centre for Travel and Tropical Medicine. "We bring tens of thousands of animals together, crush them into these abnormal environments, poke them full of whatever and make them fatter for sale. Any microbe that enters that population is going to be disseminated to thousands of animals."[1904] Intensive poultry production diminishes the cost to the individual consumer, but may present an intolerable cost to humanity at large.

A number of prominent journalists worldwide have arrived at this idea of factory farms as potential pandemic hatcheries. Theresa Manavalan, a leading Malaysian journalist, asked us to "make no mistake, the pig is not the villain, neither is the chicken. It's actually us. And our horrible farm practices. . . . What we may have done," she warns, "is unwittingly create the perfect launch pad for an influenza pandemic that will likely kill large numbers of people across the globe."[1905] Deborah Mackenzie, from the *New*

Scientist Brussels office, wrote, "For years we have forced countless chickens to live short, miserable lives in huge, crammed hen houses in the name of intensive agriculture. In 2004, they started to wreak their revenge."[1906]

The WHO, OIE, and FAO, respectively the world's leading medical, veterinary, and agricultural authorities, all implicated industrial poultry production as playing a role in the H5N1 crisis. The World Health Organization blamed the increasing trend of emerging infectious diseases in part on the "industrialization of the animal production sector"[1907] in general, and the emergence of H5N1 on "intensive poultry production" in particular.[1908] The OIE, the World Organization for Animal Health, blamed in part the shorter production cycles and greater animal densities of modern poultry production, which result in a "greater number of susceptible animals reared per given unit of time."[1909] Said one senior FAO official, "[I]ntensive industrial farming of livestock is now an opportunity for emerging diseases."[1910]

Other experts around the world similarly placed blame at least in part on "so-called factory farming,"[1911] "intensive poultry production,"[1912] "large industry poultry flocks,"[1913] "intensive agricultural production systems,"[1914] or "intensive confinement."[1915] "We are wasting valuable time pointing fingers at wild birds," the Food and Agriculture Organization stated, "when we should be focusing on dealing with the root causes of this epidemic spread which . . . [include] farming methods which crowd huge numbers of animals into small spaces."[1916]

In October 2005, the United Nations issued a press release on bird flu, stating: "Governments, local authorities and international agencies need to take a greatly increased role in combating the role of factory-farming, commerce in live poultry, and wildlife markets which provide ideal conditions for the virus to spread and mutate into a more dangerous form."[1917]

Emeritus professor Kennedy Shortridge was awarded the highly prestigious Prince Mahidol Award in Public Health, considered the "Nobel Prize of Asia,"[1918] for his pioneering work on H5N1.[1919] From 1977 to 2002, he advised the World Health Organization on the ecology of influenza viruses.[1920] Shortridge described how modern poultry operations have created the greatest risk scenario in history: "The industrialization is the nub of the problem," he said. "We have unnaturally brought to our doorstep pandemic-capable viruses. We have given them the opportunity to infect and destroy huge numbers of birds and . . . jump into the human race."[1921] The director of the Consortium for Conservation Medicine agreed. "The global poultry industry is clearly linked to avian influenza [H5N1]," he said. "It would not have happened without it."[1922]

COMING HOME TO ROOST

Overcrowded

What specifically about intensive production pushed the world's leading public and animal health authorities to take up arms? An industry trade journal listed some factors that make intensive poultry facilities such "ideal"[1923] "breeding grounds for disease":[1924] "poor ventilation, high stocking density, poor litter conditions, poor hygiene, high ammonia level, concurrent diseases and secondary infections."[1925]

Overcrowding is the first ingredient in the recipe to potentially increase the transmission of bird flu. Researchers have demonstrated a 100 percent contact-transmission rate of H5N1 between chickens housed at standard stocking densities, but the transmission rate was cut in half or even eliminated when the birds' living space was doubled.[1926] When a chicken experimentally infected with a highly pathogenic turkey flu virus was placed in a room with four other chickens, the infected bird died, but none of the other four fell ill. However, when the same experiment was repeated, but with thirteen chickens, five of the contact chickens in the higher-density scenario became sick and three died.[1927] In modern poultry production, the thirteen becomes tens of thousands.

In modern broiler chicken production, twenty thousand to thirty thousand day-old chicks may be placed atop coarse wood shavings or other litter material in an otherwise barren shed.[1928] As they grow bigger, quickly reaching slaughter-weight, the crowding grows more and more intense. According to a standard reference manual for commercial chicken production, "Under standard commercial conditions chickens weighing 4.5 to 6 lbs have little more than a half a square foot of living space per bird in the last two weeks of their 42–47 days of life."[1929] As one researcher reported, "[I]t looks as though there is white carpet in the sheds—when the birds are fully grown you couldn't put your hand between the birds, if a bird fell down it would be lucky to stand up again because of the crush of the others."[1930] "Obviously," Louisiana State University veterinary scientists wrote, "the potential for a disastrous epidemic is very high" under those conditions.[1931]

As I've discussed, the majority of egg-laying hens in the world are confined in battery cages[1932]—barren wire enclosures so small that each hen is allotted less space than a standard letter-sized piece of paper.[1933] A hen needs 291 square inches of space to flap her wings, 197 square inches to turn around, and 72 square inches just to stand freely.[1934] U.S. commercial battery facilities typically allow each bird an average of 64 square inches.[1935] With up to ten birds per cage and thousands of cages stacked vertically in multiple tiers, laying hen warehouses can average more than a hundred thousand chickens per shed.[1936]

The Royal Geographical Society notes, "Massive demand for chicken has led to factory (battery) farming which provides ideal conditions for viruses to spread orally and via excreta which inevitably contaminates food in the cramped conditions that most birds are kept in."[1937]

Europe has been moving away from this level of intensification, for both egg-laying chickens and chickens raised for meat. In 2007, the European Commission imposed a maximum stocking density for broiler chickens throughout Europe.[1938] In sharp contrast to the "standard commercial . . . half a square foot of living space per bird," certain organic standards in Britain already require more than 150 square feet per bird.[1939] For the health and welfare of egg-laying hens, in 2012, the European Parliament banned conventional battery-cage systems entirely.[1940] Since then, seven

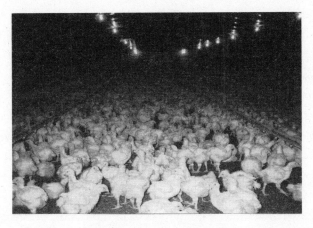

Broiler chicken shed[1941]

U.S. states have followed suit to ban or restrict the use of battery cages.[1942, 1943,1944,1945,1946,1947,1948]

In a joint consultation, the WHO, FAO, and OIE noted that the sheer number of intense contacts between birds with increasing flock density serves to spread and amplify disease agents like bird flu.[1949] This is supported by research showing that, not surprisingly, increasing chicken stocking densities result in an increased burden of infectious disease agents.[1950]

Not only does increased poultry density enable the enhanced spread of bird flu, but Webster's group considered it a "big factor" in the rise of highly pathogenic viruses in the first place. The "more hosts in close confinements" there are, the more easily the virus can mutate into a form capable of infecting humans and eventually spreading throughout the human population.[1951] The more animals there are to easily jump between, the more spins the virus may get at the roulette wheel while gambling for the pandemic jackpot that may be hidden in the lining of the chickens' lungs. Research on the evolution of antibiotic resistance, for example, has shown that "intensive production" can "vastly increase the occurrence of very rare genetic events."[1952] Influenza viruses don't just need to proliferate; they need to evolve.

In land-based birds, it may be advantageous for influenza viruses to switch from residing peacefully in the intestine to invading the respiratory tract, from being spread only through the water to also being spread through the air. To adapt, the virus must first survive by overwhelming host defenses. As shown in earlier examples, when animals are spread apart, the virus is presumably constrained by needing to keep the host healthy enough, long enough, to spread to another. Under extreme crowding conditions, though, natural biological checks and balances on virulence may no longer apply. Anthropologist and author Wendy Orent explained this to the *Los Angeles Times*:

> *H5N1 has evolved great virulence among chickens only because of the conditions under which the animals are kept—crammed together in cages, packed into giant warehouses. H5N1 was originally a mild virus found in migrating ducks; if it killed its host immediately, it too would die. But when its next host's beak is just an inch away, the virus can evolve to kill quickly and still survive.[1953]*

With tens of thousands, if not hundreds of thousands, of susceptible hosts in a single chicken shed, the virus can rapidly cycle from one bird to the next, accumulating adaptive mutations. French scientist C. J. Davaine was one of the first to demonstrate the concept of "serial passage." How much anthrax-infected blood, he wondered, would it take to kill a rabbit?

Davaine showed that it took ten drops of blood swarming with anthrax to infect and kill a rabbit. Fewer than ten drops and the rabbit survived. But, when he took blood from the first rabbit and infected another, the second required a smaller infectious dose. The anthrax germ was learning. Passing from rabbit to rabbit, the anthrax adapted to its new host to become more and more deadly. By the fifth rabbit, instead of requiring ten drops to kill the rabbit, it only took 1/100th of a single drop to kill. By the fifteenth passage, the pathogen became so well adapted that it only took 1/40,000th of a single drop. After passing through twenty-five rabbits, just 1/1,000,000th of a drop could be fatal. One one-millionth of just one drop could kill.

Indeed, when a pathogen passes into a new environment, species, or even host, it may start out with low pathogenicity, but when it passes from animal to animal, it can learn to become a more proficient killer.[1954] Forget twenty-five hosts: Broiler chicken sheds offer an average of 25,000 captive hosts and some egg-laying hen sheds 250,000.[1955]

Once the virus burns through a chicken shed, its survival is again jeopardized—unless it can find new victims. Depending on the ambient conditions, influenza virus can only endure in wet manure for weeks at most.[1956] The virus no longer has the luxury of being sheltered for months, lurking in the depths of some Canadian lake. It has very little time to find its way into another flock, so the virus hitches a ride on whatever it can find: footwear, clothing, tires, trucks, cages, crates, insects, rodents, or even the wind, blown out into the countryside by the colossal fans that ventilate the sheds. Mink fur farms are crowded enough to suffer influenza outbreaks, but unless there are multiple farms to which the virus can travel, the virus seems to inevitably fizzle out.[1957]

When spatial analyses were carried out of the spread of H5N1 in Asia, outbreaks corresponded to areas with the greatest numbers of chickens per square mile. When researchers overlaid a poultry density map of a country on a map of outbreaks, the maps lined up with statistical significance.[1958] So, within a shed, on a farm, or even across an entire region, as the WHO's Asian director put it at the time, "outbreaks of avian influenza correspond to where [poultry] population density is very high."[1959]

Large, crowded populations may be the only way a short-lived virus like influenza has been able to exist for millions of years. Viruses tend to have one of two "viral life strategies."[1960] There are persistent viruses like herpes, which have survived through the ages because they can hide within the body, only peeking out for a transient blistering rash in order to spread before going back underground to hide from the body's defenses. Then there are the acute viruses like influenza, which have no place to hide. They only have a matter of days to spread before they kill the host or, likelier, the host kills them. Therefore, without a vast, dense population of susceptible hosts, the virus would quickly disappear.

Even in wild waterfowl, influenza is transient. There is no evidence that ducks carry the virus for more than a few weeks at a time, so the virus seems to rely on the fact that for a hundred million years, aquatic birds like ducks and geese have gathered in mass congregations. Combined with efficient waterborne transmission, this rather unique circumstance of a densely crowded yet mobile population makes waterfowl essentially the only host in the animal kingdom thought able to continuously support such a short-lived infection.[1961] Bats may play a parallel role for coronaviruses.[1962]

In 1989, a bird flu virus jumped straight into horses in China, killed 20 percent of a herd, and then quickly disappeared.[1963] Such epidemics seem necessarily self-limited since the population is restricted in size and not rapidly replenished with new hosts.[1964] Unless we start circulating tens of thousands of horses through crowded megabarns, horse flu has little chance of taking root and, presumably, even less chance of posing a human threat. Only, perhaps, when the poultry population and density reached a critical mass—and one that was continuously repopulated—could chickens act as harbingers of viruses like H5N1.[1965]

Stressful

Overcrowding may also increase the vulnerability for each individual animal. Frederick Murphy, dean emeritus of the School of Veterinary Medicine at the University of California–Davis, noted how these changes in the way we raise animals for food "often allow pathogens to enter the food chain at its source and to flourish, largely because of stress-related factors."[1966] The physiological stress created by crowded confinement can have a "profound" impact on immunity,[1967] predisposing animals to infection.[1968] Diminished immune function means diminished protective responses to vaccinations. "As vaccinal immunity is compromised by factors such as . . . immunosuppressive stress," wrote a leading[1969] USDA expert on chicken vaccines, "mutant clones have an increased opportunity to selectively multiply and to be seeded in the environment."[1970] Studies exposing birds to stressful housing conditions provide "solid evidence in support of the concept that stress impairs adaptive immunity in chicken."[1971]

Chickens placed in overcrowded pens develop, over time, "increased adrenal weight"—a swelling growth of the glands that produce stress hormones like adrenaline—while, at the same time, experiencing "regression of lymphatic organs," a shriveling of the organs of the immune system.[1972] This is thought to demonstrate a metabolic trade-off in which energies invested in host defense are diverted by the stress response,[1973] which can result in "extensive immunosuppression."[1974] Europe's Scientific Veterinary Committee reported that one of the reasons Europe phased out battery cages for egg-laying hens is that evidence suggests caged chickens may have higher rates of infections "as the stresses from being caged compromise immune function."[1975]

Leading meat industry consultant Temple Grandin, an animal scientist at Colorado State University, described the stresses of battery-cage life in an address to the National Institute of Animal Agriculture. "When I visited a large egg layer operation and saw old hens that had reached the end of their productive life, I was horrified. Egg layers bred for maximum egg production . . . were nervous wrecks that had beaten off half their feathers by constant flapping against the cage."[1976] Referring to egg industry practices in general, Grandin noted, "It's a case of bad becoming normal."[1977]

Under intensive confinement conditions, not only may the birds be unable to comfortably turn around or even stand freely, but the most basic of natural behaviors such as feather preening may be frustrated, leading to additional stress.[1978] Overcrowding may disrupt the birds' natural pecking order, imposing a social stress that has been shown for more than forty years to weaken resistance to viral infection[1979] and, more recently, a multitude of other disease challenges.[1980] Industry specialists concede it "proven" that "high stress levels, like the ones modern management practices provoke," lead to a reduced immune response.[1981]

We see the similar stressors in the pig industry. "Forget the pig is an animal," an industry journal declared decades ago. "Treat him just like a machine in a factory."[1982] And, indeed, breeding sows, as I've discussed, are typically confined in barren metal stalls or crates so narrow they can't turn around. Prevented from performing normal maternal behavior (and, clearly, physical behavior), the pigs produce lower levels of antibodies in response to an experimental challenge.[1983] "Studies suggest," reads a review, "that the stress of lying on bare concrete may reduce resistance to respiratory disease leading to increased infection risk."[1984] German researchers found specifically that straw bedding was linked to decreased risk of infection with the influenza virus.[1985]

Another source of stress for many birds raised for meat and eggs is the wide variety of mutilations they may endure. Bits of body parts of unanesthetized birds—such as their combs, their spurs, and their claws—can be cut off to limit the damage of often stress-induced aggression. Sometimes, toes are snipped off at the first knuckle for identification purposes.[1986] University of Georgia poultry scientist Bruce Webster described the broiler chicken at an American Meat Institute conference as "essentially an overgrown baby bird, easily hurt, sometimes treated like bowling balls."[1987]

Most egg laying hens in the United States are "beak-trimmed."[1988] Parts of chicks' beaks are sliced off, often with a hot blade, an acutely painful[1989] procedure shown to impair their ability to grasp and swallow feed.[1990] Already banned in some European countries as unnecessary,[1991] the procedure is viewed by some poultry scientists as no more than a "stop-gap measure masking basic inadequacies in environment or management."[1992]

A National Defense University Policy Paper on agricultural bioterrorism specifically cited mutilations in addition to crowding as factors that increase stress levels to a point at which the resultant immunosuppression may play a part in making U.S. animal agriculture vulnerable to terrorist attack.[1993] University of Guelph Animal and Poultry Science Department University professor emeritus Ian Duncan has been outspoken about the animal and human health implications of these stressful practices for decades. "All these 'elective surgeries' involve pain," Duncan has written, "perhaps chronic pain. No anesthetic is ever given to the birds. These mutilations are crude solutions to the problems created by modern methods of raising chickens and turkeys."[1994]

The former head of the Department of Poultry Science at North Carolina State University described how turkeys start out their lives. Newborn turkey chicks are:

> squeezed, thrown down a slide onto a treadmill, someone picks them up and pulls the snood off their heads, clips three toes off each foot, debeaks them, puts them on another conveyer belt that delivers them to another carousel where they get a power injection, usually of an antibiotic, that whacks them in the back of their necks. Essentially, they have been through major surgery. They have been traumatized.[1995]

Research performed at the University of Arkansas' Center of Excellence for Poultry Science suggests that the cumulative effect of multiple stressors throughout turkey production results in conditions like "turkey osteomyelitis complex," where decreased resistance to infection leads to a bacterial invasion into the bone, causing the formation of abscessed pockets of pus throughout the birds' skeletons. The stress of catching and transport alone has been shown to induce the disease.[1996]

If modern production methods make animals so vulnerable to illness, why do they continue? The industry could reduce overcrowding, thereby lowering mortality losses from disease, but, as poultry scientists explain, "improving management may not be justified by the production losses."[1997] In other words, even if many birds die due to disease, the current system may still be more profitable in the short run. "Poultry are the most cost-driven of all the animal production systems," reads one veterinary textbook, "and the least expensive methods of disease control are used."[1998] It may be cheaper to just add antibiotics to the feed than it is to make substantive changes, but relying on the antibiotic crutch helps foster antibiotic-resistant superbugs and does nothing to stop bird flu.

The leading poultry production manual explains the economic rationale for overcrowding: "[L]imiting the floor space gives poorer results on a bird basis, yet the question has always been and continues to be: What is the least amount of floor space necessary per bird to produce the greatest return on investment."[1999] What remains missing from these calculations is the cost in human lives, which for poultry diseases like bird flu, could potentially run into the millions.

Filthy

In intensive confinement production, crowding, stress, and filth go hand in hand in hand. The USDA points out that a single gram of manure (approximately the weight of a paper clip) from an infected chicken can contain "enough virus to infect 1 million birds."[2000] A twenty-thousand-bird broiler flock produces more than a ton of droppings every day.[2001]

They are literally sitting in it. By the end of their lives, many of the birds can no longer stand. "The birds are bred for such size that their legs become so weak that they often cannot support the weight of their bodies," explained a USDA poultry specialist. "They therefore spend much of the time squatting on the floor in the litter."[2002] That's where they eat, sleep, and defecate. At just six weeks old, chickens raised for meat are so heavy and the stress on their hips and legs so great that they spend more than three-quarters of their time lying in their own waste.[2003] Temple Grandin wrote: "Today's poultry chicken has been bred to grow so rapidly that its legs can collapse under the weight of its ballooning body. It's awful."[2004] By the time they are slaughtered, all their carcasses show evidence of gross fecal contamination.[2005] Small wonder modern poultry products represent such prime carriers of foodborne illness,[2006] especially since, unlike with cows and pigs, the skin may be eaten with the meat.[2007]

The putrefying feces generate several irritating chemicals, including hydrogen sulfide (the "rotten egg" gas), methane, and ammonia.[2008] "Ammonia in a poultry house is nauseating to the caretaker, irritates the eyes, and affects the chickens," states one poultry science textbook.[2009] Given the extreme stocking density, the litter can get so saturated with excrement that birds may develop sores or "ammonia burns" on their skin, known as breast blisters, hock burns, and footpad dermatitis, all of which have become significantly more common and serious over the last several decades.[2010] The ammonia burns the birds' eyes and lungs, as well.

Studies have shown that high levels of ammonia increase the severity of respiratory disorders like pneumonia,[2011] in part by directly damaging the respiratory tract, predisposing them to infection.[2012] A massive study involving millions of birds from nearly one hundred commercial farms across multiple countries found that ammonia levels increased the excretion of the stress hormone corticosteroid, a potent immune depressant.[2013]

Besides the role chronic irritative stress plays, ammonia also directly suppresses the immune system.[2014] Ammonia gets absorbed into the birds' bloodstreams, where it interferes with the action of individual white blood immune cells.[2015] Although airborne aerosol spread of H5N1 still remains relatively inefficient, even among birds,[2016] the ammonia damage associated with intensive poultry production may facilitate the virus acquiring so-called pneumotropic, or "lung-seeking," behavior.[2017]

The air within industrial broiler chicken sheds is thick with fecal dust, presumably making disease spread effortless for the influenza virus. Increased stocking density leads to higher concentrations of aerial pollutants, which then leads to increased respiratory disease challenge to the birds' immune systems.[2018] In addition to fecal material, the airborne dust in such facilities has been found to contain bacteria, bacterial toxins, viruses, molds, nasal discharge, feather and skin debris, feed particles, and insect parts.[2019] Poultry confinement buildings can average more than a million bacteria floating in every cubic yard of air.[2020]

In addition to adding to airway irritation, these dust particles clog up the birds' lungs, overwhelming the lungs' clearance mechanisms. Researchers demonstrated decades ago that exposing a chick to a normally harmless strain of E. coli in an environment clouded with dust or ammonia can cause disease.[2021] The very air birds breathe while in intensive confinement may predispose them to infection with influenza.

Every day, another ton of droppings is dropped. In the United States, chickens raised for meat are slaughtered at about forty-five days and a new flock of chicks is brought in from the hatchery. Unbelievably, the sheds may not be cleaned between flocks. So, newly hatched chicks may be placed directly on the tons of feces that have already been layered down, and the cycle continues. "European growers visiting U.S. production facilities inevitably find this practice shocking," admitted poultry specialist Frank Jones at the Department of Poultry Science at North Carolina State University.

Veterinary experts have also been critical of this practice. As specified in the journal of the World Organization for Animal Health, fecal waste should be removed from the shed before adding a new flock.[2022] Placing day-old chicks in sheds contaminated with "built-up" litter is said to expose the birds to "a wide range of poultry pathogens."[2023] The Advisory Committee on the Microbiological Safety of Food reported that the most significant source of

Campylobacter infection in chickens—infection that goes on to sicken millions of Americans[2024]—is "the environment of the industrial broiler house."[2025] The poultry industry suspects that "general farm hygiene could reduce the numbers [of *Campylobacter* bacteria-contaminated carcasses] by around 40%." But, a "zero tolerance" policy is impractical, the industry emphasizes, "because it is impossible to achieve at reasonable cost."[2026] Leaving the caked layer of fecal material is another example of "least cost production," not least risk.

Low-cost poultry housing often means dirt floors.[2027] Every time the shed is cleaned, some of the dirt is scraped up, eventually requiring replacement with more dirt. Concrete floors are easier to clean more frequently, but are more expensive. "We're really locked into the system we've got," Jones said. "It would cost dearly to change it now."

In a specially commissioned feature on preventing disease to celebrate *Poultry International*'s forty-year publishing history, the trade magazine noted: "Replacing used litter between flocks is a standard practice worldwide, but it will not gain acceptance in the United States." The investment would evidently not be worth the return. "[U]nless federal regulations force drastic changes," the article concluded, "nothing spectacular should be expected."[2028]

No Sunlight

When poultry sheds are eventually scooped out, some of the scrapings—about one million tons per year—are fed to American cattle,[2029] and some are spread upon cropland as fertilizer. Out in the open air, combined with the sanitizing rays of the sun, the tons of manure rapidly dry and the fecal microbes rapidly die.[2030] Inside dimly lit sheds, however, human pathogens like *Salmonella*[2031] and *Campylobacter*[2032] thrive in the moist litter. So may viruses like H5N1.

Transmission experiments with chickens reveal that the spread of H5N1 is predominantly via the fecal-oral route rather than in respiratory droplets. H5N1 can survive in wet feces for weeks, but, at ambient temperatures, it is inactivated as soon as the feces dry out.[2033] In an outdoor, free-range setting, then, the spread of bird flu viruses like H5N1 would be expected to be relatively inefficient.

In countries like Thailand, the combination of tropical heat and crowded confinement necessitates "evaporative cooling" in poultry sheds, which uses large fans and a water mist to cool down the birds during the hot season. Although this reduces heat stress, the high level of humidity ensures that the litter is kept moist, which may facilitate the spread of pathogens like bird flu. These "evap houses" increase flock survival, but may increase virus survival as well.[2034]

Farther north in China, some poultry flocks may be outdoors most of the year but taken inside during the cold winter months, offering researchers a unique opportunity to compare bird flu activity in flocks confined indoors versus those let outside. Indeed, bird flu outbreaks are likelier to occur when the birds are crammed inside. Although this may be due to other factors, such as increased viral survival at colder temperatures, the FAO blames in part the winter confinement.[2035] Increased crowding indoors with suboptimal ventilation,[2036] combined with less solar radiation across the Earth's surface,[2037] may be one of the reasons why the human flu season flips every year between the northern and southern hemispheres following the winter.

"Birds that are housed indoors year-round should be considered more susceptible to infectious diseases," an avian virus textbook reads, "because of decreased air quality, the accumulation of pathogens in a restricted environment, and the lack of exposure to sunlight. These factors function collectively to decrease a bird's natural resistance to disease."[2038]

The absence of adequate ventilation and sunlight inherent to intensive confinement is a powerful combination for the spread of influenza. Perhaps the best studied illustration of the danger of crowded enclosed spaces in human medicine was a commercial airline flight in 1977 that was stuck on a tarmac for more than four hours due to a mechanical failure—while a young woman lay prostrate in the back of the cabin feverishly coughing with the flu. Within three days, nearly three out of four of her fellow passengers were destined to share in her pain.[2039] Laboratory studies on animals show the same thing: Decreased air exchange is strongly associated with increased influenza infection rate.[2040]

Lessons can be learned from past pandemics. In 1918, as Boston hospitals filled beyond capacity, a tent hospital was set up in nearby Brookline. Though exposing ailing patients to the chilly Boston autumn was condemned by Bostonians as "barbarous and cruel," it turned out that the fresh breeze and sunshine seemed to afford the overflow patients far better odds of survival than those inside the overcrowded, poorly ventilated hospitals.[2041]

A study of the 1957–58 pandemic demonstrated the potential role of sunlight. Ultraviolet rays damage genetic material. That's why we get a sunburn. The ultraviolet light in the sun's rays damages DNA in our skin, triggering the inflammation that manifests as redness and pain.[2042] Ultraviolet lights, then, have been used in tuberculosis wards to kill off some of the TB bugs coughed into the air. To see if influenza could be killed in the same way, researchers compared influenza rates in patients in TB buildings with UV lights to patients in TB buildings without UV lights during the pandemic. In the rooms without UV, 19 percent got the flu; in rooms with the UV lights only 2 percent became infected, a statistically significant difference.[2043] This suggests that sunlight may help sanitize influenza virus from the air, highlighting the increased risk of crowding poultry indoors. For flocks raised outdoors, according to the FAO, the natural UV rays of the sun may "destroy any residual virus."[2044]

If sunlight has such a disinfectant quality, why doesn't the industry install windows to allow some natural sunlight to perhaps cut down on airborne fecal pollutants? More light means chickens become more active, which means, as one poultry industry trade journal describes, "birds burn energy on activity rather than on growth and development." Natural lighting has a negative impact on "feed conversion."[2045] In other words, the animals "waste" energy on moving instead of just growing fatter to reach slaughter weight faster. According to *Broiler Industry*, "It is obvious that the light supplied by sunshine during the day and normal darkness at night is the most inferior of any lighting program."[2046]

Bred to Be Sick

Immune competence among modern poultry strains may be at an all-time low. Breeding for production traits, like increased breast muscle in birds raised for meat or increased laying ability in egg breeds, seems to necessarily mean breeding for decreased immune function. Given the intensive breeding-out of immune functionality, almost all modern commercial chickens may be "physically compromised" in a way that would facilitate wild waterfowl viruses taking hold. "[D]omestic poultry have been bred to be plump and succulent rather than disease-resistant," a senior virologist at the Australian Animal Health Laboratory pointed out. "[T]hey're sitting ducks, so to speak, for their wild cousins' viruses."[2047]

It wasn't until well into the twentieth century that the poultry industry began segregating chicken breeds—some for meat and others for eggs.[2048] Once maximum productivity became the emphasis, these two traits became mutually exclusive. For broiler chickens, "meat output per chick" is considered the most important goal,[2049] so the bigger the better.[2050] In contrast, the industry wants laying hens to be small. Big eggs from small bodies ensures that more of the feed goes into the egg rather than being "wasted" on the upkeep of the rest of the animal.[2051]

In the egg industry, "feed conversion," the conversion of feed into eggs, is considered the trait with the single biggest "impact on profitability." Modern egg-laying hens are bred to be so scrawny that it's not profitable to raise male chicks for meat. Since they can't lay eggs, male chicks are an unwanted by-product of the industry. It makes more economic sense to kill them shortly after hatching by the hundreds of millions[2052]—grinding them up alive, gassing them, or throwing them into a dumpster to suffocate or dehydrate[2053]—than to waste feed on them.[2054]

So, in the interest of maximizing productivity, two different lines of chickens were created, one for meat and another for eggs. As one historian noted, by the end of the 1950s, the "era of the designer chicken" had arrived.[2055] The results have been extraordinary. Selective breeding over time is, after all, what turned the wolf into a poodle. Ancestors to the modern-day chicken laid only about twenty-five eggs a year.[2056] Today's laying hens produce more than ten times that number,[2057] leading to increasing problems with uterine prolapse[2058] and broken bones due to critical weakening, as skeletal calcium is mobilized to form shells for the eggs.[2059]

The "essence"[2060] of broiler chicken production, as poultry scientists describe it, is "turning feed stuffs into meat."[2061] Chicken ancestors grew to be about two pounds in four months.[2062] In the 1950s, the industry could raise a five-pound chicken in less than three months. Due mostly to selective breeding (in addition to growth promoting drugs), this now takes an average of forty-five days.[2063] Broiler chickens now grow more than twice as large in less than half the time. To put the growth rate of today's broiler chickens into perspective, the University of Arkansas Division of Agriculture reported, "If you grew as fast as a chicken, you'd weigh 349 pounds at age two."[2064] In one century, as one historian relates, "the barnyard chicken was made over into a highly efficient machine for converting feed grains into cheap animal-flesh protein."[2065]

Interestingly, this transformation in chickens was considered such an "outstanding example of the contribution of breeding work"[2066] that many of the earliest poultry scientists helped form the American Breeders' Association,[2067] which went on to lead the human eugenics movement.[2068] Leading U.S. poultry scientist and eugenics pioneer Charles B. Davenport spoke of poultry breeding efforts as akin to "race improvement"[2069] and "purification."[2070] Likewise, Heinrich Himmler's experience with chicken breeding has been noted for having shaped his views on the subject.[2071]

The "improvement" of poultry over the last century has been deemed "quite profitable,"[2072] but the industry admits to the downsides. The editor of industry trade journals *WATT PoultryUSA* and the *Poultry Tribune* wrote, "Ongoing efforts to increase breast-meat yield, for example, have created a higher propensity for musculoskeletal problems, metabolic disease, immunodeficiency, and male infertility, primarily because the extra protein going to breast muscle production comes at the expense of internal organ development."[2073]

Today's broiler chickens grow so fast that they outpace their cardiovascular system's ability to keep up, leading to forms of heart failure like Sudden Death Syndrome (also known as "flip-over syndrome"). Heart failure is an increasingly[2074] major[2075] cause of mortality among commercial flocks, even though the birds are only a few weeks old. An industry journal reported that "broilers now grow so rapidly that the heart and lungs are not developed well enough to support the remainder of the body, resulting in congestive heart failure and tremendous death losses."[2076]

Mortality rates of broilers are up to seven times that of chickens not bred for fast growth.[2077] This tradeoff is accepted if the increased mortality is compensated for by an increase in meat yield or feed conversion. To maximize profits, commercial broiler producers accept a mortality rate of 5 percent.[2078]

Chickens aren't dying just because their circulatory systems are collapsing under the strain. Chickens bred for unnaturally developed muscles (meat) have unnaturally underdeveloped immune systems. Broiler chickens selected for accelerated growth suffer from weakened immunity, which increases mortality[2079] by making them "more susceptible to a variety of infectious diseases."[2080] When you breed for one characteristic, you may lose another. The modern tomato, for example, may be perfectly round and make it to market less bruised, but it also may be tough, pink, and tasteless compared to heirloom varieties. Just as purebred poodles tend to have problems with their hips, modern-day purebred chickens tend to have problems with their immune systems.

Even excluding heart failure, studies show that the highest mortality is seen in the fastest-growing chickens and the lowest mortality in the slowest-growing chickens. Researchers conclude, "It appears that broilers with faster growth rate are under physiological and immunological stress that makes them more sensitive to infectious diseases."[2081] This has been shown for both viral[2082] and bacterial[2083] pathogens. In one study, broiler chickens were intentionally infected with E. coli and 40 percent of the fast-growing, heavier birds died, compared to only 8 to 20 percent mortality for slower-growing breeds. The scientists commented, "These results indicate that rapid growth rate substantially reduces broiler viability."[2084]

Research with turkeys shows the same thing, despite the president of the National Turkey Federation's claim that "[r]ealty [sic] is that in this country the poultry industry treats the health of the birds as the number one issue."[2085] Lighter and slower-growing turkey breeds, in contrast to those conventionally used, have better immune performance[2086] and therefore are more resistant to stress[2087] and disease.[2088] Researchers have observed that in natural outbreaks of disease like fowl cholera,[2089] turkeys bred for increased egg production and those selected for increased body weight had significantly higher mortality rates.[2090] Slower-growing, lighter breeds of turkeys also have greater adaptability to the stresses associated with production, such as overcrowding.[2091] USDA researchers at the University of Arkansas went so far as to suggest in a paper in *Poultry Science* that "fast growth in modern turkey lines" may result in stress responses "incompatible with the severe stressors that sometimes occur during commercial poultry production."[2092]

The turkey industry has so altered the natural order that the enormous breast meat mass of commercial breeds has resulted in the birds being physically incapable of mating.[2093] "One hundred percent artificial insemination," researchers note in *Livestock Production Science*, "allowed for the continuation of intense selection for body weight in male lines."[2094] Female turkeys are inseminated by tube or syringe.[2095]

Selection has been so intense that commercial turkeys, like broiler chickens, can barely support their own weight. A staff editor of the leading U.S. livestock feed industry publication wrote that "turkeys have been bred to grow faster and heavier but their skeletons haven't kept pace, which causes 'cowboy legs.' Commonly, the turkeys have problems standing . . . and fall and are trampled on or seek refuge under feeders, leading to bruises and downgradings as well as culled or killed birds."[2096] One group of researchers concluded, "We consider that birds might have been bred to grow so fast that they are on the verge of structural collapse."[2097]

Many do collapse and spend much of their time lying in their own waste. Similar to broiler chickens, most turkeys in commercial production are overcrowded in warehouse-like sheds and the majority[2098] suffer from ulcerative contact dermatitis, from breast blisters to bedsore-like hock burns.[2099] These painful lesions add to the stress that may impair overall immune performance. USDA researchers conclude: "Selection of poultry for fast growth rate is often accompanied by a reduction in specific immune responses or increased disease susceptibility."[2100]

Slower growth is costly, but so are disease outbreaks. Why doesn't the industry select for birds with improved immune responses? They've tried. Early in the industry's history, rather crude methods were used to try to breed for resistance. Breeders would take baby chicks and challenge their immune systems by exposing them to adults with Marek's disease, a poultry disease caused by a cancer-causing herpes virus. Those who lived through the exposure went on to create the next generation, one that would presumably be more resistant to the disease.[2101] No one wants to bite into a tumor at KFC.

Sometimes the chicks didn't get infected by casual exposure, though. Breeders found that by dripping virus-laden blood from infected chickens into the eyes of baby chicks, they were able to guarantee infection, but this produced mortality rates between 30 and 60 percent. It was not considered economical to kill more than half the chicks. "Challenge by intraperitoneal injection of whole blood or suspensions of fresh tumorous gonads from clinically sick birds was also tested," poultry scientists report, "but later discontinued because the mortality rates exceeded the optimum of 50%." The intent was to kill off half the chicks, but injecting ground-up tumorous sex organs into the abdomens of baby chicks turned out to be a little too fatal.[2102]

Challenge tests continue in poultry breeding, but on a much smaller scale.[2103] This kind of direct selection is considered "inconvenient" in intensive production systems due to the costs involved.[2104] Breeders have tried selecting for antibody response directly, but poultry scientists have found that those with the best antibody responses consistently had significantly lower weights at all ages.[2105] Research dating back several decades shows that chickens bred to be disease-resistant have lower body weight and produce smaller eggs.[2106] Studies suggest that immune defects may actually enhance poultry performance.[2107] Seems like you can have one or the other—immunity or growth—and the industry chooses growth.

This happens across species. Growth and disease susceptibility have been shown to go hand in hand in pigs,[2108] cattle,[2109] and dairy cows. Over the past century, genetic manipulation of dairy cows through selective breeding has tripled the annual milk yield to eighteen thousand pounds of milk per cow. It took the first half of the last century to force the first ton increase, but since the 1980s, the industry has managed to add extra tons every eight or nine years.[2110] Turning cows into milk factories has taken a toll on their immune systems,[2111] increasing their risk of mastitis,[2112] infections of the udder. Mastitis may be painful for the animal and spike the milk supply with increasing levels of somatic (pus) cells, but decreased cow immunity, as opposed to decreased chicken immunity, is unlikely to aid and abet in the killing of millions of people.

Why is immunity reduced when production is maximized? Our best understanding is the "resource allocation theory." There is only a certain amount of energy, protein, and other nutrients coming into an animal's system at any one time. Those resources can go to build muscle or to host defense, like a national budget in which money is divided between the country's infrastructure and homeland security. So dairy cows, for example, have been bred to "redirect resources from the maintenance of an adequate immune system to milk production in order to maintain advantages in milk yield," reads one dairy science textbook.[2113] This is a trade-off between production traits and immunocompetence.[2114]

Studies show that old-fashioned, slower-growing chicken breeds have larger[2115] and better developed[2116] antibody-producing immune organs. Instead of being bred to transfer the bulk of resources to build breast meat while neglecting other needs, these slower-growing breeds had sufficient resources to foster a more functional antibody response system.[2117] Antibodies are critically important for vaccine effectiveness, particularly in animals like broiler chickens who are killed after only a handful of weeks of life and don't have time to acquire a set of their own immune memories. "Those animals which are intensively reared and slaughtered young," notes one agricultural microbiologist, "will have the greatest potential for carrying pathogens."[2118]

One of the reasons that 1 to 4 percent of broiler chickens die from "acute death syndrome"[2119] (in which chickens suddenly lose their balance, violently flap their wings, go into spasms, and die of acute heart failure) is that the metabolic demand for oxygen created by the increasing muscle mass leaves the rest of their body short of oxygen.[2120] Forget immunity—many modern broiler chickens can hardly keep up with breathing and can outgrow their lungs, hearts, and immune systems.

The maintenance of an effective immune system is metabolically very costly.[2121] The "big eater" macrophage immune cells burn through almost as much energy as maximally functioning heart muscle.[2122] Antibodies are made out of protein. When the body is churning out thousands of antibodies per second, there is less protein available for growth. Studies show that chickens capable of mounting a decent antibody response have lower weight and lower weight gain than chickens with suboptimal antibody production.[2123]

Germ-free chicks raised in germ-free environments grow faster than chickens in unsanitary environments.[2124] Even minute exposures to the normal microbial flora of the gut are enough of an immune stimulus to significantly reduce growth rates.[2125] Though there's no tissue damage and no evidence of disease, just the normal day-to-day functioning of the immune system diverts energy from maximal growth.[2126] That's why you can feed germ-free chickens in a sanitary laboratory environment all the antibiotics you want and there will be no change in growth rates, whereas commercially confined chickens fed antibiotics demonstrate a remarkable spurt in growth.[2127] By breeding for maximum production, the industry seems to be breeding for minimum immunity.

The reason that selecting for growth impairs immunity is the same reason that human AIDS and tuberculosis patients waste away. Fighting off infection requires a remarkable demand for energy and nutrients. The body shifts resources away from nonessential anabolic (meaning growth, as in "anabolic steroids") and maintenance processes toward bolstering life-or-death defenses.[2128] This redistribution of resources makes sense from an evolutionary point of view. What use is long-term growth when short-term survival is threatened? Not only are the body's construction projects halted, but they start to be torn down for raw materials. People with severe infections can lose up to one-third of their body weight as the body starts eating away at itself to feed more fuel into the immune machine.[2129]

Even relatively insignificant challenges to the immune system can significantly affect growth. Simple vaccinations can result in a greater than 20 percent decline in daily weight gain for farm animals and increase protein demands as much as 30 percent,[2130] demonstrating the perverse balance between growth and immunity. The poultry industry can't have it both ways.

Before domestication, natural selection chose strong immune systems for survival.[2131] After domestication, though, "[a]rtificial selection concentrated on improvement of production traits with little attention to resistance to disease,"[2132] reads one poultry breeding textbook. The industry seems more interested in the survival of the fattest, not the fittest.[2133]

Animals are preprogrammed by evolution to grow at the near optimal rate. The faster a juvenile animal grows to maturity in the wild, the faster he or she would presumably be able to win out over competing suitors to mate and produce more offspring. This would tend to select for maximum growth rates, but resource allocation is not the only reason Mother Nature puts on the brakes. Even in a germ-free environment, cells cannot divide and grow while simultaneously performing at peak efficiency.

Faster-growing fish, for example, swim less efficiently than slower-growing fish.[2134] Faster-growing rainbow trout have been shown to have significantly impaired swimming performance.[2135] Salmon genetically engineered to grow more than twice as fast by length as control fish have half the critical swimming speed, meaning the control fish swim twice as fast.[2136] Not only do broiler chickens bred for accelerated growth have smaller immune organs, but what little immunity they do have may not be functioning effectively.

The budgetary analogy, therefore, is imperfect. It's not that there is just a certain amount of resources to go around and every dollar spent on infrastructure is a dollar not spent on defense. It's worse than that. By forcing broiler chickens to divert the lion's share of resources to fast growth, not only is host security left to hold bake sales, but immune defenses may be actively undermined, too.

The industry has tried to shore up the imposed deficiencies with feed restriction programs, improved sanitation, and chemoprophylactic treatments.[2137] As USDA researchers note in a *Poultry Science* article, "Much of the progress seen in intensive poultry production over the past 50 yr has been possible due to the availability of very effective and inexpensive antibiotics which have prevented stress-induced opportunistic bacterial disease and allowed efficient production even as density and growth rate increased." The researchers go on to show displeasure that human health concerns are pressuring the industry away from such crutches.[2138]

Despite drugs and new vaccines, the head of the prestigious Wageningen University Animal Production Systems group reached the sobering conclusion long ago that a modern broiler chicken "still cannot cope adequately with its pathogenic environment."[2139] There is only so far we may be able to subordinate chicken biology to the dictates of industrial production before running into unintended consequences.[2140] "We are severely changing the way these animals grow," remarked one poultry geneticist in "High Yielding Broiler Production: The Big Trade-Off," an article in *Broiler Industry*. "I believe the time is rapidly approaching when management alone won't be able to overcome the genetic problems because of the metabolic stresses that are being put on these birds."[2141] Or, as Rachel Carson put it nearly sixty years ago, "Nature fights back."[2142]

The history of industrial agriculture in general is replete with technological fixes associated with unforeseen consequences, such as DDT. An academic history of the broiler industry views intensive poultry production as paradigmatic in this regard. The author writes:

> Virtually every effort to further industrialize broiler [chicken] biology
> has resulted in the emergence of new risks and vulnerabilities. Intensive
> confinement combined with increased genetic uniformity has created new
> opportunities for the spread of pathogens. Increased breast-meat yield has
> come at the expense of increased immunodeficiency. And, of course, widespread
> recourse to antibiotics has created a niche for the proliferation of resistant
> bacteria.[2143]

In an industry whose bottom line is *the* bottom line, though, it all makes good business sense.

The poultry industry accepts the fact that broilers with the fastest growth rates start suffering from heart failure as they reach slaughter-weight and may just keel over dead, even after they have "already consumed almost all of their feed allowance and therefore taking the largest possible slice out of the profit."[2144] But not only is that readily factored into the equation, it may be welcomed as a sign of good breeding. As one chicken farmer wrote, "Aside from the stupendous rate of growth . . . the sign of a good meat flock is the number of birds dying from heart attacks."[2145]

An interesting proviso is added by leading poultry breeding expert Gerard Albers. Although "decisions in the poultry industry are largely and increasingly driven by economic considerations," Albers notes, "the psychological impact of flock morbidity and mortality on the farmer cannot be ignored. Mortality rates above a certain psychological threshold are unacceptable." The excess mortality may just become too disturbing. Albers is not optimistic, though, that breeding for "increased livability" will take precedence over selection for "more profitable" traits.[2146]

The same attitude pervades the egg industry. In an article titled "Industrial Perspective on Problems and Issues Associated with Poultry Breeding," laying hen breeding corporations insist that "[e]gg production per hen housed will continue to be the single most important trait under selection."[2147]

In the broiler chicken industry, the costs of production diseases are estimated at 10 to 20 percent of total production costs,[2148] a small price to pay for jumbo-sized birds. It is simply not in the financial interest of the industry to fully mitigate disease rates. As poultry researchers have asked, "Is it more profitable to grow the biggest bird and have increased mortality due to heart attacks, ascites [heart failure], and leg problems, or should birds be grown slower so that birds are smaller, but have fewer heart, lung, and skeletal problems?" Their answer? "A large portion of growers' pay is based on the pound of saleable meat produced, so simple calculations suggest that it is better to get the weight and ignore the mortality."[2149] In the face of bird flu viruses like H5N1, though, the deaths of chickens aren't the only mortalities the industry may be ignoring.

The industry could breed for improved immunity even though it has "been shown to result in decreased body weight,"[2150] but openly admits that "disease resistance will not be selected for if the cost in a loss of genetic improvements in other traits is too great." The industry prefers to externalize, or pass along, disease costs to the human population. "For example," an industry breeding text reads, "to select for effective resistance to *Salmonella* would currently cost so much in performance that it would be totally unfeasible."[2151] It doesn't seem to matter that *Salmonella* continue to plague poultry in the United States,[2152] nor that hundreds of Americans die from *Salmonella* every year.[2153] Let the consumers sterilize their meat thermometers and be extra careful not to drip a drop of fecal fluid on their kitchen floor so as not to risk killing their toddler.

Europe has been reconsidering its breeding program. The European Commission's Scientific Committee broiler report stated that its "most important recommendation" was that "[b]reeders should give a considerably higher priority to health variables in the breeding index, if necessary at the expense of the selection pressure for growth and feed conversion."[2154] Meanwhile in the United States, growth rates continue to be pushed faster every year.[2155] One poultry specialist mused, "Mathematically, it is evident that the present rate of improvement in growth cannot be continued for more than a couple of decades, or the industry will be faced with a bird that virtually explodes upon hatching."[2156]

H5N1 ought to have been the wake-up call to industry breeders that myopic breeding schemes prioritizing growth over health threaten the continued viability of their industry.[2157] The message does not seem to have gotten through. "In broilers," poultry researchers wrote, "part of the immune response seems to dysfunction due to the genetic selection on bodyweight and feed conversion. Nevertheless, broilers seem to be able to survive with this immune response in the present husbandry systems."[2158] Five percent tend not to last six weeks, but enough do survive to economically justify the system. Their dysfunctional immune systems may make them convenient viral fodder, though, for the initiation and spread of bird flu viruses with human pandemic potential.

Monoculture

A handful of corporations supply most of the breeding stock for all the world's poultry. As much as 95 percent of the world's poultry was provided by four turkey breeding companies, five egg-laying chicken breeders, and five broiler breeder companies.[2159] Soon, the industry predicted, there may essentially only be three poultry breeders in the world.[2160] A single pedigree cockerel can potentially give rise to two million broiler chickens.[2161]

Mass consolidation has positive and negative aspects. On the plus side, selection decisions can be propagated across the entire world in a matter of years. If the industry decided to prioritize selection for stronger immunity, in three or four years, practically the entire global flock could be replaced with the improved disease-resistant variety. The flip side is that further emphasis on production traits with detrimental effects on immunity are distributed at the same speed.[2162] Another downside is the increasing genetic uniformity of poultry worldwide, which alone may increase the susceptibility of the global flock to disease.[2163]

According to the FAO, over the last century, a thousand farm animal breeds—about one-sixth of the world's cattle and poultry varieties—have disappeared.[2164] Breeds continue to go extinct at a rate of one or two every *week*. More than a thousand breeds—one out of four of all livestock varieties—are facing extinction.[2165] The greatest threat to farm animal diversity, according to the FAO, is the export of high-producing breeding stock from industrialized to developing countries that dilutes, or completely displaces, local native breeds.[2166]

This erosion of biodiversity has human public health consequences. The American Association of Swine Veterinarians explained why the genetic bottlenecking created by narrowly focused breeding schemes may be a main reason for the mounting concern over human zoonotic diseases: "As genetic improvement falls into the hands of fewer companies and the trend towards intense multiplication of a limited range of genotypes (monoculture, cloning) develops, there is mounting concern that large populations may have increasingly uniform vulnerability to particular pathogens."[2167] This is the risk posed by any type of agricultural mono-cropping.

We can learn from past mistakes. In the early 1970s, for example, the U.S. corn industry developed "Tcms" corn, a highly profitable strain adapted for large-scale farming. Only after 85 percent of the nation's seed corn acreage was covered with the new variety did the industry realize that the strain also happened to be particularly susceptible to a rare form of leaf blight fungus that then wiped out areas of the U.S. corn belt.[2168]

Turkey producers have the option of rearing heritage breeds and so "may be able to improve both disease resistance and the safety of their poultry products," University of Arkansas poultry scientists point out, "by choosing slower growing commercial lines."[2169] There may not be sufficiently slow-growing commercial lines of broiler chickens from which to choose at present, but they could be created if sufficient political will were directed at such a task.

The American industry began injecting genetic diversity from native Chinese lines of heirloom chickens in hopes of strengthening the immunity of the U.S. flock. "Some of the Chinese chickens have been shown to be very disease resistant," explained one Hong Kong University zoologist. "Because they have not been under heavy selective breeding, in general their disease resistance is very high."[2170] Given the inverse relationship between immunity and accelerated growth, though, the industry may not go far enough.

In response to the stalemate between disease resistance and short-term profitability, the industry has been experimenting with creating a transgenic "superchicken," genetically engineered to be resistant to avian influenza.[2171] This is reminiscent of the cattle industry's attempt to invent mad cow disease–resistant cattle. Might it not be more prudent to simply stop feeding slaughterhouse waste to natural herbivores? Prudent, perhaps, but hardly economical.

Biodiversity is biosecurity. Even the most virulent of diseases typically do not kill all infected individuals, in part due to natural inborn genetic variability. In the wild, natural selection takes advantage of this variation to pass disease-resistant qualities to the next generation.[2172] The diversity in nature tends to ensure that some individuals will survive whatever comes along. Artificial selection for production qualities undermines Mother Nature in two ways: by inbreeding unnaturally elevated egg production and fleshiness over fitness, and by reducing the genetic diversity that can act as resistance insurance against present and unforeseen threats of disease.[2173]

Acquired Immunodeficiency Syndromes

The relationship between immune-weakening poultry viruses and bird flu was first proposed by University of Hong Kong zoologist Frederick Leung and later expanded upon by anthropologist and agroecologist Ronald Nigh.[2174] Leung noted a speculative correlation between Hong Kong chicken farms that had suffered outbreaks of an immunodeficiency virus known as infectious bursal disease virus (IBDV) in 1996 and the subsequent initial outburst of H5N1 about six months later in 1997.[2175]

The bursa is a specialized avian organ responsible primarily for the development of a bird's immune system.[2176] That's how human antibody-producing "B-cells" got their name, since they were first discovered in chickens.[2177] Just as HIV in humans replicates in white blood cells called *T-helper cells,* leading to their destruction and the body's subsequent immunodeficiency, IBDV in birds infects B-cells, crippling the immune system and leaving survivors immunosuppressed for life.[2178] With a "severely impaired"[2179] ability to produce antibodies, surviving birds respond poorly to vaccinations[2180] and are susceptible to a wide variety of viral, bacterial, and parasitic diseases.[2181]

Beginning in the 1980s—a couple of decades after IBDV was identified[2182]—the United States started seeing a dramatic increase in chickens suffering from various respiratory infections. Vaccines no longer seemed to be working as effectively.[2183] Investigators discovered that a new hypervirulent strain had arisen in the most concentrated poultry production area in the world,[2184] the Delmarva peninsula, incorporating corners of Delaware, Maryland, and Virginia.[2185] The Delaware variant, as it was called, started its march around the world in the late 1980s,[2186] thanks in part to a "high concentration of poultry in close proximity."[2187] There is even evidence that IBDV of domestic chickens has been detected in Emperor penguins in the Antarctic, an example of industrial animal agriculture's "pathogen pollution" to the farthest reaches of the globe.[2188]

There has also been a dramatic increase in the virulence of another viral affliction—Marek's disease (MD), first described a century ago[2189]—since the 1960s.[2190] Besides tumors in the skin, muscles (meat), nerves, and abdominal organs of chickens, the Marek's disease herpes virus also causes immunosuppression.[2191] A major scientific review describes the evolution of virulence in what is now a familiar story:

> Poultry production up to the mid 1900s mainly comprised backyard farming with very low population densities of birds . . . with low growth rates and low egg production. In this environment, MD was not considered as a major disease even though outbreaks of MD were reported in different parts of the world. However, since the 1960s there have been major changes in poultry production practices. Today poultry production has become a major global industry operating in very high population densities under highly intensive management conditions aimed at higher rates of growth and productivity . . . Until about 1960, when the poultry production was not on an intensive scale, both the virus and the hosts were able to achieve a state of balanced

*co-existence. However, the transformation of the poultry industry into the
intensive production practices from the early 1960s saw a shift in this balance
greatly in favor of the virus. The continuous availability of large populations
of genetically susceptible naïve hosts, usually in an overcrowded environment,
enabled the virus to spread rapidly, encouraging their rapid evolution towards
greater virulence. This was evident when huge MD outbreaks swept through
poultry flocks in the 1960s, wiping out large populations all around the
world.*[2192]

The first wave of evolution in the late 1950s shifted the virus from
"mMDV" (mild Marek's disease virus) to "vMDV" (virulent Marek's disease
virus). Due in part to continued and escalating industrial practices, "vMDV"
became "vvMDV." Presently, the world is dealing with "vv+MDV."[2193] The
industry created yet another monster.

Other immunosuppressant viruses include chicken infectious anemia virus (CIAV) and a virus that causes hemorrhagic enteritis in turkeys.[2194] CIAV
was first described in 1979[2195] and has since spread throughout the world
to become ubiquitous in egg and meat-type chickens worldwide.[2196] CIAV
destroys immune precursor cells, undermining the immune system before
it can even develop.[2197] Immunosuppression associated with CIAV is considered to be a factor in "many of the disease problems in flocks raised under the
high-density conditions of modern poultry production."[2198]

These immunodeficiency viruses can interact with each other to syn-
ergistically further predispose the global chicken flock to infection. CIAV
infection, for example, can boost the virulence of Marek's virus,[2199] and
co-infection between IBDV and CIAV can result in an even more profound
vulnerability to additional infectious disease agents.[2200] A poultry scientist
working for Tyson described the U.S. poultry industry as being "in a constant battle with immunosuppressive diseases."[2201]

The unhygienic conditions under which commercial poultry are confined
conspire to spread these viruses. Infection with Marek's disease occurs when
a chicken inhales infected dust in a poultry shed saturated with virus flaking
directly off the chickens' skin.[2202] The emergence of new strains of IBDV has
also been blamed in part on "improper cleaning and disinfection."[2203] One
reason why the industry *doesn't* clean and disinfect sheds more frequently
is that they want young breeding chickens to get infected with viruses like
CIAV early on in the hopes they will clear the infection before egg laying

leads to progeny with "poorer performance."[2204] Immunodeficiency diseases like Marek's cost the poultry industry more than a billion dollars a year,[2205] but cleaning up its act might cost even more. One animal science textbook explains that "compromise inevitably must be struck because animal agriculture is a business, and providing the best environment possible may be unprofitable."[2206]

None of these viruses affect humans directly, but with the threat of bird flu, anything that leads to immune suppression in chickens may now be an issue of human public health importance. The same factory farming conditions that facilitated the emergence of killer viruses like H5N1 are leading to the emergence—and spread—of immunodeficiency viruses that may themselves be partially responsible for H5N1 and may midwife even deadlier pandemic strains into the world.

GUARDING THE HENHOUSE

Chicken Run

Clearly, stressful and overcrowded confinement in industrial poultry facilities facilitates immune suppression in birds already bred with weakened immunity, offering viruses like bird flu ample opportunities for spread, amplification, and mutation. Placing inbred birds into these kinds of unsanitary environments without a breath of fresh air or a ray of sanitizing sunshine seems the perfect crucible for the evolution of the next superflu strain of pandemic influenza. Why then has there been concern about the opposite: free-range flocks?

Sociography scholar Mike Davis blames the international corporate poultry sector for launching a global offensive to blame small producers,[2207] the hundreds of millions of farmers raising a dozen or so birds in their backyards.[2208] The commercial poultry industry boasts of "biosecurity," described as the industry's "buzzword du jour,"[2209] arguing that keeping birds confined indoors year-round protects them from exposure to wild birds and any diseases they might be carrying.[2210] The U.S. National Pork Board defends large-scale pig confinement using the same rationale.[2211]

After the Hong Kong outbreak, Webster wrote that hypothetically, past outbreaks of high-grade viruses "could probably have been prevented if domestic poultry had been raised in ecologically controlled houses that maintained a high standard of security and limited access."[2212] This makes sense, but only in theory. In practice, whether trying to stem the spread of H5N1 or prevent outbreaks of highly pathogenic bird flu in the first place, locking birds in industrial confinement operations may increase the public health risk on a global scale.

The Thai poultry industry has used bird flu as an excuse to further industrialize its production systems. Thai poultry baron billionaire Dhanin Chearavanont, a leader in the "Tysonization" of Southeast Asia, convinced the government that his factory farms were the safest way to raise chickens,[2213] effectively forcing thousands of small farmers out of business. The government started yoking peasants under contract to corporate "chicken farming estates"[2214] and mandated that only owners of closed farms would receive compensation for restocking flocks culled for disease control.[2215] But H5N1 has wiped out birds on "closed" farms, too. One of Chearavanont's own farms containing more than a hundred thousand birds became infected.[2216] Likewise, despite millions of free-range chickens in France[2217] and Nigeria,[2218] the first outbreaks in Europe and Africa, respectively, involved a farm confining more than eleven thousand turkeys[2219] and a battery cage egg facility in which forty thousand chickens died.[2220]

Neighboring Cambodia and Laos present case studies for comparison. While Thailand industrialized production so heavily that it became the fourth largest poultry exporter in the world,[2221] the majority of poultry production in Cambodia and Laos had remained extensive (rather than intensive) and comprised largely of farmers with small outdoor flocks. In which countries did bird flu spread to the greatest extent? In the countries where most birds were intensively confined indoors, or in those where most of the chickens were raised outdoors? According to the Food and Agriculture Organization, "Evidence suggests that HPAI [Highly Pathogenic Avian Influenza] did not become established in Cambodia to the extent that it did in Vietnam and Thailand," the two countries on either side of Cambodia. "This may be attributable in large part to the primarily extensive nature of the poultry industry (poultry density in Cambodia is much lower (less than 30%) than in Thailand and Vietnam)."[2222]

The USDA reported a similar phenomenon in Laos, the other country sandwiched between Thailand and Vietnam. Of the few outbreaks that did occur in Laos, more than 90 percent broke out in commercial poultry operations, not free-ranging flocks.[2223] Past outbreaks of bird flu offer further hindsight.

In 2004, while H5N1 was blasting across southeast Asia, a highly pathogenic H7N3 outbreak swept through Canada's Fraser Valley east of Vancouver.[2224] Dozens of poultry workers involved in the gassing and incineration of the nineteen million chickens culled developed symptoms of infection.[2225] Laboratory-confirmed bird flu infections in two workers[2226] prompted the World Health Organization to raise Canada's "pandemic preparedness level" to the same as those Asian countries affected by H5N1.[2227] Canadian agricultural interests in government seemed no better than their Asian counterparts in terms of transparency: The Canadian Food Inspection Agency not only initially denied the existence of human infections to the public but also withheld the information from the provincial Centre for Disease Control, an omission the Centre said "could have had severe consequences."[2228] Thankfully, both infected workers and all other presumed human cases resolved without reported complication.[2229]

The backyard chicken farmers blamed the commercial industry for the outbreak[2230] and the industry blamed the small farmers.[2231] An industry spokesperson not only denied that high-density broiler chicken sheds played a role in the outbreak, but challenged the assertion that the sheds were overcrowded at all. "Anything that creates a better environment for our birds," the spokesperson said, "basically makes our industry stronger."[2232]

"Only healthy animals produce" is a common defense used by proponents of factory farming. Profitability does depend on productivity, but productivity is not measured on a per-animal basis. "Productivity," according to University of California–Davis poultry specialist Joy Mench, "is often measured at the level of the unit (e.g., number of eggs or egg mass per hen-housed), and individual animals may be in a comparatively poor state of welfare even though productivity within the unit may be high."[2233] Some of the worst problems are created by some of the most profitable practices, such as breeding for accelerated growth rates,[2234] which, as I've discussed, leaves many birds crippled, brittle-boned, bloated from heart failure, and scarred with ammonia burns after squatting in their own waste and that of countless others. Industry insiders admit that the "success of the modern poultry industry has also created an environment very favourable to highly contagious agents."[2235]

Publicly, the industry denies culpability. Internally, it admits to "the growing realization that viruses previously innocuous to natural host species have in all probability become more virulent by passage through large commercial populations."[2236] An article in the trade journal *Poultry International* offers a concise explanation of the role of large-scale production:

> The AI virus lives harmlessly in the ducks popular in Asia to control insect pests and snails in rice paddies. If this duck flu passes to chickens kept nearby, it can mutate into a deadly and highly contagious strain that speeds rapidly with accompanying high mortality. The larger the flocks and the more intensive the production level, the more scope there is for the disease to spread for genetic changes to the virus.[2237]

The same conclusion was reached by many in the Canadian scientific community. University of Ottawa's Earl Brown explained to the Canadian press: "If you get a [H5 or H7] virus into a high-density poultry operation and give it a period of time, generally a year or so, then you turn that virus into a highly virulent virus. That's what always happens."[2238] Canada's National Manager of Disease Control within the Food Inspection Agency seemed to agree: "Just passing the virus to 3,000 or 4,000 chickens is enough to change a harmless virus into something more pathogenic."[2239] "It is high-density chicken farming that gives rise to highly-virulent influenza viruses," Brown concluded. "That's pretty clear."[2240]

These conclusions were based on the best available science. The Canadian outbreak first erupted not in a backyard flock or free-range farm, but at an entirely enclosed, "sophisticated" industrial facility. It then jumped from broiler shed to broiler shed, largely skipping free-range farms.[2241] The spread of the virus was traced mainly to the human lateral transmission of infective feces via equipment or some other fomite moved from farm to farm.[2242] This may also explain how the virus was first introduced into the industrial broiler houses to begin with. Chickens don't need to come in direct contact with ducks to get infected; they just need contact with the virus, which can be walked into a "biosecure" operation on someone's clothing.[2243]

In the end, epidemiological analyses placed commercial flocks in the 2004 Canadian outbreak at 5.6 times likelier to be infected than backyard flocks. Infected backyard flocks were discovered *after* nearby commercial flocks were infected, suggesting that the virus spread from the industrialized operations to free-range poultry, and not vice versa.[2244] Yes, birds kept outdoors are likelier to come into contact with wild waterfowl, but they also come into regular contact with sunlight, space, and fresh air. Lower stress levels may help their bodies better resist the initial infection, and, since they don't live on layers of their own waste while cramped into poorly ventilated sheds by the tens of thousands, the virus may not spread effectively enough to mutate into a killer. Instead of blaming backyard flocks, attention should be turned, as a former *Vancouver Sun* editor put it, to the factory farms, the "profitable vulnerabilities built into our food supply."[2245]

The largest outbreak of avian influenza before H5N1 exploded in 2004 was the 2003 outbreak of highly pathogenic H7N7 in the Netherlands that laid to waste thirty million birds,[2246] infected more than a thousand people,[2247] and killed an investigating veterinarian.[2248] In an article titled "Why Factory Farms and Mass Trade Make for a World Where Disease Travels Far and Fast," the Consumer Affairs correspondent for *The Guardian* wrote that the disease "spread like wildfire through the country's intensive poultry industry," blanketing hundreds of operations[2249] and expanding into Belgium and Germany.[2250] Despite biosecurity control measures, it was found to be impossible to contain and only seemed to stop once it had burned through the boundaries of dense poultry production.[2251]

While some blame the rise in factory farming for this outbreak, others blame the rise in free-range farming.[2252] Free-range flocks were not, however, found to be at increased risk during the outbreak.[2253] According to a review in *World Poultry,*

> A notable feature of the Dutch epidemic was that large, densely-stocked flocks were worst affected. Some extensively managed [as opposed to intensively managed] flocks were infected by the virus without showing significant illness of either birds or people. This does not mean that everyone should return to high-cost, low-output, production systems . . . but it does mean that some producers might usefully soften housing and management systems which put excessive strain on birds in terms of stocking density, air quality, group size, population instability and general vitality.

After the article goes on to admit to concern that intensive confinement systems may be critically weakening the birds' immune systems and putting the entire poultry industry at risk, it ends by declaring that "a chain is only as strong as its weakest link!"[2254]

Although the Dutch virus did kill one person, most of the symptoms it caused were mild and hundreds of those infected showed no symptoms at all. However, some who did develop symptoms were able to pass the virus to others in their households. Adapting to chickens seems to have adapted the virus to humans.[2255] The outbreak in the Netherlands not only showed that intensive chicken farms may brew a virus capable of human-to-human transmission, but that such a strain can arise in an advanced industrialized country with modern, high-tech poultry facilities.[2256]

With intensive confinement operations spreading around the globe, southern China may lose its distinction as the purported pandemic epicenter of the world.[2257] In Chile in 2002[2258] and in Italy and Mexico in the 1990s, the same scenario played out. A low-grade waterfowl virus found itself locked inside a building with thousands of chickens, leading to the "now predictable mutation to a highly pathogenic virus."[2259]

In Mexico, a low-grade H5N2 virus causing no more than mild respiratory symptoms in chickens found its way into industrial poultry facilities outside Mexico City and turned deadly,[2260] eventually affecting nearly a billion birds throughout the country.[2261] The "informative, but frightening"[2262] lesson to be learned from the Mexico outbreak is that once a harmless waterfowl virus is introduced into millions of domestic poultry,[2263] it can "accumulate multiple mutations and become a highly pathogenic strain that causes high mortality."[2264]

The Italian outbreak in 1999–2000 among "intensively reared poultry" caused the deaths of more than thirteen million birds in three months and evolved into a virus with 100 percent morbidity and 100 percent mortality[2265]—meaning that once the virus gets into a flock, every bird catches it and every bird dies. Over the preceding twenty years, the Italian poultry industry had grown and industrialized dramatically, particularly in the Veneto and Lombardia regions, precisely where the 1999 epidemic broke out.[2266]

The epidemic wiped out both broiler chicken and egg-laying operations. At the time, World Organization for Animal Health veterinary officials in Italy wrote, "To date, HPAI [highly pathogenic avian influenza] has affected virtually all intensively reared avian species regardless of age or housing system."[2267] The virus spread faster in broiler chicken sheds than within battery-cage egg facilities. Caged hens would all eventually succumb to the virus, but it had to spread from cage to neighboring cage, whereas it was able to blast its way throughout the broiler shed in one fell swoop, infecting chickens living directly on their own waste. The investigating scientists suspected then that the behavior of viral spread "was probably related to the amount of infected feces in direct contact with the birds."[2268] This suggests that outdoor flocks may be the least at risk since droppings may quickly dry in the sun and open air, rapidly killing any virus contained within.[2269]

Wishful Thinking

Outbreaks within and between modern, fully-enclosed, "biosecure" confinement facilities around the world have begged the question of how a virus from wild waterfowl gets inside in the first place. As we know, the virus itself may literally fall from the sky in the droppings of migratory waterfowl. Ducks crisscross virtually every continent in the world, potentially dive-bombing the countryside with virus[2270] from a theoretical height of up to twenty thousand feet.[2271] A single duck can drop billions of infectious doses of virus in a single day.[2272] The most comprehensive sampling of North American waterfowl found that up to 60 percent of juvenile ducks heading south from Canada were infected[2273] and able to actively excrete virus for as long as thirty days.[2274] With decreased and downgraded wetlands in North America[2275] and elsewhere,[2276] waterfowl may be forced to congregate in greater numbers, which would be expected to push infection rates even higher.[2277]

Once on the ground outside, the virus may quickly dry up and die unless it is transported to an environment more favorable for survival. The prime conduit for mechanical transfer of infective feces has historically involved contaminated poultry workers or equipment.[2278] Although, even without human involvement, "You have a lot of everything," remarked one USDA poultry microbiologist. "A lot of birds, a lot of manure, a lot of moisture, a lot of dust. Everything that walked into that house—every two- and four- and six-legged creature—is a potential vector for moving it around."[2279]

Rodents, insects, and wildlife could all be vectors ferrying the virus into confinement facilities.[2280] Experimental evidence shows that rats and mice, both huge problems in the poultry industry,[2281] may carry H5N1.[2282] An outbreak in Australia established that starlings and sparrows are also potential spreaders of bird flu viruses,[2283] and other wildlife species found in waterfowl habitat and on poultry farms, such as skunks, ground squirrels, and raccoons, have been shown capable of harboring bird flu viruses.[2284] DNA fingerprinting studies of *Campylobacter* suggest contact between housed poultry and wild birds[2285] who may be drawn to the bounty of free food available inside broiler sheds. In trying to describe why wild migratory birds are attracted to poultry operations, Ellen Silbergeld, an esteemed professor at the Johns Hopkins University Bloomberg School of Public Health, explained, "You rob a bank because that's where the money is—this is where all the food is, so of course they're going to try to get inside."[2286]

Flies may even carry the contagion. Just as up to 50 percent of the copious[2287] flies captured near poultry houses have been found carrying the poultry fecal bacteria *Campylobacter*,[2288] the deadly H5N2 virus was isolated from garbage flies[2289] during the 1980s outbreak in Pennsylvania.[2290] Influenza viruses may even seep into the water supply, with surface water from contaminated ponds potentially leaching into nearby groundwater supplies for confined poultry.[2291] A North Carolina State University poultry health management professor wrote in an industry trade journal that, understandably, "high biosecurity and proper monitoring are still wishful thinking in many areas of intensive poultry production."[2292]

Increasing intensification has made it even more wishful. The World Organization for Animal Health (OIE) has pointed out that the changes in the global poultry industry over the last decades make infectious diseases "significantly more difficult to control because of the greater number of susceptible animals reared per given unit of time and to the difficulties in applying adequate biosecurity programmes."[2293] The OIE noted that biosecurity measures may be simply incompatible with modern high-density rearing systems.[2294] "When an outbreak of avian influenza occurs in an area with a high [poultry] population density," OIE officials wrote, "the application of rigorous biosecurity measures might not be possible."[2295] The industry and USDA researchers[2296] have confessed that this is one of the disadvantages of the U.S. system. As I've discussed, poultry operations have ratcheted up in scale so dramatically that not only are twenty thousand to twenty-five thousand broiler chickens typically confined in a single shed, but there may be up to sixteen sheds at a single facility,[2297] and some egg-laying operations have the capacity to cage more than four million hens in a single complex.[2298] And, when sheds and farms are situated close enough to one another, we know that the virus may be able to spread through the wind.[2299]

Even assuming that all poultry workers, staff, and visitors paid perfect attention to biosecurity protocols—such as scrubbing footwear in disinfectant every time they stepped into a shed and washing their hands three separate times before entering (as instructed by the USDA's instructional video *Biosecurity: For the Birds*[2300])—a stray barn swallow or housefly could theoretically carry contagion in or out of an intensive confinement facility. And studies show that attention to biosecurity protocol is a far cry from perfect.

The U.S. poultry industry claims to have the "best biosecurity system in the world,"[2301] but academic and governmental investigations have uncovered widespread disregard for biosecurity precautions among large and small domestic producers.[2302] In 2002, University of Maryland researchers sent questionnaires about biosecurity practices to commercial broiler facilities throughout the Delmarva Peninsula, where more than a hundred million broiler chickens of various ages are at any given time. Fewer than half of the facilities returned the survey, and those that did admitted to severe lapses in biosecurity. The researchers concluded that U.S. broiler flocks "are constantly at risk of infection triggered by poor biosecurity practices."[2303]

In a moment of candor from the industry, Charles Beard, acting as U.S. Poultry and Egg Association vice president, admitted that relying on biosecurity measures to protect the U.S. poultry industry "could appear naïve."[2304] "After all," he wrote, "biosecurity is mostly a 'people' thing." The University of Maryland surveys show biosecurity "enthusiasm" to be lacking, and the "convictions" of poultry corporations like Tyson have leaned more toward twenty felony violations for illegal dumping of untreated wastewater into the nation's rivers[2305] than toward a desire to practice biosecurity. In fact, Tyson Foods, the largest chicken-producing corporation in the world,[2306] found itself before the Supreme Court in 2005 for refusing to pay workers for time spent donning protective clothing at a poultry plant. The Court ruled unanimously against Tyson.[2307]

Breaches in biosecurity occur in modernized facilities around the world.[2308] The European Food Safety Authority has recognized that when this happens in a densely populated poultry area, these breaches can result in "massive spread."[2309] The bottom line, according to animal disease control experts, is that biosecurity measures are costly for the industry[2310] and "not easy to sustain in the long term."[2311] Emeritus veterinary poultry professor Simon M. Shane, author of the *Handbook on Poultry Diseases,* even notes a "decline in the standards of biosecurity in an attempt to reduce costs in competitive markets." The decline is a contributing factor, Shane concludes, in the frequency and severity of disease outbreaks.[2312]

In *Poultry Digest,* longtime industry insider and avian health expert Ken Rudd wrote a candid article titled "Poultry Reality Check Needed," in which he laid out in stark terms the industry's skewed priorities:

> *An examination of virtually all the changes made in the past decade shows that they've come in the guise of convenience and efficiency, but they are, in fact, cost-cutting measures. Few, if any, decisions have been made solely for the sake of avian health or the long-term protection of the industry. The balance between the two has been lost; the scale is now weighted almost entirely on the cost-cutting side. And, therefore, on the side of microorganisms—much longer on this earth than humans!*[2313]

Specifically, Rudd criticized the profitable yet risky practice of reducing the duration of downtime between flocks and the trend of not cleaning poultry houses between flocks. He pleaded with his industry to "consider the cost of catastrophe."[2314]

One need look no further than other widespread viral disease outbreaks, like foot and mouth disease in Europe, to understand the vulnerability of modern animal agriculture.[2315] In the United States, within three years of the emergence of the highly virulent "Delaware variant" of IBDV, the immunodeficiency virus, virtually the entire broiler chicken industry east of the Mississippi was affected.[2316] If this is the "best biosecurity system in the world," then the global industry may need to fundamentally rethink how it raises birds for meat and eggs. The United States, the country that pioneered industrialized poultry production, has reported more bird flu than any other country in the world.[2317]

Made in the USA

Bird flu viruses have been detected every year in the United States since the mid-1960s.[2318] In just the last five years, the United States has suffered more than two hundred outbreaks of highly pathogenic avian influenza viruses, including H5N1, H5N2, H5N8, H7N8, and H7H9, resulting in the deaths of more than fifty million chickens and turkeys.[2319] The 2014 autumn bird migration from the Pacific flyway appeared to bring an H5N8 virus from Asia[2320] that descended from the original H5N1 virus,[2321] which then mixed with a variety of North American strains[2322] to create the most explosive and expensive animal disease outbreak in U.S. history.[2323] In response to a call to condition future indemnification payments on a requirement that poultry operations reduce their bird-stocking densities, the USDA admitted that "the impact of an HPAI outbreak is amplified where poultry production is highly concentrated" and will "encourage farmers to consider reducing the number of birds in poultry houses," but they're "not going to adopt this type of governmental restriction at this time."[2324] In other words, they're going to leave it up to the poultry industry while continuing to reimburse—with taxpayer dollars—the same operations whose intensive confinement practices helped incubate and spread disease in the first place.[2325]

The second largest outbreak in U.S. history was the 1983 Pennsylvania eruption that spread down through Maryland and Virginia[2326] and led to the deaths of seventeen million domestic birds[2327] at a cost to the nation of more than $400 million.[2328] (The 2015 outbreaks cost the United States an estimated $3.3 billion.[2329])

Investigators speculate that the H5N2 virus responsible for the outbreak may have started out in a flock of wild ducks that landed in a pond on a chicken farm in eastern Pennsylvania.[2330] Duck feces on the boots of a farmer may have first brought the virus inside the broiler sheds.[2331] The virus, like essentially all wild waterfowl viruses, started out benign, causing a drop in egg production or mild upper respiratory symptoms, but soon started "racing though giant commercial chicken warehouses."[2332] The resident director of the University of Pennsylvania's poultry laboratory explained that "with that many opportunities to mutate under those intensive conditions," the virus changed from one that gave chickens the sniffles to the "bloody Jell-O" virus Webster called "chicken Ebola," causing birds to hemorrhage throughout their bodies.[2333]

Webster's team performed genetic analyses of the H5N2 virus before and after it turned lethal. To their surprise, the two differed by only a single amino acid. Amino acids are building blocks strung together in chains that make proteins. The H5 hemagglutinin protein is more than five hundred amino acids long.[2334] All it took was a tiny point mutation in the viral genetic material to change the thirteenth amino acid in the H5 chain from an amino acid named *threonine* to one called *lysine*—a mutation that, in Webster's words, "change[d] that benign virus into one that was completely lethal."[2335] "That such a tiny change in the virus could enable it to wreak so much havoc," Webster and colleagues later wrote, "was an awesome discovery."[2336]

The U.S. Department of the Interior's U.S. Geological Survey (USGS), created by an act of Congress in 1879, represents the nation's leading governmental authority on the biological sciences.[2337] Reflecting on the evolution of low-grade to high-grade strains of bird flu, the USGS echoes other world authorities in implicating industrial poultry practices not only as providing an "excellent opportunity" for rapid spread (particularly when "poultry are housed at high densities in confined quarters"), but also playing in part an "ideal" role in possibly sparking the next human pandemic.[2338]

H5N2 resurfaced two years later in low-grade form in Massachusetts, New Jersey, Ohio, and again in Pennsylvania,[2339] traced back to live poultry markets in New York City each time. A survey of live markets in 1986 found forty-eight harboring the virus,[2340] suggesting to investigators that live poultry markets may have been the critical mixing point between ducks or geese and chickens that triggered the original Pennsylvania epidemic.[2341]

Efforts to purge bird flu viruses from live poultry markets over the years have been largely unsuccessful,[2342] despite periodic quarantine, depopulation, cleaning, and disinfection. In 2004, an outbreak of highly pathogenic H5N2 was discovered in a flock of seven thousand broiler chickens in Texas after the owner introduced a chicken from a live poultry market in Houston into his flock.[2343] Considering the Hong Kong outbreak and other U.S.[2344] and Italian outbreaks were traced back to live poultry markets,[2345] USDA poultry researchers describe live bird markets as the "missing link in the epidemiology of avian influenza."[2346]

The first human case of bird flu infection in the United States was in 2002. An H7N2 virus caused more than two hundred outbreaks in chicken and turkey operations across a mass poultry production area first in Virginia and then into West Virginia and North Carolina, leading to the destruction of almost five million birds.[2347] It was a low-pathogenicity virus and only suspected in one human infection,[2348] but genetic analyses show that it is mutating toward greater virulence.[2349]

In 2003, a person was admitted to a hospital in New York with respiratory symptoms and was confirmed to have been infected with the H7N2 bird flu virus. Despite a serious underlying medical condition, the patient recovered and went home after a few weeks.[2350] By that year, the virus had swept through millions of egg-laying hens in huge battery-cage facilities in Connecticut and Rhode Island,[2351] outbreaks that the industry admits "confirm the vulnerability of egg production units."[2352] OIE expert Ilaria Capua has described it as "very difficult" to keep an industrial battery-cage egg facility clean and prevent spread from farm to farm via eggs, egg trays and equipment. "In our opinion," she told the Fifth International Symposium on Avian Influenza, "when the infection gets into a circuit, it will spread within that circuit. It finds its way to spread."[2353]

The way H7N2 was found to spread in the United States was via live poultry markets. The markets were suspected in the outbreaks in Pennsylvania (1996,[2354] 1997, 1998, 2001, and 2002[2355]), Virginia (2002),[2356] Connecticut and Rhode Island (2003), and Delaware (2004).[2357] The Delaware outbreak in a broiler operation confining more than eighty-five thousand chickens spread to Maryland before being stamped out by killing more than four hundred thousand birds.[2358] In two cases, direct epidemiological evidence links the presence of trucks hauling birds to live poultry markets at affected farms within a week before the appearance of clinical disease.[2359] The trucks deliver birds from the farms to the markets, pick up the empty dirty crates, and then return to the farms. The "most likely scenario," according to USDA scientists, is that the crates or trucks were not completely disinfected of the potential billions of infectious particles present with any infectious fecal contamination.[2360]

The U.S. live poultry market system has been described by the University of Georgia Southeastern Cooperative Wildlife Disease Study as an "intricate web of retail markets, poultry auctions, wholesale dealers, and farm flocks." The study notes that in this system, "birds may change hands up to five times before reaching the consumer," increasing exposure and decreasing trackability.[2361]

Scientists have watched H7N2 since its emergence in live poultry markets in the United States in 1994. As mentioned earlier, the virus's fail-safe mechanism that shackles it from becoming too dangerous in its natural waterfowl host is the hemagglutinin activation step that limits viral replication to "safe" organs in the body, like the intestine. Once placed in a land-based host like a chicken, though, viral mutants that can infect all the victim's organ systems may have a selective advantage since easy waterborne spread is no longer possible. H5 and H7 viruses can transform by accruing basic (as opposed to acidic or neutral) amino acids in the hemagglutinin protein cleavage site, where the enzymes of the host activate the virus. Once the virus accumulates approximately five basic amino acids, it may transform from a low-pathogenicity virus to a highly pathogenic virus.

The earliest H7N2 isolates in U.S. live poultry markets in 1994 already had two basic amino acids in the critical cleavage site. By 1998, the virus was up to three. Then, in 2002, H7N2 viruses were found with four. Only one more tiny mutation and the virus could have become deadly.[2362] Even though the virus was technically still an LPAI virus, the federal government could see the writing on the wall and stepped in to stamp out H7N2 wherever it escaped—and indemnify the industry.[2363]

Efforts to eradicate the virus at the source—in live poultry markets—had failed. According to the USDA Animal and Plant Health Inspection Service, "Despite educational efforts, surveillance, and increased state regulatory efforts, the number of [virus] positive markets has persisted and increased." In 1998, 30 percent of the markets were infected with H7N2, particularly in the New York metropolitan area. New York has more live markets than all other states in the Northeast combined.[2364] By 2001, inspectors could find the virus at 60 percent of markets at any one time.[2365]

The states were failing to control the problem. With the virus dangerously close to potentially locking in that final mutation, the USDA had to intercede, coordinating a system-wide closure of all retail live poultry markets throughout the northeastern United States in 2002. Following the mass closure, all birds were sold off or killed, and all markets were cleaned and disinfected, left empty for days, and then repopulated with birds only from closely monitored source flocks confirmed to be negative for all avian influenza viruses. Then they watched and waited. Within five weeks, H7N2 was back.

It is unknown whether the virus somehow persisted in the markets or was reintroduced. Regardless, despite their best efforts at eradication and control, it seems clear that live poultry markets represent a public health risk. Writing in the *Journal of Virology*, USDA researchers concluded that "the rampant reassortment of AIVs [avian influenza viruses] in the LBMs [live bird markets] could increase the risk of species crossover because it would increase the chances of the occurrence of the correct constellation of genes to create a virus that replicates efficiently in mammals."[2366] In 2006, the virus was supposedly eradicated from the live bird market system,[2367] but in 2016, hundreds of cats in New York City fell ill with an H7N2 influenza that was 96 to 98 percent identical with the live bird market viruses.[2368] A shelter worker[2369] and an attending veterinarian became infected, underscoring the mammalian adaptation of the virus.[2370]

The mass market closure and disinfection did seem to knock the virus back a step, though, back to three basic amino acids.[2371] Still, unless all live poultry markets are closed, H7N2 could presumably continue its march toward virulence. As the director of the virology lab at Cornell University's Animal Health Diagnostic Center put it, "It is two major mutations away from becoming a virus that could kill a lot of chickens and become much more pathogenic to people."[2372] The H7N2 virus that was circulating in live bird markets in the Northeastern United States has been found to possess an affinity for the alpha-2,6 linkages found in human lungs.[2373] Some of the isolates were also found resistant to the antiflu drug amantadine.[2374] Even more concerning, the bird flu virus that infected the New Yorker was found to experimentally transmit animal-to-animal via direct contact,[2375] something H5N1 has not yet been shown able to do.[2376]

Many suspected that H5N1 would beat H7N2 to the pandemic punch, but, were it not for H5N1, the betting might be more on live poultry markets in New York City—not Hong Kong—to deliver the next killer superflu virus. According to the USDA's Agricultural Research Service,

> The U.S. currently has the largest, most genetically homogeneous and, thus potentially, the most disease-susceptible population of food animals in the history of mankind . . . The emergence of a new disease or a slight shift in the epidemiology of an existing disease could lead to immediate and disastrous results for American livestock producers and consumers.[2377]

Concluded researchers at the Johns Hopkins School of Public Health: "There is substantial evidence challenging the assumption that industrialized operations are more biosecure and biocontained."[2378] The Virginia outbreak in 2002 that led to the deaths of millions of birds and found its way onto hundreds of farms exemplified this vulnerability. Based on the rapid spread of bird flu in the United States in 2002, leading USDA poultry researchers have stated the obvious: "[B]iosecurity on many farms is inadequate."[2379] And that was before the 2015 outbreak that hit hundreds of commercial operations across nine states.[2380] The executive editor of *Poultry* magazine and professor of poultry science at Mississippi State has editorialized, "If WHO is right and a pandemic brings human AI to the United States, will you be able to look your family and neighbors in the eye and say you've done all you can to stop the spread? Having to answer that question alarms me!"[2381]

III. Pandemic Preparedness

COOPING UP BIRD FLU

Taming of the Flu

The only way to truly stop a pandemic, it has been suggested, is to stamp it out at its source.[2382] Once it starts, as noted the editorial board of the journal of the Canadian Medical Association, "School closure, quarantine, travel restrictions and so on are unlikely to be more effective than a garden hose in a forest fire." But every forest fire starts with a spark. Some experts believe that, at least theoretically, if caught early enough, a pandemic ember could be extinguished. It's like a spark and a squirt gun, suggested the director of the U.S. National Vaccine Program. "If you aim properly you can get the spark and be done with it. If you miss, though, the fire is going to spread and there is nothing you can do to stop it."[2383]

Two independent mathematical models—one out of the Imperial College of London[2384] and another from Emory[2385]—suggested that, under the right conditions, a pandemic outbreak might be able to be snuffed at the source in a matter of months. If their approach worked, instead of half the world becoming infected, fewer than 150 individuals might succumb.[2386] The strategy—called "ring-fencing"—would be to surround the outbreak at its source and smother it by blanketing everyone in the area with antiviral drugs.[2387] "Basically," wrote one of the lead biostatisticians, "you contain it at the source or you fail."[2388]

There are caveats. The models assumed that the outbreak would be rapidly detected and reported while still in limited human clusters restricted to a small geographical area. The virus would have to be caught before it got highly contagious.[2389] No one could be allowed in or out.[2390] And, of course, we'd have to have effective antiviral drugs available.

That's the computer model. In the real world, odds are the outbreak would not be detected in time. Countries in Southeast Asia, for example, tend to have poor surveillance capabilities and are reluctant to admit outbreaks even when detected.[2391] "If you can't do it with the speed of a smoke alarm and a fire truck, you don't have a chance in hell of stopping this," Osterholm told a reporter.[2392]

The biggest chink in our armor may be lack of clinical surveillance and rapid detection.[2393] To even theoretically stop a pandemic, the Imperial College model necessitates discovering the incipient pandemic when there are just thirty human cases. In the Emory model, the world would have about twenty-one days to intervene.[2394] "The chances of that happening," admitted Secretary Leavitt, "are not good."[2395] The National Academy of Medicine has concluded that there is "no single example, in the United States or elsewhere, of a well-functioning zoonotic disease surveillance system integrated across human and animal health sectors."[2396]

When bird flu first emerged in Vietnam, for example, the country's leading analytical center—the National Institute of Hygiene and Epidemiology in Hanoi—had no safety cabinets, freezers, centrifuges, or incubators and had to turn to the WHO for a loan. Simple blood tests had to be shipped out of country for results.[2397] "We did not even have masks and gloves," said one virologist at the Institute.[2398] Some countries like Laos had never even had a virology lab.[2399]

The World Health Organization, the World Organization for Animal Health, and the Food and Agriculture Organization of the United Nations came together in 2005 to put out an international plea for funds to help control the disease in poultry populations and detect the disease in human populations. They called for a minimum of $100 million.[2400] "Countries in Asia are doing their best to control the virus but they cannot and should not be expected to do this job on their own," said the FAO's chief veterinary officer.[2401] "The coming influenza pandemic will cut huge swathes in the world community," professor John Oxford warned, "and history will look back with a jaundiced eye should governments hesitate and not join in this war, and place monetary priorities elsewhere."[2402]

Samuel Jutzi, the top FAO official at the time, said, "There is an increasing risk of avian influenza spread that no poultry-keeping country can afford to ignore."[2403] Worse than ignoring, countries have actively covered it up. Even if countries could afford proper facilities, many Asian countries have admitted to concealing outbreaks, in part, to protect poultry industry interests. "An obvious major weak spot in global surveillance," the director of the Australian National Centre for Epidemiology and Population Health pointed out, "is the tendency of national governments to deny or suppress information."[2404] Thailand presents a good case study.[2405]

Thai Curry Favor with Poultry Industry

With thirty thousand to fifty thousand birds commonly found in each unit on intensive poultry farms, mass culling means significant financial loss.[2406] Some facilities in Thailand have reported to each have more than ten million chickens.[2407]

According to the Thai Broiler Association, Thailand was the world's fourth largest poultry exporter before bird flu hit,[2408] producing more than a million tons of meat every year and generating four billion in U.S. dollars in revenue.[2409] At the center of the meltdown of Thailand's poultry industry is multibillionaire Dhanin Chearavanont, profiled in *Time* magazine's "The Families That Own Asia,"[2410] who brought the U.S.-style industrial chicken farming pioneered by Tyson to Thailand[2411] nearly forty years ago, transforming a small family business into a multinational corporate empire.[2412] Chearavanont was the Thai tycoon caught making an illegal $250,000 donation to the U.S. Democratic National Committee in 1996. Not to be partisan, he was accused of slipping George H. W. Bush a quarter million dollars as well.[2413]

In November 2003, chickens started dying across Thailand. Senator Malinee Sukavejworakit, a medical doctor and representative of one of the worst affected provinces, became concerned. The government assured her that it was just chicken cholera—a disease with no human health implications—and therefore nothing to worry about. The third week of January, she got a call from a physician colleague about a local butcher dying with classic bird flu symptoms. The senator visited him in the hospital. "He told me he'd been butchering chickens on a farm and he'd come across a whole lot of birds with insides like he'd never seen," she said. "They smelled rancid." She visited the devastated farm. "[W]hatever this is," the farmer told her, "it isn't cholera." When the Public Health Department refused to release the butcher's test results, she decided to go public.[2414]

As chief advisor for the Senate Committee on Public Health, Sukavej-worakit convened a meeting and held a press conference the next day. For her efforts to expose the truth, the Deputy Agriculture Minister accused her of being "irresponsible to the motherland." The Prime Minister himself dismissed the idea of a bird flu epidemic as "fantasy and imagination," warning that such "exaggeration will damage the country's poultry exports and leave chicken farmers and workers in the field to suffer."[2415]

Chearavanont wasn't suffering, though. Throughout the crisis, while birds were dying, corporate processing plants were working overtime. "Before November we were processing about 90,000 chickens a day," trade unionists explained to the *Bangkok Post* after the scandal broke. "But from November to January, we had to kill about 130,000 daily. It's our job to cut the birds up. It was obvious they were ill: their organs were swollen. We didn't know what the disease was, but we understood that the management was rushing to process the chickens before getting any veterinary inspection. We stopped eating [chicken] in October."[2416]

Later it was divulged that the nation's veterinary scientists had been detecting and reporting H5N1 for months to Thailand's Livestock Department, but as one senator alleges, "All the academics and experts had to shut up due to political interference."[2417] The Bangkok press found evidence that the government had been colluding with Big Poultry[2418] to hide the epidemic to give exporters time to process and sell diseased inventory.[2419] An editor at the *Bangkok Post* later explained to a group of journalists why the press didn't pick up on the cover-up sooner. "Our tendency is just to report what people are saying and rely too much on the government," she said. "As it turned out, the government was suppressing the truth."[2420]

The international community was not surprised. "The bottom line is, economic considerations are what dictate the responses of the governments trying to ensure the consequences of avian outbreak is minimized," said WHO's representative in Thailand. "That's understandable, but it's more important that sufficient measures are taken to prevent humans from catching the disease."[2421] The first to die of H5N1 in Thailand was a six-year-old boy.

"The government knew," his father said, "so why didn't they tell the public so that we could protect ourselves?"[2422]

This scenario was repeated throughout the region. An outbreak in Japan was concealed by poultry company officials—two of whom later committed suicide[2423]—and only came to light thanks to an anonymous tip. *The Japan Times* editorialized that the factory farm—one of the largest in the area—was apparently "concerned more about profit than safety."[2424] After Indonesia's national director of animal health disclosed to *The Washington Post* that pressure from the poultry industry forced the government to hide its outbreak for more than a year, she was fired. When UN officials complained about the dismissal, the Agriculture Minister replied, "The thing is, we don't want to publicize too much about bird flu because of the effect on our farms. Prices have dropped very drastically."[2425] He withheld information, he explained, because "we did not want to cause unnecessary losses through a hasty decision."[2426]

The deputy director of Focus on the Global South, a nonprofit advocacy organization, summed up the Thailand scandal:

> *The government handling of the bird flu is a saga of cover-ups, incompetence, lies and extremely questionable decisions: the long delay before admitting the existence of the bird flu both in animals and in humans, the selective measures taken to stop the spread of the epidemic and most spectacularly, the massive public relations campaigns to convince Thai citizens that eating chicken was nothing less than a patriotic act.*[2427]

The director was referring to numerous PR stunts across the region. The Thai government gathered celebrities[2428] for free "chicken eating festivals,"[2429] and Kentucky Fried Chicken in Thailand gave away fifty thousand pieces of chicken.[2430] In China, the executive vice minister of health—a vegetarian—ate chicken for the first time in thirty years to proclaim its safety. China's main propaganda unit acknowledged that the staged meals suggested an official shift "from traditional propaganda to Western-style political communications skills to handle crises."[2431] The strategy was perhaps made most famous by the British Minister of Agriculture who was shown on television feeding a hamburger to his four-year-old daughter while reassuring the public with the blanket statement that eating beef was "perfectly safe," a few short years before young people started dying from mad cow disease.[2432]

Not all such media events had the desired effect. At a cull ceremony at a pig farm in Indonesia, the Minister of Agriculture showed up in a special white outfit complete with gloves and mask, surprising the staffers, reporters, and hundreds of locals who wore no protective gear at all. "Don't blame me if you get bird flu because you don't wear a mask. This is very dangerous, you know, as the virus can be transmitted through the air," he warned reporters through his mask.[2433]

The official state cover-ups surrounding bird flu reminded many of the SARS debacle in China. All occurrences of infectious disease outbreaks were considered official state secrets; physicians or journalists caught disclosing SARS-related information to their friends were arrested under the official State Secrets Law.[2434] By the time China finally admitted there was a problem—months after the first discovered case—hundreds of people were already infected.[2435] In general, said a WHO spokesperson, "Economics and agriculture are weighing too heavily in decisions taken by governments, and more concern should be given to the risk to human health."[2436]

In the case of COVID-19, patient zero may have been infected in November 2019,[2437] but local officials were apparently able to successfully conceal the epidemic from central authorities, effectively delaying national action until well into January 2020.[2438] Modeling funded by the Bill & Melinda Gates Foundation suggests that if China would have acted even one week earlier, they could have prevented two-thirds of subsequent cases. Had they not acted at all, though, the epidemic could have been sixty-seven times worse.[2439]

This is one of the reasons that the prospect of ring-fencing a pandemic in time is so remote. "If they would have acknowledged this [SARS] early, and we could have seen the virus as it occurred in south China, we probably could have isolated it before it got out of hand," explained one infectious disease expert. "But they completely hid it. They hide everything. You can't even find out how many people die from earthquakes."[2440] The foundation of the theoretical models is openness and cooperation for rapid detection of outbreaks of influenza. "Would they admit to it if it was here?" one Asian diplomat asked. "That's the big question, since they deny everything left, right and center."[2441]

Reluctance to share data seems a universal phenomenon. In an article in the journal *Science* titled "Flu Researchers Slam U.S. Agency for Hoarding Data," international scientists claim that getting data from the CDC is somewhere between "extremely difficult and impossible."[2442] "The CDC is not the CIA," the director of the Federation of American Scientists' project on government secrecy said. "Withholding data is not just bad public policy, it is bad science."[2443]

During a 2004 outbreak of low-grade bird flu in Delaware and Maryland, state authorities refused to release the identity of the affected poultry operations. "The stigma attached to having an infectious disease is real," explained one North Carolina State University veterinarian in *Poultry International*,[2444] "and often leads people to keep this information from others." A spokesperson for the group Common Cause in Delaware, however, disagreed with the policy. "When you're talking about a worldwide problem, you really can't keep things secret even if you think it's good public policy. People want to know, and they want their government agencies to be honest, open and transparent."[2445]

Even when governments try to do the right thing, the populace may not go along. When H5N1 hit turkeys in Turkey, the order "Bring your poultry to the town square this evening for slaughter" blared from town hall speakers. "Failure to comply could mean up to six months in jail."[2446] When authorities went to forcibly round up ducks and chickens in the region, they were reportedly met by hostile farmers armed with pitchforks and axes.[2447]

Part of the problem may be that existing international law on infectious disease control is archaic, formed many decades ago, long before mass global travel. The World Health Organization, for example, can only issue "soft law" recommendations, rather than binding obligations. This outmoded system of international relations in general dates back to the seventeenth-century Peace of Westphalia ending the Thirty Years War. The Westphalian system is built upon the principle of absolute national sovereignty.[2448] "Many governments see it [disease prevention] as an internal business," said the WHO's director-general. "There is a basic gut feeling that this is my problem, I will deal with it in my way. Now, in a globalized world, any disease is one airplane away. It is not a provincial or national issue, it's a global issue."[2449]

The World Trade Organization has more powers than the World Health Organization.[2450] Analogous to FEMA during the Hurricane Katrina crisis, the WHO also lacks the authority to investigate outbreaks without an invitation.[2451] For SARS, though, the WHO did issue its first ever travel advisory in fifty-five years.[2452] The ensuing political backlash over lost trade and tourism may explain some of the deference to member nations in somewhat downplaying the immediacy of the current pandemic threat.[2453] In the understated fashion typical to international law journals, one review concluded, "The soft law process on infectious disease control has not been working well."[2454]

> *"We have as much chance of stopping a pandemic as we would of putting a curtain around Minnesota and keeping out winter."*
>
> —MICHAEL OSTERHOLM[2455]

Even assuming that countries had the resources for proper surveillance and reported outbreaks promptly, no antiviral stockpile existed to carry out the ring-fencing strategy to stop H5N1. The WHO only had 120,000 courses of antivirals, whereas millions may have been necessary.[2456] The WHO sent 2,500 treatments to Vietnam, 500 to Cambodia,[2457] and a few hundred courses divided among forty-four hospitals in Indonesia; many received no more than a handful.[2458] Countries at risk, like Sri Lanka, reported they don't have a single dose.[2459] "I think the take-home message," said an epidemiologist at Harvard at the time, "is that the current stockpile is very unlikely to be adequate to stop anything."[2460]

Meanwhile, the Western world continued in its "narcissistic planning,"[2461] as described in a medical journal editorial, ignoring pleas from the World Health Organization to pour resources into Southeast Asia.[2462] The United States may have spent $1 billion to domestically stockpile antiviral drugs,[2463] more than ten times the entire health budget for Vietnam. In Cambodia, the total annual budget for a campaign to encourage citizens to report suspected cases of bird flu was about $3,000.[2464] In a *New Yorker* interview, a senior public health official pondered the question of whether countries in the West might send their resources to combat the flu in Southeast Asia. He told the reporter, "Who are you kidding?"[2465]

In the end, mathematical models remain just that—mathematical models. Even assuming that the models are valid, they are so qualified with conditional assumptions as to potentially render them useless under real world conditions. Public health experts point out that the odds are vanishingly slim of early detection of a small cluster in a rural area with little public health infrastructure, followed by the distribution of an antiviral stockpile that doesn't yet exist—all within a three-week period.[2466] Michael Oster-holm, disease control expert and responsible for leading the single-largest containment campaign in U.S. history to control a meningitis outbreak,[2467] is skeptical that influenza can be stopped: "To believe that you can contain this locally is to believe in fairy tales."[2468]

Even if the human pandemic could be successfully quashed, might we still have faced a "reloading" problem? Experts speculate that H5N1 could be so endemically entrenched within multiple globe-trotting migratory species of birds that its eradication must be regarded as impossible, presenting a constant pool of mutant virus ready to pop up somewhere else. In bird populations, we are dealing with a moving target.[2469] The genie cannot be put back in its bottle.

Given these considerations, a microbiologist at Chinese University summed up the bottom line: "[O]nce H5N1 becomes easily transmissible in humans, it will be the end," he said. "We can do nothing to control this spreading."[2470]

RACE AGAINST TIME

| *"He who desires, but acts not, breeds pestilence."*

—WILLIAM BLAKE

For years, scientists have requested detailed operational blueprints—country by country down to neighborhood by neighborhood—on how best to make it through twelve to twenty-four months of a pandemic.[2471] "If the greatest pandemic in history is indeed on the horizon," wrote the editorial board of *Lancet* in 2005, "that threat must be met by the most comprehensive public-health plan ever devised."[2472] "We have only one enemy," CDC director Ger-berding said repeatedly, "and that is complacency."[2473]

Unfortunately, no country has prepared.[2474] In policy journals like *Foreign Affairs,* senior officials admitted that planning for what they called "the most catastrophic outbreak in human history" was "abysmally inadequate."[2475] Despite repeated warnings over the years that a new pandemic is inevitable and repeated prods by the WHO for countries to draw up preparedness plans, only about fifty of more than two hundred countries did so.[2476] Some of those "plans" were as stunted as a single page,[2477] and most, as described in the science journal *Nature,* were "very sketchy."[2478] The WHO called for countries to "put life in these plans" by carrying out practice simulations. "One has to be very vigilant, honest and brave," asserted Margaret Chan, the WHO's chief of pandemic preparedness. "Sometimes you need to make unpopular, difficult recommendations to political leaders which may have a short-term impact on the economy and on certain sectors."[2479] As the Los Angeles County Disaster Preparedness Task Force motto reads, "The only thing more difficult than preparing for a disaster is trying to explain why you didn't."[2480]

Fewer than 10 percent of the countries with plans took the necessary further step of translating the plans into national law.[2481] Concerned about the state of U.S. preparedness, then chair of the Infectious Disease Society of America's Pandemic Influenza Task Force said, "Although many levels of government are paying increased attention to the problem, the United States remains woefully unprepared for an influenza pandemic that could kill millions of Americans."[2482] Osterholm was, as usual, more direct. "If it happens tonight," Osterholm said at a forum sponsored by the Council on Foreign Relations, "we're screwed."[2483]

Osterholm laid it out on *The NewsHour with Jim Lehrer*: "We can predict now 12 to 18 months of stress, of watching loved ones die, of potentially not going to work, of wondering if you're going to have food on the table the next day. Those are all things that are going to mean that we're going to have to plan unlike any other kind of crisis that we've had in literally the last 80-some years in this country."[2484]

The U.S. pandemic preparedness plan has been long in the making. The planning process started in 1976, only to become one of the longest-standing incomplete processes in Washington.[2485] Various drafts emerged in 1978 and 1983, but were reshelved and forgotten until the latest effort to update and implement such a plan began in 1993.[2486] The Government Accountability Office, the watchdog arm of Congress, scolded the Department of Health and Human Services on six separate occasions for failing to develop a national response plan despite many years of "process."[2487]

In October 2005, a draft of the plan was obtained by *The New York Times.* The "preparedness plan" highlighted how poorly prepared the country was for a pandemic. The headline read, "U.S. Not Ready for Deadly Flu, Bush Plan Shows."[2488] In *The Boston Globe,* Massachusetts Senator Edward Kennedy noted that other nations like Canada, Britain, and Japan had completed their plan a year or years before. "They're putting their plans into action right now," Kennedy wrote, "while we're waiting to read ours for the first time. America deserves better."[2489] Senator Arlen Specter agreed. "We need a better way of finding out what the hell is going on."[2490]

One of the factors blamed for the twenty-nine-year delay in producing a plan was the difficulty of interdepartmental coordination. A pandemic would impact all agencies of government, but they don't all have the same priorities. Senior policy analysts described the Department of Agriculture and the Department of Health and Human Services, for example, as "not exactly good bedfellows." The USDA's traditional mission to defend the economic interests of the agricultural industry sets up a natural tension with agencies prioritizing broader concerns.[2491] Experts predicted the economic impact on U.S. agriculture would be nothing compared to the havoc wreaked by the virus more generally.[2492]

The official plan was finally released in November 2005. The CDC planners did not mince words: "No other infectious disease threat, whether natural or engineered, poses the same current threat for causing increases in infections, illnesses, and deaths so quickly in the United States and worldwide."[2493] In terms of preparedness, though, *The New York Times* editorialized that it "looks like a prescription for failure should a highly lethal flu virus start rampaging through the population in the next few years." The editorial noted that experts found the plan "disturbingly incomplete," particularly because it "largely passes the buck on practical problems" to state and local authorities, "none of which are provided with adequate resources to handle the job."[2494] Columbia University's Irwin Redlener called it "the mother of all unfunded mandates."[2495] We saw how unprepared we were for even a relatively mild pandemic like COVID-19. Laurie Garrett of the Council on Foreign Relations has long advocated an integrated public health infrastructure. "If such an interlaced system did not exist at a time of grave need it would constitute an egregious betrayal of trust," she wrote in a book bearing the same name, *Betrayal of Trust: The Collapse of Global Public Health.*[2496]

Chicken Little Gets the Flu

Another impediment to progress may have been the reluctance of authorities to appear as though they were sowing undue panic among the populace. At

that point, the U.S. government had not yet involved the public to any significant degree.[2497] Many of the Congressional briefings on H5N1 and pandemic
preparedness have been classified as "Top Secret/Sensitive Compartmented
Information," which does not sit well with Redlener. "This is old-fashioned cold
war secrecy being applied to a public-health issue," he said, "a very bad idea."[2498]

Bureaucratic tendencies toward condescension are not limited to the
United States. *The London Times* ran a story describing an emergency meeting
of twenty-five European states to deal with the threat of H5N1 at which they
urged citizens not to be panicked by bird flu.[2499] In response, the leading
public health blog dealing with avian influenza wrote, "I don't know about
you, but the one thing that makes me want to panic is when the leaders of
25 countries meet in emergency session and tell me not to panic."[2500] Similar
attempts to placate the public were made a century ago.

A year after California Senator Hiram Johnson coined the famous phrase,
"The first casualty when war comes is truth,"[2501] public officials were publicly
lying to downplay the 1918 pandemic so as not to undermine the war effort.[2502] One of the leading pandemic historians notes how this resulted in a
public backlash:

> *People could see while they were being told on the one hand that it's ordinary*
> *influenza, on the other hand they are seeing their spouse die in 24 hours or*
> *less, bleeding from their eyes, ears, nose and mouth, turning so dark that*
> *people thought it was the black death. People knew that they were being lied*
> *to; they knew that this was not ordinary influenza.*[2503]

According to historians, the first reaction of most authorities during the
1918 pandemic was "just flat-out denial."[2504] The Chief Health Officer of
New Zealand told the papers to "tell your readers not to get upset." Rome's
Chief Sanitation Officer belittled the flu as a "transitory miniscule phenomenon." Poland's Public Health Commission and Rhodesia's Medical Director issued the identical bromide: "There is no cause for alarm."[2505] Toronto's
Medical Officer said, "There is absolutely no necessity for anxiety," even as
the plague arrived on their doorsteps,[2506] echoing the Health Commissioner
of New York City: "The city is in no danger of an epidemic. No need for
our people to worry."[2507] The resulting mistrust of government officials only
added to the climate of fear, a scenario officials were in danger of repeating
in the face of the H5N1 pandemic threat.[2508] "That men do not learn very

much from the lessons of history," Aldous Huxley once said, "is the most important of all the lessons that history has to teach."[2509]

One factor that may have affected U.S. officials in particular is memories of the "swine flu debacle" of 1976, in which tens of millions of Americans were vaccinated against a supposed pandemic strain of influenza that never materialized. Not only was the CDC left with ninety million useless doses of vaccine,[2510] but several people who were vaccinated suffered life-threatening side effects[2511] resulting in thousands of lawsuits being filed, hundreds of which were settled for a total of millions of dollars.[2512] The resulting political fiasco led to the firing of the heads of the CDC and the Department of Health.[2513]

What made the threat of H5N1 different from the presumed threat of swine flu in 1976? How could U.S. officials be certain that bird flu was not another Chicken Little scenario? The critical difference was the global scientific consensus that H5N1 may represent a genuine pandemic threat. Back in 1976, authorities throughout the world—including the World Health Organization—disagreed with the United States that the death of a single soldier from a swine influenza virus warranted universal vaccination. They thought America was overreacting.[2514] With H5N1, though, the world's authorities were in agreement. As summarized by Lee Jong-wook, the late director-general of the World Health Organization, viruses like H5N1 represent a "grave danger for all people in all countries."[2515]

This is a role public health officials don't relish. "I do not want to be right," said the WHO's Lee. "We're not scare-mongering here," avowed Canada's top expert, head of the national microbiology lab. "We're not crying wolf," he said. "There is a wolf. We just don't know when it's coming."[2516] In reference to public health officials who feared they would be accused of alarming people unnecessarily, one risk communications expert reminded a reporter, "They forget that in the actual Boy Who Cried Wolf story, the wolf finally showed up."[2517]

Lee insisted that every country must have not only a national pandemic response plan, but also a communications strategy to keep the public informed as to what is happening and what they can do without causing panic.[2518] Communicating public health risks, though, is like driving with both feet, according to Osterholm. "You're putting one foot on the gas and the other on the brake. You want to motivate on the one hand, and not cause panic on the other."[2519]

On behalf of Trust for America's Health and Columbia University's Mailman School of Public Health, researchers conducted one-on-one interviews with TV, radio, and print journalists who cover public health issues. Numerous respondents said they had purposefully toned down their coverage or passed on pandemic flu stories altogether so as "to present the news without inducing panic." The study suggested that the reporters were very knowledgeable but "fear that passing along too much of this knowledge to their readers will lead to panic."[2520]

Public complacency, according to the dean of the Harvard School of Public Health, is the biggest roadblock to pandemic preparedness.[2521] The American public wants to see more in-depth reporting on the subject.[2522] This patronizing attitude revealed in the study suggests that some journalists may be holding back instead of providing the full story which might otherwise motivate people to action.

One media participant in the study explained their dilemma:

> I don't want to panic anyone, but I do want to prepare my audience. I have personally told my family to get 90 days worth of supplies together, in case they need to stay away from other people for a while. I don't tell my readers that, because our editors think that may be ineffective and will cause panic. But the world is a scary place. People need to understand what could happen so that they can be ready. [2523]

Not wanting to cause panic is admirable, but in a country somewhat accustomed to being alerted in response to formless terrorist threats, it would seem appropriate to inform about threats that are considered both real and imminent.[2524] One CDC's communications director expressed skepticism that it was possible to effectively motivate people to take appropriate precautions against health risks without making them feel at least some level of concern or anxiety. "This is like breaking up with your boyfriend without hurting his feelings," the director said. "It can't be done."[2525]

WHO risk communication specialists considered "don't be afraid to frighten people" to be a key principle in communicating risks such as H5N1 with integrity.[2526] At the time, UN Secretary-General Kofi Annan counseled, "If other pandemics have taught us anything, it is that silence is deadly."[2527]

It is true that when people are already terrified, scaring them further may push them into denial. In general, however, public opinion polls showed that the population remained too apathetic about the threat of bird flu.[2528] A poll in Europe showed that the majority of the population believed that their governments could somehow protect them in the event of a pandemic.[2529] In a WHO publication, the communication experts concluded, "We can't scare people enough about H5N1."[2530] I can only hope the COVID-19 crisis has woken people up to taking pandemic threats more seriously.

One reason bird flu may sound apocryphal is that we don't want to believe there's something that modern medical science can't handle.[2531] Said Alberta's Health Minister, "What worries me most is the ignorance of people in the public who assume that if they get sick there'll be something there for them, and they don't realize the devastation this could be."[2532] Seeing how overwhelmed certain hospitals became just during a presumed Category 2 pandemic with COVID-19 should help dispel that notion.

The prospect of a more severe pandemic might also just be too disturbing to consciously consider. The same disbelief existed in 1918. From fancy dress balls in the Johannesburg City Hall in Spanish costume emblazoned with "Spanish flu" to Londoners holding "sneezing parties" with a bottle of champagne given as prize to the lustiest sneeze, the citizens of the world in early 1918 ridiculed as a joke the threat of "Spanish Influenza."[2533] They were not laughing for long.

Media messages about H5N1 were mixed. Until fall 2005, news of the impending pandemic was practically nonexistent in North America.[2534] Editorial pages slowly started to take notice of the gravity of the situation. *The Philadelphia Inquirer* editorialized in August that "the U.S. policymakers remain amazingly passive about pandemic preparations."[2535] In September 2005, though, bird flu hit prime time. The ABC News *Primetime* special started with these words: "It could kill a billion people worldwide, make ghost towns out of parts of major cities, and there is not enough medicine to fight it. It is called the avian flu."[2536] Finally, the issue started getting the coverage it deserved.

Then, the media backlash began. Headlines like "No Local Threat from Avian Flu"[2537] or "Bird Flu Not Expected to Affect Arkansas"[2538] downplayed the global reach by misunderstanding the capacity of the virus to mutate into a human transmissible form. It was framed as strictly a threat to chickens and a few peasant farmers. Meat industry officials the world over said things such as: "We care about a pandemic. We do care. But so far, there is no scientific evidence of human-to-human transmission."[2539] Of course, by then it will be too late.

"It's still seen by many capital cities in the West as basically a lot of chickens dying and chicken farmers, so they think, where is the urgency?" explained the FAO of the United Nations. "Our reply is, if this develops into an uncontrollable pandemic in a year, it won't be farmers dying in the paddy-fields of Vietnam. People will be dying in Washington, New York, London and Paris."[2540] Countries, however, continued to bury their heads in the sand,[2541] and the United States was no exception, claimed Osterholm, who doubled in his professional life as both director of the Center for Infectious Disease Research and Policy and associate director for the Department of Homeland Security's National Center for Food Protection and Defense. "This to me is akin to living in Iowa," Osterholm said, "and seeing the tornado 35 miles away coming. And it's coming. And it's coming. And it's coming. And it keeps coming."[2542]

"I worry that too many policy leaders dance around this issue fearful that somehow they will either offend or frighten the public," Osterholm said, answering critics who complained about his dire warnings. "Our job is not to upset people or to calm people. Our job is to tell the truth."[2543] "I am not trying to scare people out of their wits," he said. "I am trying to scare them into their wits."[2544]

Our Best Shot

In 2005, two months following the Hurricane Katrina disaster, President Bush proposed a multibillion-dollar spending plan to address the pandemic, allotting much-needed funds to boost antiviral stockpiles and give domestic vaccine production a shot in the arm to improve vaccine technology.[2545] In an unclassified Congressional briefing, Gregory A. Poland of the Mayo Clinic and the Infectious Diseases Society of America said, "We and the entire world remain unprepared for what could arguably be the most horrific disaster in modern history." He emphasized, "The key to our survival, in my opinion, and to the continuity of government is vaccination.[2546]

Officials understood that waiting for the pandemic strain to arise before starting vaccine production would mean a six- to eight-month delay and untold numbers of deaths. Instead of waiting, many experts advocated making a human vaccine to the bird-adapted H5N1 in hopes that the current strain would be sufficiently similar to the virus that eventually "went human" for the vaccine to afford at least some protection. The vaccine industry was not quick to act on that recommendation. In 2004, the editorial board of science journal *Nature Medicine* asked, "Why have we waited so long to develop a human vaccine against avian flu despite evidence—dating back to 1997—of human infection?"[2547] A year earlier, after another man in Hong Kong died from H5N1, Robert Webster put it flatly: "We've had H5N1 since 1997, yet we don't have a vaccine on the shelf. That is a black eye for WHO and the system. What the hell have we been doing?"[2548]

Despite years of lost lead time, the development of an H5N1 vaccine was announced in 2005. *The New York Times* ran an exclusive in its Sunday edition trumpeting, "Avian Flu Vaccine Called Effective in Human Testing." The story of a human H5N1 vaccine was picked up by the Associated Press and echoed with titles like "Vaccine Appears to Ward Off Bird Flu."[2549] These feel-good "hope is on the way" stories may have led to a nationwide collective sigh of relief. Unfortunately, the story was effectively retracted days later[2550] as details emerged.[2551]

The announcement had been based on a small clinical study showing that healthy volunteers injected with a vaccine made from a single Southeast Asian strain of H5N1 did seem to make antibodies against the virus. However, the H5N1 strain used was not the one that escaped from China into Russia and winged its way to Western Europe. What's more, the response unfortunately did not necessarily translate into protection from disease. Other experimental influenza vaccines had similarly raised antibodies, but, paradoxically, they led to increased severity of disease and mortality in vaccinated animals in laboratories.[2552] Even if the vaccine could effectively reduce mortality from the avian strain utilized *and* the imminent human pandemic virus, the researchers discovered that the dose required to elicit the immune response was so huge that it made global production impractical.[2553] To Osterholm, the results suggested that the world was even less prepared than previously thought.[2554] "You know how you creep, then you walk, then you run?" Osterholm asked. "We're still on our knees."[2555]

Annual flu vaccines typically only require a single shot of 15 micrograms (μg) of killed virus protein, since people already have a low level of pre-existing immunity to similar strains from past flu seasons.[2556] Essentially no one, though, has any natural immunity to H5 viruses.[2557] The researchers reported that a massive vaccination dose—two separate injections of 90μg—would be required. Twelve times the standard dose of regular flu vaccine means twelve times fewer vaccine doses can be produced. "Needing two doses of 90μg is the worst-case scenario," noted a leading virologist. "You are not going to get very far with that."[2558]

At the time, the U.S. production capacity for seasonal flu vaccines was 180 million doses. Two doses of 90μg would mean that if the entire U.S. production system devoted itself entirely to making pandemic vaccine, it could only produce enough to protect fifteen million people, barely 5 percent of the U.S. population.[2559] Globally, the situation was worse. At the concentration required, the world's vaccine producers, straining at full capacity, would only be able to cover about 1 percent of the planet's population. "There is now a tremendous anxiety among scientists—including me—about this," said Professor Peter Dunnill, chair of the Advanced Centre for Biochemical Engineering at University College, London, at the time. "Instead of providing protection for up to a billion people across the world, we will be lucky to get enough doses to vaccinate a few dozen million."[2560] A WHO official asked, "Who's going to get the limited antivirals and vaccines that do become available? And how do we live with people who don't? What do we say to them?"[2561]

"The good news is, we do have a vaccine," Secretary Leavitt told CBS News' *The Early Show*.[2562] "It doesn't matter if we have a vaccine now or not," Osterholm exclaimed in a telephone interview. "We can't make it."[2563] It's not enough to produce a vaccine; it must be mass produced.[2564] Anthony Fauci, director of the U.S. National Institute of Allergy and Infectious Diseases, described the "critical issue" as: "Can we make enough vaccine, given the well-known inability of the vaccine industry to make enough vaccine?"[2565] "For those of us who do this and think about it every day, all day," Fauci continued, "even if we could and wanted to and made the decision—this is what we need—the capacity's not there."[2566] This begged the question, *why not?* Why weren't there more dedicated factories? Why did the vaccine distribution system allegedly remain "broken, both technically and financially?"[2567] Why was the manufacturing process—as an expert summed up in one word—"lousy?"[2568]

Two-time Pulitzer Prize–winning journalists Donald L. Barlett and James B. Steele have been called by *The Washington Journalism Review* "almost certainly the best team in the history of investigative reporting."[2569] They took on those questions for the seasonal flu shots in a *New York Times* editorial and laid blame on the privatization of vaccine production. "Preventing a flu epidemic that could kill thousands," they wrote, "is not nearly as profitable as making pills for something like erectile dysfunction."[2570] Bringing a vaccine to market may cost drug companies close to $1 billion;[2571] that's how much money Viagra alone brings in every year.[2572] Ideally, vaccines are "one shot deals," unlike medications more profitably taken long-term.[2573] "It's basically the corporate model working," said a flu expert at the University of Michigan. "You put your money where the blockbusters are."[2574]

Industry insiders agree. David Fedson, a former director of medical affairs for a major vaccine manufacturer, noted, "We have a toxic mixture in America of a corporate culture that is inappropriate for producing vaccines for national security and a political culture that is unwilling to accept government responsibility for ensuring it is achieved." "Our corporate culture demands a 15–25% annual net return on sales," he said, "which life-saving commodity products such as vaccines never attain."[2575]

Lacking adequate domestic vaccine production, the fear was that Americans may have found themselves at the end of the line when the H5N1 pandemic broke.[2576] The few U.S. vaccine manufacturers produced most of their vaccine overseas in countries that could nationalize production facilities and claim first dibs.[2577] We acted in much the same way in 1976; anticipating a swine flu pandemic, the United States refused to share any of its vaccine.[2578] "It is sheer folly," one doctor wrote, "to expect overseas sourcing [of a vaccine] as an option."[2579]

The rest of the world would be left even worse off. At the time, 90 percent of production capacity for all influenza vaccines was concentrated in European and North American countries that account for only 10 percent of the world's population.[2580] "If there is an epidemic of bird flu and people start dying in the proportion people believe, I don't think goodwill is going to be an issue," said a former chairman of the Food and Drug Administration's vaccine advisory committee. "It's going to be every man for himself."[2581]

Acknowledging a "compelling national interest for a vaccine manufacturing capacity to exist," the Bush administration's answer was to provide incentives and subsidies "ranging from liability insurance to better profit margins" for the pharmaceutical giants that produce vaccines.[2582] The potential saving of millions of lives was evidently not a "compelling national interest." *Nature*'s senior reporter commented: "When the military knows it needs a fighter aircraft, it doesn't offer incentives to Lockheed Martin or Boeing. It pays them through procurement to develop the weapon to the specifications it wants."[2583]

Scientists worked on a way to decrease the required dose of H5N1 vaccine by adding a chemical adjuvant—a substance that nonspecifically irritates the immune system and may boost the immune response to the vaccine.[2584] Others pushed for more radical solutions. One new approach was cell-culture, rather than egg-based, vaccine production. One artifact of the system was that when a virus is grown in eggs for certain types of vaccines, it may adapt to the infection of eggs, rather than the infection of humans. Growing the virus directly in cultures of human cells, however, precluded that possibility.[2585] Also, according to then director of the FDA's Center for Biologics Evaluation and Review, growing vaccine virus in culture not only eliminates the need for hundreds of millions of fertile chicken eggs, but also is expected to increase the flexibility, yield, and speed of vaccine production.[2586] It was thought that President Bush's break away from pro-life forces over stem cell research may facilitate research on cell culture-based vaccines,[2587] some of which—like Sabin's famous polio vaccine—use fetal tissue.[2588]

Efforts to upgrade and expand domestic vaccine production continued in the United States, but were expected to take years to have an effect.[2589] Today, most flu vaccines are still produced using chicken eggs.[2590] Asked if it was too late to prepare for the coming pandemic, vaccine industry insider Fedson replied, "It's always too late, and it's never too soon. But we've got to start somewhere."[2591]

LESSONS UNLEARNED

"The success or failure of any government in the final analysis must be measured by the well-being of its citizens. Nothing can be more important to a state than its public health; the state's paramount concern should be the health of its people."

—FRANKLIN DELANO ROOSEVELT [2592]

The "better late than never" Bush proposal of billions to improve domestic antiviral and vaccine capacity was not without its critics. The head of the UN

Food and Agriculture Organization questioned why the United States wasn't helping more with efforts to monitor and control the disease in Southeast Asia. "It doesn't look to us quite rational," he said, "that we would be ready to spend so much money on the second line of defense and then on the first line of the combat field, we're not putting even $100 million."[2593] Once it hit, paltry antiviral stockpiles in rich countries, as the Canadian Medical Association put it, would provide no more than a pandemic "speed bump."[2594] But even if, on a global scale, antivirals did turn out just to be a "Band-Aid," as the dean of Drexel University's School of Public Health noted, they would stop some of the bleeding.[2595]

Putting all our bird flu eggs in one Tamiflu basket might not have been the wisest allocation of U.S. funds. A better solution may have been to revitalize our critical public health infrastructure, which had been crippled, according to the National Academy of Medicine, by "grave underfunding and political neglect."[2596] As one senior senator admitted, "The decline in preparedness and effectiveness of the nation's first-line medical defense systems can be traced to these ill advised budget cuts which forced the termination of essential and research and training programs."[2597] Quoting from a 1988 Institute of Medicine report, "We have let down our public health guard as a nation and the health of the public is unnecessarily threatened as a result."[2598] A 2002 updated Institute report concluded that the U.S. public health system "that was in disarray in 1988 remains in disarray today."[2599]

The general director of the conservative Mercatus Center suggested a budget-neutral switch of most of the $10 billion that was going into developing anti-ballistic missile defense, in part to help bolster local public health system preparedness.[2600] Unfortunately, the opposite trend seemed to be happening. Just as President Bush repeatedly underfunded the New Orleans levees[2601] before Hurricane Katrina hit, funding for local and state public health departments continued to be cut. For fiscal 2005, the administration proposed a $100 million *cut* for state and local public health preparedness[2602] and $129 million in proposed cuts for 2006.[2603] House Democratic Leader Nancy Pelosi criticized these cuts as leaving "our state and local health agencies without the resources they need to protect communities in the event of a pandemic."[2604] The president of the National Association of County and City Health Officials agreed. "Critical funding is shrinking," he said, "just as public health agencies are being required to expand their work in pandemic influenza preparation and response."[2605]

After 9/11, the Department of Homeland Security spent billions preparing for disasters, but most of it was concentrated on acts of terrorism.[2606] "No one cares about disasters until they happen," lamented one emergency management expert. "That is a political fact of life."[2607] The president of the National Academy of Medicine and former dean of the Harvard School of Public Health described nature as the worst terrorist one can imagine.[2608]

The Trump Administration's firing of the U.S. pandemic response team to cut costs[2609] is a continuation of this theme. The day before the dissolution became public, one of the officials on that team, the director of medical and biodefense preparedness at the National Security Council, was speaking at a symposium to mark the one hundredth anniversary of the 1918 influenza pandemic. "The threat of pandemic flu is the number one health security concern," she reportedly told the audience. "Are we ready to respond? I fear the answer is no."[2610]

> "Don't need a weatherman to know which way the wind blows."
>
> —Bob Dylan

In the White House Rose Garden press conference that triggered a surge of bird flu media coverage, President Bush addressed the pandemic. "The people of the country ought to rest assured," Bush said, "that we're doing everything we can."[2611] Iowa Senator Tom Harkin was not assured. "'Trust us' is not something the administration can say after Katrina," he said in an interview. "I don't think Congress is in a mood to trust. We want plans. We want specific goals and procedures we're going to take to prepare for this."[2612]

Hurricane Katrina hit just days after Bush reportedly finished reading the classic historical text on the 1918 pandemic during his August vacation on his ranch. John M. Barry's *The Great Influenza: The Epic Story of the Deadliest Plague in History*[2613] details how the U.S. government, in the words of a 2005 report by the National Academy of Medicine, "badly handled" the situation.[2614] This combination may have spurred the administration's sudden interest. Redlener called it the "post-Katrina effect." He said, "I don't think politically or perceptually the government feels that it could tolerate another tragically inadequate response to a major disaster."[2615]

As Secretary Leavitt toured hurricane emergency shelters after Rita, the hurricane that hit just a few weeks after Katrina, it hit him how catastrophic the pandemic would be. "What if it weren't just New Orleans?" he recalled thinking. "What if it were Seattle, San Diego, Corpus Christi, Denver, Chicago, New York? Make your own list."[2616] "We have learned in the past weeks," Secretary Leavitt told reporters, "that bad things can happen very fast."[2617]

He also should have learned the folly of ignoring the warnings of experts. Whether it was the *Challenger* disaster, 9/11, or Katrina, there were experts who cautioned that these particular tragedies might happen. The U.S. Army Corps of Engineers had been warning about the levees in New Orleans for years, and New Orleans' major newspaper ran a five-part series in 2002 that accurately predicted not only the inevitable blow from a major storm, but also the nightmarish aftermath.[2618] "The danger of a major hurricane hitting New Orleans was ignored until it was too late," said Senator Kennedy. "We can't make the same mistake with pandemic flu."[2619] Though senior public health scientists described an H5N1 pandemic with soundbites like "Hurricane Katrina a thousand times over,"[2620] a former FEMA director in October 2005 described the level of federal preparation for the pandemic as "zero."[2621]

In a Category 5 pandemic, there would be no cavalry.[2622] During Katrina, the nation's resources were mobilized to aid three states. Imagine every city as New Orleans. "We could be battling 5,000 different fronts at the same moment. Any community that fails to prepare with the expectation that the federal government will come to the rescue will be tragically wrong," Secretary Leavitt told state public health officials.[2623] In Chicago, public health officials ran through a mock influenza pandemic scenario. The simulation showed the public health system breaking down almost immediately.[2624] The chief medical officer of the Department of Homeland Security warned, "The federal government will not be there to pick you off your roof in a pandemic."[2625] "If the avian flu were to hit here, it would be like having a Category 5 viral hurricane hit every single state simultaneously," said the director of Trust for America's Health.[2626] "We're not prepared. It's the ugly truth."[2627]

George Mason University's Mercatus Center concluded that we must "[r]ealize that the federal government will be largely powerless in the worst stages of a pandemic and make appropriate local plans."[2628] Each individual community should be responsible for preparing its own pandemic plan— preparation begins with each family, each circle of friends, each neighborhood, each business, each township. "Someday," Osterholm wrote in the public policy journal *Foreign Affairs,* "after the next pandemic has come and gone, a commission much like the 9/11 Commission will be charged with determining how well government, business, and public health leaders prepared the world for the catastrophe when they had clear warning. What will be the verdict?"[2629]

According to the Holbert C. Harris chair of economics at George Mason University and general director of the University's Mercatus Center, the administration's multibillion-dollar initiative to begin preparations may have been too little, too late. "[I]f a pandemic came in 2006," he said, "American efforts would be statistically indistinguishable from zero preparation."[2630] Osterholm explained, on behalf of the Center for Infectious Disease Research and Policy:

> If we were to begin a Manhattan Project–type response tonight to expand vaccine and drug production, we wouldn't have a measurable impact on the availability of these critical products to sufficiently address a worldwide pandemic for at least several years. What we need to do right now is focus on what will get us through a pandemic without counting on drugs. We just don't have a supply chain that can manufacture enough vaccine and antivirals to make a meaningful dent in what we'd need if the pandemic hits in the next two or three years. We need to think about things like food supplies, health care workers and facilities, essential services. We're wasting time.[2631]

IV. Surviving the COVID-19 Pandemic

PUMPING THE BRAKES

Slowing an Outbreak

Regardless of where the COVID-19 virus SARS-CoV-2 came from, now that it's spreading from human to human, what can we do about it?

MERS could be stopped because of its relatively low "basic reproduction number," abbreviated as R_0. (That's the *R naught* you may have heard about.) R_0 is a measure of how contagious a new pathogen is. More specifically, it represents the number of people a single infected individual is expected to pass the disease to in a susceptible population. For MERS, the R_0 was only 1, so each MERS patient tended to transmit the disease to only one other person.[2632] You can imagine how much easier a disease like that can be stopped compared to a virus with the potential to spread exponentially, viruses like the SARS or COVID-19 coronaviruses, with an R_0 of 2 or greater. In the case of a virus with an R_0 of 2, for example, unless stopped, one infected person could become two, then four, then eight, and so on. The coronavirus that causes COVID-19 may be able to latch onto receptors in the human respiratory tract better than the coronavirus that caused SARS[2633] and also replicate better in the upper airways,[2634] but the primary reason there may have been more cases of COVID-19 in the first month of reporting[2635] than

SARS ever caused revolves less around how contagious it is and more around *when* it is contagious.[2636]

The three characteristics of microbes "most likely to cause pandemics and global catastrophes" are: (1) novelty, so there's no preexisting immunity; (2) respiratory spread (respiratory tract infections are humanity's fourth-leading killer even outside a pandemic);[2637] and (3) transmission before symptom onset.[2638] The last four airborne pandemics were caused by new flu viruses, each of which fit all three of those criteria. SARS, however, was not considered a pandemic, despite spreading to twenty-nine countries and regions. Why did the World Health Organization only consider SARS a "Public Health Emergency of International Concern," and how were we able to stop it within just a few months at only 8,096 cases and 774 deaths?[2639] Though it was a brand-new virus spread via respiratory droplets, SARS largely lacked the third necessary characteristic: significant spread before symptoms arise.

For SARS, the average incubation period—the time between first becoming unwittingly infected after sufficient exposure to the virus and first coming down with symptoms—was around five days.[2640] It took another six to eleven days, however, for viral loads to fully ramp up in upper respiratory tract secretions coughed or sneezed from one person to the next.[2641] So, even after falling ill, patients with SARS weren't very infectious in the first five days or so.[2642] Since viral loads peaked about ten days *after* people started feeling sick,[2643] you can see how easily human-to-human transmission could be staunched if patients could be isolated within the first few days after the onset of symptoms.[2644] And that's exactly what happened. A massive international effort spearheaded by the WHO was able to identify all the cases by their symptoms, isolate the patients, and trace all their contacts.[2645] We were able to similarly eradicate smallpox from the planet because that disease was also only contagious after you knew who had it.[2646]

Fever screening at airports helped stop the global spread of SARS in its tracks. You didn't become particularly infectious until after symptoms started, and 100 percent of SARS patients developed a fever.[2647] In a way, SARS was a disease designed to be stopped. Similarly, with MERS, 98 percent of its patients got a fever.[2648] In the case of COVID-19, though, as many as 36 percent do not present with fever at the onset of symptoms,[2649] and, more seriously, patients may be infectious during the incubation period without any symptoms at all. The viral loads in the nose and throat of asymptomatic patients with COVID-19 have been similar in some cases to those of symptomatic patients, as many as fifteen million viral copies within every quarter teaspoon of snot.[2650] Like the flu, you can potentially spread the disease days before you know you have it,[2651] even while you're feeling perfectly fine.[2652] That's a disease that's hard to stop. To slow the spread of that kind of disease, you have to try isolating everyone.[2653]

Slowing a Pandemic

Closing nonessential businesses, canceling gatherings, and encouraging people to shelter in place at home all attempt to break every possible chain of transmission. China was condemned for its early response, sanctioning critics[2654] and denying the extent of the crisis (referring to it as "preventable and controllable"[2655]), but later lauded for that same authoritarian approach when it came to successfully enacting extreme quarantine measures. A top WHO official praised China's efforts as "probably the most ambitious, and I would say, agile and aggressive disease containment effort in history."[2656]

It was, however, too little, too late to contain the disease locally.[2657] By the time authorities banned travel out of Wuhan, more than a third of the fourteen million residents had already left the region, whether for the Chinese New Year holiday or to flee before the lockdown of the city went into effect on January 23, 2020.[2658] One could argue that had local officials not wasted weeks silencing whistleblowers and releasing false epidemic reports, the world could have been spared this pandemic,[2659] but the aggressive actions China subsequently did take may have indeed bought us all some time.[2660]

Enacting so-called wartime control measures,[2661] China initiated the largest community containment effort in history,[2662] affecting an estimated 760 million people.[2663] Borders were closed, cities were sealed off, and people were confined to their homes. Unlike "lockdowns" other countries started instituting that still allowed residents to venture freely outside as long as they respected a certain personal distance, in China, citizens were restricted with permission cards that only allowed them to leave their home every second day for a maximum of thirty minutes.[2664] The policy was criticized by human rights advocates,[2665] but it worked. The epidemic immediately started decelerating.[2666]

Chinese authorities achieved what many public health experts didn't think was possible—the relative containment of the spread of a widely circulating respiratory infection.[2667] Within two months, Hubei Province, ground zero where the disease first emerged, reported its first day of no new local cases.[2668] "I will praise China again and again because its actions actually help in reducing the spread of the novel coronavirus to other countries," the director-general of the World Health Organization said.[2669] "In many ways, China is actually setting a new standard for outbreak response. It's not an exaggeration."[2670]

The day Hubei Province reported no new cases, though, is the day the world confirmed its two hundred thousandth case.[2671] Would the rest of the world be willing to enact rules one global health policy specialist called "astounding, unprecedented, and medieval"?[2672] The command-and-control authority of the Chinese government allowed them to enforce a resource-intensive containment strategy that involved costs to trade, travel, and liberty that many doubted democracies would be able to stomach.[2673] Thankfully, successful strategies in countries such as Singapore and South Korea showed that such draconian measures may not be necessary.

All the nations that were able to get the disease under control quickly relied on a foundation of testing and tracing. In other words, identify all cases through mass testing and then trace every possible contact each patient had to break as many chains of transmission as possible through isolation and quarantine.[2674] South Korea had a test approved the first week of February[2675] and ramped up to test as many as eighteen thousand people a day through dozens of fast, free, drive-through testing stations.[2676] With such expansive, well-organized testing, countries like South Korea were able to control the epidemic without resorting to locking down its populace.[2677] The World Health Organization took notice. "We have a simple message for all countries," the director-general declared, "test, test, test."[2678]

The United States did not appear to get the message in time. By mid-March, South Korea had already tested more than a quarter million of its citizens, more than fifty times more per capita than the United States.[2679] Hamstrung by FDA red tape[2680] and a series of blunders,[2681] sufficient U.S. testing capacity failed to materialize before the window on containment closed.[2682] It's humbling to realize that the United States and South Korea recorded their first cases on the same day,[2683,2684] yet the ensuing epidemics took very different courses.

Once containment fails, the strategy then shifts to suppression and mitigation. If you don't know who's infected, all you can do is try to prevent everyone from coming into contact with anyone. By mid-March, one in four Americans were being told to stay home to try to curb the spread.[2685] As Dr. Fauci told policy-makers and the public, "If it looks like you're over-reacting, you're probably doing the right thing."[2686]

Closing nonessential businesses and encouraging people to stay inside to limit social contacts are efforts taken in an attempt to "flatten the [epidemic] curve" before it flattens us—in other words, to slow the spread of the illness to more evenly distribute the cases over time.[2687] This would give health systems time to scale up and respond effectively, not only to treat COVID-19 but to maintain overall care continuity.[2688] During the recent Ebola crisis in West Africa, for example, deaths increased from other causes as well, due to the saturation of the health-care system (as well as the death of health-care workers).[2689]

School closures are more controversial, as they could threaten the availability of the 29 percent of health-care providers in households with young children. One model suggested that school closures might have to reduce COVID-19 cases by more than 25 percent to make up for the loss of health-care workers in terms of a net reduction in COVID-19 mortality.[2690] This may be achievable for pandemic influenza,[2691] a disease in which children may play a critical role in community transmission,[2692] but children don't appear to be the main drivers of the transmission of COVID-19.[2693]

Until an effective vaccine is widely available, likely not until 2021 at the earliest,[2694] population lockdowns can help rob the virus of susceptible hosts. Once such measures are relaxed, though, the disease could come roaring back.[2695] In the pandemic of 1918, for example, some U.S. cities experienced a second peak in mortality following the lifting of social-distancing measures.[2696] By periodically pressing the brake with flattening-the-curve strategies like shelter-in-place ordinances to slow community transmission, the hope is that we can turn the initial tidal wave of cases into a series of smaller successive waves our health-care capability can more safely ride out.[2697] If not, more intensive care units in U.S. hospitals may become overwhelmed just as they did in Italy,[2698] and doctors will have to make triage decisions as to who lives and who dies. It's better to be six feet apart than six feet under.

Proposed triage protocols have already been published in the journal of the American College of Chest Physicians. First in line for ventilators are those who are most likely to survive both in the short term and over the subsequent year. Then the priority goes to children and adults under the age of fifty. Those fifty to sixty-nine are in the next tier, followed by those aged seventy to eighty-four, and, finally, eighty-five and older. If there's a tie, lifesaving ventilation may be allocated based on "some form of lottery," like flipping a coin.[2699] In *The New England Journal of Medicine*, a preeminent group of medical ethics experts wrote, "[W]e believe that removing a patient from a ventilator or an ICU bed to provide it to others in need is also justifiable and that patients should be made aware of this possibility at admission," adding, "the decision to withdraw a scarce resource to save others is not an act of killing and does not require the patient's consent." To relieve frontline clinicians of the burden, they suggest the designation of "triage officers" to make the decisions.[2700]

The countries that were able to mobilize the fastest and have been best able to control COVID-19 were those that had learned hard lessons from previous outbreaks. China, Hong Kong, Singapore, and Taiwan bear the memories of SARS.[2701] More recently, South Korea suffered a MERS outbreak in 2015, triggered by a businessman returning from the Middle East.[2702] The countries' test-and-trace infrastructures were in place and their populations primed to sacrifice for the promise of containment.[2703] Maybe COVID-19 is the dry run we needed, the fire drill to awaken us from our complacency. If outbreaks involving dozens or even hundreds of deaths can rally countries to a state of pandemic preparedness, perhaps the thousands or even millions of deaths from COVID-19 will orient the countries of the world to the mission of pandemic prevention.

That's what this book is about. But first, what can each of us do individually to ride out the current pandemic?

TREATING AND AVOIDING COVID-19

The Clinical Course of COVID-19

With an average incubation period calculated at about five days, we have almost a week between the moment we get sufficiently exposed to the virus and the moment we start showing symptoms. In those five or so days, we can be infected—and potentially infectious—before we know it. About 98 percent of those who are going to start showing symptoms do so by day twelve,[2704] which explains why people are typically quarantined for two weeks after a potential exposure.[2705] After infection, viral shedding may continue for more than a month[2706] (with an average of twenty days), though it's not clear how contagious survivors are during that extended time period.[2707]

The most common symptoms are fever and cough, eventually experienced by about 90 percent and 70 percent of patients, respectively, based on an analysis of more than fifty thousand COVID-19 patients.[2708] Only about four in ten may experience fatigue, three in ten cough up phlegm, and two in ten experience muscle aches. Only about one in ten appear to suffer either from gastrointestinal symptoms, such as nausea, vomiting, or diarrhea, or common cold–type symptoms like runny or stuffy nose, headache, or a sore throat.[2709] This is consistent with the regional concentration of ACE2—the receptors the virus latches onto—in the lungs, rather than the nose or throat.[2710] (In pangolins, ACE2 is found on their flicking anteater tongues.[2711]) The only symptom found predictive of a more severe course was difficulty breathing, which resulted in more than six times the odds of eventually having to be admitted into the ICU.[2712]

The notion that the course of about 80 percent of cases are "mild" is derived from an analysis by the Chinese Center for Disease Control and Prevention that was based on nearly forty-five thousand confirmed cases. While there are certainly mild and even asymptomatic cases, it's important to understand what "mild" means to the Chinese CDC. Its definition of mild included those with "walking pneumonia," meaning pneumonia not dire enough to require supplemental oxygen or hospitalization but pneumonia nonetheless—certainly not the common cold–type courses people might think of when they hear the word mild, though the cases were at least mild enough that people should be able to treat themselves at home. The remaining 20 or so percent of confirmed cases were classified as either severe (about 15 percent), which involved difficulty getting enough oxygen, or critical (5 percent), encompassing respiratory failure, septic shock, and multisystem organ failure. About half of the critical cases died.[2713]

The severity of COVID-19 varies widely based on preexisting conditions. Those with high blood pressure are at twice the odds of suffering a severe course and those with cardiovascular disease three times the odds.[2714] Those with either condition are about four times likelier to end up in the ICU.[2715] Those with COPD—chronic obstructive pulmonary diseases like emphysema—appear to be at the highest risk with six times the odds of a severe course for COVID-19 and nearly eighteen times the odds of ICU admission.[2716]

A history of air pollution exposure may increase susceptibility,[2717] but, ironically, the number of lives saved by the decreased air pollution in China, thanks to its lockdown, may exceed the number of people killed by the virus,[2718] averting as many as twenty-four thousand to thirty-six thousand premature deaths a month.[2719] This means China's air quality was so bad that COVID-19 may have ended up saving lives in China.

As with the other two deadly coronavirus diseases, SARS[2720] and MERS,[2721] those with diabetes also appear to be at higher risk,[2722] though based on a retrospective SARS analysis, optimal blood sugar control during treatment may improve prognosis.[2723] Excess body fat alone seems to be a risk factor independent of diabetes.[2724] Those with severe obesity (weighing more than 215 pounds at the average American's height of five foot six) have seven times the odds of ending up on a ventilator.[2725] But even just being overweight puts you at risk. Those with a body mass index (BMI) of 28 or more (about 175 pounds at the average height) appear to be at nearly six times the odds of suffering a severe COVID-19 course.[2726] In the United States, the average BMI exceeds 29.[2727]

The excess risk from the excess body fat may arise from greater systemic inflammation,[2728] fat covering the heart itself,[2729] or the restriction of breathing caused by excessive fatty tissue in the upper body.[2730] Even without taking weight into account, most American adults over the age of fifty suffer from a "comorbidity" that may put them at risk.[2731]

HOLDING ALL THE ACES?

A history of smoking is a risk factor for COVID-19 disease progression,[2732] though, surprisingly, active smoking may[2733] or may not be.[2734] This seeming paradox may provide a clue as to why those with hypertension appear to be at higher risk.

It's easy to imagine why those with heart disease are at higher risk of crashing from COVID-19. Lung infections can put a tremendous strain on the heart. Up to nearly 30 percent of patients hospitalized for regular pneumonia develop cardiovascular complications.[2735] About one in thirty-five suffer cardiac arrest,[2736] and those who don't are still at up to a four times higher risk of a heart attack or stroke within the first thirty days after being released from the hospital.[2737] But why is just having high blood pressure a COVID-19 severity risk factor?

Under certain circumstances, those hospitalized for regular pneumonia with hypertension may do *better.* Investigators speculated this may be due to the anti-inflammatory effects of a common class of high blood pressure drugs called *ACE inhibitors*[2738] (like lisinopril, for which there are more than a hundred million prescriptions dispensed annually in the United States alone).[2739] Indeed, people on those drugs not only appear to be less likely to die of pneumonia, they also seem to be less likely to even get pneumonia in the first place.[2740] Ironically, this same reason why those with hypertension may be protected from regular pneumonia may also be the reason why those with hypertension are at greater risk from COVID-19.

ACE inhibitor drugs may be anti-inflammatory, but they may also upregulate the expression of ACE2,[2741] which, as you may remember, is the enzyme the COVID-19 virus latches onto in our lungs to infect our cells and spread. So, perhaps the reason those with hypertension seem to be doing worse is that so many of them are on this class of drugs, which may be making them more susceptible to viral attack. ACE2 expression is increased in comorbid conditions like hypertension,[2742] but the drug connection has yet to be verified.[2743] Certainly, those who are on these ACE inhibitor drugs for heart failure, or for severe or uncontrolled hypertension, should not just stop taking them. (You definitely do not want to have a stroke when ICUs are overwhelmed.) However, the vast majority taking these drugs do so to treat well-managed mild hypertension, and for these patients, physicians may want to consider temporarily discontinuing them for those at high risk of contracting COVID-19.[2744]

Early on, I recommended that people consider not taking ibuprofen unnecessarily,[2745] as it is another drug thought to boost ACE2 expression.[2746] While the concern remains theoretical, no drug is completely benign. (Drugs like ibuprofen cause intestinal-lining damage in as many as 80 percent of users, for example.[2747]) So, *no* drug should be taken unnecessarily. Furthermore, ibuprofen-like drugs are strongly advised against in lower respiratory tract infections, as it has been associated with higher complication rates in both children and adults with pneumonia. [2748] In fact, fever may actually be beneficial and probably shouldn't be routinely treated by any means, including with non-ibuprofen-type drugs like Tylenol.[2749] Those prescribed low-dose aspirin for cardiovascular disease, however, should continue their treatment.[2750]

To bring this full circle to our original question, the ACE2 connection may also offer some insight into the inconsistent findings between current and past smokers. Nicotine can *down*regulate ACE2.[2751] So, while it's always a good idea to quit smoking, this may explain why active smokers may or may not necessarily be at significantly higher risk of COVID-19 progression.[2752]

Advanced age is also a key risk factor for COVID-19 progression.[2753] Although the disease has afflicted newborns only a few days old through seniors in their nineties, most patients (nearly 90 percent in one large case series) are between thirty and seventy-nine.[2754] The severity of disease, however, disproportionately affects older individuals. In China, the average age of those requiring intensive care was sixty-two, compared to the non-ICU cases, which had an average age of forty-six.[2755] In the United States, even without underlying conditions or other risk factors, those aged sixty-five and older appear to be hospitalized or end up in the ICU at approximately three times the rate of those aged nineteen to sixty-four.[2756]

Though the media has capitalized on stories of young, healthy individuals suffering severe or even fatal outcomes, people under sixty-five without known underlying, predisposing medical conditions account for only about 1 percent of all COVID-19 deaths.[2757] Of confirmed cases in South Korea, only about one in a thousand died in their thirties and forties, but that rose to closer to one in one hundred and fifty of those patients in their fifties, one in fifty of those in their sixties, one in fifteen in their seventies, and one in five patients in their eighties.[2758] Though the relative lack of testing makes U.S. data less reliable, based on the first few thousand American cases, these age-related death risks are similar.[2759] The vulnerability of our seniors to the pandemic was exemplified by ground zero of the first major U.S. outbreak, a nursing home in Washington State. Of the home's 130 or so residents, 101 became infected, and more than a third lost their lives.[2760]

On autopsy, the respiratory surface of the lung under a microscope appears obliterated by scar tissue.[2761] Pulmonary fibrosis (lung scarring) is expected to become one of the long-term complications among survivors of serious COVID-19 infection.[2762] A six-month follow-up of SARS survivors found about one in three showed evidence of scarring on chest x-rays, and one in six suffered a significant impairment in lung function.[2763]

Death from COVID-19 comes from progressive "consolidation" of the lung, meaning your lungs start filling up with something other than air. In the case of regular pneumonia, it's largely pus. In COVID-19 pneumonia, postmortems show you drown in lungs that are "filled with clear liquid jelly."[2764]

How to Treat COVID-19

At the time I am writing this in April 2020, there is no specific, proven therapy for COVID-19. More than four hundred clinical treatment trials are under way,[2765] but we should not expect a vaccine or effective antiviral drug to be available anytime soon.[2766]

Many have asked me for advice on what they can eat to help bolster their immune system. "How Not to Die from Infections" is, after all, the title of chapter 5 of my book *How Not to Die*,[2767] and I do have more than a hundred free videos online at NutritionFacts.org that reference immune function.[2768] There are amazing studies—like randomized double-blind trials showing, for example, that eating broccoli sprouts can reduce viral loads for influenza, decrease virus-induced inflammation,[2769] and boost our antiviral natural killer cell activity.[2770] But this isn't the flu.

I certainly support general, commonsense advice to stay healthy during the crisis, put forth by such trusted authorities as the World Health Organization and the American College of Lifestyle Medicine. Such guidance includes getting sufficient sleep (seven to nine hours), keeping active, reducing stress, staying connected—albeit remotely—to friends and family, and eating healthfully (a diet centered around whole plant foods).[2771,2772,2773] However, I have resisted the urge to jump on the snake-oily spamwagon of *foods to boost your immune system* given our near-total ignorance of the immunological aspects of this new disease. Enhancing specific arms of the immune system could hypothetically even make things worse.

The assumption that the elderly are more susceptible to serious COVID-19 due to the waning of their immune system with age may not be correct. Young children have relatively immature immune systems and normally suffer disproportionally from viral infections such as the flu,[2774] but not, apparently, from COVD-19—or SARS or MERS, for that matter.[2775] Likewise, immunosuppressed patients are normally at greater risk of severe complications from respiratory viruses, but, again, that may not be the case with COVID-19 or the other two deadly coronaviruses. Take the example of a married couple as described in a Swiss medical journal. They were the same age and admitted to the hospital on the same day with same COVID-19 infection. Tragically, the wife was immunocompromised, because she was in chemotherapy treatment for breast cancer, while her husband had an intact immune system. The wife did fine, though, and was out of the hospital in less than a week, whereas the husband ended up in intensive care.[2776] How is it possible that the immunocompromised patient did better? Because our own immune response may be the main driver of lung tissue damage during coronavirus infection.[2777]

One theory as to why children seem protected suggests that greater preexisting exposure to common cold coronaviruses offer kids some cross-protection against the new virus.[2778] Ironically, a competing theory suggests it's their *lack* of exposure to similar viruses that's safeguarding them.[2779] There's a phenomenon known as *ADE,* antibody dependent enhancement. In most cases, the antibodies our bodies make to target pathogens neutralize them or, at the very least, tag them for removal. Sometimes, though, antibodies can actually facilitate viral infection and exacerbate disease. This may be the case with SARS, where antibodies generated against the viral spike proteins were sometimes found to promote infection.[2780] In monkeys, an experimental SARS vaccine resulted in aggravated lung damage.[2781] Vaccine developers are well aware of this phenomenon and would work to ensure any commercial vaccine would be free from this failing,[2782] but it has been used to venture a guess to account for the unusual age distribution of severe COVID-19 cases.

Perhaps similar coronaviruses circulated silently decades ago, and those old enough to have been exposed to them are now experiencing exaggerated responses to COVID-19.[2783] I'm not suggesting this speculation is true. I just use it to illustrate the complexity of our immune interactions. Pathogens attack, we counterattack, and then pathogens sometimes evolve to use our own counterattack in their favor. Just a word of caution before trying to specifically boost some element of our immune system before understanding the full scope of a new threat: Given the uncertainties, the best strategy is not to get infected in the first place, especially not until effective treatments—and a functioning health-care system—are available.

WHAT ABOUT ZINC?

I did look into zinc as a potential treatment after the fact-checking site Snopes validated that a noted virologist did indeed make a February 2020 recommendation to "Stock up now with zinc lozenges."[2784] He based his supposition on the efficacy of zinc for common colds, up to 29 percent of which are caused by coronaviruses.[2785] There is a sweet backstory: A three-year-old girl undergoing chemotherapy for leukemia (a disease marked by low zinc levels[2786]) refused to swallow a zinc supplement. Immunosuppressed, she had just started getting a cold. Instead of swallowing the supplement, she just let it dissolve in her mouth, and the cold seemed to disappear within hours.[2787] This observation led her own father to conduct the first randomized double-blind placebo-controlled trial on zinc lozenges.[2788]

There have since been more than a dozen randomized controlled trials published. Overall, researchers have found that zinc is indeed beneficial in reducing both duration and severity of the common cold when taken within the first twenty-four hours of symptom onset.[2789] Zinc lozenges appear to shorten colds by about three days,[2790] with significant reductions in nasal congestion and discharge, hoarseness, and cough.[2791]

The common cold results for zinc are often described as "mixed," but that appears to be largely because some studies used zinc lozenges containing ingredients like citric acid that strongly sequester zinc, so little or no free zinc is actually released.[2792] Lozenges containing around 10–15 mg of zinc as either zinc acetate or zinc gluconate without zinc binders such as citric acid, tartaric acid, glycine, sorbitol, or mannitol[2793] taken every two waking hours for a few days starting immediately upon symptom onset may work best.[2794] Best for the common cold, but what about COVID-19?

There are at least three purported mechanisms for the protection afforded by zinc.[2795] The first is that it interferes with the attachment of rhinoviruses, the most common cause of the common cold, to our cells.[2796] This presumably wouldn't help us in the case of COVID-19 since SARS-CoV-2 utilizes a different docking receptor. Zinc also appears to slow rhinovirus replication, at least in a petri dish,[2797] which was also found with the original SARS coronavirus, but that was in conjunction with a chemical that ferried zinc inside the cells.[2798] There are natural dietary compounds that may play a similar function,[2799] but even if viral replication were able to be slowed in the throat where the lozenge is, the COVID-19 virus is thought to propagate primarily in the lungs, not the throat.[2800]

The third mechanism by which zinc may help seems more promising: boosting our own antiviral immunity. For example, giving zinc pills to children with severe pneumonia has been shown to reduce mortality[2801] as much as threefold over placebo, but those studies were done in countries like Uganda,[2802] India,[2803] and Ecuador[2804] where there may have been preexisting zinc deficiencies.[2805] It's unclear if similar benefits could be had in higher-income countries with better population-wide micronutrient status.

I doubt zinc is going to be helpful for COVID-19 in well-nourished individuals, but taken as directed it shouldn't hurt, though zinc supplements and lozenges can cause nausea,[2806] especially when taken on an empty stomach. And one should never put zinc in their nose. There are intranasal zinc gels, sprays, and swabs sold commercially that have been linked to the potentially permanent loss of one's sense of smell.[2807]

(Happy ending: That three-year-old girl beat the cancer, never relapsed, and grew up to become a scientist herself.[2808])

How to Avoid COVID-19

Governments can only do so much. Preliminary evidence from Japan suggests the cancellation of events, gatherings, and meetings may slow the spread of COVID-19 by as much as 35 percent, but that has not been enough to contain the outbreak.[2809] During the unbridled phase of a pandemic, the best thing we can do may be to shelter in place, staying home to reduce contact with those outside our households as much as possible.[2810] You can't just wait until you hear it's in your area. By the time a single death occurs in your community, hundreds or even thousands of cases are likely present.[2811]

Those of us who need to leave our homes to provide essential services, from direct care to food delivery, should strive to keep a safe distance from others and sufficiently sanitize our hands every time we touch a public surface before we touch our mucous membranes, meaning our eyes or the inside of our nose or mouth. Once the pandemic is more under control, ample testing is in place, and the health-care system is no longer overrun, these social distancing precautions may start to be relaxed at least for less vulnerable individuals.[2812]

You can't infect others if you're not infected, and you can't get the virus unless the virus can get to you.

The COVID-19 virus is thought to be transmitted from one person to the next via respiratory droplets coughed out by the infected, propelled through the air, and then landing up the nose, in the mouth, or perhaps even on the eyes of a person nearby. Indirect avenues of spread involve infecting yourself by touching your eyes, nose, and mouth with hands contaminated by a virus-laden object or surface, such as rubbing your eyes or picking your nose after shaking someone's hand or touching a public surface like an elevator button, handrail, gas pump, or toilet handle.[2813] The levels of virus swarming in the snot of COVID-19 sufferers can reach close to a million per drop,[2814] which explains how easy it is for them to so thoroughly contaminate their surrounding environment.

The presence of the COVID-19 virus in stool samples suggests another way toilets may potentially transmit infection.[2815] Modern flush toilets aerosolize a plume of up to 145,000 droplets of toilet water into the air,[2816] which can remain floating around for at least thirty minutes.[2817] This may be one of the ways poliovirus is transmitted.[2818] So, put a lid on it. Close the lid before you flush and then, of course, thoroughly wash your hands.

During the SARS outbreak, traces of the virus were not only found on items handled directly by patients (like TV remote controls) and surfaces touched by those who interacted with the patients (like a refrigerator door at a nurses' station) but also floating in air samples taken from an infected patient's hospital room, suggesting the possibility of more robust airborne transmission than just coughed droplets.[2819] A similar study initially performed in a COVID-19 patient's hospital room found the virus on the majority of sampled surfaces, but all the air samples were negative.[2820] Since then, we've learned differently.

Studies performed at the Nebraska Biocontainment Unit and the National Quarantine Unit found the majority of air samples tested positive for traces of the COVID-19 coronavirus—even in the hallways outside of patients' rooms. However, the researchers were unable to verify if the airborne virus was infectious, given the extremely low concentration, less than a hundred copies per cubic foot of air.[2821] Nevertheless, because the virus can remain viable for hours when experimentally misted into the air,[2822] special care should certainly be taken during aerosol-generating medical procedures.

How long does the virus last on contaminated surfaces? Coronaviruses are "enveloped" viruses, wrapped in a stolen swath of our own cell membranes. As they bud out of infected cells, they cloak themselves in the outer layer of our cells. That oily coating helps them hide from immune surveillance, but it also makes them susceptible to disinfection and environmental inactivation. Non-enveloped viruses like poliovirus can persist for weeks outside of the body, whereas enveloped viruses tend to only be able to survive for days.[2823] As enveloped viruses go, though, coronaviruses tend to be relatively resistant.[2824]

There is a coronavirus that infects pigs that can last for a month on non-porous surfaces[2825] like metal, plastic, or glass, but human coronaviruses only make it about a week at most.[2826] On copper and brass, coronaviruses may not be able to survive longer than a few hours.[2827,2828] Different corona-viruses have different environmental stability. SARS-CoV, the SARS virus, lasts more than six days dried on plastic, whereas one of the common cold coronaviruses can't even make it three days.[2829] SARS-CoV also lasts up to four days in water or soil,[2830] but it survives for just minutes after drying on paper or cotton when lightly soiled or up to a day when heavily contami-nated.[2831] But what about SARS-CoV-2?

The COVID-19 virus appears to be more stable on cardboard than the SARS virus, with infectivity extinguished only after twenty-four hours at the same viral load that led to the SARS virus becoming inactive after eight hours.[2832] The COVID-19 virus appears to survive for less than three hours on printing paper, though.[2833] Its half-life on steel or plastic is about six hours, so about 99 percent is gone by forty-eight hours, but it may take as long as ninety-six hours for all infectivity to disappear.[2834] On cloth, SARS-CoV-2 may only last for one day, but, on the outer layer of surgical masks, it can survive for seven days.[2835]

The virus can only infect you, however, if it can get inside you. Having the virus on your fingers is only a problem if you then inoculate yourself by transferring that virus to your eyes, mouth, or nose, which connects down to your lungs. It's not your face in general—touching your forehead, cheek, or chin is presumably no more dangerous than touching your elbow. The virus can't pass through your skin. (The virus can only replicate in live cells, as I've discussed, and the outer layer of your skin is covered by protective strata of dead skin cells.) To get into your lungs, the virus has to find its way to your mucous membranes, the moist lining of your eyes, nostrils, or mouth. How can a virus get from your eyes to your lungs? The reason your nose starts to run when you cry is that tears drain though tiny channels that tunnel through the nasal bone and spill into your nostrils, and viruses in your eye can travel the same route.[2836]

As long as you don't touch your face, why does it matter if surfaces are contaminated? Because you *do* touch your face. The oft-repeated twenty-three-times-an-hour statistic is an overestimate, since most of the touches recorded in the cited study on university students were just to the skin on the face, but ten touches an hour were to the eyes, nose, or mouth.[2837] Adults videotaped in an office-type setting did worse, each touching their nostrils, eyes, or lips an average of nearly sixteen times an hour.[2838]

What about doctors? Physicians and other paramedical professionals were covertly observed during Grand Rounds at a hospital. About 40 percent picked their nose at least once.[2839] In family medicine offices, clinicians and staff touched their eyes, nose, or mouth an average of nineteen times in two hours (with a range from zero to one hundred and five touches).[2840] More concerning in terms of patient safety, however, was the finding that doctors only wash their hands about 30 percent of the times they should—even in intensive care units.[2841] And, even when medical personnel did wash their hands, it was only for an average of less than nine seconds.[2842]

How to Inactivate COVID-19

Because it's so difficult for people to keep themselves from unconsciously touching their faces, it's critical to be able to disinfect your hands. This can be accomplished by properly washing your hands with soap and water. The CDC recommends sudsing up for at least twenty seconds.[2843] It's not clear why they chose that duration.[2844] Unsurprisingly, there is evidence that washing with soap for twenty seconds is preferable to washing without soap for five seconds,[2845] but most of the published soap-to-soap studies compare fifteen seconds to thirty seconds and have found there does not appear to be a meaningful difference.[2846] The twenty-second recommendation was likely made to encourage sufficient hand coverage. Researchers have found the most frequently missed areas when washing include the fingertips, thumbs, and backs of hands.[2847] Artificial nails are discouraged, as they've been shown to interfere with handwashing efficacy.[2848]

Should you use hot water? No need. Contrary to popular belief,[2849] studies going back more than eighty years show no benefit in germ removal when using hot water over cool water,[2850] and frequent handwashing with hot water may increase the risk of skin irritation.[2851] (The false belief that warm or hot water is preferable may also add an additional million metric tons of carbon through energy usage to the atmosphere from the United States alone every year.[2852]) The use of lotions or creams has been shown to help protect hands from the minor skin damage associated with frequent handwashing at any temperature.[2853]

For health-care professionals, both the World Health Organization[2854] and the Centers for Disease Control and Prevention[2855] recommend using alcohol-based hand sanitizer, whether gel, foam, or spray, over handwashing for routine hand disinfection—that is, when hands are not visibly soiled. Part of the reason is enhanced compliance. Just as we cannot rely on people not to touch their faces, we cannot rely on people to wash their hands properly. In a family medicine clinic, fewer than one in ten handwashings met even a ten-second version of the CDC standards. In contrast, more than eight out of ten instances of disinfections with alcohol-based cleansers, which simply entails rubbing the hands together until the alcohol covers all surfaces of the hands and waiting for product to dry completely, hit the mark.[2856]

Normally cheap and ubiquitous at dollar stores everywhere, hand sanitizer was one of the first items to disappear from store shelves and internet inventories as the COVID-19 crisis loomed. Anyone heeding my decade-old advice on pandemic preparedness to stock up should already be well supplied, but, if not, you can make your own. Although 40 percent alcohol (either ethanol, regular drinking alcohol, or isopropyl, found in rubbing alcohol) has been found to topically kill some enveloped viruses like SARS or MERS, others, like hepatitis C and ebolavirus, require 60 percent alcohol or more, as measured on a volume rather than weight basis.[2857] That's why recommended alcohol concentrations in hand sanitizers range from 60 percent[2858] to 80 percent,[2859] because they want to account for a wide variety of pathogens. But what do we need specifically for COVID-19?

On Snopes, the social media meme that a "homemade hand sanitizer made with Tito's Vodka can be used to fight the new coronavirus" was ruled as false, since most vodkas (including Tito's) only contain 40 percent alcohol and Snopes cited the CDC's 60 percent minimum rule.[2860] However, the CDC has since published evidence by a respected team of researchers funded by the European Commission and German government that the COVID-19 coronavirus could be inactivated within thirty seconds by just *30* percent alcohol (either ethyl or isopropyl).[2861] In that case, a variety of hard liquors could indeed be repurposed for use as hand sanitizers for COVID-19, either straight or even diluted to a certain extent.

Most vodka, rum, brandy, gin, and whiskey exceed 30 percent alcohol by volume. So, from a COVID-19 standpoint, bottles of hand sanitizer can still be found on the shelves—of liquor stores, if not at drugstores. Past guests in my home were surprised to see so many big plastic bottles of cheap, 120-proof vodka in my wine rack (especially for someone who doesn't drink at all). I stocked up a decade ago, following my own pandemic prep guidelines to make extra DIY, budget-friendly hand sanitizer for the next outbreak. And, with the COVID-19 virus, it looks like I may be able to cut it 50:50. Note that 30 percent alcohol isn't enough to kill many other pathogens, so I would still recommend 60–80 percent alcohol products if you can get them. But, in a pinch during this crisis, it can be comforting to know there may be some alternatives.

The WHO[2862] and interim FDA[2863] guidelines for those making their own hand sanitizer include the use of an emollient (1.45 percent by volume glycerine, also spelled as *glycerin* and known as *glycerol*) to help keep the alcohol from drying the skin, as well as a preservative (0.125 percent by volume of the standard 3 percent hydrogen peroxide) to kill any contaminating bacteria spores. What's important for inactivating the virus, though, is the alcohol content.

Assuming 30 percent alcohol is sufficient and you had all the ingredients, you could make a gallon of COVID-19 hand sanitizer by combining twelve cups of an 80-proof liquor (40 percent alcohol by volume) with a quarter cup of glycerine and a teaspoon of regular-strength (3 percent) hydrogen peroxide and then just filling the rest of the gallon container with water. You could also quarter the recipe to make a quart (3 cups liquor, 1 tablespoon glycerine, ¼ teaspoon hydrogen peroxide, and water). For this particular virus, however, the easiest method would be to just use the 80-proof liquor straight up as a hand-sanitizing rub. Pour it into a squirt or spray bottle and apply enough to completely cover all surfaces of your hands and then rub together until they are dry. The addition of a gelling agent like aloe vera is not recommended, as it might compromise antiviral efficacy.[2864]

On inanimate surfaces, bleach is recommended for disinfection (1 part household bleach diluted in 49 parts water, so about 1 teaspoon bleach per cup of water).[2865] A more typical 1:100 dilution of bleach as sometimes recommended by manufacturers may not be sufficient, based on data from another human coronavirus.[2866] Note that the 1:50 recommendation is for standard (5 percent sodium hypochlorite) bleach. Read the label: If you have 2.5 percent hypochlorite bleach, you'd have to use 2 teaspoons per cup, and if you have 10 percent hypochlorite bleach, the equivalent would be ½ teaspoon per cup.

The bleach solution can be used within a month of preparation if stored in a closed, opaque container at room temperature.[2867] Though it's recommended that you leave it on the surface you're disinfecting for at least ten minutes,[2868] when put to the test, five minutes at that concentration was found to wipe out SARS-CoV-2.[2869] Note that surfaces grossly contaminated by bodily secretions may require a stronger bleach solution (1 part household bleach to 9 parts water left for ten minutes).[2870]

WARNING: Don't Mix It Up

Never mix bleach with any other cleanser. Bleach reacts with ammonia, which is found in many glass cleaners, to create hazardous gases called *chloramines*. Bleach also reacts with acids like vinegar (and some toilet bowl, drain, and automatic dishwashing detergents) to create chlorine gas, which is also toxic.[2871]

Alcohol can be used on surfaces that aren't suitable for bleach, such as metal, which bleach can stain or even corrode.[2872] Povidone-iodine (7.5 percent), chloroxylenol (0.05 percent), chlorhexidine (0.05 percent), and benzalkonium chloride (0.1 percent), which are found in a variety of commercial disinfectant products, have also been shown to clear the COVID-19 virus within five minutes, but a soap solution (1 part hand soap, 49 parts water) appeared to take as long as fifteen minutes to kill it.[2873] Dishwashing detergent appears to work faster, at least against the SARS virus, with the same 1:50 dilution of dish soap to water working within five minutes.[2874]

Within thirty seconds, Lysol disinfectant spray and a 1:64 dilution of Pine-Sol destroy murine hepatitis virus, a mouse coronavirus that's used as a potential surrogate for human coronaviruses (since it's safer to handle in the lab), but they have yet to be tested against the COVID-19 coronavirus.[2875] In a pinch, wine vinegar (6 percent acid) was shown to destroy more than 99.9 percent of the SARS virus at least, within sixty seconds.[2876] Although the EPA suggests common quaternary ammonium compounds found in a variety of household cleansers should be effective,[2877] I found an old paper that reported they were "virtually useless" as a sole disinfectant against viruses dried onto surfaces, including one of the common cold human coronaviruses,[2878] though benzalkonium chloride has been found to be effective against SARS-CoV-2 (at 0.1 percent for five minutes).

There do not seem to be any published cases of infection from grocery deliveries or restaurant takeout, but out of an abundance of caution, after unpacking food at home, discard disposable bags and cardboard packaging, wash or sanitize hands, and disinfect the counters or other surfaces any bags or boxes touched.[2879] Reheating food even just to the temperature of hot tea (70°C or 158°F) can inactivate the virus within five minutes.[2880] As always, thoroughly wash fruits and vegetables under running water before consumption.[2881]

The most macabre decontamination advice I found was published in the *Journal of the Chinese Medical Association*: "Corpses should be burned or buried deep."[2882]

What to Do If You Come Down with COVID-19

Ideally, once you became infected, you would be safely quarantined away from your family in a "fever clinic," a dedicated facility designed to assess, test, treat, and triage patients, so you don't put the people you live with at risk. Fever clinics were one of the strategies used to bring the outbreak in China under control by preventing clusters of family infections.[2883] In lieu of such innovations, the best choice is to try to recover at home, isolated as much as possible from your housemates. Preferably, you should avoid contact with both people and pets and be cordoned off in a "sick room" with a separate bathroom, if possible.[2884]

CAN PETS BECOME INFECTED?

In rare cases, dogs have been found infected with the new coronavirus.[2885,2886] However, the virus replicates poorly in canines, they don't seem to get sick, and they don't appear to be able to pass the virus along to others.[2887] Dogs also tested positive during the SARS outbreak, but no dog-to-human transmission was reported.[2888]

The COVID-19 coronavirus has been shown to reproduce efficiently in cats, though, who are able to experimentally transmit the virus to other cats in separate cages, presumably via respiratory droplets even though they may not themselves become sick.[2889] After the COVID-19 outbreak, a survey of 102 cats in Wuhan province found evidence of infection in 15 of them, presumed to be cases of human-to-animal transmission, as with the pet dogs.[2890] In the United States, the first confirmed case of animal infection was a sickened tiger at the Bronx Zoo.[2891]

To reduce the risk of spreading the disease, cover your nose and mouth with a tissue when you cough or sneeze, throw the used tissue in a lined trash can, and then immediately sanitize your hands. Don't share personal household items, such as eating utensils, towels, or bedding. Wash your hands often. Routinely disinfect all high-touch objects in your sick room and bathroom yourself, such as phones, doorknobs, and toilet surfaces, and have someone else clean and disinfect the rest of the house.[2892] Running the exhaust fan in the bathroom,[2893] using an air purifier,[2894] opening the windows in the sick room to enhance ventilation,[2895] and, based on data from surrogate coronaviruses, using a humidifier if the air is dry may also cut down on the viral circulation.[2896] During the SARS outbreak, hospital wards with larger ventilation windows appeared to harbor significantly lower infection risk for health-care workers.[2897]

If you must be in the same room with someone else, you should wear a face mask.[2898] That's what masks were originally designed for, so-called source control, rather than self-protection.[2899] They are meant to protect others from you, rather than you from others. Common cold coronaviruses (as well as flu and rhinoviruses) can be detected in exhaled breath, not just coughing and sneezing, and surgical masks can cut down on the amount of virus you exhale out into the world.[2900] We don't yet know if this is true of COVID-19, but the head of the Standing Committee on Emerging Infectious Diseases and 21st Century Health Threats at the National Academy of Sciences told the White House that "[c]urrently available research supports the possibility that SARS-CoV-2 [the COVID-19 coronavirus] could be spread via bioaerosols generated directly by patients' exhalation."[2901]

This shouldn't be surprising. After all, respiratory droplets are not just sneezed gobs of mucus. When your breath fogs when you're outside on a really cold day, that's an illustration of respiratory droplets. That plume of vapor coming out of your mouth is made up of tiny droplets of water straight from your lungs. On a warm day, you can imagine yourself breathing out that same cloud—you just can't see it. Err on the side of caution and assume the virus is in the breath.

Should Everyone Wear Masks in Public?

If infected individuals are exhaling virus before they even know they have it, perhaps everyone should be covering their faces in public. The CDC initially resisted such a measure, a decision the director-general of the Chinese CDC considered "a big mistake."[2902] The U.S. CDC relented on April 3, 2020, and recommended "wearing cloth face coverings in public settings where other social distancing measures are difficult to maintain," such as at grocery stores or pharmacies.[2903] The 180-degree shift is probably best exemplified by the U.S. surgeon general's swing from tweeting "Seriously people— STOP BUYING MASKS!"[2904] to being featured in a video weeks later demonstrating how to improvise masks out of a bandana and rubber bands.[2905] The CDC now has easy no-sew instructions at bit.ly/CDCDIY.

Even though face coverings are intended to protect others from the wearer rather than the wearer from others, masks were recommended for self-protection during the last pandemic for those at high risk in unavoidably crowded settings.[2906] In hospital settings, mask wearers appeared to have been comparatively protected from contracting SARS.[2907] However, even three or four layers of cloth (cotton handkerchiefs) only filter a fraction of what a simple surgical mask can block.[2908] Improvised masks didn't seem to help people from getting infected in 1918, attributed to the fact that to get the necessary protective filtration, so many layers of gauze had to be used that breathing was difficult and air leaked around the edges.[2909]

The World Health Organization still doesn't think routine mask-wearing in public is necessary, expressing concern that it might lead to a false sense of security and neglect of more important measures, such as hand hygiene and social distancing.[2910] On the other hand, one could imagine how wearing a mask might prompt people to avoid touching their faces. Gloves could play a similar role. Seeing bright purple gloves on your hands can serve as a constant reminder. Yes, you can still breathe in the virus while wearing a mask and you can still contaminate yourself with gloved fingers, but anything that keeps you constantly conscious about the position of your hands to stop you from touching your face could potentially help.

Speaking of being self-conscious, if everyone wore masks in public, then symptomatic patients who definitely should be wearing them wouldn't fear being singled out for stigma.[2911] Of course, universal use of face masks in public during a pandemic could only be considered if supplies permit. Sadly, inadequate preparation, misuse, and hoarding have led to a critical shortage of personal protective gear for those on the front line.[2912] That's why the CDC is recommending "cloth face coverings" instead of surgical masks for people who are not health-care workers or other medical first responders.[2913] (You know things are getting desperate when an editorial in the *Journal of the American Medical Association* entitled "Sourcing Personal Protective Equipment During the COVID-19 Pandemic" includes as a proposed solution "coffee filter masks."[2914])

Cloth coverings are no substitute for masks, but they may be better than nothing.[2915] A study testing the efficacy of various homemade masks found that scarves, pillowcases, and 100 percent cotton T-shirts were probably the most suitable household materials, blocking various bacteria and viruses about 60 percent as well as surgical masks. Vacuum cleaner bags worked better, right up there alongside surgical masks, but were considerably harder to breathe through.[2916] Compared to N95 respirators, at the particle size at which N95s block more than 95 percent, a mask made out of a T-shirt only blocks about 10 percent, a scarf about 20 percent, a sweatshirt about 30 percent, and a towel closer to 40 percent.[2917] Engineers at the University of Cambridge suggest a single sock pressed tight against the nose and mouth might make a good emergency mask substitute.[2918] Regardless of what you use, cloth face coverings should be washed regularly.[2919]

Surgical masks are still advised for those who are sick and necessarily exposed to others, as well as when disinfecting a residence that may have been exposed to the virus. You would also want to wear disposable gloves, open all the windows while mopping the floor and cleaning all surfaces with a disinfectant solution, and wash all linens and the clothes you wore cleaning with detergent. Make sure to hold soiled linens away from your body, and don't shake them before they are washed. And, as always, take care not to touch your eyes, nose, and mouth when removing your mask, and carefully wash your hands afterward.[2920]

What About N95 Respirators?

Surgical masks are usually made out of paper with a gelatinous layer and should be changed every four hours or when they become wet with saliva or other fluid, whichever comes first.[2921] As the name implies, surgical masks are typically meant to protect others (that is, the patient opened up on the operating table). However, N95 respirators, those cuplike masks that fit tighter to the face, are intended to protect the wearer.[2922] The *N* in N95 stands for *NIOSH*—the U.S. National Institute for Occupational Safety and Health—and *95* reflects the filtering efficiency of the mask, effectively filtering out 95 percent of particles of a certain size.[2923]

The WHO and CDC have conflicting guidelines as to what health-care workers should wear during routine care of patients with COVID-19. The CDC, along with its European counterpart, recommends respirators, whereas the WHO suggests surgical masks are sufficient.[2924] While part of the WHO's reluctance to endorse N95s may be out of a sensitivity to the global scarcity of such resources, the underlying transmission dynamics of COVID-19 remain largely unknown, so it's impossible at this time to say which recommendation is right with any certainty.[2925]

The relative importance of direct respiratory spread for COVID-19 versus indirect contact via contaminated objects is unclear. For other viral respiratory illnesses like the common cold, breathing appears more important than touching.[2926] For example, in one rhinovirus experiment, only 50 percent of those touching contaminated coffee cup handles became infected.[2927] For the flu, the relative importance of transmission continues to be debated.[2928]

Note that N95 respirators only work at peak efficiency if they conform completely to the face. For example, they are not suitable for people with facial hair.[2929] Even one to two days of beard growth can undermine the necessary seal.[2930] They also must be used properly. In a laboratory setting, N95 respirators have been found to be very effective, but out in the real world, a review of the best science on preventing the spread of respiratory viruses found "no evidence that the more expensive, irritating and uncomfortable N95 respirators were superior to simple surgical masks," perhaps due to poor compliance.[2931] I still remember how uncomfortable they were from years ago when I was working with tuberculosis patients.

Even with the perfect mask sealed over your mouth and nose, your eyes are still exposed, leading to a suggestion that medical workers wear goggles.[2932] Monkeys can be infected by the COVID-19 coronavirus dripped into their eyes,[2933] but a retrospective study of SARS at least found no documented cases of transmission to health-care workers attributed to the lack of eye protection.[2934]

Until we know more about the transmission of the COVID-19 coronavirus, it would seem prudent for those in close contact with coughing patients to err on the side of caution and use both eye protection (like at least a face shield) and N95 respirators. During the SARS outbreak in North America, regular surgical masks were initially recommended, but the advice switched to respirators after doctors started dying.[2935]

Most people who contract COVID-19 spontaneously recover without the need for medical intervention. If you come down with it, protect those around you, get rest, stay hydrated, and monitor your symptoms. If serious problems arise, such as difficulty breathing or persistent pain or pressure in the chest, seek medical attention, but call your doctor or emergency room first before heading in, since they may have special instructions for suspect cases in your area.[2936]

The CDC advises that once your symptoms start getting better, you've been fever-free for three full days off fever-reducing medicines, *and* it's been at least a full week since your symptoms first appeared, then you can start relaxing your home isolation.[2937] The World Health Organization is more conservative, however, recommending self-quarantine for a full fourteen days for anyone with symptoms or anyone living with anyone having symptoms.[2938]

HOW COVID-19 ENDS

Will COVID-19 just go away naturally as warmer weather approaches? We shouldn't count on it. Though the common cold coronaviruses follow a seasonal pattern like the flu, peaking every winter,[2939] there are other respiratory virus infections that peak in the spring or summer.[2940] In fact, MERS-CoV, the last deadly coronavirus to cause an epidemic, peaked in August in the sweltering heat and blistering sun of the Arabian Peninsula.[2941]

The mechanisms underlying the seasonality of viral respiratory infections remain a subject of scientific debate. It's likely a combination of factors involving the virus itself (for example, viral viability at different temperatures and humidity), host immunity (such as vitamin D status and the drying of our airways), and host behavior (like crowding together indoors).[2942] However, the near-universal susceptibility to novel pandemic viruses may supersede these seasonal factors.[2943] All recent flu pandemics emerged in the spring or summer months in the northern hemisphere,[2944] though secondary waves did tend to hit during the following winter.[2945] Even if the contagiousness of COVID-19 drops this summer due to warmer, wetter weather, it is not expected to make a large dent in the pandemic curve.[2946]

What would stop the pandemic is herd immunity, having a critical portion of the populace immune to the virus. An infection can only burn through a population if there are enough susceptible individuals for the viral sparks to jump from one person to the next. Immune individuals who can't get or transmit the virus act as firebreaks to slow the spread or like control rods in a nuclear reactor to break the chains of transmission. Ideally, this is accomplished through mass vaccination. Vaccines are a way to fight fire with fire, using the virus to fight the virus by generating the benefits of infection (immunity) without the risks (disease and death). Without a vaccine, herd immunity is only achieved the hard way—through mass infection.

The proportion of the population that needs to acquire immunity to stop a pandemic can be roughly estimated from the basic reproduction number I alluded to before, the number of people a single infected individual tends to go on to infect. The basic equation is $P_{crit} = 1 - 1/R_0$, where R_0 is the basic reproduction number and P_{crit} is the minimum proportion of a population needed to be vaccinated or have recovered with subsequent immunity to smother the outbreak within that population.[2947] So, if every COVID-19 case leads to two others becoming infected, half the population may need to be vaccinated or infected before the pandemic dies down $(1 - 1/2 = 0.50)$. But, if each person on average infects four others, then one would need closer to three-quarters of the population to be immune to stop it $(1 - 1/4 = 0.75)$. This is an overly simplistic model[2948] but offers a rough ballpark approximation.

Based on R_0 estimates for the COVID-19 virus from large outbreaks in affected countries, the minimum population immunity required ranges from about 30 percent (based on South Korea's R_0 estimate of 1.43) to more like 80 percent (based on an early R_0 estimate from Spain that was closer to 5).[2949] This is why it's so important to enact curve-flattening measures like social distancing to reduce the number of contacts and drive down the basic reproduction number as low as possible. We don't want to have to wait until 80 percent of the population is infected.

Of course, this is all working under the assumption that people who recover from COVID-19 acquire immunity to reinfection. So far, it works in rhesus monkeys. Scientists rechallenged two recovered monkeys with the virus and were unable to successfully reinfect them a month later.[2950] We don't yet have a definitive answer as to whether humans become immune after infection, but the fact that at least a small study reported potential treatment benefit from "convalescent plasma," the transfusion of blood products from a recovered patient into an ailing patient, suggests the buildup of at least temporary immunity.[2951]

We have three lines of defense against viral reinfection: circulating antibodies that can neutralize the virus, memory B cells that can create new antibodies upon reexposure (the reason people can remain immune from the chickenpox virus for fifty or more years, for example), and memory T cells that can help hunt down virus-infected cells. The benefit of convalescent plasma derives from the antibodies, but a six-year follow-up study of patients recovered from SARS found that about 90 percent (twenty-one out of twenty-three) no longer had any detectable anti-SARS antibodies in their bloodstreams. But that's okay because their memory B cells could just make more, right? Unfortunately, not a single SARS-specific memory B cell was found in any of the former SARS patients. About 60 percent (fourteen out of twenty-three) were able to mount a memory T cell response, though it's not clear if that alone would be able to protect them from reinfection.[2952] At the rate immunity wanes to the common cold coronaviruses, a Harvard modeling group suggested prolonged or intermittent social distancing may need to be maintained into 2022.[2953]

Unlike HIV, which keeps parts of itself hidden to evade the immune system and establish a long, latent infection, the COVID-19 coronavirus appears to take more of a smash-and-grab approach. It brazenly displays its array of spike proteins in a presumed attempt to better bind to its victim but counts on jumping ship before immunity develops by quickly being coughed onto a new host. This effrontery bodes well for both the post-recovery acquisition of immunity and the prospects of vaccine development.[2954] A trait the COVID-19 coronavirus does share with HIV, however, is its rapid mutation rate.[2955]

As I've discussed, one reason RNA viruses like HIV, coronaviruses, and flu viruses represent a higher pandemic threat than those that use DNA as their genetic material is that viral RNA replication can be sloppy.[2956] Every copying cycle can result in multitudes of variants, most of which probably aren't even viable. But the flip side of this intrinsic inefficiency is that rare deviants may arise from the mutant swarm that comes exploding out of each infected cell that are either better adapted to the current host or tailored toward new ones.[2957]

The high mutation rate of coronaviruses may help explain their proclivity to jump across species barriers in the first place,[2958] but the question we face now is what the COVID-19 coronavirus will do next. The genetic sequences of the viral copies recovered from COVID-19 patients around the world have already diverged as much as 15 percent as different strains spread around the globe.[2959] In the SARS epidemic, certain early mutants went on to dominate, which led to the supposition that genetic adaptation to humans was helping to drive the outbreak,[2960] but that remains to be substantiated. Though the COVID-19 viral mutations to date don't yet offer insight into the direction of its evolution,[2961] we cannot rule out the possibility that the virus could transform in the near future to becoming even more transmissible or dangerous.[2962]

V. Surviving the Next Pandemic

OUR HEALTH IN OUR HANDS

Coming Soon to a Theater Near You

Regarding future pandemics, one authority was quoted as saying, "Short of obtaining [antiviral] drugs, there's not really much we can do to prepare."[2963] That's hardly true. We know from the COVID-19 pandemic we can still practice defensive strategies, such as social distancing, respiratory etiquette, and other hygiene measures like hand sanitization. No one just comes down with the flu. You catch the virus from someone else or, more precisely, someone else's virus catches you.

In 1918, half of the world's population became exposed to the virus.[2964] The half-empty interpretation means seeing this as an unthinkably transmissible contagion. The half-full view recognizes that half of the global populace was able to hide from the virus. The question then becomes, *how does this other half live? How can you better the odds that you'll fall into the lucky half?*

Social distancing has been described as avoiding any "unnecessary contact of people."[2965] Since COVID-19 and influenza are communicable diseases spread from one person to the next, it makes sense that the fewer people you come in contact with, the fewer chances you have of catching it. On a personal level, social distancing means staying in one's home, not going to work, and avoiding crowds like the plague, especially in enclosed spaces. On a community basis, this may mean closing schools, churches, and other public gatherings.[2966] "Most Americans take for granted their freedom," reads one legal review of the hygiene laws that were imposed in 1918, "to associate with others in a variety of social settings."[2967]

In 1918, at the recommendation of the Surgeon General of the U.S. Public Health Service,[2968] entire states reportedly shut down public gatherings of any kind, including funerals.[2969] The American Public Health Association agreed that "[n]onessential gatherings should be prohibited." Laws "regulating coughing and sneezing" were also deemed desirable.[2970] Huge signs in New York streets warned: "It is unlawful to cough and sneeze." Violators faced up to a year in jail.[2971] Within days, more than five hundred New Yorkers were hauled into court. Chicago's Health Commissioner told the police department, "Arrest thousands, if necessary, to stop sneezing in public."[2972] Signs read, "Spit Spreads Death."[2973]

Across America, there were cities of masked faces. People were afraid to talk to one another, eat with one another, kiss one another. The country held its breath.[2974] Some cities made it a crime to shake hands.[2975] Hundreds were rounded up for not wearing masks and thrown in jail for up to thirty days.[2976] Civil libertarians and Christian Scientists, with support from some business sectors, formed the Anti-Mask League in protest. Tobacconists complained that sales were down because people couldn't smoke with their masks on. Shop owners worried that compulsory masks would discourage people from Christmas shopping.[2977] Due to business pressure, some cities closed down all schools, churches, and theaters, but kept the department stores open,[2978] perhaps giving a whole new meaning to the phrase "shop 'til you drop."

The closing of schools and other public institutions was not universally accepted.[2979] A 1918 editorial in the British Medical Journal read, "[E]very town-dweller who is susceptible must sooner or later contract influenza whatever the public health authorities may do; and that the more schools and public meetings are banned and the general life of the community dislocated the greater will be the unemployment and depression."[2980] Echoes of that same your-money-or-your-life sentiment are certainly being heard today. That may be a false dichotomy, though, as cities in 1918 that took more aggressive measures appeared to recover economically as fast or even faster.[2981] The closing of schools may have been especially useful in stemming the spread.[2982]

Though the role children play in community transmission of COVID-19 is still unknown,[2983] as I've discussed, they have been the primary vectors for the spread of pandemic influenza.[2984] Evidence from a variety of sources mark kids as the major transmitters of influenza in general in a given community.[2985] A real-time surveillance system set up at Boston's Children's Hospital found that school-aged children may actually drive each winter's flu epidemic. Preschoolers in particular are considered "hotbeds of infection."[2986] Not only might they be likelier to pick their noses and not cover their sneezes, but children are able to shed flu virus for up to six days prior to showing any symptoms. That means that for almost a week before anyone suspects, they are infected and can be spreading the virus to others.[2987]

In this way children play a central role in disseminating influenza. Studies suggest that they pick up the virus mixing with other kids at school and then become the major entry point for the virus to gain access to the household.[2988] And each flu season, children kill their grandparents. Japan experimented with its flu vaccine strategy in the 1970s and 1980s and showed that by targeting children for flu shots, hospitalization and death in the elderly could be reduced.[2989]

It's easier for some than others to stay away from crowds and kids, but avoiding influenza is a difficult task for all.[2990] Exhaled into the air and surviving for hours on solid surfaces like metal or plastic, influenza is notoriously transmissible.[2991] Another expert noted at a conference on pandemic influenza, "I know how to avoid getting AIDS, but I do not know how to avoid getting influenza."[2992]

To avoid the disease completely would mean a divorce from society. A realistically stark description of a coming pandemic at a Council on Foreign Relations forum convinced one audience member "to get in my car and move to Montana or something." He was told, "It won't help."[2993]

Webster told *The New Yorker*: "We have to prepare as if we're going to war and the public needs to understand that clearly . . . if this does happen, and I fully expect it will, there will be no place for any of us to hide. Not in the United States or in Europe or in a bunker somewhere. The virus is a very promiscuous and efficient killer."[2994]

The Power of One

In 1918, it took only one stranger to bring death to an entire community, even in the farthest-flung parts of the world. In China's remote Shanxi province, the spread of the pandemic was traced to a single woodcutter, tramping from village to village. In Canada, the virus wore the uniform of a stubborn Canadian Pacific Railways official who flouted quarantine, dropping off infected repatriate soldiers from Quebec all the way west to Vancouver. An entire port city in Nigeria was infected by fewer than ten persons.[2995]

Social distancing, taken to its logical extreme, would mean total isolation from the outside world. True, becoming a hermit living in a cave would presumably preclude one from dying during the pandemic, but this is easier said than done. No man is an island . . . but what if he lived on one?

Pandemic influenza first reached the Pacific Islands in 1830 on the *Messenger of Hope,* a ship carrying the first load of Christian missionaries. Fast forward to November 7, 1918. The SS *Taline* pulls into Apia Harbor in the New Zealand colonial island of Western Samoa from Auckland at 9:35 a.m. Despite many Spanish influenza–infested passengers aboard, the captain tells the island medical officer that no one is sick. With a clean bill of health, the yellow flag of quarantine is lowered, and the ship is docked.[2996]

Just miles away lay American Samoa, an island governed by the U.S. Navy. Word spreads of the outbreak on Western Samoa. The American Commander offers to send volunteer medical personnel to help. Western Samoa's administrator stubbornly refuses, disconnecting the telegraph and later explaining that he "didn't like Americans."[2997] A week later, the New Zealand army lieutenant colonel in charge of Western Samoa orders all communications between the islands cut, furious over American Samoa's refusal to let any ships come near its island.[2998]

The U.S. Naval Administration shut off American Samoa from the outside world for eighteen months, extending into 1920, refusing even mail delivery.[2999] Because of its precautions, American Samoa remained the only country in the world in which not a single person died during the pandemic of 1918.[3000] In neighboring Western Samoa, just a few miles away, more than one-fifth of the entire population died,[3001] probably the highest percentage of any country in the world.[3002]

Simple quarantine does not work, because healthy-appearing people can spread the disease. But the U.S. Navy showed that isolation, in which one excludes both sick and healthy people, can. While Western Samoans died by the thousands, American Samoan records continued to reveal the normalcy of Samoan life, logging rare deaths from "eating shark's liver" or from "a falling coconut."[3003]

Two other islands also escaped unscathed—St. Helena in the South Atlantic, famed as Napoleon's exile,[3004] and Yerba Buena Island right in the San Francisco bay. As the pandemic raged along the California coast, the U.S. Naval training base stationed on Yerba Buena clamped down with a policy of total seclusion of its four thousand inhabitants and practiced such preventive measures as literally blowtorching drinking fountains sterile every hour.[3005]

Total exclusion is more difficult on mainlands than on islands, but portions of northern and eastern Iceland[3006] and one town in Alaska also successfully hid throughout the pandemic.[3007] Coromandel, a resort town in New Zealand, cut itself off from the rest of the world using a rotating roster of shotgun-wielding vigilantes. It worked.[3008]

The only town in the continental United States to even come close was the remote mining settlement of Gunnison, Colorado.[3009] While surrounding mining towns were being devastated[3010] and the situation in Denver was described as "full of funerals all day and ambulances all night,"[3011] the residents of Gunnison blockaded off the two mountain pass approaches with armed men[3012] and escaped with one of the lowest reported infection rates in the country.[3013] Similarly, U.S. Army commands tried to isolate entire military units. They "failed when and where [these measures] were carelessly applied," but "did some good . . . when and where they were rigidly carried out."[3014]

Island nations like New Zealand considered similar measures in the face of an H5N1 outbreak, examining the feasibility of the immediate blockading of all people and imports—even food and medicine—when the pandemic hits. "To do that," a New Zealand microbiologist realized, "all those people overseas on holiday would not be allowed in either. It sounds a good idea, but I would find it interesting to see whether it could ever be done."[3015]

Mike Davis, author of *The Monster at Our Door: The Global Threat of Avian Flu,* was asked in an interview what he and his family planned to do when the pandemic hit. "There is the run-for-the-hills strategy, quite frankly," he said, though he acknowledged this may not do much good. "Living in an unpopulated area may work for a handful of people. Maybe some survivalists can do this. But odds are that at least a quarter of Americans will be infected [and fall ill] in a pandemic flu."[3016] America's purple mountain majesties cannot fit 330 million people.

Coughs and Sneezes Spread Diseases

Practicing social distancing techniques not only protects you from the crowds, it protects the crowds from you. If one actually falls ill, the best thing to do from a public health standpoint may be to self-quarantine at home to prevent the spread of the virus.[3017] We are getting a taste of this with COVID-19, but with a more dangerous pathogen, you could be visiting a potential death sentence on everyone you meet if you do go out. The extreme lethality of a virus like H5N1 may actually work in humanity's favor—people may become so ill and succumb so quickly that they are unlikely to get out of bed and spread it to others outside their households. However, experts expect the virus may ratchet down its lethality in the interest of being more effectively spread. And of course, if we do become infected, it may be a day or two or even longer before we know it, so all but essential personnel should consider preparing for a prolonged "snow emergency"–type isolation at home in the event of a pandemic.[3018] Instead of a snow "day," though, Osterholm compared it to preparing for a worldwide "12- to 18-month blizzard,"[3019] although each wave may only last a matter of weeks.[3020] Everyone should also begin getting into the habit of practicing what infectious control experts refer to as proper "respiratory etiquette."[3021]

Most people know to cover their nose and mouth when they cough or sneeze, but most people are not doing it right. You shouldn't cough or sneeze into your hand. You should only cough into the crook of your arm or into a tissue.[3022] Covering our nose and mouth can somewhat limit the dispersal of contaminated respiratory droplets, but when we cough into our hand, it becomes coated with virus that can then be transferred to everything from elevator buttons and light switches to gas pumps and toilet handles.[3023] One study found that the flu virus could be recovered from more than 50 percent of common household and day care center surfaces during flu season.[3024] This is not surprising, given that up to five infectious viral doses have been measured in every drop of nasal secretions.[3025] Coughing into the inner elbow area of the arm or sleeve prevents the contamination of your hands.[3026] This takes practice to get used to it, though, so we have the COVID-19 pandemic to thank for getting us all to start rehearsing now. The Mayo Clinic has a slogan: "The 10 worst sources of contagion are our fingers."[3027]

Fomite is the technical term for a contaminated physical object, like the archetypal doorknob, that can transmit disease among people. It comes from the Latin *fomes,* meaning "tinder."[3028] This sparking of an infectious blaze can be prevented through disinfection. At room temperature and humidity, influenza virus can survive intact for up to forty-eight hours on nonporous surfaces like metal or plastic and up to twelve hours on cloth, paper, or tissues,[3029] but can be killed easily with a simple solution of household bleach. Influenza viruses can be killed by a much more dilute solution of bleach than was required for the COVID-19 virus. One tablespoon of chlorine bleach mixed in a gallon of water should be sufficient for the flu virus. This diluted bleach solution can be sprayed on potentially contaminated common surfaces and left to sit for at least five minutes. Frequently used but infrequently disinfected objects, such as refrigerator handles and phone receivers, should not be missed.[3030] The bleach solution can also be used to wash contaminated clothes and bedding, as research has shown that a shaken contaminated blanket can release infectious viral particles into the environment.[3031] It must be *chlorine* bleach, meaning it should contain a chlorine-based compound like sodium hypochlorite. So-called color-safe bleaches should not be used as disinfectants for influenza or COVID-19.

Wrapped in a stolen fatty coat from our cells, flu and coronaviruses can potentially lie in wait for days under the right conditions, patiently twiddling their thumbs until someone grasps the same doorknob. As I've noted, the virus still needs to bypass the skin barrier and find a way into the body, though. This is why we should get into the habit of avoiding touching our eyes, noses, and mouths whenever possible in public until we can wash or sanitize our hands.[3032] The power of this simple intervention is illustrated by a study that showed that children aged four to eight taught to avoid touching their noses and eyes essentially halved their risk of contracting cold infections.[3033] Although viruses like influenza can go airborne, studies of outbreaks at nursing homes suggest that this direct physical contact may play a significant role in its spread.[3034]

Washing Your Hands of the Flu

The causal link between contaminated hands and infectious disease transmission in general is considered to be one of the best-documented phenomena in clinical science.[3035] Eighty percent of all infectious diseases are transmitted by touch—from the common cold to "flesh-eating" bacteria and Ebola. A director of Clinical Microbiology at New York University considered proper handwashing as serious a public health issue as smoking cessation.[3036] Proper handwashing certainly seemed to work during the SARS epidemic. Those at high risk who washed their hands were found to be ten times less likely to contract the disease.[3037] That oily envelope stolen from our cells makes both coronaviruses and influenza viruses especially sensitive to being washed away by the detergent quality of ordinary hand soap. As we learned in medical school, while soap may not kill a virus, the "solution to pollution is dilution." Handwashing is meant to decrease viral counts below an infectious threshold. According to the former influenza program officer of the National Institute of Allergy and Infectious Diseases, without a vaccine the "single most important step people can take to help prevent getting the flu is to wash their hands."[3038]

People don't wash their hands as often as they should—or even as often as they think they do. Ninety-five percent *say* they wash their hands after using a public toilet, yet the American Society for Microbiology published a survey of almost eight thousand people across five U.S. cities and found the true number to be only about two-thirds. Chicago topped the list at 83 percent; in New York City, the actual number fell to less than half.[3039]

Doctors are no exception. Though about a hundred thousand Americans die every year from infections they contracted in the hospital[3040] and handwashing is considered the single most important measure to prevent such infections,[3041] studies have shown that less than half of doctors follow proper hand-washing protocols in the hospital. A sample of doctors working in a pediatric intensive care unit of all places were asked how much they *thought* they washed their hands. The average self-estimate of their own hand-washing rate was 73 percent, with individual responses ranging from 50 to 95 percent. These doctors were singled out and followed. Their actual hand-washing rate? Nine percent.[3042]

From an editorial in *The New England Journal of Medicine*: "It seems a terrible indictment of doctors that practices and protocols must be developed to take the place of something as simple . . . as handwashing. Perhaps an even bigger concern for current medical practice, and one which should lead us all to do some soul searching, is that careful and caring doctors can be extraordinarily self-delusional about their behavior."[3043] The top excuses doctors use for not washing hands are: being too busy and dry skin.[3044]

As I've discussed, when doctors do wash their hands, studies show that they only wash for an average of nine seconds.[3045] Proper handwashing, according to then director of clinical microbiology at Mount Sinai, involves lathering with plenty of soap for twenty to thirty seconds (about the time it takes to sing the "alphabet song" three times at a fast tempo), rinsing, and then repeating for another twenty to thirty seconds.[3046] CDC guidelines are similar ("at least 20 seconds"[3047]), with additional reminders to wash between fingers and under the nails, and to soap into the creases around knuckles.[3048] There is little evidence, as I've mentioned, suggesting that hot (or even warm) water is better at sanitizing hands. On the contrary, the colder the water is, the less skin damage is done by the detergents in the soap after repeated handwashing. Washing with warm or tepid water may be more comfortable, but one need not find hot water to wash effectively.[3049]

Most Americans profess to washing their hands after changing a diaper or before handling food, but most don't even claim to wash after coughing or sneezing.[3050] At a minimum, experts advise, hands should be washed after *every cough, every sneeze,* and *every time* we shake hands with anyone. It would be even better if hand-shaking were to go the way of hand-kissing. These simple recommendations may decrease the number of colds we get every year, the number of work days we miss, and the number of days we are laid up in bed. During a pandemic, they may even save your life.[3051]

There's the Rub

Views on hand sanitation have been evolving rapidly. Starting in 2005, World Health Organization consensus recommendations now favor the use of alcohol-based sanitizing rubs or gels over handwashing for routine hand disinfection throughout the day. Products containing between 60 to 80 percent alcohol were found more effective than soap in every scientific study available for review, and, as I've discussed, enveloped viruses such as coronaviruses and influenza are especially susceptible to topical alcohol sanitizers. Alcohol solutions not only were found to be more effective at eliminating germs, but require less time and cause less irritation than handwashing. Handwashing still has a place when hands are dirty or visibly contaminated with bodily fluids like respiratory secretions or blood, but for routine decontamination, alcohol-based products may be the preferred method for hand sanitation.[3052]

Feeling industrious? You can make a cheaper, more effective version at home that fits the greater-than-60-percent-alcohol recommendation:

Recipe for Alcohol Sanitizer Rub

4 cups 70 percent rubbing (isopropyl) alcohol

4 teaspoons glycerin

Mix to make approximately one quart (liter).

The glycerin acts as a humectant, or moisturizer.[3053] Glycerin is preferred since it's nontoxic, cheap, nonallergenic, and widely available. Vegetable glycerin can typically be found in natural food stores or online, and bulk rubbing alcohol can be found in drugstores in convenient 32-ounce (4-cup) bottles. During a pandemic crisis, all forms of alcohol are expected to sell out quickly, but made in advance, this recipe could easily yield enough low-cost hand sanitizer solution for a whole neighborhood. Additionally, liquid alcohol sanitizer solutions have been found to be better at disinfecting hands than the alcohol gel products and can be just as conveniently stored in small squirt bottles.[3054]

Instead of using isopropyl alcohol, which can be acutely toxic if ingested,[3055] one can substitute a 140-proof scotch whiskey. An additional advantage to using booze is that stockpiled liquor, along with cigarettes, gasoline, water, guns, canned vegetables, and, oddly, cosmetics, has historically been among the most highly valued barter items in crisis situations.[3056] As I mentioned before, a group of respected researchers published evidence that the COVID-19 coronavirus could be inactivated by half that alcohol concentration, but for an all-purpose pandemic sanitizer—one rub to rule them all—I would recommend sticking with the advice of the CDC to shoot for an alcohol concentration between 60 and 95 percent.[3057]

Although there have been cases of serious alcohol intoxication in patients who drank bottles of alcohol sanitizer gel, only a negligible amount of alcohol is absorbed directly through the skin when properly used topically.[3058] Alcohol gels and rubs are flammable, though, so they need to be kept away from flames and hot surfaces. There is a case in the medical literature of a U.S. health-care worker who applied alcohol gel to her hands, immediately stripped off a polyester isolation gown, and touched a metal door before the alcohol had evaporated. The removal of the polyester gown created so much static electricity that an audible static spark was generated that ignited the unevaporated alcohol on her hands. This unlikely series of events can be avoided by following proper sanitizer protocol by rubbing one's hands together upon application until the alcohol has evaporated completely and the hands are dry.[3059]

In October 2005, a campaign involving a dozen countries was organized to launch a secret weapon against bird flu: instructions to improve hand hygiene by urging people to wash their hands and carry around a small plastic bottle of alcohol sanitizer.[3060] Similar education campaigns need to be spread worldwide, convincing people to increase their standard of hygiene to the highest possible level by practicing safe coughing and sneezing practices, and sanitizing their hands before touching their faces after contact with others or with public surfaces.[3061] And if people ever needed another reason to quit smoking or avoid secondhand smoke, now is the time. Keeping the respiratory lining healthy can help prevent respiratory viruses from taking hold. "Adhering to simple measures," said a state deputy health commissioner, "may mean the difference between life and death."[3062]

Masking Our Ignorance

What is the best use of masks and the best mask to use? San Francisco is one of the cities in 1918 that made mask wearing compulsory. Citing a slogan the Italian Supreme Command had printed on every gas mask—"Who leaves this mask behind, dies"—the San Francisco mayor threatened to arrest anyone unmasked.[3063] Within thirty-six hours, the SFPD had hauled in 175 "mask-slackers."[3064]

The main mode of coronavirus and influenza virus transmission may be coughed and exhaled respiratory droplets of virus-laden mucus and saliva. Conversational speech alone can produce thousands of these tiny droplets,[3065] which tend to settle out of the air within minutes, extending a few feet into the person's immediate environment.[3066] Since, as I've discussed, infection occurs when one of these droplets lands on the surface of another person's eye, in his mouth, or up her nose, or is planted in one of these three places with contaminated hands,[3067] wearing a mask may not only thwart droplet contact with mucus membranes, but it may also remind the mask wearer not to touch their face.[3068]

I talked about the pitfalls of not lowering the toilet lid before flushing in "Treating and Avoiding COVID-19." Fecal fog, anyone? Live virus was isolated from the diarrhea of a child dying from H5N1, raising the possibility that virus could be spread from human to human via a fecal-oral route as well. Experiments using fluorescent-stained water have demonstrated that not only are toilet seats significantly contaminated, but a flume of aerosolized toilet water—reaching the standing height of a child—is created when a toilet is flushed.[3069]

During a pandemic crisis, if we are forced to venture out for any reason, wearing masks in public restrooms—and in all crowded public areas—may be prudent.

I also discussed surgical masks, N95 respirators, and homemade cloth masks in "Treating and Avoiding COVID-19." Although they do not have N95's filtration capacity or resilience, the advantage of surgical masks is better breathability—causing less thermal and physical discomfort and fatigue[3070]—and better affordability. Before the COVID-19 pandemic hit, surgical masks were sold at pharmacies for pennies; N95 masks were available at hardware stores for a dollar or more each. Whether either mask would provide sufficient protection in an influenza pandemic, though, is a matter of controversy.[3071]

There is no doubt that surgical masks can filter out some larger respiratory droplets. During the SARS outbreak, high-risk personnel wearing surgical masks seemed fifteen times less likely to contract the disease.[3072] Because droplets are the primary means by which influenza spreads, authorities such as the U.S. Department of Health and Human Services settled upon surgical masks as amply protective,[3073] especially given their cost-effectiveness.[3074]

Although droplet spread is the principal method, true airborne transmission of influenza virus in particles too small to be filtered out by surgical masks has been documented.[3075] Yes, respiratory droplets settle to the ground, but sweeping the floor as much as a day later can agitate tiny desiccated particles of virus back into the air, which may pass through surgical masks and have been shown to be infectious in a laboratory setting.[3076] N95 masks are made out of a special, nonwoven polypropylene fabric that generates static electricity to trap tiny particles.[3077] No mask provides a perfect barrier, but N95 masks would be expected to provide greater protection to airborne virus than surgical masks.[3078] "N100" masks, which are even more expensive, filter out an estimated 99.7 percent of fine particles.[3079]

Whichever masks are used, they need to be worn and disposed of properly. A gap between face and mask of even a few millimeters can render a mask ineffective.[3080] In occupational settings, facial hair is shaved and N95 masks are meticulously fitted to match each individual's face for size and shape and often tested using bitter-tasting test aerosols to double check for an airtight seal. In a household setting where fit-testing is not possible, the best option might be to duct-tape the entire periphery of the mask to one's clean-shaven face.[3081]

Handling or reusing worn masks risks hand contamination.[3082] If need be, masks may be reused by the same person unless they become damaged, wet, dirty, or hard to breathe through.[3083] Ideally, though, all masks should be used only once[3084] and properly disposed of using gloves.[3085]

None of these masks protects the eyes. Those in contact with infected persons should consider practicing the "m3g" approach popularized during SARS[3086]—mask, gown, gloves, and goggles.[3087] Gowns should ideally cover the body and arms, and be tucked into the gloves at the wrist. Surgical or examination gloves are designed for single use and disposal. Washing or disinfecting gloves can cause deterioration of the thin material. Proper utility gloves, on the other hand—the rubber gloves used for housekeeping chores—can be decontaminated and reworn.[3088] And silicone-seal swimming goggles are the recommended eyewear. Already wear glasses? Tightly fitting safety goggles with tape over air vents will help protect your eyes.

Even with these precautions, influenza is so contagious that exposure to crowded public settings or contact with potentially infected persons should be kept to an absolute minimum. During a massive bird flu outbreak in the Netherlands in 2003, investigators could not demonstrate a protective effect on poultry workers of masks and safety goggles. The official government account suspected that workers became infected by taking their contaminated overalls off *after* they had removed their masks and goggles.[3089] Considering the Netherlands outbreak and given the lack of data from 1918 showing that compulsory masking was an effective public health strategy, the World Health Organization has been permissive but not encouraging of national laws enforcing mask wearing by decree in national pandemic response plans.[3090] Currently, the WHO recommends masks only for asymptomatic individuals if they are taking care of someone suspected of infection with the COVID-19 coronavirus.[3091]

In terms of individual strategies, the best recommendation may be what finally shook out of the SARS crisis:[3092] in public, surgical masks for the sick and N95 masks for the healthy.[3093] Of course, that's only in a perfect world where there are enough masks to go around. If you had followed my advice from fifteen years ago to buy a personal cache of N95 masks and are not in need of them to take care of a loved one, I would encourage you to donate them to frontline medical professionals fighting for their own lives as they fight to save others. Contact your local hospital or a nonprofit such as GetUsPPE.org.

In the face of a pandemic, the CDC has encouraged all hospitals, physicians' offices, and other health-care providers to issue surgical masks to all incoming patients showing any evidence of a respiratory illness as part of "universal respiratory etiquette." In Japan, that was already routinely practiced. When people in Japan with a cold or cough need to go out into a public setting, they often wear a surgical mask. This civic mindedness is a practice worth emulating.[3094]

Effective masks are not easily replicated at home. When mask prices shot through the roof in Asia during the SARS epidemic,[3095] some strapped bras to their faces.[3096] Improvised masks made out of woven material, such as cotton cloth or gauze, however, offer little protection from airborne pathogens (but do remind the wearers not to touch their faces in public before decontaminating their hands and can cut down on the respiratory droplets you spew out into the environment), as I discussed in "Treating and Avoiding COVID-19."

Some countries stocked up on masks.[3097] No such stockpile had been planned in the United States, though, leaving it up to individuals to arrange for their own safety. The North American investment firm BMO Nesbitt Burns underscored the need to take personal responsibility in its report on pandemic planning. "Face masks would fly off the shelves and restocking would be impossible," its global economic strategist wrote. "Black markets in face masks (as an example) would develop and crime would become a serious problem. The military and National Guard, as well as police and firefighters, would be needed to maintain the peace, and yet their ranks will be depleted by illness."[3098] Having the tools on hand (and face) to practice simple hygiene measures may improve one's chances of falling into the half lucky enough only to watch others become ill.

BE PREPARED

Home Health Aid

If, despite our best precautions, we fall ill, how can we take care of ourselves at home if the health-care system breaks down?

I've talked about the symptoms of COVID-19. What about the next pandemic? Presumably by the time it hits your area, the constellation of symptoms for the particular virus should be well known. Typically for the flu, onset is sudden. The French call it *la grippe,* conjuring images of being seized by disease. People describe it as "like being hit with a truck." The flu generally strikes with sudden fever and chills, cough, muscle aches, fatigue, and weakness such that it's hard to get out of bed. It is hard to miss.

Although high fever in children for any reason can cause them to vomit, gastrointestinal symptoms are rare with influenza.[3099] The so-called twenty-four- or forty-eight-hour "stomach flu," with nausea, vomiting and diarrhea, is an unfortunate misnomer. As mentioned in "Livestock Revolution," the "twenty-four-hour flu" is most often a case of food poisoning (viral foodborne gastroenteritis), not influenza.[3100]

The common cold, in contrast to influenza, is more of a localized, sniffly-sneezy-sore-throat-stuffy-nose phenomenon, lacking the systemic flu symptoms of extreme fatigue, fever, and severe aches and pains. Cough, headache, and chest discomfort can accompany either, but tend to be more severe in influenza.[3101]

With or without antivirals, the foundation of treatment for influenza becomes rest and fluids. Fatigue, weakness, and muscle aches are your body's way of telling you to stay in bed. Your body is no dummy. Not only will you be less likely to spread the disease to others, but bed rest lets your body proportion more energy to mobilize initial defenses.[3102] Avoiding exertion also reduces the likelihood of gasping virus further into the lungs with deep inhalation.[3103] In fact, one guess as to why more young men than young women died in 1918 "may be due to the tendency of many men, out of necessity or masculine impulse, to continue working rather than resting when they were sick."[3104]

Next to antivirals, the best thing one can typically do to survive the flu is to keep properly hydrated by sipping at least one cup of water, tea, juice, soup, or other nonalcoholic beverage every waking hour. That's two to four quarts of liquid a day, which loosens pulmonary secretions to help rid the body of the virus[3105] and prevent the dehydration that accompanies fever.[3106] If you or the person you are nursing isn't eating, electrolytes can be added to the rehydration solution.

Recipe for Rehydration Solution

1 quart (or liter) drinking water
2 tablespoons sugar
¼ teaspoon salt
¼ teaspoon baking soda

Mix to make approximately one quart

If available, adding an additional half cup of orange juice, coconut water, or a mashed ripe banana would add potassium. If baking soda is unavailable, substitute another quarter teaspoon of salt.[3107] If a person is too sick to drink, fluid can be given literally drop by drop until the patient recovers.[3108] Treating influenza outside of a medical setting is less a matter of feeding or starving a fever than it is of drowning it.

Fever reduction is a controversial subject. Fever may be uncomfortable, but it has a beneficial effect on the course of many infections. Elevated temperatures have been shown to inhibit influenza virus replication. Again, our body usually knows best.[3109] Artificially breaking a fever with drugs like acetaminophen (Tylenol) or ibuprofen (Motrin, Advil) may make us feel better, but we may be undermining our body's ability to fight. A cool cloth on the forehead may also help and can do so without lowering our internal virus-fighting fever. Drugs should be considered, though, when the febrile discomfort or muscle aches interfere with sleep, which is also important for recovery. High fevers—above 104°F—should definitely be treated. A combination of acetaminophen and ibuprofen, both taken at the same time, and tepid water sponge-baths should successfully bring down almost any high fever. Aspirin should *never* be given to a child because of the risk of a rare but serious side effect known as *Reye's syndrome*.[3110] Chicken soup might be out of the question during a bird flu pandemic, but warm liquids in general can relieve symptomatic congestion and may also beneficially raise the temperature of the respiratory passageways.[3111]

The lay press has touted the anti-viral benefits of a chemical compound found naturally in grapes called *resveratrol*.[3112] In laboratory experiments performed on infected mice, injection with resveratrol did indeed seem to enhance survival,[3113] but the researchers used massive doses in a non-oral route in nonhuman subjects.[3114] The human equivalent would mean drinking four gallons of red wine's worth of the compound daily.[3115] So, while resveratrol may hold some future pharmacological potential, grape juice may be no better than any other hydrating liquid. No combination of questionable remedies touted over the internet has been shown to trump bed rest and fluids to improve survival.

Collateral Damage

Surviving the disease is only one part of surviving the pandemic. Prominent financial analysts predicted that a pandemic with a virus like H5N1 could trigger an unprecedented global economic collapse.[3116] The chief of Pediatric Infectious Disease at Winthrop University said it colorfully in the 2005 *Pediatric Annals*: "Two masters of suspense, Alfred Hitchcock and Stephen King, may have been closer to the truth than they ever would have believed. Both birds and a super flu could bring about the end of civilization as we know it."[3117]

The U.S. National Intelligence Council's 2020 Project "Mapping the Global Future" identified a pandemic as the single most important threat to the global economy.[3118] Realizing that the prospects for preventing the pandemic are practically nonexistent, chief scientists like Osterholm worked with the business community to help ensure an infrastructure for survivors of what is being predicted in policy journals as the "shutdown of the global economic system."[3119] Speaking as associate director of the National Center for Food Protection and Defense for the Department of Homeland Security to a conference of agricultural bankers, Osterholm laid it out: "This [H5N1] is going to be the most catastrophic thing in my lifetime. When this situation unfolds, we will shut down global markets overnight. There will not be movement of goods; there will not be movement of people. This will last for at least a year, maybe two."[3120] These could well be years characterized by "utter chaos,"[3121] he said; "panic would reign."[3122]

The major North American brokerage firm BMO Nesbitt Burns was the first to describe the global economic implications, suggesting that a pandemic could set off a catastrophic downturn akin to the Great Depression. "A pandemic would be even worse," its report read, "in that many would avoid homelessness and soup lines having paid the ultimate price."[3123] The firm's chief economist pointed out a big difference between a pandemic crash and the Great Depression. "We won't have 30% unemployment," she said, "because frankly, many people will die."[3124]

Attempts were made to calculate the costs. An Oxford University group estimated the cost of a mild pandemic at trillions of dollars,[3125] which appears to be the unfolding case with COVID-19,[3126] but considered it impossible to guess the price tag of a more virulent pandemic that could leave the world economy in shambles for years.[3127] SARS only caused a few dozen deaths in Canada and, according to the Minister of State for Public Health, the entire economy "went to its knees."[3128] Experts noted that we were "very lucky that SARS was SARS" and not something like pandemic influenza, which would make SARS "look like a vacation."[3129]

Part of the economic paralysis would arise from the fear of contagion. Laurie Garrett is the first reporter ever to win all three of journalism's top "P" awards—the Peabody, the Polk, and the Pulitzer. At a Council on Foreign Affairs meeting, she tried to ground the dialogue by discussing the possible implications for a city like Washington, D.C. "An influenza virus like H5N1," she said, "loves doorknobs. It loves the poles in the Metro. It loves every entrance, every common surface that we touch." She described the environmental persistence of the virus:

> So all of Washington, D.C., is full of commonly touched surfaces, and all of a sudden you would see this city utterly paralyzed. Government would stop. You could not imagine any way that people would feel safe commuting in and out of the District, going to government offices, getting on the Metro, all the things that are of the essence of how you keep this place moving around. All I'm saying is that if you amplify your imagination of what this would mean to Washington, to all the most important hubs of the global economy, you easily can see the impact this would have on the global economy.[3130]

Similar descriptions were made of the Big Apple shaken to its core. As associate dean of Columbia University's School of Public Health, Irwin Redlener had been working with New York City officials to ready the metropolis for a coming pandemic. Redlener expected that attempts would be made to lock down entire sections of the city under quarantine. "The city," he said, "would look like a science fiction movie."[3131]

As with Hurricane Katrina, it's not enough to ride out the storm; we also have to weather the aftermath—the shortages, the loss of essential services, and the ensuing social chaos. With supply chains broken as borders slam shut,[3132] major global shortages are expected for everything from soap, paper, and light bulbs to regular medications, gasoline, and parts for repairing military equipment and municipal water supplies.[3133] At a pandemic preparedness conference, Garrett sat quietly through presentation after presentation on the various facets of avian influenza. "Well yes," she asked when the Q & A period finally arrived, "but how will we eat?"[3134]

We were much more self-sufficient in 1918.[3135] Since our global economy is now built upon just-in-time inventory control, companies have minimal stockpiles of raw materials or finished goods.[3136] Modern corporations no longer have warehouses brimming with months' worth of inventory. Grocery stores rarely have more than a few days' supply of popular goods stored, and the Grocery Manufacturers Association has been pushing for even tighter inventory restrictions. The chief executive of the Council of Supply Chain Management Professionals told *The Wall Street Journal* that food retailers "can't afford a just-in-case inventory."[3137] The threat of a bad winter storm can lead to regional shortages of key commodities;[3138] imagine those shortages dragging on for months.[3139]

With COVID-19, though the toilet paper supply may have been wiped, food has continued to flow. Pandemic modeling suggests that it would just take a 25 percent reduction in labor availability to create widespread food shortages.[3140] In a more serious pandemic, Congress was informed by an occupational health specialist that not only would grocery stores be empty, but we might also lose power, water, and phone service. A World Economic Forum simulation suggested that the internet would shut down within two to four days.[3141] Osterholm told Oprah, "Go ask the city of Chicago, 'How much chlorine do they have?' Many of the world's cities may have no more than five to seven days of chlorine on hand to actually use and purify their water supply."[3142] We might be forced to endure deep winter with no heat.[3143] The crumbling of critical infrastructure could be a result, in part, of rampant absenteeism.[3144] "Billions would fall sick," a WHO spokesperson explained, "billions more would be too afraid to go to work, leading to a collapse of essential services."[3145] Top-level UN pandemic catastrophe simulations suggested that maintaining water, power, and provision of food for the healthy may save more lives than focusing on treatment of the sick.[3146]

Like many police in New Orleans after Hurricane Katrina, even essential workers such as doctors simply might not show up for work.[3147] Would they be asked to operate in overflow "hospitals"—gymnasiums, arenas, armories—anywhere the sick could be warehoused? Garrett predicted that these makeshift sickbays may deteriorate into post-Katrina Louisiana Superdome squalor.[3148] Under those conditions, Osterholm wondered, "Would *you* show up to work? . . . Would your loved ones show up to work if they were being exposed to a life threatening infection with virtually no protection?"[3149]

During the COVID-19 pandemic, medical workers the world over have heroically risked exposure and stayed true to the original 1847 American Medical Association Code of Ethics obligation: "When pestilence prevails, it is [physicians'] duty to face the danger, and to continue their labors for the alleviation of suffering, even at the jeopardy of their own lives." That requirement was removed from the code in 1977, but the AIDS epidemic restored some of that duty, to provide medical care "even in the face of greater than usual risks to physicians' own safety, health, or life." For those in their thirties or forties, the risk of dying from COVID-19 may be only about one in a thousand.[3150] Would doctors still show up if it were one in two?

Corpse Management

Disposal of the dead, referred to in crisis management circles as "corpse management,"[3151] presents special problems for public health officials. "We talk about how people should bury their dead in their backyards, how far from the septic systems," explained the director of the King County public health department in Seattle. "In case you're wondering, it's $20 apiece for high-quality body bags."[3152]

A half century ago, the average time from when a coffin was constructed to when it was buried in the ground was months. These days, it's under three weeks[3153]—much faster, so Osterholm predicts, "We will run out of caskets overnight."[3154] Crematorium capacity is equally limited.[3155] There will be no place for the dead.[3156]

"In our lifetime, we have not seen a disease sweep through a community and people die so fast that there's no one to take care of them at the hospital and there's no one to bury them," said Greg Poland, M.D., chair of the Vaccine Research Group at the Mayo Clinic. "That's what will happen in a [severe] pandemic. It would be more deaths than all the world's wars in all of human history. All within the space of 6 to 18 months."[3157] Even in a pandemic as mild as COVID-19, ice rinks[3158] and refrigerated trucks[3159] have had to be temporarily commandeered for the purpose. In some countries, bodies have been left in the streets.[3160] In New York City, some COVID-19 victims ended up in mass graves.[3161]

In the United Kingdom, officials had scoured the countryside for suitable sites for mass graves as part of "Operation Arctic Sea," the British government's emergency pandemic simulations.[3162] Their preparedness plan considered creative solutions such as mobile inflatable mortuaries big enough to hold hundreds of bodies.[3163] In Australia, officials realized that even with mandatory cremations and all their crematoria working twenty-four hours a day, seven days a week without disruption, bodies still may pile up. If so, the plan is then to have Army engineers with refrigerated trucks dispose of bodies in "communal burials." The government realized that this may raise a "multitude of issues in our multicultural community." A spokesperson for the Health Department pleaded, "We need all religious societies to respect the fact they may need to be buried communally in mass graves."[3164]

Bird Flu Vultures Lining Up

According to public opinion polling, the people most concerned about a bird flu pandemic were those with salaries higher than $100,000. Further analysis suggested that was not due to higher education levels, but that "[p]eople with higher incomes . . . have more to lose."[3165] Investment banking firms like Citigroup, though, saw a sterling silver lining—the opportunity to profoundly profit from a pandemic.

Think about the real estate deals. "Soaring death rates would puncture the housing bubble and create vast housing oversupply," predicted one banking firm. "To the extent that a disproportionate share of 20- to 40-year-olds would die, housing markets would weaken in response to excess supply. . . . Property values would fall, and some would be had later at bargain-basement prices."[3166]

Foreign exchange speculators would make a killing. "Negative news," a senior foreign exchange dealer explained, "is a chance to make a profit."[3167] While stock in life insurance companies was not considered a good bet, *An Investor's Guide to Avian Flu* read, "Certainly there would be winners, such as funeral homes and other 'death-related' businesses."[3168] Citigroup Investment Research recommended selling off stock in shopping malls, air travel, and luxury goods, but picking up shares of cleaning-product makers like Clorox, home entertainment, and telecommunications. The defense sector was also heralded as a long-term winner.[3169]

If history truly is a good teacher, we would expect opportunistic advertising. In 1918, Colgate toothpaste swore that "good teeth" meant "good health."[3170] InfoWars founder Alex Jones was more direct, claiming his toothpaste "kills the whole SARS-corona family at point-blank range."[3171] We would expect price gouging. In 1918, undertakers tripled coffin prices.[3172] During the COVID-19 pandemic, one seller offered fifteen N95 face masks on Amazon for $3,799.[3173]

Many states have laws prohibiting price gouging during national emergencies. During a blackout, for instance, it is against the law to suddenly spike the price of flashlights in certain states. The Mercatus Center, the corporate-funded[3174] think tank at George Mason University, was in favor of all price-gouging prevention laws being repealed in preparation for the pandemic. The Center argued that price gouging is an effective way to prevent shortages and apparently imagined some sort of trickle-down benefit of effectively restricting critical supplies to the wealthy. "We should not obsess," the Center's general director wrote in its official report *Avian Flu: What Should Be Done,* "over whether 'the rich' or 'the poor' are obtaining a greater share of treatment or prevention."[3175]

All will not be roses for the wealthy who survive. "[M]any of the comforts of our daily life," one expert explained, "lettuce in winter, light bulbs, new sneakers, are grown for us or made for us by people who live in developing countries. If their workforces are decimated, we will feel the knock on effects."[3176]

Describing the "implications for all this" as "really fascinating," one of Canada's foremost economists predicted that "[c]learly at the end of the crisis there would be many bargains to be had."[3177] But people would need to be in a financial position to exploit the situation. BMO Nesbitt Burns published a report instructing the six-figure income set on how to best play their cards. Those who could hoard cash would "ultimately benefit by buying real estate, farms, businesses, and stocks at extraordinary prices." The banking conglomerate admitted that this may sound "rather callous," but rationalized that this was the way it had always been done. In the lead-up to the Great Depression, went its explanation, those with liquid assets were able to "scoop up the property of those who were heavily indebted."[3178] The pandemic could be good for the 1 percent.

The 1918 pandemic was followed by the Roaring Twenties when, we were reminded, among the lucky survivors "there were hordes of newly-rich people . . . and many of the Old Rich had become fabulously rich." With the right pandemic portfolio, investment firms advised, survivors of the pandemic would not need to rely on luck "to take advantage of the wide array of cheap assets."[3179]

Post-pandemic wages may rise, thanks to the "accompanying negative shock to population and the labor force." The same boon evidently followed the Black Plague, with some historians arguing that rents dropped and wages rose. A financial analysis of 1918 claimed that the pandemic had a "large and robust positive effect" on per capita income growth, calculating exactly how much positive economic growth could be attributed to each additional death.[3180] During the 2005 Council on Foreign Relations Conference on the Global Threat of Pandemic Influenza session titled "What Would the World Look Like After a Pandemic?" bioterrorism expert Yanzhong Huang, the director of Center for Global Health Studies at Seton Hall University, remarked, "I want to point out that this negative shock to the population growth is not necessarily a negative thing."[3181]

There was some financial advice in those pandemic investment reports applicable to the general public. Commonsense appeals not to worsen one's personal debt seemed like sound advice,[3182] but other recommendations appear less valid. The president of Global Trends Investments, for example, recommended fallback to precious metals and hard currency,[3183] but with so many deaths expected, large-scale estate liquidations of jewelry might undercut the gold market.[3184] A lesson from Hurricane Katrina was that local economies might revert to systems of barter.[3185] Money, one expert from the British Institute for Animal Health asserted, "would be meaningless."[3186] Should the worst-case scenario come to pass, the president of investment research firm WBB Securities declared (perhaps only half jokingly), "the best bets may be canned goods and shotgun shells."[3187]

"We have learned very little that is new about the disease, but much that is old about ourselves."

—FREDERICK C. TILNEY, ON THE 1916 POLIO
EPIDEMIC IN NEW YORK[3188]

Major crises can bring out the best in people, and the worst. "We need to take steps so that people who are spared by the pandemic influenza virus aren't done in by starvation, cold, chronic diseases, or contaminated water," wrote one prominent risk management specialist.[3189] "We don't want people who are spared by the virus done in by riots either."

Civil society is expected to disintegrate, triggering violent social disturbances as populations attempt to flee contaminated areas or engage in mass looting.[3190] After Katrina hit, it took only forty-eight hours for 20 percent of New Orleans' police force to disappear and drug addicts in withdrawal to claim the streets with gunfire.[3191] FEMA director Brown said his agency was forced to work "under conditions of urban warfare."[3192] And that was only one city in crisis.

Experts fear that civil unrest could be a tipping point for instability in a number of governments around the world "as their economies implode."[3193] There is a concern that even early on in unaffected countries, panic and chaos could erupt as the world media reports the daily advance of the pandemic.[3194]

In 1918, orderly life in America began to collapse. Families stopped taking care of each other. In its 1919 *An Account of the Influenza Epidemic,* the Red Cross reported that "people [were] starving to death not from lack of food but because the well were panic stricken and would not go near the sick."[3195] Social services begged neighbors to take in children whose parents lay dying or dead. A historian reported, "The response was almost nil."[3196] Victor Vaughn, Surgeon General of the U.S. Army, described as "a careful man, a measured man, a man who did not overstate to make a point," warned, "Civilization could have disappeared within a few more weeks."[3197]

In 1918, the social order broke down. The chief diagnostician in the New York City Health department summarized the impact of the pandemic on the mental state of its victims: "Intense and protracted prostration led to hysteria, melancholia, and insanity with suicidal intent."[3198] Violence erupted. In San Francisco, a Health Department inspector shot a man for refusing to wear a mask. In Chicago, a worker shouted, "I'll cure them my own way!" and then proceeded to cut the throats of his wife and four children.[3199]

Riots broke out. The War Department, overwhelmed by the pandemic, was unable to assist in controlling the civic disorder at home.[3200] All levels of government were severely crippled, affecting public services across the board.[3201] Undertakers had to hire private armed guards around their valuable coffins.[3202]

The official U.S. pandemic preparedness plan predicted many of the same scenarios developing in the face of a severe pandemic,[3203] which didn't surprise researchers in the field. Asked one,

What happens when people in South Side Chicago or Compton or the Bronx see people dying of this, while others get the care they need? What happens if the hospitals which traditionally serve the needs of the inner city begin to run out of beds? Do we think that people will sit pat in the projects and poor neighborhoods of our country and watch as their family and friends, their very communities, die? I don't see why there wouldn't be civil unrest.[3204]

When Chinese villagers realized that information had been withheld by provincial leaders during the SARS outbreak, they rioted against proposed quarantine centers that were being prepared to isolate outsiders. Asked why information had been withheld from the villagers, one bureaucrat told a news correspondent, "They just won't understand."[3205] Open communication is considered vital to maintaining trust. As former senator Sam Nunn said, playing the U.S. president in Dark Winter, a smallpox bioterrorist exercise,[3206] "The federal government has to have the cooperation from the American people. There is no federal force out there that can require 300 million people to take steps they don't want to take."[3207]

This means the national debate needs to be start immediately. Who should get the ventilator, the vaccine, the hospital bed—the 70-year-old grandparent, the 30-year-old mother of two children, or the children themselves? "People in America are not used to that kind of rationing," a CDC economist told *Science*.[3208] The chief of clinical bioethics at the U.S. National Institutes of Health published a suggestion that proved controversial with those in the medical field.[3209] He proposed that children should be given precedence, even if just prioritizing doctors might save more lives, based on what's been called the "fair innings" principle[3210] that "each person should have an opportunity to live through all the stages of life."[3211] The time for that discussion is *before* a pandemic begins.[3212]

Social psychologists describe a chilling effect on human nature, values, and motivations visited upon us by plagues throughout history. A chronicler of the Black Death wrote in 1348, "Father abandoned child, wife husband, one brother another. . . . And no one could be found to bury the dead for money or friendship." He himself was forced to bury his five children with his own hands.[3213] According to a distinguished medical historian, the general attitude could be summed up by a line from Ben Jonson's *The Alchemist* in which, during a plague outbreak, one character tells another, "Breathe less, and farther off!"[3214]

This base human tendency, born of fear and distrust, can fester into a *Lord of the Flies* social pathology of hate.[3215] The bubonic plague led to violent attacks upon minorities such as the Jews, especially after one Jew famously "confessed" (under torture) to poisoning wells across Europe.[3216] This led to further spread of the disease as persecuted peoples fled affected areas en masse. Dominant social groups seized the situation to further socially conservative agendas, under the flag of "God's punishment for sin."[3217] During the COVID-19 crisis, attacks and harassment targeted against Asian Americans reportedly skyrocketed.[3218]

Scapegoating is endemic throughout medical history. Since the early sixteenth century, for example, syphilis has been called *morbus gallicus* (the "French pox") in Italy, *le mal de Naples* (the "disease of Naples") in France, the "Polish disease" in Russia, the "Russian disease" in Siberia, the "Portuguese disease" in India, the "Castilian disease" in Portugal, and the "British disease" in Tahiti.[3219]

In 1918, the rich blamed the poor and the poor blamed the rich for the emergence of the "Spanish Lady"—itself a xenophobic, misogynistic label. Swedish socialists staged a general strike proclaiming "Flu Avenges the Workers." The poor areas of the world did suffer disproportionately, but in some cities such as London, the death rate was "as high in prosperous Chelsea and Westminster as in the slums of Bermondsey and Bethnal Green" for the first time in the history of public health records.[3220] As one expert noted, "[I]nfluenza's very very democratic."[3221]

The 1918 pandemic was fodder for racists and anti-Semites. In Baltimore under Jim Crow segregation, the hospitals were closed to African Americans at their moment of greatest need. Once the pandemic passed, Baltimore officials then defended the city's poor public health performance by attributing the city's elevated mortality rate to its proportion of black residents.[3222] The Poles blamed the Jews, whom they called "a particular enemy to order and cleanliness."[3223] As reviewed in *The New England Journal of Medicine,* this was "sadly neither the first nor the last, of the social scapegoating that is one of the most common, ugly, and unproductive features of epidemics in human society."[3224]

Victims of infectious disease are blamed and shunned to this day. During the SARS epidemic, artists of Chinese descent were denied access to a middle school in New Jersey.[3225] Some of the employees of the company that fell prey to the first anthrax case were doubly victimized. Family physicians refused to see them, and their kids were turned away from schools.[3226]

The religious intolerance and victim blaming of 1918 was repeated in 2005 following Hurricane Katrina.[3227] Founder of the Christian Coalition of America and former presidential candidate Pat Robertson linked both Katrina and terrorist attacks to legalized abortion.[3228] The director of the fundamentalist Christian organization Repent America prayed, "May this act of God cause us all to think about what we tolerate in our city limits, and bring us trembling before the throne of Almighty God."[3229] A Christian leader within New Orleans agreed that it was God's mercy that purged New Orleans. "New Orleans now is abortion free," he said. "New Orleans now is Mardi Gras free."[3230]

The pandemic of 1918 brought out the worst in people, but it also brought out the best. "White and colored worked side by side then," recalled one survivor from Louisiana. "Had we the cooperation between races today that we had during that epidemic it would be a blessing."[3231] The U.S. Homeland Security Council National Strategy for Pandemic Influenza relied on this goodwill: "Institutions in danger of becoming overwhelmed will rely on the voluntarism and sense of civic and humanitarian duty of ordinary Americans."[3232] A month after the World War I armistice, the German bacteriologist famous for inventing the test for syphilis wrote from Berlin: "For me there are no Germans, no Englishmen—only men who suffer and must be helped." As the fateful year wound down, a Greek daily summed up the evolving spirit of the times with the line: "Today all nations sneeze as one."[3233]

"In the absence of a pandemic, almost any preparation will smack of alarmism, but if a pandemic does break out, nothing that has been done will be enough."

—TONY ABBOTT, AUSTRALIAN MINISTER FOR HEALTH[3234]

What should we do when the whole world gets sick? "From my perspective," Osterholm said, "we pray, plan, and practice . . . We have to plan as if this will happen tonight."[3235]

Just as past experience with SARS may have helped countries like Singapore and Taiwan better deal with COVID-19, hard lessons from the coronavirus pandemic will hopefully translate into global readiness for the next one. Pandemic planning needs to be on the agenda of every institution, including every school board, every food distributor, every mortuary, every town hall, and every legislature.[3236] The corporate world seemed to have been the first to have awakened to the pandemic threat long before COVID-19 erupted. Corporations from Boeing to Microsoft to Starbucks started mobilizing continuity plans back in 2005,[3237] though details were considered "privileged company information."[3238] Microsoft reportedly distributed bottles of hand sanitizers to all of its sixty-three thousand employees worldwide.[3239] The national U.S. preparedness plan, however, still remained to be employed across the country.

The paradox of a pandemic is that it is worldwide, but intensely local. Nobody is "outside" the pandemic to send help.[3240] "Communities, in large part, will be on their own," predicted the executive director of the National Association of County and City Health Officials.[3241] The same may have been said of individuals. The president of the College of General Practitioners laid out the bottom line: "Self-management and self-reliance will be the cornerstone."[3242]

Every family must draft and implement its own plan and discuss that plan with friends.[3243] Every organization one is affiliated with—schools, clubs, work, places of worship—must be pushed to initiate its own plans.[3244] "We must hang together," Ben Franklin is attributed as saying, "or assuredly we shall all hang separately."

As the H5N1 pandemic threat started looming more than a decade ago, Health and Human Services Secretary Leavitt criticized Americans for not preparing sufficiently. "People have not exercised adequate personal preparedness," he said, "to last more than three or four days in their normal environment without going to the store."[3245]

According to WHO risk communication experts, these grave public warnings are useful on four different levels. First, people will hopefully take responsibility for preparing themselves logistically. Second, they may help spur their communities into greater preparedness. Third, people may be more supportive of their governments' planning efforts, and, fourth, when the pandemic begins, the advance notice will have given people time to get used to the idea emotionally, feel less panicky, and take a more active role in protecting themselves, their families, and their communities.[3246]

In that case, why didn't we hear more from public officials urging individuals to prepare for what experts declared was a coming pandemic? One reason is that officials did not want to panic the populace. "What I've found is that, behind the scenes, many public health officials are distancing themselves from this global-health-crisis rhetoric," said a former chief medical officer of Ontario. "It's not like terrifying someone about smoking or HIV, where you're actually asking them to do something about it."[3247] "Scaring people about avian influenza accomplishes nothing," he said, "because we're not asking people to do anything about it." The mistake didn't lie in scaring people, though; it was in failing to realize and communicate just how much the public could do to prepare.[3248]

"How Scared Should We Be?" asked the title of a *Time* magazine story on bird flu. The subtitle answered: "Scared Enough to Take Action."[3249] Long before COVID-19 erupted, we should have immediately started getting into the habit of practicing proper hand hygiene and respiratory etiquette. We should have prepared our family's pandemic preparedness kit. Now that we're in the throes of a pandemic, though, we should finally commit to taking these critical steps before the *next* outbreak—and actually following through as soon as we can.

The kit should contain everything one might need to stay at home for a period that could last from days to months with or without running water and electricity.[3250] Everyone's checklist will differ based on individualized family needs, but once COVID-19 is over, you can start the list by writing down what necessities are used as they come up on a day-to-day basis.[3251] The New Zealand government took the additional step of including in the back of all the nation's phone books a list of instructions as to what to do when the pandemic struck and items to stock in one's "B-ready kit."[3252]

In a remarkable speech at a conference in Wyoming, Health and Human Services Secretary Leavitt said:

> When you go to the store and buy three cans of tuna fish, buy a fourth and put it under the bed. When you go to the store to buy some milk, pick up a box of powdered milk. Put it under the bed. When you do that for a period of four to six months, you are going to have a couple of weeks of food, and that's what we're talking about.[3253]

Though critics dismissed his comments as a bit fishy—comparing it to "duck and cover" during a nuclear attack[3254]—he was at least on the right track. Shortly afterward, the Department of Health and Human Services released guidelines for a more varied menu. After all, "Powdered milk and tuna?" Jay Leno quipped. "How many would rather have the bird flu?"[3255]

Launched late in 2005, the official U.S. government website pandemic flu.gov morphed into quite a useful resource for those with access to the internet, listing downloadable pandemic planning checklists and guides for schools, businesses, and community groups. Unfortunately, it has been taken down and moved to an archived page on the CDC website that hasn't been updated since 2016. The following is adapted directly from its preparedness guidelines for individuals and families.

PANDEMIC FLU PLANNING CHECKLIST

You can prepare for an influenza pandemic now. You should know both the magnitude of what can happen during a pandemic outbreak and what actions you can take to help lessen the impact of an influenza pandemic on you and your family. This checklist will help you gather the information and resources you may need in case of a flu pandemic.

1. To plan for a pandemic:
   - Store a supply of water and food. During a pandemic, if you cannot get to a store or if stores are out of supplies, it will be important for you to have extra supplies on hand. This can be useful in other types of emergencies, such as power outages and disasters.
   - Have any nonprescription drugs and other health supplies on hand, including pain relievers, stomach remedies, cough and cold medicines, fluids with electrolytes, and vitamins.
   - Talk with family members and loved ones about how they would be cared for if they got sick, or what will be needed to care for them in your home.
   - Volunteer with local groups to prepare and assist with emergency response.

- Get involved in your community as it works to prepare for a pandemic.
2. To limit the spread of germs and prevent infection:
   - Teach your children to wash hands frequently with soap and water, and model the correct behavior.
   - Teach your children to cover coughs and sneezes with tissues, and be sure to model that behavior.
   - Teach your children to stay away from others as much as possible if they are sick. Stay home from work and school if sick.
3. Items to have on hand for an extended stay at home:

   Examples of Food and Non-perishables
   Canned or Tetra Pak beans, soups, and milks
   Canned and frozen fruits and vegetables
   Apples, sweet potatoes, and winter squash
   Pasta and canned or jarred tomatoes
   Whole grains
   Dried legumes
   Freeze-dried meals
   Protein bars or fruit bars
   Dry cereal or granola
   Nuts and nut butters
   Whole-grain crackers
   Dried fruit and trail mixes
   Canned or Tetra Pak juices
   Bottled water, tea
   Canned or jarred baby food and formula
   Pet food

   Examples of Medical, Health, and Emergency Supplies
   Prescribed medical supplies
   Soap and alcohol-based hand sanitizer
   Disposable gloves
   N95 and surgical masks
   Thermometer
   Medicines for fever
   Antidiarrheal medication
   Vitamins

Fluids with electrolytes

Cleansing agents, disinfectant cleaners

Flashlight and batteries

Portable radio

Manual can opener

Garbage bags

Toilet paper and tissues

Disposable diapers

The family food checklist focuses on nutritious staples that can be stored without refrigeration and eaten without cooking, such as ready-to-eat canned goods,[3256] but includes hearty options for milder pandemics as well. Other possibilities include instant packaged mixes like instant oatmeal, mashed potatoes, and cup soups. There's even a cookbook—*Apocalypse Chow*—a humorous yet serious attempt at palatable "pantry cuisine," using jarred, canned, and freeze-dried foods.[3257]

How much food is enough? Dr. Fauci recommended stockpiling "a few weeks' worth of water, a few weeks' worth of non-spoilable foods."[3258] Osterholm told Oprah, "Everyone should have enough food today so that they could basically be in their homes for four or five weeks."[3259] Expert Webster has a three-month store of food and water in his home.[3260] That's what the U.S. State Department suggested: "[C]urrent guidance notes that families should be prepared to 'shelter-in-place' for up to twelve weeks, and maintain sufficient food and water supplies to accommodate that entire period."[3261] (Though, after flu bloggers pointed out the discrepancy between this three-month stockpiling recommendation and the two weeks cited by the Department of Health and Human Services,[3262] the three-month guideline mysteriously vanished from U.S. consulate websites.[3263])

Some have recommended locating a rural refuge, if possible, to ride out the storm away from population centers and any ensuing civil unrest. When asked what people could do to protect themselves before a vaccine would be available, Webster replied, "If they have a house in the hills, then go for it—and stay there for three months. And have enough food there already so you can stay as far away from your neighbors as possible."[3264] Rural states like Vermont expected their populations to as much as double to accommodate urban refugees. Vermont officials reserved freezer space from Ben and Jerry's to store overflow corpses.[3265]

Food and water might also be more easily obtained in the countryside.[3266] In case of "complete infrastructure breakdown," the State Department advises stockpiling a gallon of fresh water per person per day,[3267] as does FEMA,[3268] with additional allowances for any household pets. For a family of three, that would involve storing a ton of water—literally. Webster has a better suggestion. "So you are advocating that people stockpile food and medicine?" "Absolutely," Webster replied. "Most of us can afford to buy dry food for three months. One bottle of Clorox is enough to purify all the water you need out of the local river."[3269]

According to FEMA, one can disinfect water (sourced from a freshwater stream or lake) by keeping it at a rolling boil for a full minute or, if unable to boil it, by using water-purifying tablets found in camping stores or using bleach.

Recipe for Water Purification

1 quart (liter) clear water

10 drops an unscented liquid household chlorine bleach that is 1 percent sodium hypochlorite *or* 2 drops for 4 percent to 6 percent sodium hypochlorite bleach *or* 1 drop per quart for 7 to 10 percent bleach

Mix well and let stand for 30 minutes before drinking. Double the amount of bleach for cloudy or colored water, or water that is extremely cold. The water should have a slight chlorine odor after purification. If not, repeat dosage of bleach and let stand an additional 15 minutes. If the chlorine taste is too strong, try pouring the treated water back and forth from one clean container to another several times.[3270] Following this method, a single bottle of bleach would purify all the water you need to shelter-in-place for twelve weeks or more.

The Boy Scout motto, "Be prepared," begged the question, *Be prepared for what?* The founder of the Scouts replied, "Why, any old thing."[3271] With another pandemic inevitable, the best we can do is mediate the consequences. This means doing our best to avoid falling ill, developing contingency plans to survive the infection, and making all necessary preparations to endure social chaos. "The objective of pandemic preparedness can only be damage control," said top WHO flu expert Klaus Stöhr. "There will be death and destruction."[3272]

VI. Preventing Future Pandemics

TINDERBOX

Trojan Duck

Pandemics may be inevitable, but the emergence of Ebola-like superstrains may be preventable. As porous as U.S. biosecurity is, the American system offers some distinct advantages.[3273] Avian influenza tests are provided free of charge by the USDA to the poultry industry, so more than a million tests have been carried out every year.[3274] That's a small percentage of the nine *billion* birds slaughtered annually for human consumption in the country,[3275] but is probably the best national surveillance in the world.[3276] Many poultry-raising countries cannot afford to test millions of birds, and, as a result, low-pathogenic viruses can asymptomatically seed themselves undetected far and wide before additional mutations may make the disease hard to miss.[3277]

Confinement systems can also make the systematic culling of infected populations easier once the disease is found.[3278] More and more countries moved toward killing entire flocks infected with any H5 or H7 viruses—low-grade or not—to prevent the viruses from mutating into highly pathogenic strains, "but this is only feasible," experts asserted, "if there is financial support from local or national governments."[3279] Another example of the industry attempting to externalize its costs by having the public subsidize its cleanup: the public bears the cost, and the risk.

With public assistance, though, countries with industrialized poultry production have historically been able to stop bird flu. In a country like the United States, it has spread onto hundreds of farms across more than twenty states, but by killing enough birds, the virus has been stopped. This led some to naïvely advocate that poultry farming worldwide be restricted to large-scale factory farms where infected birds can be "rapidly identified and culled,"[3280] but industrial systems also have the opposite effect.

When a virus hits an industrial facility, it hits big. "Once high density industrial poultry areas become affected infection can explosively spread within the units," the Food and Agriculture Organization of the United Nations wrote, "and the very high quantities of virus produced may be easily carried to other units, to humans, and into the environment."[3281]

The U.S. Geological Survey agreed: "Infected fowl can become virus pumps producing and shedding large quantities of infectious virus that contaminate the local environment, facilitating transmission of the virus within the population, which also increases the probability of virus spreading to sites/farms beyond the location of the original outbreak."[3282] "Clearly, eradication efforts are more successful," OIE experts have written, "if there is no massive spread into the industrial circuits of intensively reared poultry."[3283]

During the 2003 H7N7 outbreak in the Netherlands, even with the Dutch Army assisting in the culling and disposal of thirty million birds, the virus still managed to slip into two other countries and expose hundreds of people to the virus, some of whom then went home and gave it to their families.[3284] As the WHO points out, despite modern facilities in an industrialized country with a well-developed agricultural and veterinary infrastructure, the elimination of the infection in poultry was "a complex, difficult, and costly undertaking."[3285] Still, though, the infection was eliminated.

To continue to keep the price of chicken meat as low as possible, why not move all the world's chickens onto factory farms and simply ramp up surveillance? Annual distribution of sixty-nine billion or so testing kits for each bird slaughtered worldwide may seem cost-prohibitive, but it may be cheaper than breeding birds with functional immune systems and raising them at a modest stocking density in a sufficiently clean, ventilated, and low-stress environment. In the hypothetical scenario in which the global flock has been effectively Tysonized, the individual intensive confinement facilities may remain potential breeding grounds for highly pathogenic strains, but the virus would presumably be caught early enough to limit its spread. With enough resources and enough killing, the industry has shown historically that any virus could be stamped out. History changed, though, with H5N1.

No one imagined that a killer influenza virus might be able to reinfect its natural hosts without killing them; no one thought a bird flu virus could have it both ways. In its natural waterfowl reservoir, influenza is a frequent flier, flown around the world as a low-grade virus in the guts of migratory birds. In domestic poultry, the virus can grow deadly, as we've learned, but what it gains in virulence, it loses in mobility. As one poultry veterinarian put it, "Dead birds don't fly far."[3286] Any bird flu virus that grew deadly was presumed to sacrifice its power of flight, enabling industry to effectively mobilize against it. The Z+ strain of H5N1 showed that the industry presumed wrong.[3287]

Initially, wild birds were victims—not vectors—of H5N1. In 2002, H5N1 started killing off waterfowl in Hong Kong's nature parks.[3288] Thousands of bar-headed geese perished in China—up to 10 percent of the world's population of the species.[3289] Professor Shortridge speculated that H5N1 might be capable of "ecocide," wrecking the ecosystem by killing off wild bird species, creating a kind of global Silent Spring.[3290] But by early 2004, the virus was showing a trend of decreased pathogenicity in ducks, while remaining highly pathogenic in chickens and children.[3291] Forced into land-based poultry, H5N1 turned ferocious. When it next encountered waterfowl, the virus was devastating. But H5N1 gradually acquired the worst of both worlds, retaining its ability to harmlessly infect globe-trotting waterfowl while continuing to kill poultry and people.[3292]

H5N1 no longer had to start from scratch. It was caught early enough once, in Hong Kong, and destroyed. Its re-emergence in 2001 was thought to have been an independent event. Once it attained the unprecedented[3293] ability to jump back into waterfowl from poultry, though, it could become endemic in the world's wild bird population.[3294] This not only enabled the virus to spread around the world and made it virtually impossible to eradicate, it allowed for the continual ratcheting up of mutations without disruption. "We cannot contain this thing anymore," Webster told the *Los Angeles Times*. "Nature is in control."[3295]

Now that we know what bird flu viruses are capable of, we can no longer pretend that we can keep them locked up. They may come into a factory farm on a boot, in a mouse, or on a fly as a low-pathogenic virus, but may escape the same way they entered—but now as a high-pathogenic virus. During the Pennsylvania outbreak, H5N2 was found in more than a hundred wild birds and rodents in the affected area.[3296] No longer was just the neighboring farm at risk. We now know that viruses with presumed pandemic potential can escape into the global ecosystem. With that in mind, we must focus on preventing the birth of these viruses in the first place.

Both Vietnam and Thailand[3297] took steps to restrict or ban duck and goose farming, but it may have been too little, too late.[3298] Domesticated ducks were presumably likelier to transmit the virus to chickens, given their greater proximity and the continued existence of viral melting pots like live poultry markets and live animal transports. However, ending their domestication would not be expected to eliminate the risk entirely, given the presence of wild waterfowl overhead. Still, the two billion domesticated ducks farmed by people in East Asia are two billion more experimental hosts than we need allow these viruses.[3299]

The earth will be bombarded with influenza virus as long as there are wild waterfowl. But, as I've said, the viruses almost always start out harmless. They only seem to grow dangerous once they hit poultry—and seem only to grow *really* dangerous in modern-day industrial poultry farms.

One Stray Spark

Minnesota, the "land of 10,000 lakes,"[3300] is the largest brooding area for aquatic birds in the United States. More wild waterfowl hatch there every year than anywhere else in the country.[3301] In addition, it's a central flyway for migratory waterfowl flying south from Canada in the fall.[3302] Minnesota also happened to be the nation's number one turkey-producing state.[3303] That combination gave the state the dubious distinction of the avian influenza "capital of the world."[3304]

No wild turkey had ever been found infected with bird flu in Minnesota or elsewhere.[3305] Land-based birds, such as turkeys and chickens, were aberrant hosts for the virus.[3306] Only when confined in unnatural concentrations did it appear they could support viral spread that required close contact. As was shown in pigs, laboratory bird flu transmission studies on turkeys concluded that "transmission rate is markedly reduced when birds are not confined closely."[3307] In industrial confinement, each turkey is typically allotted only three square feet of living space.[3308] In the wild, turkeys may range over several square miles a day.[3309] They naturally congregate in flocks of ten to twenty.[3310] Typical confinement facilities house fifteen thousand turkeys per shed,[3311] and those penned outdoors may reach flock sizes of a hundred thousand.[3312]

With so many animals—albeit many outdoors—crowded together under skies with so many ducks, scientists counted more than a hundred separate introductions of low-grade bird flu viruses into commercial Minnesota turkey flocks since the 1970s.[3313] Yet, even with outdoor flock sizes as large as a hundred thousand birds, in the sun and open air, not a single one of those viruses mutated into a highly pathogenic strain. High-path viruses have never been known to arise in outdoor chicken or turkey flocks.[3314]

With tens of millions of ducks[3315] excreting tens of billions of viruses, it's inevitable that outdoor turkey flocks will be caught in the fly-by crossfire. But, because they are not intensively confined in the damp, poorly ventilated, and unsanitary sheds, the viruses can't seem to mutate into highly pathogenic forms. The free-range turkeys rarely suffer serious illness.

Even though the low-pathogenic viruses don't cause symptoms, the bodies of the infected turkeys mobilize resources to knock out the virus, which can result in slower weight gain or reduced egg laying, both of which present a "serious economic burden to turkey producers."[3316] So, starting in the late 1990s, Minnesota turkey farmers followed Canada's example and converted their free-range or "semi-intensive" farms to industrial confinement operations.

As in Canada,[3317] the number of avian influenza infections dropped dramatically.[3318] This may have saved the industry money in the short term, but the bill for its shortsightedness may soon fall due. Dave Halvorson is an emeritus professor and avian health specialist at the University of Minnesota. In a *Poultry Digest* review, "Avian Influenza Control in Minnesota," Halvorson wrote, "If exposed to avian influenza, those range turkeys don't usually suffer ill effects. But a nonpathogenic influenza virus, when it gets into a confinement situation, causes severe economic loss in morbidity, mortality and body weight loss."[3319] A highly pathogenic virus born of confinement may pose a human health threat as well.

In *The Monster at Our Door*, Mike Davis proposed an analogy for the roles played by indoor and outdoor poultry. "In an epidemiological sense," he wrote, "the outdoor flocks are the fuse, and the dense factory populations, the explosive charge."[3320] Birds raised outside undoubtedly have a greater exposure to aquatic birds and their viruses,[3321] but the buck seems to stop there. If there were only outdoor birds, influenza viruses would rarely have the opportunity to turn highly pathogenic.[3322] The co-existence of free-range flocks alongside intensive confinement operations, though, allows for the lit fuse to cause damage. Potential mixing at live poultry markets or via contaminated equipment or clothing could transmit low-grade viruses into confinement facilities, and an epidemic may explode.

What the turkey farmers had been trying to do was get rid of the fuses. By eliminating outdoor production, they hoped to eliminate the possibility that some neighboring producer might track some free-range manure into their local feed store. By confining turkeys indoors, there may be fewer fuses—but there is much more to detonate. With that much TNT lying around, all it takes is a spark.

In the three years following the Minnesota decision to move all the free-range turkeys indoors, more than twenty-five flocks still came up positive for bird flu.[3323] Biosecurity is never absolute. A low-grade strain of H5N1 was even found in a twenty-eight-thousand-bird turkey flock across Lake Superior in Michigan in 2002[3324]—a year before its Asian cousin H5N1 renewed killing people in Hong Kong.[3325] Since turkeys may be more susceptible to infection than chickens,[3326] the world is fortunate that turkeys are, as of yet, not raised commercially in China en masse.[3327] Up to 2020, the bird flu viruses discovered in U.S. turkey sheds had been detected in the low-pathogenic stage, but had they not been caught in time, some of them might have mutated into widespread killers.

The Food and Agriculture Organization of the United Nations understands that the probability of low-grade infection is higher for outdoor flocks, particularly those not "cooped up and fenced in,"[3328] but that the potential detrimental impact of infection within industrial operations is greater.[3329] The FAO elaborated in its FAQ, Questions and Answers on Avian Influenza:

> [C]hicken to chicken spread, particularly where assisted by intensive husbandry conditions, promotes the virus to shift (adaptation) to more severe type (highly pathogenic type) of infection. . . . Intensive production conditions favour rapid spread of infection within units and "hotting-up" of virus from low pathogenicity to a highly pathogenic types.[3330]

In the FAO diagram (figure 2), the evolution of a pandemic is traced, starting with "Increased demand for poultry products" and ending with a bird flu virus capable of human-to-human transmission.[3331]

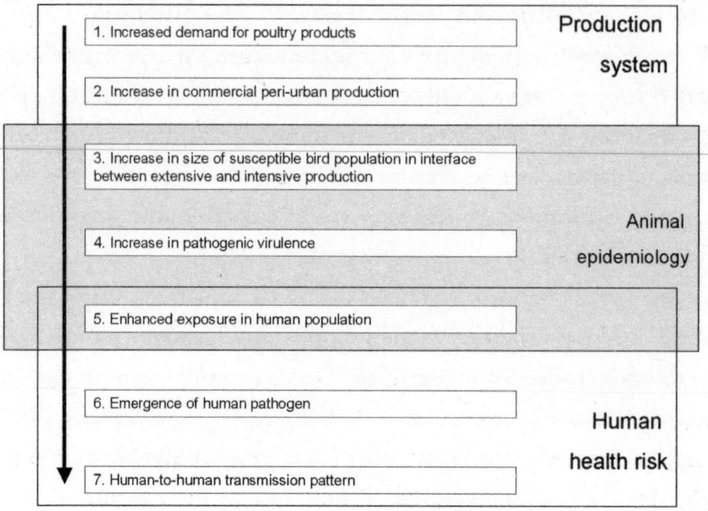

Figure 2. Tracing the evolution of a pandemic
(Courtesy of the United Nations Food and Agriculture Organization)

Minnesota turkeys had gotten fewer sniffles indoors, but turkey producers may have been tempting fate. All it takes is a stray spark—a footprint of duck dropping carried in by a rat—and the situation could explode. The April 2020 emergence of a highly pathogenic strain of H7N3 in South Carolina was in a facility confining more than thirty thousand turkeys.[3332] Just as bullets seem to find their way into unloaded guns in the household, influenza viruses littered across the countryside seem to find ways into "biosecure" sheds warehousing birds. The industry might do better to disarm completely.

To prevent the future emergence of exceptionally deadly viruses like H5N1, the global poultry industry may need to reverse its course of rushing toward greater intensification. What should poultry producers do, though, given that a virus like H5N1 has already been born? The question remained unanswered, according to veterinarian Karen Becker, senior health adviser within the U.S. Department of Health and Human Services public health emergency preparedness division.[3333] Some countries like the Netherlands placed temporary roofing over outdoor poultry yards on migration routes;[3334] others took the controversial step of forcing all poultry flocks indoors.[3335]

The organic lobby in Europe had been most vocal in resisting moves to lock outdoor flocks inside. The Soil Association, the UK's leading organic certifier, argued that disease outbreaks should instead be "minimized by the avoidance of dense stocking level or intensive housing and the promotion of positive animal health through good husbandry and free-range conditions."[3336] It's true that keeping birds in smaller numbers and lower stocking densities with access to clean pasture may provide a boost to the birds' natural immune systems, as I've discussed, but, presumably, because of prior intensive production in Asia, half of the world faces a unique situation in which an avian influenza virus that had *already* become highly pathogenic could rain from the sky.

H5N1 is not done mutating, though. Z+ H5N1 is not a pandemic virus. It would still need to change in order to acquire easy human-to-human transmissibility. That final series of mutations is less likely to happen in someone's backyard flock of ten birds. Continue to put H5N1 into sheds with twenty thousand chickens and floors covered with feces, though, and H5N1 might eventually ratchet up adaptations to the human-like epithelium lining the chicken's respiratory tract and be greatly amplified to further spill back out into the environment. While free-grazing ducks on flooded rice fields in countries like Thailand may be contributing to the spread of H5N1 through water contamination,[3337] bringing pasture-raised poultry indoors in Europe and beyond may do more harm than good, confining millions more birds in conditions that may most effectively mutate the virus further.

Presumably, the only way to significantly slow H5N1 at this late stage is to stop repopulating the sheds. Broiler chickens reach slaughter weight so quickly that if breeders stopped breeding birds and sending chicks out from the hatcheries, every broiler shed would be vacant in a matter of weeks. That would mean billions fewer opportunities for H5N1 to mutate in just one year. Instead we keep reloading.

Perry Kendall is chief medical officer of health for British Columbia and cochair of the Pan-Canadian Public Health Network.[3338] He was there during the 2004 Canadian outbreak, which, at the time, was the worst outbreak in North American history, leading to the destruction of nineteen million birds. He witnessed that birds kept indoors were *more* vulnerable than those kept outdoors. "You've got 10,000 birds all in a small shed, packed in together—they act like a Petri dish," Kendall explained in an interview. "The intensely farmed birds tend to be very genetically similar. The methods of farming result in them being actually more frail and more vulnerable to diseases, particularly since there are so many of them in such a small volume (space)." He noted how easy it remained for farm staff to trample virus indoors or for a tractor to spread it from farm to farm. "You need to ramp up your biosecurity level to what you see in a laboratory," he said, "if you really want to keep infections out of the barns."[3339]

Biosafety Level Zero

H5N1 is considered a Biosafety Level 3+ pathogen.[3340] This means that in a laboratory setting, the virus is only to be handled in unique high-containment buildings specially engineered with air locks, controlled access corridors, and double-door entries. Access is limited to competent personnel with extensive training,[3341] and showering is required upon every entry and exit.[3342] Air flow is ducted, unidirectional, single-pass filtered exhaust only.[3343] All floors, walls, and ceilings are waterproofed and sealed with continuous cove moldings.[3344] All wall penetrations—electrical outlets, phone and cable lines, and the like—are caulked, collared, or sealed to prevent any leaks.[3345] Surfaces are disinfected on a daily basis.[3346] Solid wastes are incinerated.[3347] The industrial poultry industry, in contrast, may breed the same virus at essentially a biosafety level of zero.

The intensive global poultry industry is not only playing with fire with no way to put it out, it is fanning the flames. And firewalls to contain the virus don't exist. "Unfortunately," leading USDA poultry virologist Dennis Senne told an international gathering of bird flu scientists, "that level of biosecurity does not exist in U.S. poultry production and I doubt that it exists in other parts of the world."[3348]

Further efforts could and should be made to educate poultry producers worldwide about the critical importance of biosecurity measures since the industry is no longer only gambling with its own fate, but the fate of us all. Even after seventeen million birds died as a result of the 1980s Pennsylvania outbreak, one poultry veterinarian wrote, "We must face the reality that the Egg Industry will not change its direction because of the threat of AI [avian influenza]. Industries in general change because of economic considerations."[3349] Given taxpayer subsidies for dealing with epidemic disease, the poultry industry may just factor outbreaks into the bottom line. The biosecurity measures that are practiced are better than nothing, but may not be enough to stake millions of lives upon for the sake of cheaper chicken. A pandemic of H5N1, or a comparable future bird flu, may have the capacity to spark the greatest human catastrophe of all time. It may be wiser to move away from intensive poultry production altogether or, at the very least, stop encouraging its movement into the developing world.

Massive commercial-scale poultry plants have been increasingly appearing in Thailand, southern China, Singapore, Hong Kong, Taiwan,[3350] Brazil, and India.[3351] Though they may rival the size of those in Arkansas, they may lag even further behind in hygienic standards[3352] and biosecurity.[3353] As sloppy as U.S. biosecurity has been shown to be, warehousing live birds by the millions in countries that lack comparative surveillance and control combines the worst of both worlds—the intensive confinement of the west with the impoverished infrastructure of the east and global south. Exporting our intensive production model to the developing world is a recipe for disaster.

The Food and Agriculture Organization of the UN noted that "there seems to be an acceleration of the human influenza problems over the last few decades, involving an increasing number of species, and this is expected to largely relate to intensification of the poultry (and possibly pig) production."[3354] The domestication of poultry in Asia dates back thousands of years, and live poultry markets have an extensive history in the region. What happened to bring about H5N1? At a November 2005 Council on Foreign Relations Conference on the Global Threat of Pandemic Influenza, the senior correspondent of *NewsHour with Jim Lehrer* asked that question to the "godfather of flu research,"[3355] Robert Webster:

> SUAREZ: Was there something qualitatively different about this last decade that made it possible for this disease to do something that it . . . hasn't done before . . . a change in conditions that suddenly lit a match to the tinder?
>
> WEBSTER: [F]arming practices have changed. Previously, we had backyard poultry. I grew up on a farm in New Zealand. We had a few backyard chickens and ducks. The next-door neighbor was so far away it didn't matter. Now we put millions of chickens into a chicken factory next door to a pig factory, and this virus has the opportunity to get into one of these chicken factories and make billions and billions of these mutations continuously. And so what we've changed is the way we raise animals and our interaction

with those animals. And so the virus is changing in those animals and now finding its way back out of those animals into the wild birds. That's what's changed.[3356]

Finally, the millennia-old fuses had occasion to ignite. Professor Shortridge illustrated the emergence of H5N1 in a flow chart (figure 3).[3357]

One in eight people in the world—some 900 million people—live on small farms in China where ducks and chickens and pigs are commonly found. As long as domestication continues in China and elsewhere, pandemics will presumably continue to intermittently arise.[3358] But H5N1 is like no flu virus anyone has ever seen. World War I may have showed us what the

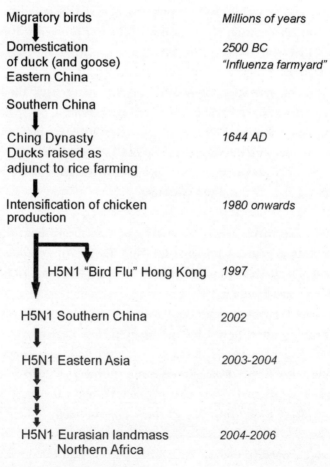

Figure 3. Charting the emergence of H5N1 (Courtesy of Kennedy Shortridge)

virus could become if it caught millions in the trenches; H5N1 may show us what happens when it catches billions.

Drawing on his thirty-seven years of experience within the industry, Ken Rudd concluded his trade publication article, "Poultry Reality Check Needed," with these prophetic words:

> *Now is the time to decide. We can go on with business as usual, hoping for the best as we charge headlong toward lower costs. Or we can begin making the prudent moves needed to restore a balance between economics and long-range avian health. We can pay now or we can pay later. But it should be known and it must be said, one way or another we will pay.*[3359]

Snowflakes to an Avalanche

Heralded by the U.S. Secretary of Agriculture's famous injunction at the time to "get big or get out,"[3360] industrial poultry production began in the 1950s,[3361] the same decade that fowl plague was discovered to be avian influenza.[3362] As the industry intensified, so did the outbreaks.[3363] There was one outbreak of highly pathogenic bird flu in the 1950s, two in the 1960s, three in the 1970s, three in the 1980s, jumping to nine in the 1990s, and then eight between 2001 and 2004, before H5N1 started its global march.[3364,3365] With the spread of H5N1, the number of outbreaks in the first few years of the twenty-first century already exceeded the total number of outbreaks recorded for the entire twentieth century. H5N1 alone has caused more than 6,500 outbreaks in more than sixty countries.[3366] Other new bird flu viruses—namely H5N2, H5N8, H7N1, H7N3, H7N4, and H7N7—have affected more than a hundred million birds across five continents.[3367,3368] In fact, as COVID-19 raged, a new outbreak of highly pathogenic bird flu broke out in South Carolina.[3369] One leading Italian flu scientist told *Science*, "We've gone from a few snowflakes to an avalanche."[3370]

Highly pathogenic bird flu is hard to miss, as it tends to wipe out entire flocks. In the past several decades, it has gone from an exceedingly rare disease in poultry to one that now crops up every year.[3371] This dramatic increase in regularity[3372] is matched by an upsurge in the scale of bird flu outbreaks. The majority of the twentieth-century outbreaks were limited in their geographic spread—some confined to a single farm or flock.[3373] In all, approximately twenty million birds were affected in the latter half of the century, compared to some two hundred million birds in just a few years in the early 2000s.[3374] In addition to H5N1 in Asia, there was, as I've mentioned, the highly pathogenic outbreak in the Netherlands in 2003 leading to the deaths of thirty million birds[3375] and the outbreak in Canada in 2004 that effectively killed nineteen million[3376] and then fifty million in the United States within just about six months in 2015.[3377] The director of the Center for Public Health Preparedness and Research at Emory University and other experts[3378,3379,3380,3381,3382] blamed the intensification of the disease on the intensification of the industry.

According to the latest global statistics, the three most common terrestrial animals slaughtered in the world are pigs, ducks, and chickens—not a good combination from a pandemic perspective. These days, about one billion pigs, three billion ducks, and sixty-nine billion chickens are slaughtered every year. Although the preceding five years saw little change in the number of rodents slaughtered for their flesh (about seventy million), the single greatest increase in slaughter was chickens, up eight billion birds. China led the world in land-based animal slaughter, killing approximately fifteen billion animals a year.[3383]

When a pandemic virus arose in China in 1968, there were five million pigs in the country and twelve million birds raised as poultry.[3384] Now there are nearly seven hundred million pigs and more than ten *billion* birds, nearly a one hundred thousand percent increase.[3385] Combined with more than a billion people, "Darwin could not have created a more efficient re-assortment laboratory if he tried," remarked Osterholm.[3386] Similar changes happened throughout southeast Asia,[3387] the hub of the global Livestock Revolution.[3388]

In the latter half of the twentieth century, the pig population in China grew nearly a hundredfold and the poultry population underwent a thousandfold increase.[3389] To fill the growing demand for meat, Chinese poultry facilities raised up to five million chickens at a time,[3390] and industrial pig units confined as many as a quarter million pigs in six-story concrete buildings.[3391] "As soon as you have that many animals in one spot," said the UN director of Animal Production and Health, "you are likely to get into trouble with disease."[3392]

A study published in the *Bulletin of the World Health Organization* reported five different strains of influenza circulating in chickens in Hong Kong and China as far back as 1982.[3393] Why did it take until 1997 for bird flu to go on the rampage? A professor of virology at University College in London answered, "We've had nothing like this gigantic chicken breeding in the world before."[3394]

The chicken industry became the fastest-growing land-based meat sector in the world.[3395] Between 1990 and 1997, the developing world saw an 85 percent increase in the millions of tons of poultry produced.[3396] In Asia, raising chickens stopped being just a backyard activity. Since its start in the late 1980s, poultry production has quadrupled in Thailand and Vietnam, and increased sevenfold in Indonesia and China.[3397] A dozen egg farms in Thailand produced about two-thirds of the country's egg market by caging more than a million hens each.[3398]

In 1980, nearly all chickens in China were still being raised in traditional backyard systems[3399]; seventeen years later, when H5N1 emerged in Hong Kong, approximately half of the ten billion poultry[3400] in China were intensively confined[3401] in more than sixty thousand broiler chicken facilities, with a few operations raising more than ten million chickens at a time.[3402] Perhaps only a change this great—from small, outdoor, backyard flocks to intensive confinement in ten-million-bird mega farms—could account for the dramatic shifts that occurred in the ecology and epidemiology of avian influenza during this same period. "One of the things we're very worried about in today's situation versus 1918," Osterholm said, speaking on a Council on Foreign Relations panel, "is that, in fact, we have so many new hosts available, that virus can transmit between those billions and billions of chickens in one year more so today than it used to be able to do in a whole century."[3403]

The head of the Asian office of the World Health Organization blamed the emergence of viruses like H5N1 in part on our "[o]ver-consumption of animal products."[3404] Not long ago, a Chinese family would slaughter a chicken only on special occasions. That changed to a chicken every week. "This means we're hastening the probability of the emergence of a truly lethal flu strain," said then Council on Foreign Relations senior fellow Garrett in an interview.[3405]

Clearly, the majority of the world's pork and poultry is now produced on large-scale industrial animal factories,[3406] with further intensification predicted for the foreseeable future.[3407] Already by the turn of the century, China's fast-food industry had a $24-billion turnover with the market sector growing 20 percent annually. McDonald's had 400 restaurants in China; Kentucky Fried Chicken had 681.[3408]

H5N1 has further accelerated the intensification of the industry, forcing into bankruptcy as many as 90 percent of smaller Asian poultry producers who lacked the reserve to stomach a loss of markets for months at a time.[3409] Giant U.S. chicken corporations like Tyson and Perdue could afford expensive control measures and rapidly expanded into China.[3410] Cargill, a U.S.-based transnational corporation with annual sales at the time exceeding $60 billion,[3411] eradicated, at its own expense, all bird species, including wild ducks, in and around the poultry facilities it owned or contracted across twenty-two Chinese provinces.[3412] With only the larger corporate producers left standing, the greater number of birds in intensive confinement may have provided fertile fodder for viruses like H5N1 to gain greater virulence. "We are offering this virus every opportunity," Osterholm said. "Every day is an evolutionary experiment going on in Asia, every minute, every second."[3413]

Worst of Both Worlds

Increasing outbreaks among chickens over the past two or three decades have seemed to go hand in hand with increasing human transmissibility in both high- and low-grade bird flu viruses. Not long ago, human infection with avian influenza was almost unheard of. Since the emergence of H5N1 in 1997, however, more than a dozen other bird flu viruses have jumped the species barrier[3414] to infect thousands of people in more than twenty countries.[3415] H9N2 infected children in China in 1999 and 2003; H7N2 was found infecting persons in New York and Virginia in 2002, 2003,[3416] and 2016;[3417] H7N3 infected poultry workers in Canada in 2004[3418] and Mexico in 2012;[3419] and then there was H7N7 in Italy,[3420] H10N7 in Australia[3421] and Egypt, H6N1 in Taiwan, and H5N6, H7N4, H7N9, and H10N8 with infections up through 2019.[3422] It's like snowflakes to an avalanche in people, too.

Before H7N9 ascended in 2013, the largest human outbreak from bird flu in history was the 2003 disaster in the Netherlands. One of the most densely populated countries in the world, the Netherlands squeezed sixteen million people, eleven million pigs, and more than ninety million poultry[3423] into a country no more than twice the size of New Jersey.[3424] Little surprise, then, that such conditions fostered the bird flu epidemic that led to the deaths of an unprecedented (at the time) thirty million birds.[3425]

A shocking government report released the following year revealed that the outbreak of H7N7 in the Netherlands had not only infected more than a thousand people,[3426] but the virus had passed from human to human. Symptomatic poultry workers passed the virus to a "whopping" 59 percent of their household family members.[3427] Fortunately, only one person died—a veterinarian involved in the cull.[3428] It was a relatively wimpy virus, typically causing, at most, mild flu symptoms. Dutch experts realize, though, how close their poultry industry had come to potentially preempting H5N1 by sparking the next human pandemic. According to experts from the country's National Institute of Public Health:

> Although we launched a large and costly outbreak investigation (using a combination of pandemic and bioterrorism preparedness protocols), and despite decisions being made very quickly, a sobering conclusion is that by the time full prophylactic measures were reinforced . . . more than 1,000 people from all over the Netherlands and from abroad had been exposed. Therefore if a variant with more effective spreading capabilities had arisen, containment would have been very difficult.[3429]

Bird flu viruses previously required freak lab accidents to directly infect people; now infection occurs with frightening and increasing regularity. There was an almost eighty-year lag between the time a wholly avian flu virus seemed to grow fatal in 1918 and when a bird flu virus acquired enough virulence to kill again in Hong Kong in 1997. Although industrial poultry production was invented in the 1950s, intensive production has truly gone global only fairly recently. Shortridge concluded in the academic text *Avian Influenza: Prevention and Control*: "The intensification of the poultry industry worldwide seems to be a key element in causing influenza viruses of aquatic origin to undergo 'more rapid' adaptation to land-based poultry."[3430] We have dug WWI-type trenches for billions of birds all around the world.

With unprecedented numbers of chickens intensively confined at record density,[3431] we have been seeing bird flu viruses adapt to humans in ways never seen before. The reason the 1918 virus killed fewer than 5 percent of its victims may have been because it was essentially restricted to the lungs. The spitting of blood and blackening of limbs were a result of the slow-motion drowning the virus triggered by choking the lungs with fluid. For H5N1, "[i]t's worse than that," said Osterholm. "[I]t also goes in and begins to shut down all your vital organs. It's a domino effect. Your kidneys go down, then your liver goes down, you have all this destruction through necrosis of your lungs and your internal organs. Everything goes."[3432] Never before had a bird flu virus learned to activate itself throughout the human body until H5N1.[3433]

By adapting to chickens, bird flu viruses hit an evolutionary jackpot. And, by adapting to chickens, the viruses may be adapting to the human race—another multibillion-host bonanza for the virus.[3434] But there need not be billions of chickens. We don't need to keep repopulating broiler and layer sheds. No scientist is naïve enough to think that humans will stop eating poultry or eggs in the near term. Even if the worst-case scenario is one day realized, KFCs may very well be rebuilt with the rest of human civilization. Until, perhaps, the day chicken flesh can be safely grown economically in a lab,[3435] humanity may continue to face influenza pandemics. Ending chicken consumption may be little more than a hypothetical, but ending the riskiest practices, the most intensive forms of industrial poultry production, seems an attainable goal.

With the emergence of H5N1, the fate and future of chickens became inexorably tied up with our own. The disease resistance of chickens may need to be considered a critical public health issue. No longer may it remain a simple business decision of counting carcasses and seeing if the per-bird profits of the survivors compensate for the mortality within the chicken industry. It may be a matter of global health how the industry breeds and rears birds, or whether they should be breeding and rearing them at all.

Humanity may decide that eating chicken is worth weathering the occasional pandemic, but is cheaper chicken worth risking viruses like H5N1? The best that free-range poultry seem able to pull off appears to be the 1918 2.5 percent mortality, and it may have needed World War I as an accomplice to do it. As hard as it is to imagine a virus more ominous than H5N1, intensive poultry production on a global scale is a relatively new phenomenon. As poultry consumption continues to soar in the developing world, there is no biological reason that bird flu could not evolve and mutate into an even deadlier niche.

All pandemic precursor strains continue to exist in the natural waterfowl reservoir, lying in wait for an opportunity to break out.[3436] As The New York Times put it, "Somewhere, in skies or fields or kitchens, the molecules of the next pandemic wait."[3437] H5N1 showed that chickens can breed a flu virus of unparalleled human lethality, and the Dutch H7N7 outbreak showed that chickens can produce a virus that directly jumps from human to human.[3438]

Even if H5N1 never developed the capacity to go pandemic, it may only be a matter of time before the new poultry factories of the world breed the deadliest of combinations.

REINING IN THE PALE HORSE

"Extreme remedies are most appropriate for extreme diseases."

—HIPPOCRATES[3439]

The chief of virology at Hong Kong's Queen Mary Hospital believed that "the cause and solution [of H5N1] lies within the poultry industry."[3440] Figure 4, from a U.S. Department of the Interior report on the bird flu threat,[3441] illustrates the key role domestic poultry play in the development of pandemic influenza.[3442] As I've discussed, all avian influenza viruses start in waterfowl, but there does not seem to be direct spread from the natural duck reservoir directly to mammals or humans; domesticated fowl are required as the stepping-stone. The most a wild duck virus seems to be able to do to a person is cause a mild case of pinkeye.[3443]

The scientists who unsuccessfully tried to infect human volunteers with wild duck viruses in the lab even tried passing the virus from one person to the next to enhance human infectivity. They squirted a million infectious doses up the first person's nose, then inoculated a second person with the first per-

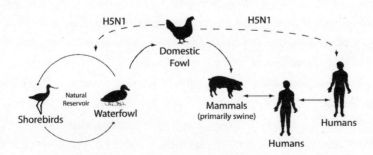

Figure 4. Domestic poultry's role in the development of pandemic influenza
(Courtesy of the U.S. Department of the Interior)

son's mucus, and continued down the line. Despite the high doses used and five person-to-person passages, the virus still could not grab hold. A study published in *Clinical Infectious Diseases* found that pig farmers are up to thirty-five times likelier to show evidence of swine flu exposure than those with no occupational contact with pigs,[3444] but studies of Canadian wildlife personnel consistently found them negative for waterfowl virus infection.[3445] Influenza viruses found in their natural undisturbed state do not seem to pose a human threat.

Duck viruses may not be lucky enough to catch twenty thousand people in one big elevator, but stumbling upon twenty thousand chickens squeezed into an enclosed space is not only possible, it happens all the time. When a duck virus gains that kind of all-access pass, this overcrowding allows for millions of passages of viruses through cells and susceptible hosts who have nowhere to run. In this way, the virus can be amplified[3446] and perhaps adapt to humans by proxy. Thanks to that evolutionary quirk of nature—the striking molecular resemblance of the respiratory tract of a chicken to our own—as the virus gets better and better at infecting and killing chickens, it may be getting better and better at infecting and killing us.

According to a senior molecular virologist at the University of Cambridge, "Chickens provide a bridge between the wild bird population where avian influenza thrives and humans where new pandemic strains can emerge. Removing that bridge will dramatically reduce the risk posed by avian viruses to humans."[3447] If domestication of poultry is the bridge,[3448] it's a bridge that can be burned.

The domestication and captivity of birds have created biohazards like *Salmonella, Campylobacter,* Psitticosis (parrot fever), and avian tuberculosis. Most seriously, it brought us influenza.

If the development of animal agriculture marked the "start of the era of zoonosis," as the dean of Michigan State's veterinary school asserted, then the scaling back of animal agricultural production may hasten its end.[3449] In the hopes of severing the link from the viral reservoir, some at the FAO have suggested that domestic duck farming be abolished.[3450] Ducks were domesticated 150 generations ago,[3451,3452] a blink in human evolution.[3453] While ending the domestication of ducks would not alleviate the current crisis, since viruses like H5N1 and H7N9 have already flown the coop, it may help prevent future ominous viruses from arising.[3454]

"Prevention of H5N1 avian influenza in humans is best achieved by controlling infection in poultry," advised the WHO.[3455] As noted by the dashed lines in the Department of the Interior's diagram, though, not only had H5N1 jumped directly from chickens to humans, it pulled off one of its greatest tricks yet—a homecoming of sorts—reinfecting waterfowl. By retaining its lethality for chickens and humans, while remaining relatively harmless for migratory birds, the Z mutant of H5N1 created a monster, enabling the presumably factory-farmed virus to wing itself around the world. That's how one of its descendants was able to wipe out fifty million chickens and turkeys in the United States just a few years ago.[3456] At this stage, the prospect of eradication seems remote.[3457]

A leading flu authority at Mount Sinai School of Medicine remarked that if you eliminated the ducks in the world, you'd essentially eliminate pandemic influenza.[3458] "But you can't kill all the ducks and aquatic birds of the world—that would be absurd," said Webster. "It makes you realize that influenza is a noneradicable disease."[3459] The influenza virus itself, as it exists in nature, may be "noneradicable," but we don't care what happens naturally inside the guts of wild ducks—and the ducks don't seem to either. It's the human pandemic variety we want to get rid of, which may be possible if we remove the stepping-stones by which the virus hops from the rice paddies of Asia to children hop-scotching in Europe.

According to the U.S. Geological Survey, "Currently there is no evidence that humans have been affected with H5N1 influenza virus through contact with wild birds. All reported human infections have been associated with contact with domestic poultry."[3460] In theory, then, the solution to preventing future pandemics, and maybe even stopping the potentially impending pandemic in mid-flight, is to kill all the chickens.

H5N1 has been stopped before. "It was fairly obvious," Shortridge said, recounting Hong Kong in 1997, "the chickens had to go."[3461] And it worked—killing all the chickens in the territory eliminated the virus. Genetic analyses of the H5N1 strain that arose four years later showed that it emerged independently, jumping again from the natural duck reservoir to chickens. Hong Kong tried killing all the chickens once again, but it was too late. Leading scientists advocated ridding the entire territory of chicken farms, banning imports, and closing down poultry markets, but H5N1 had already escaped.[3462]

Dutch virologist Jan de Jong, the first to make the discovery of H5N1 human infection, scoffed at the limited culling of hundreds of millions of chickens as too little, too late. "These measures are really nonsense," he said in a telephone interview. De Jong suggested that a near-total culling of Asia's poultry and the curtailment of poultry farming for several years would be the only way to stop the H5N1 outbreaks.[3463] Osterholm seemed to agree. "So even though we talk about having killed off 300 million chickens in trying to reduce it," he said, "we turn over billions of chickens a year in China just for food supply. Each one of those that are born and hatched are brand new incubators for the virus, too, so we keep resupplying this susceptible population, we keep allowing this."[3464] H5N1 keeps taking shots at sustained human-to-human transmission; by repopulating the global poultry flock, we keep reloading the gun. Both scientists presumably realized the economic implications that made such a solution a political impossibility.

Given H5N1's spread to Europe, the mammoth slaughter would have had to extend far beyond Asia, and because the same underlying conditions of emergence would remain, the cessation of poultry production would have to remain indefinitely. "As long as the kettle is on the fire, the water temperature will continue to rise until it reaches the boiling point," the World Health Organization's representative in Thailand explained. "The pandemic threat will not go away because we don't have a way to put out the fire yet."[3465] Yes, but we could remove the kettle. Let the flame of influenza continue to flicker in wild waterfowl, but we could in theory remove the middleman kettle of poultry production in hopes of preventing influenza from boiling over into the human population.

The logical extension of the effective 1997 Hong Kong strategy is to kill off the *entire* world's chicken flock. Lest this sound too extreme, that's already what happens to most of the world's broiler chickens every six weeks or so. Chickens raised for meat, as opposed to those raised for eggs, have been bred to grow at such accelerated speed that the global broiler flock is essentially slaughtered every handful of weeks and replaced with hatchling chicks. Logistically, killing off all commercial chickens in the world is easy. We already have them all locked up, and the slaughtering apparatus is in place and already undergoes trial runs about every month or two. If, instead of restocking, humanity raised and ate one last global batch of chickens, the viral link between ducks and humans might be severed, and the pandemic cycle could theoretically be broken for good. Maybe bird flu could be grounded.

The Centers for Disease Control and Prevention, though understanding the human health risks of the "ongoing intensification and consolidation of the food-animal industry," acknowledged the protein demands of a growing global population. The deputy director of the CDC's Office of Global Health described the dilemma simply as "we want more protein while not jeopardizing human health." However, only a trivial percentage of the world's calories and protein come from poultry.[3466,3467] Of course, there is no human nutritional need for any animal protein. In fact, according to the Harvard University School of Medicine, the healthiest sources of protein are "beans, nuts, grains and other vegetable sources of protein."[3468] One reason India was not considered a high-risk area for novel influenza strains is reportedly that a large portion of the population is vegetarian.[3469] Regardless, from a pandemic standpoint, it doesn't matter whether one switches to beans or to beef; what matters is breaking the feathered link in the chain.

Smallpox could be eradicated because there is no contemporary nonhuman animal reservoir. Unlike influenza, in which human beings are considered "irrelevant for the viruses' survival,"[3470] the smallpox virus only existed in humans and so could be vaccinated out of existence since there was no source of new genetic material.[3471] It is no coincidence that eleven out of the top dozen most dangerous bioterrorism agents are zoonotic pathogens.[3472] How else can you infect millions unless you pull something out of the animal world—a rabbit out of the hat, but in reverse? The human immune system would therefore have no prior exposure, and the infection could slip beneath our own body's radar. By cutting influenza's genetic supply lines to the animal world, presumably, no more pandemics would be possible.

What would happen to human influenza if its relationship to the avian reservoir were severed? People would still get the flu, but our bodies would be hip to it. The virus would continue its genetic drift, accumulating mutations in its outer coat so as not to be utterly routed, but no longer would there be fresh virus to swap genes with. In other words, no more viral sex. Eventually, without continued intrusions of restless alien viruses backed into new evolutionary corners, along with the presumed extinction of pandemics, we might even expect seasonal influenza to lose virulence gradually with time as it achieved more of a balance. According to Webster, it's been this "irregular infusion of avian virus genes into the human virus gene pool" that has prevented human influenza viruses from "reaching an evolutionary equilibrium with their hosts."[3473] The evidence is as easy as learning influenza's ABCs.

We've long known that there are three types of human influenza viruses: A, B, and C. Influenza A is considered the only type of influenza that can cause pandemics, because influenza A is the only type of influenza with an active link to the animal world. The influenza viruses ever bubbling forth from waterfowl are influenza A viruses that may cross over and establish themselves within poultry and pigs and people. Influenza viruses B and C are thought to have originally arisen the same way as influenza A viruses—that is, from waterfowl, centuries ago—but they've circulated and adapted to the human race for so long, for hundreds or even thousands of years, that they can no longer reassort with avian viruses.[3474] They've evolved into new species in the biological sense that they can no longer reproduce with their ancestral progenitors to create viable offspring. They are now strictly human viruses; the avian umbilical cord has been cut.[3475]

As such, influenza B and C viruses are old hat to humanity's collective immunity. They never cause pandemics and, in general, result in milder disease. Influenza C has presumably parted ways with its avian ancestors to such an extent that it rarely causes clinical disease at all.[3476] If influenza C viruses manage to cause any symptoms, the infection more closely resembles the common cold than the flu.[3477] And that is what we might expect all human influenza viruses to evolve toward in a pandemic-free world cut off from the avian reservoir.[3478] Without chickens, the worst that may bubble up from that viral volcano is a rare case of pinkeye resulting from sweeping duck manure or forgetting to turn our heads should sneezing seals not properly cover their mouths.

Things got a bit more complicated in 2011 with the discovery of the first influenza D virus in a pig in Oklahoma. Influenza D has since been found in pigs, sheep, and cattle the world over.[3479] Three-quarters of the U.S. cattle herd show evidence of exposure.[3480] So maybe reach for the bean burrito after all? Though U.S. cattle workers harbor antibodies to the virus,[3481] which suggests they've had contact with the virus, it is not yet known to cause human disease.[3482]

Instead of letting the world's chicken flock vanish, can't they all be vaccinated? As we know from our own flu shots, which have to be reformulated every year, the influenza virus may be too slippery to be stopped by vaccination because of its high rate of mutation. Vaccination can keep birds superficially healthy, but may not stop the replication and excretion of the virus.[3483] While vaccinated birds may not get sick (so profitability is not diminished), chicken sheds may remain breeding grounds for superflu viruses.[3484]

Poultry vaccination may even increase pandemic risk. In Mexico, more than a billion doses of vaccines were used by the poultry industry to try to control an H5N2 outbreak, but that led to a doubling of the viral mutation rate compared to unvaccinated chicken populations[3485] and the emergence of multiple lineages of different vaccine-resistant strains.[3486] Thankfully, only two people became infected,[3487] but the more strains that are spawned, the greater the risk of generating a new pandemic virus.[3488] Webster was particularly concerned about China's plan to vaccinate its fourteen-billion-strong poultry flock.[3489] "[P]athogens can evolve to more virulent pathotypes in vaccinated herds or flocks," reads one virology textbook, "especially when animals are held under intensive production systems."[3490]

Similarly, swine flu vaccines can prevent the drop in carcass weight associated with infection that's so bad for business, but does so without actually stopping viral shedding.[3491] The immunological pressure placed on these viruses by the vaccines may then select for viral mutants with different surface proteins, so it may select for swine flu viruses that grab human or avian genes, potentially increasing the threat to public health.[3492] The herd-of-origin of the first triple hybrid mutant discovered in the United States had been vaccinating against the classic swine flu.[3493] Maybe widespread pig vaccination in the 1990s[3494] contributed to the disruption of swine flu's eighty-year run of stability.

As long as there is poultry, there will be pandemics. It may be us or them. One consequence of the evolutionary stability of the waterfowl reservoir is that the pandemic precursors will always be waiting in the wings.[3495] Influenza viruses mutate at the same rate in wild ducks as in any other species. These duck viruses have, over millions of years, reached peak fitness such that any net change in any direction makes new mutants a little less perfect and they are selected against and nudged out of the applicant pool. The mutant swarm in aquatic birds is always correcting itself. Viral mutants continue to arise that may be just a little better at infecting chickens and humans, but are quickly outmaneuvered by the duck optimal variant. As soon as that swarm of viruses is forced into a new environment, though, any mutants for which a growth advantage exists may be quickly selected. The pandemic potential of the virus has existed, and continues to exist, ready to blast off if given the opportunity. Our role is to try to keep it in the ducks and not provide the virus an enormous lab of feathered subjects to tinker in. Noting the emergence of zoonotic diseases in general is largely a product of human activity, FAO researchers concluded that "the solution to these problems is also a matter of human choice."[3496]

Shutting Down the Flu Factories

If poultry were raised only in small outdoor flocks, influenza viruses might be robbed of the opportunity to evolve into highly pathogenic strains, but given the existence of industrial operations, small-scale farmers need to take precautions. A major 2004 USDA report on biosecurity among backyard flocks across the country found the same neglect for even basic biosecurity measures. Only about half of game fowl operations (which tend to raise cockfighting birds) were recorded as following biosecurity fundamentals such as proper attention to potentially contaminated footwear.[3497] Safety measures like disinfecting water supplies[3498] or netting the ponds found on the properties of more than one-third of U.S. small poultry operations[3499] to discourage wild waterfowl would add additional security.[3500] Some practices in Asia, like the integrated aquaculture feeding of animals' wastes and the common custom of feeding gutted chicken viscera back to the flocks, should be strongly discouraged.[3501]

Although there are measures large-scale operations could take to mediate some of the risk in minor ways—enriching environments in pig operations with straw bedding, for example[3502]—industrial production carries intrinsic dangers. A textbook on the control of avian viruses laid out the inherent contradiction between intensive confinement and healthy flocks: "The potential for a virus to be transmitted among a group of birds can be reduced by preventing overcrowding, providing maximum separation between birds, providing frequent exposure to sunlight and ensuring a constant supply of fresh air. Sunlight will destroy many viruses that are free in the environment."[3503]

To reduce the emergence of viruses like H5N1, humanity must shift toward raising poultry in smaller flocks, under less stressful, less crowded, and more hygienic conditions, with outdoor access, no use of human antivirals, and with an end to the practice of breeding for rapid growth or unnatural egg production at the expense of immunity. This would also be expected to reduce rates of increasingly antibiotic-resistant pathogens such as *Salmonella*,[3504] the number-one foodborne killer in the United States. We need to move away from the industry's fire-fighting approach to infectious disease to a more proactive preventive health approach that makes birds less susceptible—even resilient—to disease in the first place.[3505]

In light of viruses like H5N1, more and more experts have been questioning the sustainability of intensive poultry production. As UN Animal Health Officer, Peter Roeder, responsible for viral diseases at the FAO,[3506] was asked in 2003, "Could a more sustainable livestock production reduce the risk of such diseases?" Roeder answered:

> This is certainly so. . . . [T]he vulnerability to epidemic diseases of intensive, industrialized livestock farming systems is increasingly being demonstrated. This brings into doubt the viability of these systems. A high human population density in close contact with several species of intensively farmed livestock potentially provides a substrate for cross-species transmission, evolution and amplification of many pathogenic agents.[3507]

University of Philippines College of Medicine professor Romeo Quijano also judged H5N1 to be a manifestation of the inherent contradictions of industrial poultry production. "The recent outbreak of avian flu and its spread to humans in several countries," he said, "should be taken as a serious warning signal of the devastating effects of an unsustainable, environment destructive, and profit-oriented food production system."[3508] New Zealand government food safety advisor Meriel Watts declared:

> Governments should take heed of this latest food crisis and outlaw the rearing of chickens in overcrowded factory farms. Chickens can be sustainably reared in free-range, organic systems that dramatically improves the health of the birds, and consequently also dramatically reduces the risk to human health. . . . Cramming tens of thousands of birds into cramped sheds is a human health disaster in waiting.[3509]

The poultry industry disagreed. The president of the World's Poultry Science Association from Hong Kong declared that "it does not make sense to get rid of the poultry industry to get rid of the bird flu. That would be an ignorant act."[3510] FAO experts expressed concern that the strong industrial poultry sector might interfere with bird flu control efforts in general, perhaps even "hijack the agenda."[3511]

The industry bristled at the suggestion that intensive confinement causes undue stress. "Confinement rearing has its precedents," the National Live Stock and Meat Board wrote in its publication, *Facts from the Meat Board.*

"Schools are examples of 'confinement rearing' of children which, if handled properly, are effective."[3512] One agribusiness foundation wrote, "Most veal calves are kept in individual stalls similar to a baby's crib."[3513]

The industry knows how vulnerable it is to public scrutiny. Industry proponents try to deflect criticism by dismissing critiques as city-slicker ignorance.[3514] At the same time, they admit that truly informed consumers are the last thing they need. "One of the best things modern animal agriculture has going for it is that most people . . . haven't a clue how animals are raised and processed," wrote the editor of the *Journal of Animal Science* in an animal agriculture textbook.

> *If most urban meat-eaters were to visit an industrial broiler house, to see how the birds are raised, and could see the birds being "harvested" and then being "processed" in a poultry processing plant, some, perhaps many of them, would swear off eating chicken and perhaps all meat. For modern animal agriculture, the less the consumer knows about what's happening before the meat hits the plate, the better.[3515]*

This industry attitude of concealment extended to bird flu. Industry reaction to the 2002 outbreak of H6N2 in poultry in Southern California is instructive. A study published by the National Institute of Medicine provides the background:

> *Millions of birds shedding viruses traveling in trucks easily spread the infection to farms along the route. That is when the Turlock region, which is bound by three major roads, became known as the Triangle of Doom: a bird couldn't enter the region without becoming infected with H6N2. Tens of millions of birds in California became infected with this H6N2 virus during a four-month period beginning in March 2002.[3516]*

The industry covered it up. Corporate producers used their own veterinarians and did not release the diagnoses—not to the state, not to neighboring states, not to the World Organization for Animal Health, and not even to neighboring farms, even though the information might have let them better protect their flocks. According to the 2005 National Institute of Medicine report *The Threat of Pandemic Influenza: Are We Ready?*, the emergence of the "Triangle of Doom" was kept quiet "by corporate decision-makers who feared that consumer demand would plummet if the public knew they were buying infected meat and eggs."[3517] As with the SARS outbreak in China the following year, economic interests trumped public health.[3518]

Public relations concerns extended to questioning research directions. At a 2004 avian influenza symposium, when a medical epidemiologist and pediatrician in the Influenza Branch at the CDC insisted that further studies on H7N3 viruses in the U.S. poultry industry needed to be done, a poultry representative seemed more concerned about the industry's public appearance. Eric Gonder, a spokesperson for the National Turkey Federation, the North Carolina Poultry Federation, and one of the nation's largest pig producers[3519]—all at the same time[3520]—responded, "How would you suggest we conduct these studies without getting into a negative perception of agriculture?"[3521]

Europe took the lead in opposition to the trend of intensification in animal agriculture. David Burne, as the European Commissioner for Health and Consumer Protection, said at a Public Health Risks from Emerging Zoonotic Diseases conference in 2004, "Let me say a final word on animal rearing practices":

> In the agricultural sector, greater account needs to be taken of the implications of intensive animal husbandry practices. Public health policy needs to have a much greater role to ensure human health protection. Policies need to encourage a shift away from intensive rearing and to ensure the adequacy of risk management measures at farm and production unit level. These are issues that we also need to pursue at international level.[3522]

Wrote the official French Agency for Food Safety:

> The never-ending quest for better productivity and profit, the constantly evolving technologies in animal farming and the ever-increasing exchanges in a market now open to the world, might favor exposure to hazards. New and largely unexpected so-called production or "man-made" diseases will come along after those we already experience.[3523]

The French Food Safety Agency's Network for the Prevention and Control of Zoonoses, comprised of sixteen European partners and more than three hundred scientists, focused blame in part on "the growing trade in meat, milk and other animal products."[3524] In reaction to the spate of emerging animal diseases, and to the dismay of the industry,[3525] the Chancellor of Germany called for an end to factory farming[3526] and "a new politics that stands for consumer protection, improved food safety and natural, environmentally-friendly farming."[3527]

In 2001, the World Bank made a surprising reversal of its previous commitment to fund large-scale livestock projects in developing nations. In its new livestock strategy, the Bank acknowledged that as the sector grew, "there [was] a significant danger that the poor are being crowded out, the environment eroded, and global food safety and security threatened."[3528] This reflected the multiplicity of issues in addition to zoonotic disease pointed out by "factory farming" opponents. Critics argued that production profitability should not be the sole consideration in animal agriculture,[3529] and, in addition to human and animal health[3530] and welfare,[3531] other factors should be taken into account, such as soil heath,[3532] biodiversity,[3533] climate change,[3534] social justice,[3535] equity,[3536] good governance,[3537] and environmental stewardship.[3538]

In the United States, the American Public Health Association (APHA) is among those advocating for "radical" (from the Latin *radix*, for "root"[3539]) change. As I mentioned in "Tracing the Flight Path," in 2003, the APHA passed a "Precautionary Moratorium on New Concentrated Animal Feed Operations," in which it urged all federal, state, and local authorities to impose an immediate moratorium on the building of new factory farms—including industrial turkey, laying hen, broiler chicken, and duck facilities.[3540] In November 2019, it reiterated its stance, publishing a new policy statement calling once again for a moratorium on new factory farms, as well as a moratorium on the expansion of existing ones.[3541]

The industry claimed that intensification is driven by consumer demand for cheap meat.[3542] In response to the lead 2005 *New Yorker* story on the threat of bird flu, staff writer Michael Specter was asked if, based on his research, we would "have to rethink such things as large-scale poultry farming?" He replied:

> *Well, I can't imagine a better prescription for killing large numbers of animals with a single disease than packing tens of thousands of them into factory farms where they are lucky if they have 15 inches of personal space. Still, the economic incentives toward factory production of food are huge—we want cheap meat. So it's going to be very difficult to change.[3543]*

According to one economic analysis, transitioning to slower-growing breeds of broiler chickens with improved immunity might be expected to cost consumers no more than a dollar or two a year.[3544] The proportion of household income Americans spend on food is low compared to other countries, though this may be more a reflection of American wealth than the actual price of U.S. groceries.[3545] And the true cost may not be reflected on the label. According to a team of food policy experts, our current industrial model of animal agriculture "may deliver cheap food (defined as food accounting for a reduced proportion of household expenditure) but it has an unfortunate tendency to disguise or add to the environmental health bill"[3546]—and the public health bill, too. Agricultural economists have suggested "true cost" pricing and labeling schemes to educate consumers about their choices in the marketplace.[3547]

Lonnie King was the dean of Michigan State University's College of Veterinary Medicine and president of the American Veterinary Epidemiology Society. He is also a member of the National Academy of Sciences and the former administrator of the USDA's Animal and Plant Health Inspection Service.[3548] King was instrumental in creating an advisory panel within the World Organization for Animal Health to address emerging zoonoses.[3549] His talk at the 2004 meeting of the USDA National Agricultural Research, Extension, Education and Economics Advisory Board was titled "Emerging Threats and Opportunities in Animal Agriculture."[3550]

King set out to explain the root causes behind the Third Age of human disease, which "began about 1975 with the emergence or reemergence of zoonotic diseases." He described the factors leading to the creation of this "microbial perfect storm" as "anthropogenic," meaning human-caused. "As climate changes and ecosystems are destroyed, pathogens will become ubiquitous, constantly mixing and mutating to find new animal hosts and new avenues of infection."[3551]

King told the USDA Advisory Board that animal agriculture has reached a "strategic inflection point" where the "old rules and lessons no longer apply." He characterized this paradigm shift as moving from agriculture as "a trusted provider" to agriculture as "a part of the problem." King agreed with the National Research Council and Government Accountability Office reports that advised the USDA to shift its focus away from increased production and toward other priorities, such as environmental sustainability.[3552]

Veterinary scientists at the University of Georgia published a review in the journal *Clinics of Laboratory Medicine* in which they wrote, "Watching the steady stream of new and emerging diseases, one is reminded of the carnival game 'Whack-a-mole.'" Instead of just responding to each new crisis as it arises, they proposed a more proactive strategy of addressing the underlying causes of disease emergence.[3553] Council on Foreign Relations' senior fellow for Global Health Garrett concluded, "Ultimately, humanity will have to change its perspective on its place in Earth's ecology if the species hopes to stave off or survive the next plague."[3554]

Facing the Red Queen

Scientists like Joshua Lederberg don't think this is mere rhetoric. He should know. Lederberg won the Nobel Prize in medicine at age thirty-three for his discoveries in bacterial evolution. Lederberg went on to become president of Rockefeller University. "Some people think I am being hysterical," he said, referring to pandemic influenza, "but there are catastrophes ahead. We live in evolutionary competition with microbes—bacteria and viruses. There is no guarantee that we will be the survivors."[3555]

There is a concept in host-parasite evolutionary dynamics called *the Red Queen hypothesis,* which attempts to describe the unremitting struggle between immune systems and the pathogens against which they fight, each constantly evolving to try to outsmart the other.[3556] The name is taken from Lewis Carroll's *Through the Looking Glass* in which the Red Queen instructs Alice, "Now, here, you see, it takes all the running you can do to keep in the same place."[3557] Because the pathogens keep evolving, our immune systems have to keep adapting as well just to keep up. According to the theory, animals who "stop running" go extinct.

So far, our immune systems have largely retained the upper hand, but the fear is that given the current rate of disease emergence, the human race is losing the race.[3558] In a *Scientific American* article titled "Will We Survive?" one of the world's leading immunologists wrote:

Has the immune system, then, reached its apogee after the few hundred million years it had taken to develop? Can it respond in time to the new evolutionary challenges? These perfectly proper questions lack sure answers because we are in an utterly unprecedented situation [given the number of newly emerging infections].[3559]

The Johns Hopkins team who wrote *Beasts of the Earth* concluded, "Considering that bacteria, viruses, and protozoa had a more than two-billion-year head start in this war, a victory by recently arrived Homo sapiens would be remarkable."[3560]

Lederberg ardently believed that emerging viruses may imperil human society itself. Said NIH medical epidemiologist David Morens:

When you look at the relationship between bugs and humans, the more important thing to look at is the bug. When an enterovirus like polio goes through the human gastrointestinal tract in three days, its genome mutates about two percent. That level of mutation—two percent of the genome— has taken the human species eight million years to accomplish. So who's going to adapt to whom?

Pitted against that kind of competition, Lederberg concluded that the human evolutionary capacity to keep up "may be dismissed as almost totally inconsequential."[3561] To help prevent the evolution of viruses as threatening as H5N1, the least we can do is take away a few billion feathered test tubes in which viruses can experiment, a few billion fewer spins at pandemic roulette.

The human species has existed in something like our present form for approximately two hundred thousand years. "Such a long run should itself give us confidence that our species will continue to survive, at least insofar as the microbial world is concerned. Yet such optimism," wrote the Ehrlich prize–winning former chair of zoology at the University College of London, "might easily transmute into a tune whistled whilst passing a graveyard."[3562]

Apocalypse Now?

When it comes to the next pandemic, the question is never *if*, but *when*— and how bad? It's been more than twenty years since the first human death from H5N1. If the H5N1 influenza were able to trigger a human pandemic, wouldn't it have done so by now? Some evidence suggests that the 1918 flu virus that triggered the greatest medical disaster in history "smouldered" for at least eleven years before it went pandemic.[3563] We simply don't know enough about the ecology of these viruses to accurately estimate a timeline. H3N8, for example, circulated in horses in North America for nearly *forty* years before jumping into dog populations and triggering the canine flu that grabbed headlines in 2005.[3564] With regards to H5N1, a World Health Organization and USDA research team concluded that "[i]t is probably dangerous to rely on the 'if it were going to happen it already would have' argument."[3565]

John Oxford, PhD, wrote the book on influenza—literally. He co-authored the standard textbook *Influenza: The Viruses and the Disease* (along with the more general textbook *Human Virology*). In his generous review of my book on pandemic prevention in the prestigious science journal *Nature,* he answered why we should concern ourselves with the few hundred human deaths to date:

> *Well, go back to 1916, to Etaples in northern France, where a form of flu causing heliotrope cyanosis (a characteristic lavender coloration of the face) with a case fatality of 60% was beginning to spread. There were 145 cases. At some point in the next two years it mutated to become more infectious and 30 times less virulent. Then it killed 50 million people. Doesn't this ring a nasty bell?[3566]*

According to the director of the National Center for Disaster Preparedness at Columbia University, most scientists remain convinced that "we most certainly will encounter a deadly H5N1 global pandemic at some time in the future."[3567]

But a spate of new bird flu viruses are infecting humans. As one FAO consultant described it, they are "now lining up across factory farms like tropical depressions in the ocean."[3568] The first to make landfall may be H7N9. Emerging in 2013, this new bird flu strain apparently combined one gene from domestic ducks, one from wild birds, and the other six genes from domestic poultry[3569] to create a virus that has since infected more than fifteen hundred people in China and caused more than six hundred deaths.[3570] It surpassed the number of H5N1 human infections by 2015,[3571] and reports of limited human-to-human transmission started to be published by 2017.[3572,3573] According to the CDC, H7N9 currently represents our gravest pandemic flu threat.[3574] With an apparent case fatality rate of nearly 40 percent—two in five people—it is one of the deadliest human pathogens ever described, and, as a flu virus, has the potential to blanket the globe. One published estimate of the impact of an H7N9 pandemic could have on the United States suggests that millions of Americans could die.[3575]

In a Flap

The poultry industry started to wake up to the pandemic threat, but seemed more concerned about how the disease will affect business. Big Chicken in the United States looked forward to the "export market opportunities for U.S. chicken and turkey to replace lost poultry production" due to the global spread of H5N1,[3576] but was worried about what bird flu might mean for poultry consumption in general. An article in *Poultry International* pointed out that "[p]reviously known and documented flu pandemics . . . almost certainly originated in poultry. Because the connection was either not appreciated at the time and/or not widely publicized, there was little or no impact on public confidence in poultry products. The poultry industry," concluded author Terry Mabbett, "is unlikely to get off so lucky next time around."[3577]

The poultry industry acknowledged that public health implications could be serious, but had other concerns as well. USDA researchers voiced fear that "[i]f this virus [H5N1] were to become established in the human population, it has the additional potential to cross back to chickens from humans and cause a severe influenza outbreak in poultry."[3578] The industry was concerned that if there was a human H5N1 pandemic, it could disseminate the virus over long distances and lead to "further infections of poultry."[3579]

Some in the industry confessed that the "emergence of zoonotic infections associated with poultry is a disquieting trend"[3580] and internally acknowledged the role of intensive confinement. "Modern day poultry production is so highly concentrated that this disease can spread so rapidly," one Maryland chicken farmer admitted. "We can't ignore this any longer." Ignorance may be blissfully more cost-effective, though, than change. One anonymous industry official of a major poultry producer was quoted acknowledging the basic principle. "It's like if one person in a crowded room coughs, more people have a chance of getting infected," the official said. "But the question is, can there be an equitable way of doing that without affecting business?"[3581]

The executive editor of *Poultry* magazine put the trade-off this way in an editorial: "The prospect of a virulent flu to which we have absolutely no resistance is frightening. However, to me, the threat is much greater to the poultry industry. I'm not as worried about the U.S. human population dying from bird flu as I am that there will be no chicken to eat."[3582]

Having Our Meat and Eating It Too

The American Public Health Association is the largest and oldest association of public health professionals in the world. As I've mentioned, they've called for a moratorium on factory farming for nearly two decades. The journal of the APHA even published an editorial entitled "The Chickens Come Home to Roost" that went beyond just calling for a deintensification of the pork and poultry industries. The editorial questioned the prudence of raising so many animals for food in the first place, given the pandemic threat they may pose:

> It is curious, therefore, that changing the way humans treat animals, most basically ceasing to eat them, or at the very least, radically limiting the quantity of them that are eaten—is largely off the radar as a significant preventive measure. Such a change, if sufficiently adopted or imposed, could still reduce the chances of the much-feared influenza epidemic. It would be even more likely to prevent unknown future diseases that, in the absence of this change, may result from farming animals intensively and killing them for food. Yet humanity doesn't even consider this option.[3583]

However, thanks to food innovations, this may be changing. Have you looked in the dairy case at the supermarket lately? Some of America's largest dairy producers have recently filed for bankruptcy due to the constellation of new consumer choices.[3584] I was peripherally involved in the largest meat recall in human history. A hidden camera investigation at a California slaughter plant for "spent" dairy cows led to the recall of nearly 150 million pounds of beef for violations of food safety rules meant to protect the public from mad cow disease. Downed dairy cows—too sick to even walk—were being dragged to slaughter with chains into the federal school lunch program.[3585] But you don't have to worry about contaminated cattle brains in your oat milk. (Plant-based milks are a no-brainer!)

Expanded options are now hitting the meat case as well. There has been a tremendous surge in interest in diversified protein sources, given the increasing consensus that reduced meat consumption is critical for addressing both the climate crisis and our burgeoning epidemics of lifestyle diseases. Eating less meat may not only help save the world, but ten million human lives a year.[3586] To their credit, in 2016, the Chinese government recommended its citizens cut their meat consumption in half to reduce their growing rates of chronic disease.[3587] A completely plant-based diet might save $30 trillion from the health benefits alone, and that would be just from the lowered rates of chronic diseases like cancer, heart disease, and type 2 diabetes,[3588] not even factoring in the decreased catastrophic pandemic risk.[3589] What we eat doesn't just affect our personal health but our global health in more ways than one.

Making healthier choices could also help mediate the next coronavirus epidemic, not only at the source by sidestepping wet markets, but by also decreasing the rates of comorbidities found to increase the risk in SARS,[3590] MERS,[3591] and COVID-19. Consider the underlying risk factors for COVID-19 severity and death—obesity,[3592] heart disease, hypertension, and type 2 diabetes[3593]—all of which can be controlled or even reversed with a healthy enough plant-based diet and lifestyle.[3594]

No longer a niche market for vegetarians, major meat producers have started blending in vegetable proteins to make hybrid meat products like Tyson's "Whole Blends" sausage links and Perdue's "next generation" chicken nuggets.[3595] Smithfield, the world's largest pork producer, recently debuted an entire line of plant-based products.[3596] How many fewer porcine viral mixing vessels are there now that Dunkin' Donuts has a meat-free breakfast sausage?[3597] How many fewer hens are caged beak-to-beak now that egg-free mayo has taken the sandwich spread sector by storm?[3598] Quorn, a brand of meat-free meat made from the mushroom kingdom, opened a single facility that can produce the meat equivalent of around twelve million chickens per year.[3599,3600]

An even more innovative approach to pandemic prevention was suggested by Winston Churchill in 1932. In an article in *Popular Mechanics* entitled "Fifty Years Hence," he predicted that "[w]e shall escape the absurdity of growing a whole chicken in order to eat the breast or wing, by growing these parts separately under a suitable medium."[3601] Indeed, in terms of efficiency, growing meat straight from muscle cells could reduce greenhouse gas emissions and water use by as much as 96 percent and lower land use by as much as 99 percent,[3602] but if you factor in pandemic risk, the benefits to human health could arguably rival those to the planet.

Food safety has been considered the primary human health benefit of a slaughter-free harvest. There has been a sixfold increase in food poisoning over the last few decades, sickening tens of millions of Americans every year, and contaminated meats and animal products are the most common cause.[3603] So, when the cultivated meat industry calls its product "clean meat,"[3604] that's not just a nod to clean energy. Food-poisoning pathogens like *E. coli, Campylobacter,* and *Salmonella* are due to fecal residue, traces of which are found on most poultry sampled in the United States and about half of retail ground beef and pork chops.[3605] They're intestinal bugs, so you don't have to worry about them if you're producing meat without intestines, just like you don't have to worry about brewing up new respiratory viruses if you're making meat without the lungs.

The APHA's "Chickens Come Home to Roost" editorial concludes: "Those who consume animals not only harm those animals and endanger themselves, but they also threaten the well-being of [future generations]. . . . It is time for humans to remove their heads from the sand and recognize the risk to themselves that can arise from their maltreatment of other species."[3606]

How we treat animals can have global public health implications. As a spokesperson for the World Health Organization has said, "The bottom line is that humans have to think about how they treat their animals, how they farm them, and how they market them—basically the whole relationship between the animal kingdom and the human kingdom is coming under stress."[3607]

The Price We Pay

"We are the original recyclers," boasted the rendering industry.[3608] Converting billions of pounds of slaughterhouse waste into cheap protein for farm animal feed seemed like a good idea at the time, a *profitable* idea. The industry got away with it for more than a hundred years.[3609] In the end, though, with the advent of mad cow disease, society realized that it wasn't worth the costs to public health and the industrial practice was banned throughout much of the world. What may be cheaper for industry may be too expensive for humanity. It was the same story with DDT and the growth hormone

DES that the poultry industry insisted on using for so many years despite the known cancer risk.

Society has determined that certain industries and practices may be too potentially damaging and has successfully scaled them back—nuclear power, clear-cutting, strip mining, to name a few. Intensive poultry production is a relatively new phenomenon of the past seventy years. In light of H5N1 and H7N9, as well as our increasing understanding of the role of poultry in pandemics, with enough political will, the industrialization in the poultry sector can be scaled back as well. We may be one bushmeat meal away from the next HIV, one pangolin plate away from the next killer coronavirus, and one factory farm away from the next deadly flu.

Senator Frist warned that H5N1 "poses an immense potential threat to American civilization."[3610] This sentiment was expressed worldwide. "It will be the worst nightmare," the president of Indonesia said in 2005. "This plague can be more dangerous than the tsunami which last year killed hundreds of thousands of people in a matter of minutes."[3611]

To help people wrap their heads around what an H5N1 pandemic could be like, Osterholm suggested that people consider the South Asian tsunami, an event that far outshadowed the devastation of Hurricane Katrina: "Duplicate it in every major urban center and rural community around the planet simultaneously, add in the paralyzing fear and panic of contagion, and we begin to get some sense of the potential of pandemic influenza."[3612] A tsunami in every city, every town, everywhere. People drowning in their own blood. That certainly helps put the COVID-19 pandemic in perspective.

I don't want to minimize the seriousness of the COVID-19 pandemic. Millions could die. But a pandemic triggered by a bird flu virus could leave *hundreds of millions* dead.[3613] "An influenza pandemic of even moderate impact," Osterholm wrote, "will result in the biggest single human disaster ever—far greater than AIDS, 9/11, all wars in the 20th century and the recent tsunami combined. It has the potential to redirect world history as the Black Death redirected European history in the 14th century."[3614] Hopefully, for humanity's sake, the direction world history will take is away from raising birds by the billions under intensive confinement so as to potentially lower the risk of us ever being in this same precarious place in the future. The silver lining of COVID-19 is that the world will be better prepared for the next global health crisis. Tragically, it may take a pandemic with a virus like H5N1 or H7N9 before the world realizes the true cost of cheap chicken.

Afterword

by Kennedy Shortridge, Ph.D., DSc(Hon), CBiol, FIBiol

Professor Emeritus Kennedy Shortridge is credited for discovering H5N1 and leading the world's first fight against the virus that would forever change our understanding of how bad pandemics could get. For his pioneering work spanning over three decades, he was awarded the highly prestigious Prince Mahidol Award in Public Health, considered the "Nobel Prize of Asia."

Horse-drawn carts piled with dead bodies circulated through the small town of Queensland, Australia. A nightmare to imagine, yet even more horrific to learn that this scene was a recurring reality throughout the world during the 1918–1919 influenza pandemic.

My mother's compelling stories about the devastating reaches of the pandemic have stayed with me since my earliest years. What started out as a spark of interest has led me to search the hows and whys of influenza pandemics through birds and mammals.

The world has seen unprecedented advances in science and technology over the past fifty years, and, with it, a phenomenal increase in the availability of food, especially meat protein, largely through the intensification of poultry production in many parts of the world, notably Asia. But at what cost?

Chicken, once consumed only on special occasions, has become a near-daily staple on dinner tables around the world as a result of animal agriculture practices that have dramatically changed the landscape of farming by confining ever greater numbers of animals in ever decreasing amounts of space. In China, the shift from small, backyard poultry rearing toward industrialized animal agribusiness began to take root in the early 1980s. In just two decades, Chinese poultry farming had increasingly intensified and an unintended by-product was developed: the prospect of an influenza pandemic of nightmarish proportions, one that could devastate humans, poultry, and ecosystems around the world.

Influenza epidemics and pandemics are not new, yet it wasn't until 1982 that the late Professor Sir Charles Stuart-Harris and I put forward the hypothesis that southern China is an epicentre for the emergence of pandemic influenza viruses, the seeds for which had been germinating for 4,500 years when it was believed the duck was first domesticated in that region. This established the influenza virus gene pool in southern China's farmyards.

Indeed, molecular and genetic evidence suggests that the chicken is not a natural host for influenza. Rather, the domestic duck is the silent intestinal carrier of avian influenza viruses being raised in close proximity to habitation.

It is the siting of large-scale chicken production units, particularly in southern China where avian influenza viruses abound, that is the crux of the problem. There, domestic ducks have been raised on rivers, waterways, and, more recently, with the flooded rice crops cultivated each year. The importation of industrial poultry farming into that same region introduced millions of chickens—highly stressed due to intensive production practices and unsanitary conditions—into this avian influenza virus milieu. The result? An influenza accident waiting to happen. The H5N1 virus signalled its appearance in Hong Kong in 1997 and made its way into dozens of countries, infecting millions of birds. It, and viruses like it, continue to threaten to trigger a human catastrophe.

Michael Greger has taken on the formidable task of reviewing and synthesizing the many factors that have brought us to the influenza threat the world now faces. Drawing upon scientific literature and media reports at large, Dr. Greger explores the hole we have dug for ourselves with our own unsavoury practices.

Indeed, while many governments and the poultry industry were quick to blame migratory birds as the source of the H5N1 avian influenza virus, and to view pandemics as natural phenomena analogous to, say, sunspots and earthquakes, in reality, human choices and actions may have had—and may continue to have—a pivotal role in the changing ecology. This book explores what those underlying conditions are.

Now that anthropogenic behaviour has reached unprecedented levels with a concomitant pronounced zoonotic skew in emerging infectious diseases of humans, H5N1 seems like a cautionary tale of how attempts to exploit nature may backfire. The use of antibiotics as farm meal growth promoters leading to antibiotic-resistance in humans or the feeding of meat or bone meal to cattle leading to mad cow disease are cases in point: profitable in the short term for animal agriculture, but with the potential for unforeseen and disastrous consequences. Intensified, industrial poultry production has given us inexpensive chicken, but at what cost to the animals and at what heightened risk to public health?

We have reached a critical point. Today's COVID-19 pandemic is just the latest in an increasingly harrowing viral storm threatening each of us. We must dramatically change the way we interact with animals for the sake of all animals.

Michael Greger has achieved much in this volume. He has taken a major step toward balancing humanity's account with other species with whom we inhabit this earth.

Acknowledgments

I am incredibly honored to have had input on an early draft from some of the true pioneers in the field—Graeme Laver, whose studies of the influenza virus over nearly six decades were instrumental in the development of antivirals and some of the earliest vaccines; Kennedy Shortridge, who first characterized the H5N1 virus at the University of Hong Kong; Earl Brown, a leading specialist in influenza virus evolution; and Katharine Sturm-Ramirez, whose expertise with HIV landed her a spot on Robert Webster's world-renowned research team. Their vital feedback was critical in shaping the arguments presented.

I must also acknowledge Mei Keyi, Men Jian Zhou, and Jin Hengli from the Beijing Bureau of Agriculture, Li Quanlu, director-general of the Beijing Livestock Veterinary Association, Li Quan Lu, secretary-general of the Beijing Animal Agriculture Association, and Deming Zhao, dean of China Agricultural University, for their endless patience answering my questions.

For scrambling to get this out into the world as quickly as possible, deep appreciation to my literary agent Richard Pine, the whole team at Flatiron Books, Miyun Park for coordinating and editing, Alissa Finley for eagle-eye fact-checking, Bowen Cho for formatting deep into the night, Marie Townsley for compiling every day, Breege Tomkinson and my mom for correcting early drafts, and Katie Schloer and the rest of the NutritionFacts.org staff for holding everything together.

Belly rubs for Melville, back scratches for Motown, and all my love to my soulmate Dr. Jen Howk.

References

1. Green A. 2020. Li Wenliang. Lancet. 395(10225):682. https://doi.org/10 .1016/S0140-6736(20)30382-2.
2. World Health Organization. 2020 Feb 7. Novel Coronavirus (2019-nCoV). Situation report—18. Geneva: WHO; [accessed 2020 Mar 23]. https://www .who.int/docs/default-source/coronaviruse/situation-reports/20200207-sitrep -18-ncov.pdf?sfvrsn=fa644293_2.
3. Page J, Fan W, Khan N. 2020 Mar 6. How it all started: China's early coro-navirus missteps. Wall Street Journal. [accessed 2020 Mar 22]; https:// www.wsj.com/articles/how-it-all-started-chinas-early-coronavirus-missteps -11583508932.
4. McNeil DG. 2003 Apr 8. Disease's pioneer is mourned as a victim. New York Times. [accessed 2020 Mar 23]; https://www.nytimes.com/2003/04/08/sci ence/disease-s-pioneer-is-mourned-as-a-victim.html.
5. Ashour HM, Elkhatib WF, Rahman MM, Elshabrawy HA. 2020. Insights into the recent 2019 novel coronavirus (SARS-CoV-2) in light of past human coronavirus outbreaks. Pathogens. 9(3):186. https://doi.org/10.3390/pathogens9030186.
6. Hui DSC, Zumla A. 2019. Severe acute respiratory syndrome: historical, epi-demiologic, and clinical features. Infect Dis Clin North Am. 33(4):869–889. https://doi.org/10.1016/j.idc.2019.07.001.
7. World Health Organization. 2004. Summary of probable SARS cases with onset of illness from 1 November 2002 to 31 July 2003. Geneva: WHO; [accessed 2020 Mar 23]. https://www.who.int/csr/sars/country/table2004 _04_21/en/.
8. World Health Organization. 2019. Middle East respiratory syndrome coronavi-rus (MERS-CoV). Geneva: WHO; [updated 2019 Nov; accessed 2020 Mar 23]. http://origin.who.int/emergencies/mers-cov/en.
9. Weber J, Alcorn K. 2000. Origins of HIV and the AIDS epidemic. MedGenMed. 2(4):1–6. http://www.medscape.com/viewarticle/408272.
10. Corman VM, Muth D, Niemeyer D, Drosten C. 2018. Hosts and sources of endemic human coronaviruses. Adv Virus Res. 100:163–188. https://doi.org /10.1016/bs.aivir.2018.01.001.
11. Chan JFW, To KKW, Tse H, Jin DY, Yuen KY. 2013. Interspecies transmission and emergence of novel viruses: lessons from bats and birds. Trends Microbiol. 21(10):544–555. https://doi.org/10.1016/j.tim.2013.05.005.

12. Mandl JN, Schneider C, Schneider DS, Baker ML. 2018. Going to bat(s) for studies of disease tolerance. Front Immunol. 9:2112. https://doi.org/10.3389/fimmu.2018.02112.

13. Zhang J, Jia W, Zhu J, Li B, Xing J, Liao M, Qi W. 2020. Insights into the cross-species evolution of 2019 novel coronavirus. J Infect. Article in press. [accessed 2020 Mar 23]. https://doi.org/10.1016/j.jinf.2020.02.025.

14. Corman VM, Muth D, Niemeyer D, Drosten C. 2018. Hosts and sources of endemic human coronaviruses. Adv Virus Res. 100:163–188. https://doi.org/10.1016/bs.aivir.2018.01.001.

15. Marty AM, Jones MK. 2020. The novel Coronavirus (SARS-CoV-2) is a one health issue. One Health. 9:100123. https://doi.org/10.1016/j.onehlt.2020.100123.

16. Memish ZA, Mishra N, Olival KJ, Fagbo SF, Kapoor V, Epstein JH, Alhakeem R, Durosinloun A, Al Asmari M, Islam A, et al. 2013. Middle East respiratory syndrome coronavirus in bats, Saudi Arabia. Emerg Infect Dis. 19(11):1819–1823. https://doi.org/10.3201/eid1911.131172.

17. Hemida MG, Alnaeem A. 2019. Some One Health based control strategies for the Middle East respiratory syndrome coronavirus. One Health. 8:100102. https://doi.org/10.1016/j.onehlt.2019.100102.

18. Willman M, Kobasa D, Kindrachuk J. 2019. A comparative analysis of factors influencing two outbreaks of Middle Eastern Respiratory Syndrome (MERS) in Saudi Arabia and South Korea. Viruses. 11(12):1119. https://dx.doi.org/10.3390/v11121119.

19. Almathen F, Charruau P, Mohandesan E, Mwacharo JM, Orozco-ter Wengel P, Pitt D, Abdussamad AM, Uerpmann M, Uerpmann H-P, De Cupere B, et al. 2016. Ancient and modern DNA reveal dynamics of domestication and cross-continental dispersal of the dromedary. Proc Natl Acad Sci U S A. 113(24):6707–6712. https://doi.org/10.1073/pnas.1519508113.

20. Müller MA, Corman VM, Jores J, Meyer B, Younan M, Liljander A, Bosch BJ, Lattwein E, Hilali M, Musa BE, et al. 2014. MERS coronavirus neutralizing antibodies in camels, Eastern Africa, 1983–1997. Emerg Infect Dis. 20(12):2093–2095. https://doi.org/10.3201/eid2012.141026.

21. Farag E, Sikkema RS, Vinks T, Islam MM, Nour M, Al-Romaihi H, Al Thani M, Atta M, Alhajri FH, Al-Marri S, et al. 2019. Drivers of MERS-CoV emergence in Qatar. Viruses. 11(1):22. https://dx.doi.org/10.3390/v11010022.

22. To KK, Hung IF, Chan JF, Yuen KY. 2013. From SARS coronavirus to novel animal and human coronaviruses. J Thorac Dis. 5(Suppl 2):103–108. https://doi.org/10.3978/j.issn.2072-1439.2013.06.02.

23. Hui DSC, Zumla A. 2019. Severe acute respiratory syndrome: historical, epidemiologic, and clinical features. Infect Dis Clin North Am. 33(4):869–889. https://doi.org/10.1016/j.idc.2019.07.001.

24. Li Q, Guan X, Wu P, Wang X, Zhou L, Tong Y, Ren R, Leung KSM, Lau EHY, Wong JY, et al. 2020. Early transmission dynamics in Wuhan, China, of novel coronavirus-infected pneumonia. N Engl J Med. 382(13):1199–1207. https://doi.org/10.1056/NEJMoa2001316.

25. Fan Y, Zhao K, Shi ZL, Zhou P. 2019. Bat coronaviruses in China. Viruses. 11(3):210. https://doi.org/10.3390/v11030210.

26. Field HE. 2009. Bats and emerging zoonoses: henipaviruses and SARS. Zoonoses Public Health. 56(6-7):278–284. https://doi.org/10.1111/j.1863-2378.2008.01218.x.

27. Malta M, Rimoin AW, Strathdee SA. 2020. The coronavirus 2019-nCoV epidemic: is hindsight 20/20? EClinicalMedicine. 20:100289. https://doi.org/10.1016/j.eclinm.2020.100289.

28. Roberton S, Trung TC, Momberg F. 2003. Hunting and trading wildlife: an investigation into the wildlife trade in and around the Pu Mat National Park, Nghe An Province, Vietnam. Nghe An (Vietnam): SFNC Project Management Unit.

29. Duckworth JW, Salter RE, Khounboline K. 1999. Wildlife in Lao PDR: 1999 status report. Vientiane: IUCN-The World Conservation Union, Wildlife Conservation Society, Centre for Protected Areas and Watershed Management. https://portals.iucn.org/library/sites/library/files/documents/2000-050.pdf.

30. Srikosamatara S, Siripholdej B, Suteethorn V. 1992. Wildlife trade in Lao PDR and between Lao PDR and Thailand. Nat Hist Bull Siam Soc. 40(1):1–47.

31. Karesh WB, Cook RA. 2005 Jul/Aug. The human-animal link. Foreign Aff. 84:38–50. [accessed 2020 Mar 23]. https://www.foreignaffairs.com/articles/2005-07-01/human-animal-link.

32. Wang H, Shao J, Luo X, Chuai Z, Xu S, Geng M, Gao Z. 2020 Mar 27. Letter to the editor: wildlife consumption ban is insufficient. Science. 367(6485):1435. https://doi.org/10.1126/science.abb6463.

33. Fan Y, Zhao K, Shi ZL, Zhou P. 2019. Bat coronaviruses in China. Viruses. 11(3):210. https://doi.org/10.3390/v11030210.

34. Wong ACP, Li X, Lau SKP, Woo PCY. 2019. Global epidemiology of bat coronaviruses. Viruses. 11(2):E174. https://doi.org/10.3390/v11020174.

35. Bell D, Roberton S, Hunter PR. 2004. Animal origins of SARS coronavirus: possible links with the international trade in small carnivores. Philos Trans R Soc Lond B Biol Sci. 359(1447):1107–1114. https://doi.org/10.1098/rstb.2004.1492.

36. Jackson W. 2003. The story of civet. Pharm J. 271(7280):859–861. https://www.pharmaceutical-journal.com/pdf/xmas2003/pj_20031220_civet.pdf.

37. Guan Y, Zheng BJ, He YQ, Liu XL, Zhuang ZX, Cheung CL, Luo SW, Li PH, Zhang LJ, Guan YJ, et al. 2003. Isolation and characterization of viruses related to the SARS coronavirus from animals in southern China. Science. 302(5643):276–278. https://doi.org/10.1126/science.1087139.

38. Tu C, Crameri G, Kong X, Chen J, Sun Y, Yu M, Xiang H, Xia X, Liu S, Ren T, et al. 2004. Antibodies to SARS coronavirus in civets. Emerg Infect Dis.10(12):2244–2248. https://dx.doi.org/10.3201/eid1012.040520.

39. Padgett DA, Glaser R. 2003. How stress influences the immune response. Trends Immunol. 24(8):444–448. https://doi.org/10.1016/s1471-4906(03)00173-x.

40. Zhao GP. 2007. SARS molecular epidemiology: a Chinese fairy tale of controlling an emerging zoonotic disease in the genomics era. Philos Trans R Soc

Lond B Biol Sci. 362(1482):1063–1081. https://dx.doi.org/10.1098/rstb .2007.2034.

41.   Wan Y, Shang J, Graham R, Baric RS, Li F. 2020. Receptor recognition by the novel coronavirus from Wuhan: an analysis based on decade-long structural studies of SARS coronavirus. J Virol. 94(7):e00127–20. https://doi.org/10 .1128/JVI.00127-20.

42.   Wan Y, Shang J, Graham R, Baric RS, Li F. 2020. Receptor recognition by the novel coronavirus from Wuhan: an analysis based on decade-long structural studies of SARS coronavirus. J Virol. 94(7):e00127–20. https://doi.org/10 .1128/JVI.00127-20.

43.   Hu B, Zeng LP, Yang XL, Ge XY, Zhang W, Li B, Xie JZ, Shen XR, Zhang YZ, Wang N, et al. 2017. Discovery of a rich gene pool of bat SARS-related coronaviruses provides new insights into the origin of SARS coronavirus. PLoS Pathog. 13(11):e1006698. https://doi.org/10.1371/journal.ppat.1006698.

44.   Qu XX, Hao P, Song XJ, Jiang SM, Liu YX, Wang PG, Rao X, Song HD, Wang SY, Zuo Y, et al. 2005. Identification of two critical amino acid residues of the severe acute respiratory syndrome coronavirus spike protein for its variation in zoonotic tropism transition via a double substitution strategy. J Biol Chem. 280(33):29588–29595. https://doi.org/10.1074/jbc.M500662200.

45.   Song HD, Tu CC, Zhang GW, Wang SY, Zheng K, Lei LC, Chen QX, Gao YW, Zhou HQ, Xiang H, et al. 2005. Cross-host evolution of severe acute respiratory syndrome coronavirus in palm civet and human. Proc Natl Acad Sci U S A. 102(7):2430–2435. https://doi.org/10.1073/pnas.0409608102.

46.   Nahar N, Asaduzzaman M, Mandal UK, Rimi NA, Gurley ES, Rahman M, Garcia F, Zimicki S, Sultana R, Luby SP. 2020. Hunting bats for human consumption in Bangladesh. Ecohealth. 17(1):139–151. https://doi.org/10.1007/s10393-020 -01468-x.

47.   Chan JF, To KK, Tse H, Jin DY, Yuen KY. 2013. Interspecies transmission and emergence of novel viruses: lessons from bats and birds. Trends Microbiol. 21(10):544–555. https://doi.org/10.1016/j.tim.2013.05.005.

48.   Baragon S. 2020 Jan 25. Live animal markets worldwide can spawn diseases, experts say. Voice of America. [accessed 2020 Apr 11]; https://www.voanews .com/science-health/coronavirus-outbreak/live-animal-markets-worldwide -can-spawn-diseases-experts-say.

49.   Zhong NS, Zeng GQ. 2008. Pandemic planning in China: applying lessons from severe acute respiratory syndrome. Respirology. 13(Suppl 1):33–35. https://onlinelibrary.wiley.com/doi/pdf/10.1111/j.1440-1843.2008.01255.x.

50.   Peeri NC, Shrestha N, Rahman MS, Zaki R, Tan Z, Bibi S, Baghbanzadeh M, Aghamohammadi N, Zhang W, Haque U. 2020. The SARS, MERS and novel coronavirus (COVID-19) epidemics, the newest and biggest global health threats: what lessons have we learned? Int J Epidemiol. [Epub ahead of print 2020 Feb 22; accessed 2020 Apr 8]. https://doi.org/10.1093/ije/dyaa033.

51.   Myers SL. 2020 Jan 25. China's omnivorous markets are in the eye of a lethal outbreak once again. New York Times. [accessed 2020 Mar 28]; https://www .nytimes.com/2020/01/25/world/asia/china-markets-coronavirus-sars.html.

52. Hui DSC, Zumla A. 2019. Severe acute respiratory syndrome: historical, epidemiologic, and clinical features. Infect Dis Clin North Am. 33(4):869–889. https://doi.org/10.1016/j.idc.2019.07.001.

53. Hemida MG. 2019. Middle East Respiratory Syndrome Coronavirus and the One Health concept. PeerJ. 7:e7556. https://dx.doi.org/10.7717/peerj.7556.

54. Fan Y, Zhao K, Shi ZL, Zhou P. 2019. Bat coronaviruses in China. Viruses. 11(3):210. https://doi.org/10.3390/v11030210.

55. Greger M. 2006. Bird flu: a virus of our own hatching. New York: Lantern Books.

56. Cheng VCC, Lau SKP, Woo PCY, Yuen KY. 2007. Severe acute respiratory syndrome coronavirus as an agent of emerging and reemerging infection. Clin Microbiol Rev. 20(4):660–694. https://doi.org/10.1128/CMR.00023-07.

57. Coronaviridae Study Group of the International Committee on Taxonomy of Viruses. 2020. The species *Severe acute respiratory syndrome-related coronavirus*: classifying 2019-nCoV and naming it SARS-CoV-2. Nat Microbiol. 5(4):536–544. https://doi.org/10.1038/s41564-020-0695-z.

58. Murdoch DR, French NP. 2020. COVID-19: another infectious disease emerging at the animal-human interface. N Z Med J. 133(1510):12–15.

59. Ting TCC. 2020 Jan 22. China real estate news. China Business Network. [accessed 2020 Mar 28]; http://www.cb.com.cn/index/show/zj/cv/cv13474141264.

60. Li Q, Guan X, Wu P, Wang X, Zhou L, Tong Y, Ren R, Leung KSM, Lau EHY, Wong JY, et al. 2020. Early transmission dynamics in Wuhan, China, of novel coronavirus-infected pneumonia. N Engl J Med. 382(13):1199–1207. https://doi.org/10.1056/NEJMoa2001316.

61. Ting TCC. 2020 Jan 22. China real estate news. China Business Network. [accessed 2020 Mar 28]; http://www.cb.com.cn/index/show/zj/cv/cv13474141264.

62. Li PJ. 2020 Jan 29. First SARS, now the Wuhan coronavirus. Here's why China should ban its wildlife trade forever. South China Morning Post. [updated 2020 Jan 29; accessed 2020 Mar 28]; https://www.scmp.com/comment/opinion/article /3047828/first-sars-now-wuhan-coronavirus-heres-why-china-should-ban-its.

63. Zhang J, Ma K, Li H, Liao M, Qi W. 2020. The continuous evolution and dissemination of 2019 novel human coronavirus. J Infect. Article in press. [accessed 2020 Mar 28]. https://doi.org/10.1016/j.jinf.2020.02.001.

64. Malik YS, Sircar S, Bhat S, Sharun K, Dhama K, Dadar M, Tiwari R, Chaicumpa W. 2020. Emerging novel coronavirus (2019-nCoV)-current scenario, evolutionary perspective based on genome analysis and recent developments. Vet Q. 40(1):68–76. https://doi.org/10.1080/01652176.2020.1727993.

65. South China Morning Post. 2020 Jan 23. Why wild animals are a key ingredient in China's coronavirus outbreak. Bangkok Post. [accessed 2020 Mar 28]; https://www.bangkokpost.com/world/1842104/why-wild-animals-are-a-key -ingredient-in-chinas-coronavirus-outbreak.

66. Schnirring L. 2020 Jan 27. Experts: nCoV spread in China's cities could trigger global epidemic. Minneapolis: Center for Infectious Disease Research and Policy; [accessed 2020 Mar 28]. http://www.cidrap.umn.edu/news-perspec tive/2020/01/experts-ncov-spread-chinas-cities-could-trigger-global-epidemic.

67. Lu R, Zhao X, Li J, Niu P, Yang B, Wu H, Wang W, Song H, Huang B, Zhu

N, et al. 2020. Genomic characterisation and epidemiology of 2019 novel coronavirus: implications for virus origins and receptor binding. Lancet. 395(10224):565–574. https://doi.org/10.1016/S0140-6736(20)30251-8.

68. Lim PL, Kurup A, Gopalakrishna G, Chan KP, Wong CW, Ng LC, Se-Thoe SY, Oon L, Bai X, Stanton LW, et al. 2004. Laboratory-acquired severe acute respiratory syndrome. N Engl J Med. 350(17):1740–1745. https://doi.org/10.1056/NEJMoa032565.

69. Andersen KG, Rambaut A, Lipkin WI, Holmes EC, Garry RF. 2020 Mar 17. The proximal origin of SARS-CoV-2. Nat Med. https://doi.org/10.1038/s41591-020-0820-9.

70. Zhou P, Yang X-L, Wang X-G, Hu B, Zhang L, Zhang W, Si H-R, Zhu Y, Li B, Huang C-L, et al. 2020. A pneumonia outbreak associated with a new corona-virus of probable bat origin. Nature. 579(7798):270–273. https://doi.org/10.1038/s41586-020-2012-7.

71. Salata C, Calistri A, Parolin C, Palù G. 2019. Coronaviruses: a paradigm of new emerging zoonotic diseases. Pathog Dis. 77(9).

72. Lu R, Zhao X, Li J, Niu P, Yang B, Wu H, Wang W, Song H, Huang B, Zhu N, et al. 2020. Genomic characterisation and epidemiology of 2019 novel coronavirus: implications for virus origins and receptor binding. Lancet. 395(10224):565–574. https://doi.org/10.1016/S0140-6736(20)30251-8.

73. Xiao B, Xiao L. 2020 Feb. The possible origins of 2019-nCoV coronavirus. ResearchGate.net. [accessed 2020 Apr 18]. https://doi.org/10.13140/RG.2.2.21799.29601.

74. Zhang YZ, Holmes EC. 2020. A genomic perspective on the origin and emer-gence of SARS-CoV-2. Cell. [Epub ahead of print 2020 Mar 26; accessed 2020 Apr 8]. https://doi.org/10.1016/j.cell.2020.03.035.

75. Lam TT-Y, Shum MH-H, Zhu H-C, Tong Y-G, Ni X-B, Liao Y-S, Wei W, Cheung WY-M, Li W-J, Li L-F, et al. 2020 Mar 26. Identifying SARS-CoV-2 related coronaviruses in Malayan pangolins. Nature. https://doi.org/10.1038/s41586-020-2169-0.

76. Zhang T, Wu Q, Zhang Z. 2020 Apr 6. Probable pangolin origin of SARS-CoV-2 associated with the COVID-19 outbreak. Curr Biol. 30:1–6. https://doi.org/10.1016/j.cub.2020.03.022.

77. Liu P, Chen W, Chen JP. 2019. Viral metagenomics revealed Sendai virus and Coronavirus infection of Malayan pangolins (*Manis javanica*). Viruses. 11(11):979. https://dx.doi.org/10.3390/v11110979.

78. Volpato G, Fontefrancesco MF, Gruppuso P, Zocchi DM, Pieroni A. 2020. Baby pangolins on my plate: possible lessons to learn from the COVID-19 pandemic. J Ethnobiol Ethnomed. 16(1):19. https://doi.org/10.1186/s13002-020-00366-4.

79. Ji W, Wang W, Zhao X, Zai J, Li X. 2020. Cross-species transmission of the newly identified coronavirus 2019-nCoV. J Med Virol. 92(4):433–440. https://doi.org/10.1002/jmv.25682.

80. Liu Z, Xiao X, Wei X, Li J, Yang J, Tan H, Zhu J, Zhang Q, Wu J, Liu L. 2020. Composition and divergence of coronavirus spike proteins and host ACE2 receptors predict potential intermediate hosts of SARS-CoV-2. J Med

Virol. [Epub ahead of print 2020 Feb 26; accessed 2020 Mar 28]. https://doi .org/10.1002/jmv.25726.

81. Xiao K, Zhai J, Feng Y, Zhou N, Zhang X, Zou J-J, Li N, Guo Y, Li X, Shen X, et al. 2020 Feb 20. Isolation and characterization of 2019-nCoV-like corona-virus from Malayan pangolins. https://doi.org/10.1101/2020.02.17.951335.

82. Lam TT, Shum MH, Zhu HC, Tong YG, Ni XB, Liao YS, Wei W, Cheung WY, Li WJ, Li LF, et al. 2020. Identifying SARS-CoV-2 related coronaviruses in Malayan pangolins. Nature. [Epub ahead of print 2020 Mar 26; accessed 2020 Apr 8]. https://doi.org/10.1038/s41586-020-2169-0.

83. Yang Y, Peng F, Wang R, Guan K, Jiang T, Xu G, Sun J, Chang C. 2020 Mar 3. The deadly coronaviruses: the 2003 SARS pandemic and the 2020 novel coronavirus epidemic in China. J Autoimmun. [accessed 2020 Mar 28]. https://doi.org/10.1016/j.jaut.2020.102434.

84. Peeri NC, Shrestha N, Rahman MS, Zaki R, Tan Z, Bibi S, Baghbanzadeh M, Aghamohammadi N, Zhang W, Haque U. 2020 Feb 22. The SARS, MERS and novel coronavirus (COVID-19) epidemics, the newest and biggest global health threats: what lessons have we learned? Int J Epidemiol. [accessed 2020 Mar 28]. https://doi.org/10.1093/ije/dyaa033.

85. Guzman J. 2020 Apr 3. Fauci: it's mind-boggling that China's wet markets are still operating during coronavirus pandemic. The Hill. [accessed 2020 Apr 11]; https://thehill.com/changing-america/well-being/prevention-cures/491025 -fauci-mind-boggling-that-chinas-wet-markets.

86. Li J-Y, You Z, Wang Q, Zhou Z-J, Qiu Y, Luo R, Ge X-Y. 2020. The epidemic of 2019-novel-coronavirus (2019-nCoV) pneumonia and insights for emerging infectious diseases in the future. Microbes Infect. 22(2):80–85. https://doi.org /10.1016/j.micinf.2020.02.002.

87. Harypursat V, Chen Y-K. 2020 Feb 24. Six weeks into the 2019 coronavirus disease (COVID-19) outbreak—it is time to consider strategies to impede the emergence of new zoonotic infections. Chin Med J (Engl). [accessed 2020 Mar 28]. https://doi.org/10.1097/CM9.0000000000000760.

88. Westcott B, Deng S. 2020 Mar 5. China has made eating wild animals illegal after the coronavirus outbreak. But ending the trade won't be easy. CNN; [ac-cessed 2020 Apr 8]. https://www.cnn.com/2020/03/05/asia/china-coronavi rus-wildlife-consumption-ban-intl-hnk/index.html.

89. Loeb J. 2020. China bans sale of wildlife following coronavirus. Vet Record. 186(5):144–145. http://dx.doi.org/10.1136/vr.m495.

90. Normile D, Yimin D. 2003. Civets back on China's menu. Science. 301(5636):1031. https://doi.org/10.1126/science.301.5636.1031a.

91. Zhou Z-M, Buesching CD, Macdonald DW, Newman C. 2020. China: clamp down on violations of wildlife trade ban. Nature. 578(7794):217. https://doi .org/10.1038/d41586-020-00378-w.

92. Yang Y, Peng F, Wang R, Guan K, Jiang T, Xu G, Sun J, Chang C. 2020. The deadly coronaviruses: the 2003 SARS pandemic and the 2020 novel corona-virus epidemic in China. J Autoimmun. [Epub ahead of print 2020 Mar 3; accessed 2020 Mar 28]. https://doi.org/10.1016/j.jaut.2020.102434.

93. Challender D, Wu S, Kaspal P, Khatiwada A, Ghose A, Ching-Min Sun N, Mohapatra RK, Laxmi Suwal L T. 2019. Manis pentadactyla (errata version published in 2020). The IUCN Red List of threatened species 2019. Cambridge (United Kingdom): International Union for Conservation of Nature and Natural Resources; [last assessed 2019 May 10; accessed 2020 Mar 28]. https://dx .doi.org/10.2305/IUCN.UK.2019-3.RLTS.T12764A168392151.en.

94. Harypursat V, Chen Y-K. 2020 Feb 24. Six weeks into the 2019 coronavirus disease (COVID-19) outbreak—it is time to consider strategies to impede the emergence of new zoonotic infections. Chin Med J (Engl). [accessed 2020 Mar 28]. https://doi.org/10.1097/CM9.0000000000000760.

95. Zhou Z-M, Buesching CD, Macdonald DW, Newman C. 2020. China: clamp down on violations of wildlife trade ban. Nature. 578(7794):217. https://doi .org/10.1038/d41586-020-00378-w.

96. Li J, Li J, Xie X, Cai X, Huang J, Tian X, Zhu H. 2020. Game consumption and the 2019 novel coronavirus. Lancet Infect Dis. 20(3):275–276. https://doi .org/10.1016/S1473-3099(20)30063-3.

97. Peeri NC, Shrestha N, Rahman MS, Zaki R, Tan Z, Bibi S, Baghbanzadeh M, Aghamohammadi N, Zhang W, Haque U. 2020 Feb 22. The SARS, MERS and novel coronavirus (COVID-19) epidemics, the newest and biggest global health threats: what lessons have we learned? Int J Epidemiol. [accessed 2020 Mar 28]. https://doi.org/10.1093/ije/dyaa033.

98. Wang H, Shao J, Luo X, Chuai Z, Xu S, Geng M, Gao Z. 2020. Wildlife consumption ban is insufficient. Science. 367(6485):1435. https://doi.org/10.1126 /science.abb6463.

99. Li J, Li J, Xie X, Cai X, Huang J, Tian X, Zhu H. 2020. Game consumption and the 2019 novel coronavirus. Lancet Infect Dis. 20(3):275–276. https://doi .org/10.1016/S1473-3099(20)30063-3.

100. Smith GD, Ng F, Li WHC. 2020 Mar 9. COVID-19: emerging compassion, courage and resilience in the face of misinformation and adversity. J Clin Nurs. [accessed 2020 Mar 28]. https://doi.org/10.1111/jocn.15231.

101. Ye ming sha, bat feces, bat dung, bat guano. 2020. Xiamen (China): Best Plant; [accessed 2020 Mar 28]. https://www.bestplant.shop/products/ye-ming-sha -bat-feces-bat-dung-bat-guano.

102. 48 Wassenaar TM, Zou Y. 2020. 2019_nCoV/SARS-CoV-2: rapid classification of betacoronaviruses and identification of Traditional Chinese Medicine as potential origin of zoonotic coronaviruses. Lett Appl Microbiol. 70(5): 342–348. https://doi.org/10.1111/lam.13285.

103. National Administration of Traditional Chinese Medicine. 2020 Feb 4. Notice on the issuance of a new coronavirus infection pneumonia diagnosis and treatment plan. Beijing: National Health Commission. Report No.: 103. http:// www.gov.cn/zhengce/zhengceku/2020-02/05/5474791/files/de44557832 ad4be1929091dcbcfca891.pdf.

104. Zhou Z-M, Buesching CD, Macdonald DW, Newman C. 2020. China: clamp down on violations of wildlife trade ban. Nature. 578(7794):217. https://doi .org/10.1038/d41586-020-00378-w.

105. Li J, Li J, Xie X, Cai X, Huang J, Tian X, Zhu H. 2020. Game consumption and the 2019 novel coronavirus. Lancet Infect Dis. 20(3):275–276. https://doi .org/10.1016/S1473-3099(20)30063-3.

106. Zhou P, Fan H, Lan T, Yang X-L, Shi W-F, Zhang W, Zhu Y, Zhang Y-W, Xie Q-M, Mani S, et al. 2018. Fatal swine acute diarrhoea syndrome caused by an HKU2-related coronavirus of bat origin. Nature. 556(7700):255–258. https://doi.org/10.1038/s41586-018-0010-9.

107. Afelt A, Frutos R, Devaux C. 2018. Bats, coronaviruses, and deforestation: toward the emergence of novel infectious diseases? Front Microbiol. 9:702. https://dx.doi.org/10.3389/fmicb.2018.00702.

108. U.S. Agency for International Development. [date unknown]. Emerging disease insights. USAID. Predict. [accessed 2020 Mar 28]. https://static1.square space.com/static/5c7d60a711f7845f734d4a73/t/5d6038708989fe00015fb309 /1566586994570/M%26A-EDI+pigs.pdf.

109. Cui J, Li F, Shi ZL. 2019. Origin and evolution of pathogenic coronaviruses. Nat Rev Microbiol. 17(3):181–192. https://doi.org/10.1038/s41579-018-0118-9.

110. Niederwerder MC, Hesse RA. 2018. Swine enteric coronavirus disease: a review of 4 years with porcine epidemic diarrhoea virus and porcine deltacoronavirus in the United States and Canada. Transbound Emerg Dis. 65(3):660–675. https://doi.org/10.1111/tbed.12823.

111. Wang Q, Vlasova AN, Kenney SP, Saif LJ. 2019. Emerging and re-emerging coronaviruses in pigs. Curr Opin Virol. 34:39–49. https://doi.org/10.1016/j .coviro.2018.12.001.

112. U.S. Government Accountability Office. 2015 Dec 15. Emerging animal diseases: actions needed to better position USDA to address future risks. Washington: GAO. Report No.: GAO-16-132. https://www.gao.gov/products /GAO-16-132.

113. Graham RL, Donaldson EF, Baric RS. 2013. A decade after SARS: strategies for controlling emerging coronaviruses. Nat Rev Microbiol. 11(12):836–848. https://doi.org/10.1038/nrmicro3143.

114. Wang Q, Vlasova AN, Kenney SP, Saif LJ. 2019. Emerging and re-emerging coronaviruses in pigs. Curr Opin Virol. 34:39–49. https://doi.org/10.1016/j .coviro.2018.12.001.

115. Vijgen L, Keyaerts E, Moës E, Thoelen I, Wollants E, Lemey P, Vandamme A-M, Van Ranst M. 2005. Complete genomic sequence of human coronavirus OC43: molecular clock analysis suggests a relatively recent zoonotic coronavirus transmission event. J Virol. 79(3):1595–1604. https://doi.org/10.1128/JVI .79.3.1595-1604.2005.

116. Corman VM, Muth D, Niemeyer D, Drosten C. 2018. Hosts and sources of endemic human coronaviruses. Adv Virus Res. 100:163–188. https://doi.org /10.1016/bs.aivir.2018.01.001.

117. Seifried O. 1931. Histopathology of infectious laryngotracheitis in chickens. J Exp Med. 54(6):817–826. https://dx.doi.org/10.1084/jem.54.6.817.

118. Ignjatović J, Sapats S. 2000. Avian infectious bronchitis virus. Rev Sci Tech. 19(2):493–508. https://doi.org/10.20506/rst.19.2.1228.

119. Cunningham CH, Spring MP, Nazerian K. 1972. Replication of avian infectious bronchitis virus in African green monkey kidney cell line VERO. J Gen Virol. 16(3):423–427.

120. Su S, Wong G, Shi W, Liu J, Lai ACK, Zhou J, Liu W, Bi Y, Gao GF. 2016. Epidemiology, genetic recombination, and pathogenesis of coronaviruses. Trends Microbiol. 24(6):490–502. https://doi.org/10.1016/j.tim.2016.03.003.

121. Wang B, Liu Y, Ji C-M, Yang Y-L, Liang Q-Z, Zhao P, Xu L-D, Lei X-M, Luo W-T, Qin P, et al. 2018. Porcine deltacoronavirus engages the transmissible gastroenteritis virus functional receptor porcine aminopeptidase N for infectious cellular entry. J Virol. 92(12):e00318-18. https://doi.org/10.1128/JVI.00318-18.

122. van der Velden VHJ, Wierenga-Wolf AF, Adriaansen-Soeting PWC, Overbeek SE, Möller GM, Hoogsteden HC, Versnel MA. 1998. Expression of aminopeptidase N and dipeptidyl peptidase IV in the healthy and asthmatic bronchus. Clin Exp Allergy. 28(1):110–120. https://doi.org/10.1046/j.1365-2222.1998.00198.x.

123. Li W, Hulswit RJG, Kenney SP, Widjaja I, Jung K, Alhamo MA, van Dieren B, van Kuppeveld FJM, Saif LJ, Bosch B-J. 2018. Broad receptor engagement of an emerging global coronavirus may potentiate its diverse cross-species transmissibility. Proc Natl Acad Sci U S A. 115(22):E5135–E5143. https://doi.org/10.1073/pnas.1802879115.

124. Liang Q, Zhang H, Li B, Ding Q, Wang Y, Gao W, Guo D, Wei Z, Hu H. 2019. Susceptibility of chickens to porcine deltacoronavirus infection. Viruses. 11(6):573. https://dx.doi.org/10.3390/v11060573.

125. Ismail MM, Cho KO, Ward LA, Saif LJ, Saif YM. 2001. Experimental bovine coronavirus in turkey poults and young chickens. Avian Dis. 45(1):157–163.

126. Boley PA, Alhamo MA, Lossie G, Yadav KK, Vasquez-Lee M, Saif LJ, Kenney SP. 2020. Porcine deltacoronavirus infection and transmission in poultry, United States. Emerg Infect Dis. 26(2):255–265. https://doi.org/10.3201/eid2602.190346.

127. Boley PA, Alhamo MA, Lossie G, Yadav KK, Vasquez-Lee M, Saif LJ, Kenney SP. 2020. Porcine deltacoronavirus infection and transmission in poultry, United States. Emerg Infect Dis. 26(2):255–265. https://doi.org/10.3201/eid2602.190346.

128. Yang Y-L, Qin P, Wang B, Liu Y, Xu G-H, Peng L, Zhou J, Zhu SJ, Huang Y-W. 2019. Broad cross-species infection of cultured cells by bat HKU2-related swine acute diarrhea syndrome coronavirus and identification of its replication in murine dendritic cells in vivo highlight its potential for diverse interspecies transmission. J Virol. 93(24):e01448-19. https://doi.org/10.1128/JVI.01448-19.

129. Xu Y. 2020. Unveiling the origin and transmission of 2019-nCoV. Trends Microbiol. 28(4):239–240. https://doi.org/10.1016/j.tim.2020.02.001.

130. Graham RL, Donaldson EF, Baric RS. 2013. A decade after SARS: strategies for controlling emerging coronaviruses. Nat Rev Microbiol. 11(12):836–848. https://doi.org/10.1038/nrmicro3143.

131. Leopardi S, Terregino C, Paola DB. 2020. Silent circulation of coronaviruses in pigs. Vet Rec. 186(10):323. http://dx.doi.org/10.1136/vr.m932.

132. Heinrich S, Wittmann TA, Prowse TAA, Ross JV, Delean S, Shepherd CR,

Cassey P. 2016. Where did all the pangolins go? International CITES trade in pangolin species. Glob Ecol Conserv. 8:241–253. http://dx.doi.org/10.1016/j .gecco.2016.09.007.

133. FAOSTAT. 2019. Livestock primary data: producing animals/slaughtered: meat, pig. Rome: Food and Agriculture Organization of the United Nations; [updated 2020 Mar 4; accessed 2020 Apr 8]. http://www.fao.org/faostat/en/#data/QL.

134. Kingsley DH. 2016. Emerging foodborne and agriculture-related viruses. Microbiol Spectr. 4(4). https://doi.org/10.1128/microbiolspec.PFS-0007-2014.

135. Corman VM, Eckerle I, Memish ZA, Liljander AM, Dijkman R, Jonsdottir H, Juma Ngeiywa KJZ, Kamau E, Younan M, Al Masri M, et al. 2016. Link of a ubiquitous human coronavirus to dromedary camels. Proc Natl Acad Sci U S A. 113(35):9864–9869. https://doi.org/10.1073/pnas.1604472113.

136. Fung S-Y, Yuen K-S, Ye Z-W, Chan C-P, Jin D-Y. 2020. A tug-of-war between severe acute respiratory syndrome coronavirus 2 and host antiviral defence: lessons from other pathogenic viruses. Emerg Microbes Infect. 9(1):558–570. https://doi.org/10.1080/22221751.2020.1736644.

137. Vijgen L, Keyaerts E, Moës E, Thoelen I, Wollants E, Lemey P, Vandamme A-M, Van Ranst M. 2005. Complete genomic sequence of human coronavirus OC43: molecular clock analysis suggests a relatively recent zoonotic coronavirus transmission event. J Virol. 79(3):1595–1604.

138. Walker PGT, Whittaker C, Watson O, Baguelin M, Ainslie KEC, Bhatia S, Bhatt S, Boonyasiri A, Boyd O, Cattarino L, et al. 2020 Mar 26. Report 12. The global impact of COVID-19 and strategies for mitigation and suppression. MRC Centre for Global Infectious Disease Analysis, Imperial College London. [accessed 2020 Apr 8]. https://www.imperial.ac.uk/mrc-global-infectious -disease-analysis/covid-19/report-12-global-impact-covid-19/

139. American Hospital Association. 2020 Feb 20. Coronavirus update: register for AHA members-only webinars on Feb. 21 and Feb. 26 related to novel coronavirus (COVID-19). Chicago: AHA; [accessed 2020 Mar 30]. https://www .aha.org/advisory/2020-02-20-coronavirus-update-register-aha-members-only -webinars-feb-21-and-feb-26-related.

140. Institute for Health Metrics and Evaluation. 2020 May 4. New IHME forecast projects nearly 135,000 COVID-19 deaths in US. Seattle: University of Washington; [accessed 2020 May 11]. http://www.healthdata.org/news-release /new-ihme-forecast-projects-nearly-135000-covid-19-deaths-us.

141. Centers for Disease Control and Prevention. 2020. COVID-19 pandemic planning scenarios. U.S. Department of Health & Human Services; [last reviewed 2020 May 20; accessed 2020 May 27]. https://www.cdc.gov /coronavirus/2019-ncov/hcp/planning-scenarios.html.

142. Centers for Disease Control and Prevention. 2007 Feb. Interim pre-pandemic planning guidance: community strategy for pandemic influenza mitigation in the United States—early, targeted, layered use of nonpharmaceutical interventions. U.S. Department of Health and Human Services; [accessed 2020 Mar 30]. https:// www.cdc.gov/flu/pandemic-resources/pdf/community_mitigation-sm.pdf.

143. Centers for Disease Control and Prevention. 2007 Feb. Interim pre-pandemic

planning guidance: community strategy for pandemic influenza mitigation in the United States—early, targeted, layered use of nonpharmaceutical interventions. U.S. Department of Health and Human Services; [accessed 2020 Mar 30]. https://www.cdc.gov/flu/pandemic-resources/pdf/community_mitigation-sm.pdf.

144. Jester B, Uyeki T, Jernigan D. 2018. Readiness for responding to a severe pandemic 100 years after 1918. Am J Epidemiol. 187(12):2596–2602. https://doi.org/10.1093/aje/kwy165.

145. Taubenberger JK, Morens DM. 2006. 1918 Influenza: the mother of all pandemics. Emerg Infect Dis. 12(1):15–22.

146. National Weather Service. [date unknown]. Saffir-Simpson Hurricane Wind Scale. Miami: National Oceanic and Atmospheric Administration. [accessed 2020 Mar 30]. https://www.weather.gov/mfl/saffirsimpson.

147. Centers for Disease Control and Prevention. 2020. COVID-19 pandemic planning scenarios. U.S. Department of Health & Human Services; [last reviewed 2020 May 20; accessed 2020 May 27]. https://www.cdc.gov/coronavirus/2019-ncov/hcp/planning-scenarios.html.

148. Verity R, Okell LC, Dorigatti I, Winskill P, Whittaker C, Imai N, Cuomo-Dannenburg G, Thompson H, Walker PGT, Fu H, et al. 2020. Estimates of the severity of coronavirus disease 2019: a model-based analysis. Lancet Infect Dis. [Epub ahead of print 2020 Mar 30; accessed 2020 Apr 8]. https://doi.org/10.1016/S1473-3099(20)30243-7.

149. Russell TW, Hellewell J, Jarvis CI, van Zandvoort K, Abbott S, Ratnayake R, CMMID COVID-19 Working Group, Flasche S, Eggo RM, Edmunds WJ, et al. 2020. Estimating the infection and case fatality ratio for coronavirus disease (COVID-19) using age-adjusted data from the outbreak on the Diamond Princess cruise ship. Eurosurveillance. 25(12):2000256. http://dx.doi.org/10.2807/1560-7917.ES.2020.25.12.2000256.

150. Gudbjartsson DF, Helgason A, Jonsson H, Magnusson OT, Melsted P, Norddahl GL, Saemundsdottir J, Sigurdsson A, Sulem P, Agustsdottir AB, et al. 2020 Apr 14. Spread of SARS-CoV-2 in the Icelandic population. N Engl J Med. [accessed 2020 Apr 18]. https://doi.org/10.1056/NEJMoa2006100.

151. Oke J, Heneghan C. 2020 Mar 17. Global Covid-19 case fatality rates. Oxford: Centre for Evidence-Based Medicine; [updated 2020 Apr 7; accessed 2020 Apr 8]. https://www.cebm.net/covid-19/global-covid-19-case-fatality-rates/.

152. World Health Organization. 2004 Apr 21. Summary of probable SARS cases with onset of illness from 1 November 2002 to 31 July 2003. Geneva: WHO; [accessed 2020 Apr 1]. https://www.who.int/csr/sars/country/table2004_04_21/en/.

153. World Health Organization Regional Office for the Eastern Mediterranean. 2019. MERS situation update, November 2019. World Health Organization. Report No.: WHO-EM/CSR/241/E. http://www.emro.who.int/pandemic-epidemic-diseases/mers-cov/mers-situation-update-november-2019.html.

154. Taubenberger JK, Morens DM. 2019. The 1918 influenza pandemic and its legacy. Cold Spring Harb Perspect Med. [Epub ahead of print 2019 Dec 30; accessed 2020 Apr 8]. https://doi.org/10.1101/cshperspect.a038695.

155. World Health Organization. 2020. Cumulative number of confirmed human

cases for avian influenza A(H5N1) reported to WHO, 2003–2020. Geneva: WHO; [updated 2020 Feb 28; accessed 2020 Apr 1]. https://www.who.int/influenza/human_animal_interface/2020_01_20_tableH5N1.pdf.

156. Institute for Health Metrics and Evaluation. 2020. COVID-19 projections. Seattle: IHME; [updated 2020 Apr 17; accessed 2020 Apr 18]. https://covid19.healthdata.org/united-states-of-america.

157. Noymer A, Garenne M. 2000. The 1918 influenza epidemic's effects on sex differentials in mortality in the United States. Popul Dev Rev. 26(3):565–581.

158. Osler W. 1904. Science and Immortality (Boston, MA: Houghton, Mifflin and Company).

159. Crosby A. Alfred Crosby on: a bad rap on Spain. Influenza 1918. Public Broadcasting System American Experience transcript. pbs.org/wgbh/amex/influenza/filmmore/reference/interview/drcrosby1.html.

160. Collier R. 1974. The Plague of the Spanish Lady: The Influenza Pandemic of 1918–1919 (New York, NY: Atheneum).

161. Greene J with Miline K. 2006. The Bird Flu Pandemic (New York, NY: Thomas Dunne Books, p. 16).

162. Editorial. 1918. Journal of the American Medical Association 71:2154.

163. Ghendon Y. 1994. Introduction to pandemic influenza through history. European Journal of Epidemiology 10:451–3.

164. Ghendon Y. 1994. Introduction to pandemic influenza through history. European Journal of Epidemiology 10:451–3.

165. Secretariat of WHO Executive Board. 2004. Avian influenza and human health. World Health Organization Executive Board report 114(6):1–5. www.who.int/gb/ebwha/pdf._files/EB114/B114_6-en.pdf.

166. American Heritage Dictionaries (ed.), 2004. The American Heritage Dictionary of the English Language, 4th Edition (Boston, MA: Houghton Mifflin).

167. Mydans S. 2005. Preparations for bird flu are urgent, Asia is warned. International Herald Tribune, October 11. www.iht.com/articles/2005/10/10/news/flu.php.

168. Deagon B. 2005. Avian flu pandemic may have big effect on U.S. businesses. Investor's Business Daily, October 12. tinyurl.com/grztq.

169. Drexler M. 2002. Secret Agents: The Menace of Emerging Infections (Washington, DC: Joseph Henry Press).

170. Bollet AJ. 2004. Plagues and Poxes: The Impact of Human History on Epidemic Disease (New York, NY: Demos Medical Publishing).

171. Collier R. 1974. The Plague of the Spanish Lady: The Influenza Pandemic of 1918–1919 (New York, NY: Atheneum).

172. Barry JM. 2004. The Great Influenza: The Epic Story of the Deadliest Plague in History (New York, NY: Penguin Books).

173. Ireland MW (ed.). 1928. Medical department of the United States Army in the World War. Communicable Diseases 9:61.

174. Barry JM. 2004. The Great Influenza: The Epic Story of the Deadliest Plague in History (New York, NY: Penguin Books).

175. Ireland MW (ed.). 1928. Medical department of the United States Army in the World War. Communicable Diseases 9:61.

176. Laver WG, Bischofberger N, Webster RG. 2000. The origin and control of pandemic influenza. Perspectives in Biology and Medicine 43(2):173–92.

177. Brem WV, Bolling GE, Casper EJ. 1918. Pandemic 'influenza' and secondary pneumonia at Camp Fremont, Calif. Journal of the American Medical Association 71:2138–44.

178. Barry JM. 2004. The Great Influenza: The Epic Story of the Deadliest Plague in History (New York, NY: Penguin Books).

179. Nguyen-Van-Tam JS, Hampson AW. 2003. The epidemiology and clinical impact of pandemic influenza. Vaccine 21:1762–8.

180. Ireland MW (ed.). 1928. Medical department of the United States Army in the World War. Communicable Diseases 9:61.

181. Grist NR. 1979. Pandemic influenza 1918. British Medical Journal 2(6205):1632–3. web.uct.ac.za/depts/mmi/jmoodie/influen2.html.

182. Grist NR. 1979. Pandemic influenza 1918. British Medical Journal 2(6205):1632–3. web.uct.ac.za/depts/mmi/jmoodie/influen2.html.

183. Cunha BA. 2004. Influenza: historical aspects of epidemics and pandemics. Infectious Disease Clinics of North America 18:141–55.

184. Harbrecht L. 2005. Doctoral student's research brings lessons, insight to a looming pandemic. AScribe Newswire, October 25.

185. Quisenberry D. 2005. Remembering the 1918 flu pandemic. Grand Rapids Press, October 30. tinyurl.com/qmev4.

186. Brem WV, Bolling GE, Casper EJ. 1918. Pandemic "influenza" and secondary pneumonia at Camp Fremont, Calif. JAMA. 71:2138–44.

187. Collier R. 1974. The Plague of the Spanish Lady: The Influenza Pandemic of 1918–1919 (New York, NY: Atheneum).

188. Drexler M. 2002. Secret Agents: The Menace of Emerging Infections (Washington, DC: Joseph Henry Press).

189. Collier R. 1974. The Plague of the Spanish Lady: The Influenza Pandemic of 1918–1919 (New York, NY: Atheneum).

190. Thayer WS. 1918. Discussion of influenza. Proceedings of the Royal Society of Medicine, November, p. 61.

191. Morrisey C. 1997. Transcript of unaired interview for Influenza 1918, American Experience, February 26. Cited in: Barry JM. 2004. The Great Influenza: The Epic Story of the Deadliest Plague in History (New York, NY: Viking, p. 235).

192. Camus A. 1948. The Plague, translated by Stuart Gilbert (New York, NY: A.A. Knopf).

193. Ward P, Small I, Smith J, Suter P, Dutkowski R. 2005. Oseltamivir (Tamiflu) and its potential for use in the event of an influenza pandemic. J Antimicrob Chemother. 55(S1):i5–i21.

194. Brainerd E, Siegler MV. 2002. The economic effects of the 1918 influenza epidemic. National Bureau of Economic Research, Inc. (Washington, DC: Summer Institute). williams.edu/Economics/wp/brainerdDP3791.pdf.

195. Taubenberger JK, Reid AH, Fanning TG. 2000. The 1918 influenza virus: a killer comes into view. Virology 274:241–5.

196. Nguyen-Van-Tam JS, Hampson AW. 2003. The epidemiology and clinical impact of pandemic influenza. Vaccine 21:1762–8.

197. Garrett L. 2005. The next pandemic? Probable cause. Foreign Affairs 84(4). www.foreignaffairs.org/20050701faessay84401/laurie-Garrett/the-next-pandemic.html.

198. Johnson NPAS, Mueller J. 2002. Updating the accounts: global mortality of the 1918–1920 "Spanish" influenza pandemic. Bulletin of the History of Medicine 76:105–15.

199. Johnson NPAS, Mueller J. 2002. Updating the accounts: global mortality of the 1918–1920 "Spanish" influenza pandemic. Bulletin of the History of Medicine 76:105–15.

200. Alexander DJ, Brown IH. 2000. Recent zoonoses caused by influenza A viruses. Revue Scientifique et Technique Office International des Epizooties 19:197–225.

201. Ungchusak K, Auewarakul P, Dowell SF, et al. 2005. Probable person-to-person transmission of avian influenza A (H5N1). New England Journal of Medicine 352:333–40.

202. Barry JM. 2004. Viruses of mass destruction. Fortune, November 1.

203. Phillips H, Killingray D. 2003. Introduction. In: Phillips H, Killingray D (eds.), The Spanish Influenza Pandemic of 1918–19: New Perspectives (London, UK: Routledge, pp. 1–26).

204. Jordan E. 1927. Epidemic Influenza, 1st Edition (Chicago, IL: American Medical Association).

205. Crosby AW. 2003. America's Forgotten Pandemic: The Influenza of 1918 (Cambridge, UK: Cambridge University Press).

206. Public Broadcasting System. Influenza 1918, Act I. American Experience transcript. pbs.org/wgbh/amex/influenza/filmmore/transcript/transcript1.html.

207. Bollet AJ. 2004. Plagues and Poxes: The Impact of Human History on Epidemic Disease (New York, NY: Demos Medical Publishing, Inc., p. 107).

208. Barry JM. 2004. The Great Influenza: The Epic Story of the Deadliest Plague in History (New York, NY: Penguin Books, p. 187).

209. Public Broadcasting System. American Experience Transcript. 1918 Influenza Timeline. pbs.org/wgbh/amex/influenza/timeline/index.html.

210. Bollet AJ. 2004. Plagues and Poxes: The Impact of Human History on Epidemic Disease (New York, NY: Demos Medical Publishing, Inc., p. 106).

211. Lehrer J. 2005. The avian flu pandemic. PBS Newshour with Jim Lehrer. October 5.

212. Barry JM. 2004. Viruses of mass destruction. Fortune, November 1.

213. Jones L. 2005. America under attack. Men's Health, November, pp. 154–9.

214. Crosby A. 1999. Influenza 1918. PBS American Experience. www.pbs.org/wgbh/amex/influenza/.

215. Crosby A. 1999. Influenza 1918. PBS American Experience. www.pbs.org/wgbh/amex/influenza/.

216. Davies P. 2000. The Devil's Flu (New York, NY: Henry Holt and Company).

217. Collier R. 1974. The Plague of the Spanish Lady: The Influenza Pandemic of 1918–1919 (New York, NY: Atheneum).

218. Apuchase L. 1982. Charles Hardy oral history tapes. June 24. Cited in: Barry JM. 2004. The Great Influenza: The Epic Story of the Deadliest Plague in History (New York, NY: Viking, p. 223).

219. Morrisey C. 1997. Transcript of unaired interview for Influenza 1918, American Experience, February 26. Cited in: Barry JM. 2004. The Great Influenza: The Epic Story of the Deadliest Plague in History (New York, NY: Viking, p. 190).

220. Collier R. 1974. The Plague of the Spanish Lady: The Influenza Pandemic of 1918–1919 (New York, NY: Atheneum).

221. Barry JM. 2004. The Great Influenza: The Epic Story of the Deadliest Plague in History (New York, NY: Penguin Books).

222. Crosby A. 1999. Influenza 1918. PBS American Experience. www.pbs.org/wgbh /amex/influenza/.

223. Barry JM. 2004. The Great Influenza: The Epic Story of the Deadliest Plague in History (New York, NY: Penguin Books).

224. Phillips H, Killingray D. 2003. Introduction. In: Phillips H, Killingray D (eds.), The Spanish Influenza Pandemic of 1918–19: New Perspectives (London, UK: Routledge, pp. 1–26).

225. 1918. Tahiti builds pyres of influenza dead. New York Times, December 25. flickr.com/photos/quiplash/34527850/.

226. Oldstone MBA. 1998. Viruses, Plagues and History (Cambridge, UK: Oxford University Press).

227. Phillips H, Killingray D. 2003. Introduction. In: Phillips H, Killingray D (eds.), The Spanish Influenza Pandemic of 1918–19: New Perspectives (London, UK: Routledge, pp. 1–26).

228. Hudson C. 1999. Something in the air. Daily Mail, August 21, pp. 30–31.

229. Crosby A. 1999. Influenza 1918. PBS American Experience. www.pbs.org/wgbh /amex/influenza/.

230. Crosby A. 1999. Influenza 1918. PBS American Experience. www.pbs.org/wgbh /amex/influenza/.

231. Fields BN, Knipe DM, Howley PM, Griffin DE. 1996. Fields Virology (Philadelphia, PA: Lippincott Williams and Wilkins). Cited in: Barry JM. 2004. The Great Influenza: The Epic Story of the Deadliest Plague in History (New York, NY: Viking, p. 102).

232. Karlen A. 1995. Man and Microbes (New York, NY: Touchstone, p. 145).

233. Public Broadcasting System. Influenza 1918, Act V. American Experience transcript. pbs.org/wgbh/amex/influenza/filmmore/transcript/transcript1.html.

234. Sacks O, Vilensky JA. 2005. Waking to a new threat. New York Times, November 16.

235. Ravenholt RT, Foege WH. 1982. 1918 Influenza, encephalitis lethargica, parkinsonism. Lancet 320(8303):860–4.

236. Almond D. 2005. Is the 1918 influenza pandemic over? Long-term effects of in utero influenza exposure in the post-1940 U.S. population. Columbia University and NBER, July. nber.org/~almond/jmp3.pdf.

237. Kolata G. 1999. Flu: The Story of the Great Influenza Pandemic (New York, NY: Simon & Schuster, Inc., p. 3).

238. Schoch-Spana M. 2000. Implications of pandemic influenza for bioterrorism response. Clinical Infectious Diseases 31:1409–13.

239. Committee on Climate, Ecosystems, Infectious Disease, and Human Health. 2001. Under the Weather: Climate, Ecosystems, and Infectious Disease (Washington, DC: National Academies Press).

240. Evans WA, Armstrong DB, Davis WH, Kopf EW, Woodward WC. 1918. Influenza: report of a special committee of the American Public Health Association. Journal of the American Medical Association 71:2068–73.

241. Evans WA, Armstrong DB, Davis WH, Kopf EW, Woodward WC. 1918. Influenza: report of a special committee of the American Public Health Association. Journal of the American Medical Association 71:2068–73.

242. Drexler M. 2002. Secret Agents: The Menace of Emerging Infections (Washington, DC: Joseph Henry Press, p. 165).

243. Bakalar N. 2003. Where the Germs Are: A Scientific Safari (New York, NY: Wiley).

244. Smith W, Andrews CH, Laidlaw PP. 1933. A virus obtained from influenza patients. Lancet 2:66–8.

245. Taubenberger J. 2005. Mission of Armed Forces Institute of Pathology. Public Broadcasting System American Experience. 1918 Influenza. pbs.org/wgbh/amex/influenza/sfeature/drjeffrey1.html.

246. Taubenberger JK, Reid AH. 2003. Archaevirology: characterization of the 1918 "Spanish" influenza pandemic virus. In: Greenblatt C, Spigelman M (eds.), Emerging Pathogens: Archaeology, Ecology and and Evolution of Infectious Disease (Oxford, UK: Oxford University Press, pp. 189–202).

247. Brown D. 2005. Back from the dead—the 1918 killer influenza. Washington Post, October 16.

248. Brown D. 2005. Back from the dead—the 1918 killer influenza. Washington Post, October 16.

249. Brown D. 2005. Back from the dead—the 1918 killer influenza. Washington Post, October 16.

250. Lockwood C. 1997. In search of the Spanish flu: scientists hope seven bodies buried in arctic ice will help solve the mystery of the 1918 pandemic. The Ottawa Citizen, October 4.

251. Lockwood C. 1997. In search of the Spanish flu: scientists hope seven bodies buried in arctic ice will help solve the mystery of the 1918 pandemic. The Ottawa Citizen, October 4.

252. Brown D. 2005. Back from the dead—the 1918 killer influenza. Washington Post, October 16.

253. Davies P. 2000. The Devil's Flu (New York, NY: Henry Holt and Company).

254. Davies P. 2000. The Devil's Flu (New York, NY: Henry Holt and Company).

255. Davis JL. 2000. Ground penetrating radar surveys to locate 1918 Spanish flu victims in permafrost. Journal of Forensic Science 45(1):68–76.

256. The Ottawa Citizen. 1998. Gravediggers begin search for 1918 flu virus in Arctic. August 23.

257. Wilford JN. 1998. Quest for frozen pandemic virus yields mixed results. New York Times, September 8.

258. Gladwell M. 1997. The dead zone. New Yorker, July 28.

259. Underwood A. 2005. Resurrecting a killer flu. Newsweek, Oct. 7.

260. Taubenberger JK, Reid AH. 2003. Archaevirology: characterization of the 1918 "Spanish" influenza pandemic virus. In: Greenblatt C, Spigelman M (eds.), Emerging Pathogens: Archaeology, Ecology and Evolution of Infectious Disease (Oxford, UK: Oxford University Press, pp. 189–202).

261. Drexler M. 2002. Secret Agents: The Menace of Emerging Infections (Washington, DC: Joseph Henry Press).

262. Davies P. 2000. The Devil's Flu (New York, NY: Henry Holt and Company).

263. Fernandez E. 2002. The virus detective. San Francisco Chronicle, February 17.

264. Fernandez E. 2002. The virus detective. San Francisco Chronicle, February 17.

265. Fernandez E. 2002. The virus detective. San Francisco Chronicle, February 17.

266. Kolata G. 1999. Flu: The Story of the Great Influenza Pandemic (New York, NY: Simon & Schuster, Inc., p. 264).

267. Gadsby P. 1999. Fear of flu—pandemic influenza outbreaks. Discover, January.

268. Martindale D. 2000. No mercy. New Scientist, October 14.

269. Koen JS. 1919. A practical method for field diagnosis of swine disease. American Journal of Veterinary Medicine 14:468.

270. Oldstone MBA. 1998. Viruses, Plagues and History (Oxford, UK: Oxford University Press).

271. Taubenberger JK, Reid AH, Lourens RM, Wang R, Jin G, Fanning TG. 2005. Characterization of the 1918 influenza virus polymerase genes. Nature 437:889.

272. Belshe RB. 2005. The origins of pandemic influenza—lessons from the 1918 virus. New England Journal of Medicine 353(21):2209–11.

273. Cohen JC, Powderly WG. 2004. Infectious Diseases, 2nd Edition (London, UK: Mosby).

274. Crawford R. 1995. The Spanish flu. In: Stranger Than Fiction: Vignettes of San Diego History (San Diego, CA: San Diego Historical Society).

275. Tumpey TM, Basler CF, Aguilar PV, et al. 2005. Characterization of the reconstructed 1918 Spanish influenza pandemic virus. Science 310(5745):77–80.

276. Webby RJ, Webster RG. 2003. Are we ready for a pandemic influenza? Science 302:1519–22.

277. Stobbe M. 2005. Researchers reconstruct 1918 flu virus. Associated Press, October 5.

278. von Bubnoff A. 2005. The 1918 flu virus is resurrected. Nature 427:794.

279. Kolata G. 2005. Deadly 1918 epidemic linked to bird flu, scientists say. New York Times, October 5.

280. Branswell H. 2005. Spanish flu bug lives again. Ottawa Sun, October 5.

281. Kolata G. 2005. Deadly 1918 epidemic linked to bird flu, scientists say. New York Times, October 5.

282. Kolata G. 2005. Deadly 1918 epidemic linked to bird flu, scientists say. New York Times, October 5.

283. Orent W. 2005. Playing with viruses: replicating this flu strain could get us burned. Washington Post, April 17, p. B01. www.washingtonpost.com/wp -dyn/articles/A58300-2005Apr16.html.

284. von Bubnoff A. 2005. The 1918 flu virus is resurrected. Nature 427:794.

285. von Bubnoff A. 2005. The 1918 flu virus is resurrected. Nature 427:794.

286. von Bubnoff A. 2005. The 1918 flu virus is resurrected. Nature 427:794.

287. Benitez MA. 2005. Ahead of the storm. South China Morning Post, April 20.

288. Russell S. 2005. Deadliest flu bug given new life in U.S. laboratory. San Francisco Chronicle, October 6.

289. Sample I. 2005. Security fears as flu virus that killed 50 million is recreated. Guardian, October 6.

290. Frist B. 2005. Manhattan project for the 21st century. Harvard Medical School Health Care Policy Seidman Lecture, June 1. frist.senate.gov/_files /060105manhattan.pdf.

291. Dhingra MS, Artois J, Robinson TP, Linard C, Chaiban C, Xenarios I, Engler R, Liechti R, Kuznetsov D, Xiao X, et al. 2016. Global mapping of highly pathogenic avian influenza H5N1 and H5Nx clade 2.3.4.4 viruses with spatial cross-validation. eLife. 5:e19571. https://doi.org/10.7554/eLife.19571.

292. World Health Organization. 2020. Cumulative number of confirmed human cases for avian influenza A(H5N1) reported to WHO, 2003–2020. Geneva: WHO; [updated 2020 Feb 28; accessed 2020 Apr 8]. https://www.who.int /influenza/human_animal_interface/2020_01_20_tableH5N1.pdf.

293. World Health Organization. 2020 Feb 10. Ebola virus disease. Geneva: WHO; [accessed 2020 Apr 19]. https://www.who.int/news-room/fact-sheets/detail /ebola-virus-disease.

294. World Health Organization. 2006. Cumulative number of confirmed human cases of avian influenza A/(H5N1). April 19. www.who.int/csr/disease/avian _influenza/country/cases_table_2006_04_19/en/index.html.

295. Branswell H. 2006. Cambodian study suggests mild bird flu cases aren't going undetected. Canadian Press, March 20. mytelus.com/news/article .do?pageID=cp_health_home&articleID=2204288.

296. 2005. U.S. a step behind bird flu. CBS Morning News, October 9.

297. 2004. Russian expert says flu epidemic may kill over one billion this year. Moscow News, October 28. www.mosnews.com/news/2004/10/28/pandemic .shtml.

298. Editorial. 2005. Bird flu outbreak could kill 1.5 billion. New Scientist, February 5. www.newscientist.com/channel/health/bird-flu/mg18524853.100.

299. 2006. Bird flu: the untold story. Oprah Winfrey Show, January 24.

300. Crawford D. 2003. The Invisible Enemy: A Natural History of Viruses (New York, NY: Oxford University Press, pg 2).

301. Greenfield CT. 2004. On high alert. Time International, January 26.

302. Davies P. 2000. The Devil's Flu (New York, NY: Henry Holt and Company, p. 76).

303. Perez DR, Nazarian SH, McFadden G, Gilmore MS. 2005. Miscellaneous threats: highly pathogenic avian influenza, and novel bio-engineered organisms. In: Bronze MS, Greenfield RA (eds.), Biodefense: Principles and Pathogens (Norfolk, UK: Horizon Bioscience).

304. Shortridge KF. 1992. Pandemic influenza: a zoonosis? Seminars in Respiratory Infections 7:11–25.

305. Sompayrac L. 2002. How Pathogenic Viruses Work (Sudbury, MA: Jones and Bartlett Publishers).

306. Ryan F. 1997. Virus X: Tracking the New Killer Plagues—Out of the Present and and Into the Future (Boston, MA: Little, Brown and Company).

307. Berdoy M, Webster JP, Macdonald DW. 2000. Fatal attraction in rats infected with Toxoplasma gondii. Proceedings of The Royal Society of Biological Sciences 7;267(1452):1591–4.

308. Revis DR. 2006. Skin, anatomy. Emedicine. February 7. emedicine.com/plastic /topic389.htmemedicine.com/plastic/topic389.htm.

309. Larson E. 2001. Hygiene of the skin: when is clean too clean? Emerging Infectious Diseases 7(2):225–30.

310. Merchant JA, Kline J, Donham KJ, Bundy DS, Hodne CJ. 2002. Human health effects. In: Iowa Concentrated Animal Feeding Operations Air Quality Study (Iowa State University and The University of Iowa Study Group, pp. 121–45).

311. Shaw J. 2005. Clearing the air: how epidemiology, engineering, and experiment finger fine particles as airborne killers. Harvard Magazine, May-June.

312. Houtmeyers E, Gosselink R, Gayan-Ramirez G, Decramer M. 1999. Regulation of mucociliary clearance in health and disease. European Respiratory Journal 13(5):1177–88.

313. Sompayrac L. 2002. How Pathogenic Viruses Work (Sudbury, MA: Jones and Bartlett Publishers).

314. Laver WG, Bischofberger N, Webster RG. 2000. The origin and control of pandemic influenza. Perspectives in Biology and Medicine 43(2):173–92.

315. Webster RG. 1998. Influenza: an emerging microbial pathogen. In: Krause RM (ed.), Emerging Infections (New York, NY: Academic Press, pp. 275–300).

316. Laver WG, Bischofberger N, Webster RG. 2000. The origin and control of pandemic influenza. Perspectives in Biology and Medicine 43(2):173–92.

317. World Health Organization Expert Committee. 1980. A revision of the system of nomenclature for influenza viruses. Bulletin of the WHO 58:585–91.

318. Oxford JS, Novelli P, Sefton A, Lambkin R. 2002. New millennium antivirals against pandemic and epidemic influenza: the neuraminidase inhibitors. Antiviral Chemistry and and Chemotherapy 13(4):205–17.

319. De Jong JC, Rimmelzwaan GF, Fouchier RAM, Osterhaus AD. 2000. Influenza virus: a master of metamorphosis. Journal of Infection 40(3):218–28.

320. Sompayrac L. 2002. How Pathogenic Viruses Work (Sudbury, MA: Jones and Bartlett Publishers).

321. Sompayrac L. 2002. How Pathogenic Viruses Work (Sudbury, MA: Jones and Bartlett Publishers).

322. Boone SA, Gerba CP. 2005. The occurrence of influenza A virus on household and day care center fomites. Journal of Infection 51(2):103–9.

323. Boone SA, Gerba CP. 2005. The occurrence of influenza A virus on household and day care center fomites. Journal of Infection 51(2):103–9.

324. Reiling J. 2000. Dissemination of bacteria from the mouth during speaking, coughing and otherwise. Journal of the American Medical Association 284(2):156.

325. Bourouiba L, Dehandschoewercker E, Bush JWM. 2014. Violent expiratory events: on coughing and sneezing. J Fluid Mech. 745:537–563. https://doi.org/10.1017/jfm.2014.88.

326. De Jong JC, Rimmelzwaan GF, Fouchier RAM, Osterhaus AD. 2000. Influenza virus: a master of metamorphosis. Journal of Infection 40(3):218–28.

327. Drexler M. 2002. Secret Agents: The Menace of Emerging Infections (Washington, DC: Joseph Henry Press).

328. Chow CB. 2004. Post-SARS infection control in the hospital and clinic. Paediatric Respiratory Reviews 5(4):289–295.

329. Sompayrac L. 2002. How Pathogenic Viruses Work (Sudbury, MA: Jones and Bartlett Publishers).

330. Sompayrac L. 2002. How Pathogenic Viruses Work (Sudbury, MA: Jones and Bartlett Publishers).

331. Sompayrac L. 2002. How Pathogenic Viruses Work (Sudbury, MA: Jones and Bartlett Publishers).

332. Sompayrac L. 2002. How Pathogenic Viruses Work (Sudbury, MA: Jones and Bartlett Publishers).

333. Sompayrac L. 2002. How Pathogenic Viruses Work (Sudbury, MA: Jones and Bartlett Publishers).

334. Sompayrac L. 2002. How Pathogenic Viruses Work (Sudbury, MA: Jones and Bartlett Publishers).

335. Overton ET, Goepfert PA, Cunningham P, Carter WA, Horvath J, Young D, Strayer DR. 2014. Intranasal seasonal influenza vaccine and a TLR-3 agonist, rintatolimod, induced cross-reactive IgA antibody formation against avian H5N1 and H7N9 influenza HA in humans. Vaccine. 32(42):5490–5495. https://doi.org/10.1016/j.vaccine.2014.07.078.

336. Sompayrac L. 2002. How Pathogenic Viruses Work (Sudbury, MA: Jones and Bartlett Publishers).

337. Sompayrac L. 2002. How Pathogenic Viruses Work (Sudbury, MA: Jones and Bartlett Publishers).

338. Seo SH, Hoffmann E, Webster RG. 2002. Lethal H5N1 influenza viruses escape host anti-viral cytokine responses. Nature Medicine 8(9):950–4.

339. Mitchison A. 1993. Will we survive? As host and pathogen evolve together, will the immune system retain the upper hand? Scientific American, September, pp. 136–44.

340. Drexler M. 2002. Secret Agents: The Menace of Emerging Infections (Washington, DC: Joseph Henry Press, p. 12).

341. Kolata G. 1999. Flu: The Story of the Great Influenza Pandemic (New York, NY: Simon & Schuster, Inc.).

342. Sompayrac L. 2002. How Pathogenic Viruses Work (Sudbury, MA: Jones and Bartlett Publishers).

343. Fraser L. 2002. Doctors fear deadly flu virus will lead to new pandemic. Daily Telegraph, September 22.

344. Taubenberger JK, Reid AH, Fanning TG. 2005. Capturing a killer flu virus. Scientific American 292(1):62.

345. 2006. Bird flu: the untold story. Oprah Winfrey Show, January 24.

346. Boccaccio G. 1350. Decameron. wsu.edu/~dee/MA/DECINTRO.HTM.

347. Public Broadcasting System. American Experience. Influenza 1918. Victor Vaughan. pbs.org/wgbh/amex/influenza/peopleevents/pandeAMEX90.html.

348. Evans WA, Armstrong DB, Davis WH, Kopf EW, Woodward WC. 1918. Influenza: report of a special committee of the American Public Health Association. Journal of the American Medical Association 71:2068–73.

349. Chan MC, Cheung CY, Chui WH, et al. 2005. Proinflammatory cytokine responses induced by influenza A (H5N1) viruses in primary human alveolar and bronchial epithelial cells. Respiratory Research 6:135.

350. Appenzeller T. 2005. The next killer flu. National Geographic, October, pp. 8–31.

351. Pedersen SF, Ho Y-C. 2020. SARS-CoV-2: a storm is raging. J Clin Invest. [Epub ahead of print 2020 Mar 27; accessed 2020 Apr 12]. https://doi.org/10.1172/JCI137647.

352. Brown D. 2005. Scientists race to head off lethal potential of avian flu. Washington Post, August 23.

353. Osterholm M, Colwell R, Garrett L, Fauci AS. 2005. The Council on Foreign Relations meeting: the threat of global pandemics. Federal News Service, June 16. cfr.org/publication.html.?id=8198.

354. Bor J. 2005. A versatile virus: an expert in infectious diseases explains why avian flu could trigger the next pandemic. Baltimore Sun, July 1.

355. Osterholm M, Colwell R, Garrett L, Fauci AS. 2005. The Council on Foreign Relations meeting: the threat of global pandemics. Federal News Service, June 16. cfr.org/publication.html.?id=8198.

356. Arnst C. 2005. A hot zone in the heartland. Little could be done to contain a deadly avian flu outbreak. Business Week, September 19. businessweek.com/magazine/content/05_38/b3951008.htm.

357. Sompayrac L. 2002. How Pathogenic Viruses Work (Sudbury, MA: Jones and Bartlett Publishers).

358. Sompayrac L. 2002. How Pathogenic Viruses Work (Sudbury, MA: Jones and Bartlett Publishers).

359. De Jong JC, Rimmelzwaan GF, Fouchier RAM, Osterhaus AD. 2000. Influenza virus: a master of metamorphosis. Journal of Infection 40(3):218–28.

360. World Health Organization. 2005. Avian influenza: assessing the pandemic threat, January 1. who.int/csr/disease/influenza/H5N1-9reduit.pdf.

361. Beck MA. 1996. The role of nutrition in viral disease. Journal of Nutritional Biochemistry 7:683–90.

362. Page RDM, Holmes E. 1998. Molecular Evolution (Oxford, UK: Blackwell Publishing).

363. Holland JJ. 1998. The origin and evolution of viruses. Microbiology and Microbial Infections 1998:12.

364. Sample I. 2004. Flu's deadly numbers game: a new pandemic looming, says Ian Sample and it's not just humans at risk. Guardian, January 29. guardian.co.uk /birdflu/story/0,14207,1133461,00.html.

365. Webster RG, Bean WJ, Gorman OT, Chambers TM, Kawaoka Y. 1992. Evolution and ecology of influenza A viruses. Microbiological Reviews 56(1):152–79.

366. Dimmock NJ, Easton A, Leppard K. 2001. Introduction to Modern Virology (Boston, MA: Blackwell Publishing).

367. Fields BN, Knipe DM, Howley PM, Griffin DE. 1996. Fields' Virology (Philadelphia, PA: Lippincott Williams and and Wilkins).

368. Barry JM. 2004. The Great Influenza: The Epic Story of the Deadliest Plague in History (New York, NY: Penguin Books).

369. Shortridge KF. 1999. Influenza—a continuing detective story. Lancet 354:siv29.

370. Davies P. 2000. The Devil's Flu (New York, NY: Henry Holt and Company).

371. McNamara TS. 2002. Diagnosis and control of zoonotic infections: pathology and early recognition of zoonotic disease outbreaks. In: The Emergence of Zoonotic Diseases: Understanding the Impact on Animal and Human Health—Workshop Summary (Washington, DC: National Academies Press, pp. 64–78).

372. Leitner T (ed.). 2002. The Molecular Epidemiology of Human Viruses (Berlin, Germany: Springer Science and Business Media).

373. Laver WG, Bischofberger N, Webster RG. 2000. The origin and control of pandemic influenza. Perspectives in Biology and Medicine 43(2):173–92.

374. Barry JM. 2004. The Great Influenza: The Epic Story of the Deadliest Plague in History (New York, NY: Penguin Books).

375. Cox NJ, Subbarao K. 2000. Global epidemiology of influenza: past and present. Annual Review of Medicine 51:407–21.

376. Center for Infectious Disease Research and and Policy. 2006. Pandemic influenza. March 22. www.cidrap.umn.edu/cidrap/content/influenza/panflu/biofacts /panflu.html.

377. Cox NJ, Subbarao K. 2000. Global epidemiology of influenza: past and present. Annual Review of Medicine 51:407–21.

378. Uniformed Services University School of Medicine. Class of 2007 USMLE Step 1 Stuff. Bugs (Blitz). usuhs.mil/2007/USMLE/Bugs%20(Blitz).pdf.

379. Underwood A, Adler J, Rosenberg D, Seno A. 2004. Scary strains. Newsweek 114(18):46–9.

380. Fouchier RA, Munster V, Wallensten A, et al. 2005. Characterization of a novel influenza A virus hemagglutinin subtype (H16) obtained from black-headed gulls. Journal of Virology 79(5):2814–22.

381. Ciminski K, Schwemmle M. 2019. Bat-borne influenza A viruses: an awakening. Cold Spring Harb Perspect Med. [Epub ahead of print 2019 Dec 30; accessed 2020 Apr 8]. https://doi.org/10.1101/cshperspect.a038612.

382. Laver WG, Bischofberger N, Webster RG. 2000. The origin and control of pandemic influenza. Perspectives in Biology and Medicine 43(2):173–92.

383. Webster RG, Bean WJ, Gorman OT, Chambers TM, Kawaoka Y. 1992. Evolution and ecology of influenza A viruses. Microbiological Reviews 56(1):152–79.

384. Mondics C. 2005. U.S. prepares for pandemic possibility. Philadelphia Inquirer, October 9.

385. von Bubnoff A. 2005. The 1918 flu virus is resurrected. Nature 427:794.

386. Kaiser J. 2005. Resurrecting the Spanish flu. ScienceNOW, October 5. sciencenow.sciencemag.org/cgi/content/full/2005/1005/2.

387. Garrett L. 2005. The next pandemic? Probable cause. Foreign Affairs 84(4). www.foreignaffairs.org/20050701faessay84401/laurie-Garrett/the-next-pandemic.html.

388. World Health Organization. 2020. Cumulative number of confirmed human cases for avian influenza A(H5N1) reported to WHO, 2003–2020. Geneva: WHO; [updated 2020 Feb 28; accessed 2020 Apr 8]. https://www.who.int/influenza/human_animal_interface/2020_01_20_tableH5N1.pdf. www.who.int/csr/disease/avian_influenza/country/cases_table_2006_04_27/en/index.html.

389. Kolata G. 2005. Deadly 1918 epidemic linked to bird flu, scientists say. New York Times, October 5.

390. Taubenberger JK, Reid AH, Lourens RM, Wang R, Jin G, Fanning TG. 2005. Characterization of the 1918 influenza virus polymerase genes. Nature 437:889–93.

391. Fehr-Snyder K. 2005. Arizona, world may not be ready for flu outbreak. Arizona Republic, October 4. www.azcentral.com/health/news/articles/1004birdflu04.html.

392. Holmes EC, Ghedin E, Miller N, et al. 2005. Whole-genome analysis of human influenza A virus reveals multiple persistent lineages and reassortment among recent H3N2 viruses. Public Library of Science Biology 3(9):e300. biology.plosjournals.org/perlserv/?request=get-document&doi=10.1371/journal.pbio.0030300.

393. Ludwig S, Stitz L, Planz O, Van H, Fitch WM, Scholtissek C. 1995. European swine virus as a possible source for the next influenza pandemic? Virology 212(2):555–61.

394. Barry JM. 2004. The Great Influenza: The Epic Story of the Deadliest Plague in History (New York, NY: Penguin Books).

395. Kennedy M. 2005. Bird flu could kill millions: global pandemic warning from WHO. Gazette (Montreal), March 9, p. A1.

396. Vong S, Coghlan B, Mardy S, Holl D, Seng H, Ly S, Miller MJ, Buchy P, Froehlich Y, Dufourcq JB, et al. 2006. Low frequency of poultry-to-human H5N1 transmission, southern Cambodia, 2005. Emerg Infect Dis. 12(10):1542–1547. https://dx.doi.org/10.3201/eid1210.060424.

397. Vong S, Coghlan B, Mardy S, Holl D, Seng H, Ly S, Miller MJ, Buchy P, Froehlich Y, Dufourcq JB, et al. 2006. Low frequency of poultry-to-human H5N1 transmission, southern Cambodia, 2005. Emerg Infect Dis. 12(10):1542–1547. https://dx.doi.org/10.3201/eid1210.060424.

398. Nasreen S, Uddin Khan S, Azziz-Baumgartner E, Hancock K, Veguilla V, Wang D, Rahman M, Alamgir ASM, Sturm-Ramirez K, Gurley ES, et al. 2013. Seroprevalence of antibodies against highly pathogenic avian influenza A (H5N1) virus among poultry workers in Bangladesh, 2009. PLoS One. 8(9):e73200. https://doi.org/10.1371/journal.pone.0073200.

399. Monamele CG, Y P, Karlsson EA, Vernet M-A, Wade A, Okomo M-CA, Abah ASA, Yann S, Etoundi GAM, Mohamadou NR, et al. 2019. Evidence of exposure and human seroconversion during an outbreak of avian influenza A(H5N1) among poultry in Cameroon. Emerg Microbes Infect. 8(1):186–196. https://doi.org/10.1080/22221751.2018.1564631.

400. Wang M, Di B, Zhou DH, Zheng BJ, Jing H, Lin YP, Liu YF, Wu XW, Qin PZ, Wang YL, et al. 2006. Food markets with live birds as source of avian influenza. Emerg Infect Dis. 12(11):1773–1775. https://doi.org/10.3201/eid1211.060675.

401. Cai W, Schweiger B, Buchholz U, Buda S, Littmann M, Heusler J, Haas W. 2009. Protective measures and H5N1-seroprevalence among personnel tasked with bird collection during an outbreak of avian influenza A/H5N1 in wild birds, Ruegen, Germany, 2006. BMC Infect Dis. 9(1):170. https://doi.org/10.1186/1471-2334-9-170.

402. Santhia K, Ramy A, Jayaningsih P, Samaan G, Putra AAG, Dibia N, Sulaimin C, Joni G, Leung CYH, Malik Peiris JS, et al. 2009. Avian influenza A H5N1 infections in Bali province, Indonesia: a behavioral, virological and seroepidemiological study. Influenza Other Respir Viruses. 3(3):81–89. https://doi.org/10.1111/j.1750-2659.2009.00069.x.

403. Ortiz JR, Katz MA, Mahmoud MN, Ahmed S, Bawa SI, Farnon EC, Sarki MB, Nasidi A, Ado MS, Yahaya AH, Joannis TM. 2007. Lack of evidence of avian-to-human transmission of avian influenza A (H5N1) virus among poultry workers, Kano, Nigeria, 2006. J Infect Dis. 196(11):1685–1691. https://doi.org/10.1086/522158.

404. Kwon D, Lee JY, Choi W, Choi JH, Chung YS, Lee NJ, Cheong HM, Katz JM, Oh HB, Cho H, et al. 2012. Avian influenza A (H5N1) virus antibodies in poultry cullers, South Korea, 2003–2004. Emerg Infect Dis. 18(6):986–988. https://doi.org/10.3201/eid1806.111631.

405. Dejpichai R, Laosiritaworn Y, Phuthavathana P, Uyeki TM, O'Reilly M, Yampikulsakul N, Phurahong S, Poorak P, Prasertsopon J, Kularb R, et al. 2009. Seroprevalence of antibodies to avian influenza virus A (H5N1) among residents of villages with human cases, Thailand, 2005. Emerg Infect Dis. 15(5):756–760. https://dx.doi.org/10.3201/eid1505.080316.

406. Ceyhan M, Yildirim I, Ferraris O, Bouscambert-Duchamp M, Frobert E, Uyar N, Tezer H, Oner AF, Buzgan T, Torunoglu MA, et al. (2010). Serosurveillance study on transmission of H5N1 virus during a 2006 avian influenza epidemic. Epidemiol Infect. 138(9):1274–1280. https://doi.org/10.1017/S0950268880999166X.

407. Schultsz C, Van Dung N, Hai LT, Ha DQ, Peiris JSM, Lim W, Garcia J-M, Tho ND, Lan NTH, Tho HH, et al. 2009. Prevalence of antibodies against

avian influenza A (H5N1) virus among cullers and poultry workers in Ho Chi Minh City, 2005. PLoS One. 4(11):e7948. https://doi.org/10.1371/journal .pone.0007948.

408. Toner ES, Adalja AA, Nuzzo JB, Inglesby TV, Henderson DA, Burke DS. 2013. Assessment of serosurveys for H5N1. Clin Infect Dis. 56(9):1206–1212. https://dx.doi.org/10.1093/cid/cit047.

409. Jang H, Boltz D, Sturm-Ramirez K, Shepherd KR, Jiao Y, Webster R, Smeyne RJ. 2009. Highly pathogenic H5N1 influenza virus can enter the central nervous system and induce neuroinflammation and neurodegeneration. Proc Natl Acad Sci U S A. 106(33):14063–14068. https://doi.org/10.1073/pnas .0900096106.

410. Branswell H. 2006. If bird flu virus becomes pandemic, high death rates possible: WHO report. Canadian Press, November 2.

411. Branswell H. 2006. If bird flu virus becomes pandemic, high death rates possible: WHO report. Canadian Press, November 2.

412. Associated Press. 2006 Dec 21. Flu pandemic could kill up to 81 million people. NBC News. [accessed 2020 Apr 8]; http://www.nbcnews.com/id/16313464 /ns/health-cold_and_flu/t/flu-pandemic-could-kill-million-people/.

413. Davis M. 2005. Avian flu: a state of unreadiness. The Nation, July 18–25, pp. 27–30.

414. Wilson Center Global Health Initiative. 2005. Emerging pandemic: costs and consequences of an avian influenza outbreak. September 19. wilsoncenter .org/index.cfm?topic_id=116811&fuseaction=topics.event_summary&event _id=142787.

415. Lo A. 2002. Millions dead, Hong Kong in chaos. How close did we come to this nightmare bird-flu scenario? South China Morning Post, December 7.

416. Davies P. 1999. The plague in waiting. Guardian, August 7. guardian.co.uk /birdflu/story/0,1131473,00.html.

417. Lo A. 2002. Millions dead, Hong Kong in chaos. How close did we come to this nightmare bird-flu scenario? South China Morning Post, December 7.

418. Hudson C. 1999. Something in the air. Daily Mail, August 21, pp. 30–31.

419. Mestel R. 2004. Bird flu haunts world's health authorities. Los Angeles Times, February 21. tinyurl.com/hzm3o.

420. Underwood A, Adler J, Rosenberg D, Seno A. 2004. Scary strains. Newsweek 114(18):46–9.

421. Mestel R. 2004. Bird flu haunts world's health authorities. Los Angeles Times, February 21. tinyurl.com/hzm3o.

422. Reynolds G. 2004. Our lives in their hands; they scour the earth for clues that could prevent millions of deaths. Independent, November 15.

423. Lo A. 2002. Millions dead, Hong Kong in chaos. How close did we come to this nightmare bird-flu scenario? South China Morning Post, December 7.

424. Drexler M. 2002. Secret Agents: The Menace of Emerging Infections (Washington, DC: Joseph Henry Press, p. 174).

425. Asthana A, Revill J, Smith AD, McLaughlan D. 2005. The killer at the door. Observer, October 16.

426. Gadsby P. 1999. Fear of flu—pandemic influenza outbreaks. Discover, January. looksmartjrhigh.com/p/articles/mi_m1511/is_1_20/ai_53501820.

427. Perez DR, Nazarian SH, McFadden G, Gilmore MS. 2005. Miscellaneous threats: highly pathogenic avian influenza, and novel bio-engineered organisms. In: Bronze MS, Greenfield RA (eds.), Biodefense: Principles and Pathogens (Norfolk, UK: Horizon Bioscience).

428. Drexler M. 2002. Secret Agents: The Menace of Emerging Infections (Washington, DC: Joseph Henry Press, p. 3).

429. Alexander DJ, Brown IH. 2000. Recent zoonoses caused by influenza A viruses. Revue Scientifique et Technique Office International des Epizooties 19:197–225.

430. Mayo Clinic staff. 2005. Bird flu (avian influenza). Infectious Disease Center, August 10. mayoclinic.com/health/bird-flu/DS00566/DSECTION=7.

431. Davies P. 1999. The plague in waiting. Guardian, August 7, Weekend page. guardian.co.uk/birdflu/story/0,1131473,00.html.

432. Brown D. 2005. Scientists race to head off lethal potential of avian flu. Washington Post, August 23, page A01.

433. Senne DA, Pearson JE, Panigrahy B. 1997. Live poultry markets: a missing link in the epidemiology of avian influenza. In: Proceedings of the 3rd International Symposium on Avian Influenza May 27–29 (University of Wisconsin, Madison, pp. 50–8).

434. Ramos SE, MacLachlan M, Melton A. 2017. Impacts of the 2014–2015 highly pathogenic avian influenza outbreak on the U.S. poultry sector. U.S. Department of Agriculture. Report No. LDPM-282-02. [accessed 2020 Apr 8]. https://www.ers.usda.gov/publications/pub-details/?pubid=86281.

435. Hofstaad MS, Calnek, BW, Helmboldt CF, Reid WM, Yoder, Jr. HW. 1972. Diseases of Poultry (Ames, IA: Iowa State University Press).

436. Davies P. 1999. The plague in waiting. Guardian, August 7, Weekend page. guardian.co.uk/birdflu/story/0,1131473,00.html.

437. McKie R, Revill J, Aglionby J, Watts J. 2004. Warning as bird flu crossover danger escalates. Observer, December 12. observer.guardian.co.uk/international/story/0,6903,1371917,00.html.

438. Capua I, Mutinelli F, Marangon S, Alexander DJ. 2000. H7N1 avian influenza in Italy (1999 to 2000) in intensively reared chickens and turkeys. Avian Pathology 29:537–43.

439. Mok D. 2002. Hong Kong's fowl problem. Time Asia, February 18.

440. Acha PN. 2003. Influenza. In: Zoonoses and Communicable Diseases Common to Man and Animals, Volume II, Chlamydioses, Rickettsioses, and Viroses (Washington, DC: Pan American Health Organization, pp. 155–71).

441. Zitzow LA, Rowe T, Morken T, et al. 2002. Pathogenesis of avian influenza A (H5N1) viruses in ferrets. Journal of Virology 76:4420–9.

442. Davis M. 2005. The Monster at Our Door: The Global Threat of Avian Flu (New York, NY: The New Press).

443. 2005. Strain Spotter. South China Morning Post, November 11, p. A17.

444. Gadsby P. 1999. Fear of flu—pandemic influenza outbreaks. Discover, January. looksmartjrhigh.com/p/articles/mi_m1511/is_1_20/ai_53501820.

445. Mestel R. 2004. Latching on to a horror. Los Angeles Times, February 18. bio-exchange.com/editorialNews.cfm?id=19668.

446. Mestel R. 2004. Bird flu haunts world's health authorities. Los Angeles Times, February 21. tinyurl.com/hzm3o.

447. Kolata G. 1999. Flu: The Story of the Great Influenza Pandemic (New York, NY: Simon & Schuster, Inc. p. 247).

448. Yuen KY, Chan PKS, Peiris M, et al. 1998. Clinical features and rapid viral diagnosis of human disease associated with avian influenza A H5N1 virus. Lancet 351:467–71.

449. Underwood A, Adler J, Rosenberg D, Seno A. 2004. Scary strains. Newsweek 114(18):46–9.

450. To K, Chan PKS, Chan K, et al. 2001. Pathology of fatal human infection associated with avian influenza A H5N1 virus. Journal of Medical Virology 63:242–6.

451. To K, Chan PKS, Chan K, et al. 2001. Pathology of fatal human infection associated with avian influenza A H5N1 virus. Journal of Medical Virology 63:242–6.

452. Davies P. 1999. The plague in waiting. Guardian, August 7. guardian.co.uk/bird flu/story/0,1131473,00.html.

453. Drexler M. 2002. Secret Agents: The Menace of Emerging Infections (Washington, DC: Joseph Henry Press, p. 176).

454. Cowen P. 2005. Avian influenza—Asia (17): Mongolia, migratory birds, H5N1, OIE. International Society for Infectious Diseases ProMED. Archive number 20050902.2597. September 2. promedmail.org/pls/promed /f?p=2400:1001:::NO::F2400_P1001_BACK_PAGE,F2400_P1001_PUB _MAIL_ID:1000%2C30272.

455. Katz JM. 2003. The impact of avian influenza viruses on public health. Avian Diseases 47:914–20.

456. Davies P. 2000. The Devil's Flu (New York, NY: Henry Holt and Company, p. 18).

457. Mestel R. 2004. Bird flu haunts world's health authorities. Los Angeles Times, February 21. tinyurl.com/hzm3o.

458. Kolata G. 1999. Flu: The Story of the Great Influenza Pandemic (New York, NY: Simon & Schuster, Inc., p. 245).

459. Shortridge KF, Gao P, Guan Y, et al. 2000. Interspecies transmission of influenza viruses: H5N1 virus and a Hong Kong SAR perspective. Veterinary Microbiology 74:141–7.

460. Altman LK. 2005. Her job: helping save the world from bird flu. New York Times, August 9.

461. Ajello R, Shepherd C. 1998. The flu fighters: how the people on the frontlines battled H5N1 to a stalemate. Not that the war is over. AsiaWeek, January 30.

462. Drexler M. 2002. Secret Agents: The Menace of Emerging Infections (Washington, DC: Joseph Henry Press, pp. 180–1).

463. Shortridge KF, Gao P, Guan Y, et al. 2000. Interspecies transmission of influenza viruses: H5N1 virus and a Hong Kong SAR perspective. Veterinary Microbiology 74:141–7.

464. Gadsby P. 1999. Fear of flu—pandemic influenza outbreaks. Discover, January. looksmartjrhigh.com/p/articles/mi_m1511/is_1_20/ai_53501820.

465. Davies P. 2000. The Devil's Flu (New York, NY: Henry Holt and Company, p. 35).

466. Fraser L. 2002. Doctors fear deadly flu virus will lead to new pandemic. Daily Telegraph, September 22.

467. Davies P. 2000. The Devil's Flu (New York, NY: Henry Holt and Company, pp. 35–36).

468. Benitez MA. 2001. Bird-flu cull "prevented pandemic"; SAR wins belated praise for halting deadly virus with slaughter of 1.6 million chickens. South China Morning Post, January 29.

469. Shortridge KF, Gao P, Guan Y, et al. 2000. Interspecies transmission of influenza viruses: H5N1 virus and a Hong Kong SAR perspective. Veterinary Microbiology 74:141–7.

470. 1998. Hong Kong's bird flu could return with a vengeance: experts. Agence France Presse, April 16.

471. 2004. Flu scientists fear massive outbreak; millions could die; Asian virus eyed. Ottawa Sun, November 18, p. 17.

472. Davies P. 1999. The plague in waiting. Guardian, August 7.

473. Brown EG, Sattar SA, Tetro J. 2006. Can we predict the nature and evolution of a H5N1 Z pandemic? A review submitted to Lancet: Infectious Diseases.

474. Rosenthal E. 2005. UN says avian flu may hit Africa next. International Herald Tribune, October 20.

475. Webster RG. 1993. Influenza. In: Morse SS (ed.), Emerging Viruses (New York, NY: Oxford University Press, pp. 37–45)

476. Shortridge KF. 2003. Severe acute respiratory syndrome and influenza. American Journal of Respiratory and Critical Care Medicine 168:1416–20.

477. Shortridge KF. 2003. Severe acute respiratory syndrome and influenza. American Journal of Respiratory and Critical Care Medicine 168:1416–20.

478. Shortridge KF. 2003. Avian influenza viruses in Hong Kong: zoonotic considerations. In: Schrijver RS, Koch G (eds.), Proceedings of the Frontis Workshop on Avian Influenza: Prevention and Control (Wageningen, The Netherlands, pp. 9–18)

479. Shortridge KF. 2003. Severe acute respiratory syndrome and influenza. American Journal of Respiratory and Critical Care Medicine 168:1416–20.

480. Shortridge KF. 1992. Pandemic influenza: a zoonosis? Seminars in Respiratory Infections 7:11–25.

481. Tempest R. 1997. Once again, researchers on the trail of a new flu strain. Morning Star (Wilmington, NC), December 15.

482. Bradsher K. 2005. China keeps secret its plans to fight bird flu. New York Times, October 16.

483. Cox JH. 2000. China livestock report. A report for Compassion in World Farming, October.

484. Cox JH. 2000. China livestock report. A report for Compassion in World Farming, October.

485. Das P. 2002. Interview: Michael Osterholm—medical detective to fighting bioterrorism. Lancet Infectious Diseases 2:502–5.

486. Cox JH. 2000. China livestock report. A report for Compassion in World Farming, October.

487. Shortridge KF, Peiris JSM, Guan Y. 2003. The next influenza pandemic: lessons from Hong Kong. Journal of Applied Microbiology 94:70–9.

488. Webster RG. 2004. Wet markets—a continuing source of severe acute respiratory syndrome and influenza? Lancet 363:234–6.

489. Nature Web. 2005. Web focus—avian flu timeline. Nature. www.nature.com /nature/focus/avianflu/timeline.html.

490. Lubroth J. 2005. Regional and global challenges of the avian influenza outbreaks in Asia and FAO's prospective. World's Poultry Science Journal 61:55–6.

491. Henley E. 2005. The growing threat of avian influenza. Journal of Family Practice 54(5):442–4.

492. Food and Agriculture Organization of the United Nations. Technical Task Force on Avian Influenza. 2005. Update on the avian influenza situation. Avian Influenza Disease Emergency News, issue 28. www.fao.org/ag/againfo/subjects /documents/ai/AVIbull028.pdf.

493. Melville DS, Shortridge KF. 2004. Influenza: time to come to grips with the avian dimension. Lancet Infectious Diseases 4:261–2.

494. 2004. Timeline: bird flu crisis unfolds. CNN, February. cnn.com/2004/WORLD /asiapcf/02/01/bird.flu.timeline/index.html.

495. MacKenzie D. 2004. Bird flu outbreak started a year ago. New Scientist, January 28.

496. Hulse-Post DJ, Sturm-Ramirez KM, Humberd J, et al. 2005. Role of domestic ducks in the propagation and biological evolution of highly pathogenic H5N1 influenza viruses in Asia. Proceedings of the National Academy of Sciences of the United States of America 102(30):10682–7.

497. Editorial. 2006. Avian influenza goes global, but don't blame the birds. Lancet Infectious Diseases 6:185. list.web.net/archives/sludgewatch-l/2006-April/001692.html.

498. 2005. Avian flu news tracker. Wall Street Journal Online, December 16. online.wsj.com/article/SB113501058739926456.html.?mod=article-outset-box.

499. Butler D, Ruttiman J. 2006. Avian flu and the New World. Nature 441:137–9.

500. Horner N. 2006. Genetic diversity keeping the bird flu at bay. Parksville Qualicum News, May 9. pqbnews.com/portals-code/list.cgi?paper=50&cat=42&i d=644011&more=

501. Henley E. 2005. The growing threat of avian influenza. Journal of Family Practice 54(5):442–4.

502. Hookway J. 2004. For rooster breeders, bird flu brings game of cat and mouse. Wall Street Journal, February 10, p. 1A.

503. World Society for the Protection of Animals. 2004. Avian influenza and humane slaughter: a dossier prepared for the World Organization for Animal

Health (OIE) conference on animal welfare. wspa-international.org/site/data
/070404_125858_Avian_flu_dossier.pdf.

504. McCord M. 2004. Grisly images lay bare shortcomings of bird flu culls.
Agence France Presse, February 1.

505. Fitzsimons E. 2003. Live hens were put into wood chippers. Union-Tribune,
April 11.

506. Mench JA, Siegel PB. 2004. Poultry. South Dakota State University Extension
and Research. ars.sdstate.edu/animaliss/poultry.html.

507. 2004. WHO warns unsafe culls increase virus mutation risk, Asia bows to
pressure. Agence France Presse, January 30.

508. World Organisation for Animal Health. 2006. Update on avian influenza in
animals (types H5 and H7). Paris: OIE; [updated 2020 Apr 8; accessed 2020
Apr 8]. https://www.oie.int/animal-health-in-the-world/update-on-avian
-influenza/2011/.

509. Fasanmi OG, Odetokun IA, Balogun FA, Fasina FO. 2017. Public health
concerns of highly pathogenic avian influenza H5N1 endemicity in Africa. Vet
World. 10(10):1194–1204. https://doi.org/10.14202/vetworld.2017.1194
-1204.

510. Brown D. 2005. Long-predicted flu finally tops agenda. Washington Post,
November 7, p. A01. www.washingtonpost.com/wpdyn/content/article/2005
/11/06/AR2005110601282.html.?nav=rss_politics.

511. World Health Organization. 2005. Cumulative number of confirmed human
cases of avian influenza A/(H5N1). November 24. www.who.int/csr/disease
/avian_influenza/country/cases_table_2005_11_24/en/index.html.

512. Stöhr K. 2005. Avian influenza and pandemics—research needs and opportunities. New England Journal of Medicine 352(4):405–7. bioon.com/biology
/UploadFiles/200501/20050129225325878.pdf.

513. Li KS, Guan Y, Wang J, et al. 2003. Genesis of a highly pathogenic and
potentially pandemic H5N1 influenza virus in Eastern Asia. Nature
430(6996):209–13.

514. Garrett L. 2005. The next pandemic? Probable cause. Foreign Affairs 84(4).
www.foreignaffairs.org/20050701faessay84401/laurie-Garrett/the-next-pan
demic.html.

515. Drexler M. 2002. Secret Agents: The Menace of Emerging Infections (Washington, DC: Joseph Henry Press, p. 180).

516. Stevens J, Blixt O, Tumpey TM, et al. 2006. Structure and receptor specificity
of the hemagglutinin from an H5N1 influenza virus. Science 312:404–10.

517. Cyranoski D. 2004. Bird flu data languishing in Chinese journals. Nature
430:995.

518. Ito T, Couceiro JN, Kelm S, et al. 1998. Molecular basis for the generation in
pigs of influenza A viruses with pandemic potential. 72(9):7367–73. pubmed
central.gov/articlerender.fcgi?tool=pubmed&pubmedid=9696833.

519. World Health Organization. Avian influenza A(H5N1)—update 28: reports of
infection in domestic cats (Thailand), situation (human) in Thailand, situation

(poultry) in Japan and China. February 20. who.int/csr/don/2004_02_20 /en/.

520. Kuiken T, Rimmelzwaan G, van Riel D, et al. 2004. Avian H5N1 influenza in cats. Science 306:241.

521. Verrengia J. 2005. Bird flu could hit U.S. next year. Associated Press, October 25.

522. Keawcharoen J, Oraveerakul K, Kuiken T, et al. 2004. Avian influenza H5N1 in tigers and leopards. Emerging Infectious Diseases 10:2189–91.

523. Thanawongnuwech R, Amonsin A, Tantilertcharoen R, et al. Probable tiger-to-tiger transmission of avian influenza H5N1. Emerging Infectious Diseases 11:699–701.

524. Kuiken T, Rimmelzwaan G, van Riel D, et al. 2004. Avian H5N1 influenza in cats. Science 306:241.

525. Ang A. 2005. WHO warns bird flu virus unstable and unpredictable, urges vigilance. Associated Press, June 10. sddt.com/News/article. cfm?SourceCode=200506101c.

526. Levy A, Scott-Clark C. 2005. Flu on the wing. Guardian, October 15. www .guardian.co.uk/birdflu/story/0,14207,1591358,00.html.

527. Smith R. 2005. Poultry has two central issues. Feedstuffs, November 14, p. 26.

528. Cookson C. 2005. H5N1 virus is hard for humans to catch. Financial Times, October 26.

529. Sipress A. 2005. Bird flu adds new danger to bloody game; cockfighting among Asian customs that put humans at risk. Washington Post, April 14.

530. United Nations Food and Agriculture Organization. 2005. Prevention and control of avian flu in small scale poultry. www.fao.org/ag/againfo/subjects /documents/ai/AI-paravets-guide.pdf.

531. Tumpey TM, Suarez DL, Perkins LEL, et al. 2002. Characterization of a highly pathogenic H5N1 avian influenza A virus isolated from duck meat. Journal of Virology 76:6344–55.

532. 2006. United States to allow processed poultry from China, despite bird flu fear. Associated Press, April 20. cp.org/english/online/full/agriculture /060420/a042042A.html.

533. 2006. Playing chicken with imports. Effect Measure, April 25. effectmeasure. blogspot.com/2006/04/playing-chicken-with-imports.html.

534. Mase M, Etob M, Tanimuraa N, et al. 2005. Isolation of a genotypically unique H5N1 influenza virus from duck meat imported into Japan from China. Virology 339:101–9. depts.washington.edu/einet/?a=printArticle&pr int=649.

535. Swayne DE. 2003. Transcript of the question and answer session from the Fifth International Symposium on Avian Influenza. Avian Diseases 47:1219–55.

536. Swayne DE, Beck JR. 2005. Experimental study to determine if low-pathogenicity and high-pathogenicity avian influenza viruses can be present in chicken breast and thigh meat following intranasal virus inoculation. Avian Diseases 49:81–5.

537. Yates VJ, Dawson GJ, Pronovost AD. 1981. Serologic evidence of avian adeno-associated virus infection in an unselected human population and among poultry workers. American Journal of Epidemiology 113:542–5.

538. Stolle A, Sperner B. 1997. Viral infections transmitted by food of animal origin: the present situation in the European Union. Archives of Virology 13:S219–28.

539. Buttner M, Oehmig WF, Rziha HJ, Pfaff E. 1997. Detection of virus or virus specific nucleic acid in foodstuff or bioproducts—hazards and risk assessments. Archives of Virology 13:S57–66.

540. Delgado C, Rosegrant M, Steinfeld H, Ehui S, Courbois C. 1999. Livestock to 2020: the next food revolution. Food, Agriculture, and the Environment Discussion Paper 28. For the International Food Policy Research Institute, the Food and Agriculture Organization of the United Nations and the International Livestock Research Institute. ifpri.org/2020/dp/dp28.pdf.

541. Adak GT, Meakins SM, Yip H, Lopman BA, O'Brien SJ. 2005. Disease risks from foods, England and Wales, 1996–2000. Emerging Infectious Diseases 11(3):365–72.

542. Adak GT, Meakins SM, Yip H, Lopman BA, O'Brien SJ. 2005. Disease risks from foods, England and Wales, 1996–2000. Emerging Infectious Diseases 11(3):365–72.

543. Stehr-Green PA, Hewer P, Meekin GE, Judd LE. 1993. The aetiology and risk factors for warts among poultry processing workers. International Journal of Epidemiology 22(2):294–8.

544. Rudlinger R, Bunney MH, Grob R, Hunter JA. 1989. Warts in fish handlers. British Journal of Dermatology 120(3):375–81.

545. Benton EC. 1994. Warts in butchers—a cause for concern? Lancet 343(8906):1114.

546. Robinson J. 1981. Cancer of the cervix: occupational risks. In: Jordon JA, Sharp F, Singer A (eds.), Pre-Clinical Neoplasia of the Cervix. Proceedings of the 9th study group of the Royal College of Obstetricians and Gynaecologists, pp. 11–27.

547. Scheurer ME, Tortolero LG, Adler-Storthz K. 2005. Human papillomavirus infection: biology, epidemiology, and prevention. International Journal of Gynecological Cancer 15(5):727–46.

548. Corrya JEL, Hinton MH. 1997. Zoonoses in the meat industry: a review. Acta Veterinaria Hungarica 45(4):457–9.

549. Swayne DE. 2005. Asian H5N1 avian influenza outbreaks and implications for food safety. International Association for Food Protection Proceedings, July 29.

550. Office of Communications, U.S. Department of Agriculture. 2005. Transcript of technical briefing regarding avian influenza, October 26. Transcript Release No. 0461.05. www.usda.gov/wps/portal/!ut/p/_s.7_0_A/7_0_1OB?contentidonly=tru%C2%AD&contentid=2005/10/0461.xml.

551. Chicken Farmers of Canada. 2005, "It is perfectly safe to eat poultry in Canada." News Release, October 19. www.chicken.ca/DefaultSite/index_e.aspx?DetailID=1124.

552. U.S. Department of State's Bureau of International Information Programs. 2005. U.N. group warns of poultry bans stemming from bird flu fear. October 28. usinfo.state.gov/gi/Archive/2005/Oct/28-602664.html.

553. Centers for Disease Control and Prevention. 2020. Foodborne germs and illnesses. U.S. Department of Health and Human Services; [last reviewed 2020 Mar 18; accessed 2020 Apr 8]. https://www.cdc.gov/foodsafety/foodborne -germs.html.

554. Schlundt J, Toyofuku H, Jansen J, Herbst SA. 2004. Emerging food-borne zoonoses. Revue Scientifique et Technique (Paris) 23(2):513–33.

555. Skirrow MB. 1998. Campylobacteriosis. In: Palmer SR, Soulsby EJL, Simpson DIH (eds.), Zoonoses: Biology, Clinical Practice, and Public Health Control (Oxford, UK: Oxford University Press, pp. 37–46).

556. Mattick K, Durham K, Hendrix M, et al. 2003. The microbiological quality of washing-up water and the environment in domestic and commercial kitchens. Journal of Applied Microbiology 94(5):842–8.

557. Centers for Disease Control and Prevention. 1990. Yersinia enterocolitica infections during the holidays in black families—Georgia. Morbidity and Mortality Weekly Report 39:45. www.cfsan.fda.gov/~mow/yersin.html.

558. World Health Organization. 2005. WHO inter-country consultation influenza A/H5N1 in humans in Asia, Manila, May 6–7. www.who.int/csr/disease /avian_influenza/H5N1%20Intercountry%20Assessment%20final.pdf.

559. Johnson JR, Kuskowski MA, Smith K, et al. 2005. Antimicrobial-resistant and extraintestinal pathogenic Escherichia coli in retail foods. Journal of Infectious Diseases 205:1040–9.

560. U.S. Department of Agriculture Food Safety and Inspection Service. 1996. Pathogen Reduction; Hazard Analysis and Critical Control Point (HACCP) Systems; Final Rule. Federal Register 61(144):38806–989, www.fsis.usda.gov /OA/fr/rule1.pdf.

561. Drexler M. 2002. Secret Agents: The Menace of Emerging Infections (Washington, DC: Joseph Henry Press, p. 87).

562. 1998. Industry Forum. Meat and Poultry, March.

563. Schlosser E. 2001. Fast Food Nation: The Dark Side of the All-American Meal (New York, NY: Houghton Mifflin Company).

564. Barbut S. 2001. Poultry Products Processing, An Industry Guide (Boca Raton, Florida: CRC Press).

565. DeWaal CS. 1996. Playing chicken: the human cost of inadequate regulation of the poultry industry. Center for Science in the Public Interest Food Safety Program, March. cspinet.org/reports/polt.html.

566. World Health Organization Regional Office for the Eastern Mediterranean. Main challenges in the control of zoonotic diseases in the Eastern Mediterranean region. www.emro.who.int/RC50/documents/DOC7.doc.

567. Duncan IJH. 1997. Killing Methods for Poultry (Guelph, Canada: Colonel KL Campbell Centre for the Study of Animal Welfare).

568. Complaint for Declaratory and Injunctive Relief. Levine v. Johanns, No. 05–4764 (N.D. Cal. filed Nov. 21, 2005).

569. Berrang ME, Meinersmann RJ, Buhr RJ, Reimer NA, Philips RW, Harrison MA. 2003. Presence of Campylobacter in the respiratory tract of broiler carcasses before and after commercial scalding. Poultry Science 82:1995–9.

570. Gregory NG, Whittington PE. 1992. Inhalation of water during electrical stunning in chickens. Research in Veterinary Science 53:360–2.

571. Raj ABM. 2004. Stunning and slaughter of poultry. In: Mead G (ed.), Poultry Meat Processing and Quality (Boca Raton, FL: CRC Press, pp. 65–85).

572. Eisnitz G. 1997. Slaughterhouse (New York, NY: Prometheus Books, p. 169).

573. Fox N. 1997. Spoiled: The Dangerous Truth about a Food Chain Gone Haywire (New York, NY: Basic Books, pp. 182–3).

574. Rusin P, Orosz-Coughlin P, Gerba C. 1998. Reduction of fecal coliform, and heterotrophic plate count bacteria in the household kitchen and bathroom by disinfection with hypochlorite cleaners. Journal of Applied Microbiology 85(5):819–28.

575. Raloff J. 1996. Sponges and sinks and rags, oh my! Where microbes lurk and how to rout them. Science News, September 14.

576. Fox N. 1997. Spoiled: The Dangerous Truth about a Food Chain Gone Haywire (New York, NY: Basic Books, p. 194).

577. Walton JR, White, EG (eds.), 1981. Communicable Diseases Resulting from Storage Handling, Transport and Landspreading of Manure (Luxembourg, Office for Official Publications of the European Communities).

578. International Food Safety Authorities Network. 2004. Highly pathogenic avian influenza H5N1 outbreaks in poultry and humans: food safety implications. INFOSAN Information Note No. 2/04—Avian Influenza.

579. U.S. Department of Agriculture. 2005. Questions and answers: avian influenza. Release No. 0458.05, October. usda.gov/2005/10/0458.xml.

580. Fox N. 1997. Spoiled: The Dangerous Truth about a Food Chain Gone Haywire (New York, NY: Basic Books, p. 25).

581. National Chicken Council, National Turkey Federation, and the Egg Safety Center. 2006. Avian influenza: protecting flocks, protecting people. avianinfluenzainfo.com.

582. Hingley A. 1999. Campylobacter: low-profile bug is food poisoning leader. FDA Consumer, September-October. www.fda.gov/fdac/features/1999/599_bug.html.

583. 2006. WHO concerned over consumption of bird flu-infected poultry. Japan Economic Newswire, May 3. tmcnet.com/usubmit/2006/05/03/1636044.htm.

584. Pinyorat RC. 2005. Thailand confirms 13th bird flu death. Associated Press, October 20. abcnews.go.com/Health/print?id=1232348.

585. Motavalli J. 1998. Nicols Fox: investigating a food supply gone haywire. E: The Environmental Magazine, May–June 1998.

586. Centers for Disease Control and Prevention. 2004. Guidance and recommendations. Interim guidance for protection of persons involved in U.S. avian influenza outbreak disease control and eradication activities. February 17.

587. International Food Safety Authorities Network. 2004. Highly pathogenic avian influenza H5N1 outbreaks in poultry and humans: food safety implications.

INFOSAN Information Note No. 2/04—Avian Influenza. www.who.int/entity /foodsafety/fs_management/No_02_Avianinfluenza_Dec04_en.pdf.

588. Van der Sluis W. 2005. Consumers and retailers demand food safety. World Poultry Salmonella and and Campylobacter Special, pp. 4–5.

589. 2005. Why not wash meat and poultry before cooking? Tufts University Health and Nutrition Letter 23:7.

590. Burgess F, Little CL, Allen G, Williamson K, Mitchell RT. 2005. Prevalence of Campylobacter, Salmonella, and Escherichia coli on the external packaging of raw meat. Journal of Food Protection 68(3):469–75.

591. Marano N (Moderator). 2004. Avian Influenza Symposium transcript. Centers for Disease Control and Prevention. November 3, p.1.

592. 1998. Chicken: What you don't know can hurt you. Consumer Reports, March, pp. 12–8.

593. Nestor F, Hauter W. 2000. Is America's meat fit to eat? (Washington, DC: Government Accountability Project, Public Citizen).

594. World Health Organization. 2005. Avian influenza: assessing the pandemic threat, January 1. www.who.int/csr/disease/influenza/H5N1-9reduit.pdf.

595. World Health Organization. 2004. Prevention and Control of Influenza Due to Avian Influenza Virus A (H5N1) (New Delhi, India: World Health Organization Press). w3.whosea.org/en/Section10/Section1027/Section1632.htm.

596. World Health Organization. 2005. Avian influenza: assessing the pandemic threat, January 1. www.who.int/csr/disease/influenza/H5N1-9reduit.pdf.

597. International Food Safety Authorities Network. 2004. Highly pathogenic avian influenza H5N1 outbreaks in poultry and humans: food safety implications. INFOSAN Information Note No. 2/04—Avian Influenza.

598. Cheng A. 2005. EU warns on raw eggs; China has new bird flu outbreak. Bloomberg, October 26. quote.bloomberg.com/apps/news?pid=10000080&si d=a2bThMk31QY4.

599. Swayne DE, Beck JR. 2004. Heat inactivation of avian influenza and Newcastle disease viruses in egg products. Avian Pathology 33:512–8.

600. Swayne DE, Beck JR. 2004. Heat inactivation of avian influenza and Newcastle disease viruses in egg products. Avian Pathology 33:512–8.

601. Mayo Clinic staff. 2005. Bird flu (avian influenza). Infectious Disease Center, October 27. ads.mayoclinic.com/health/bird-flu/DS00566/DSECTION=8.

602. National Center for Infectious Diseases, Division of Global Migration and Quarantine. 2005. Interim guidance about avian influenza A (H5N1) for U.S. Citizens living abroad. Centers for Disease Control and Prevention, October 28.

603. World Health Organization. 2005. Avian influenza: assessing the pandemic threat, January 1. www.who.int/csr/disease/influenza/H5N1-9reduit.pdf.

604. St. Louis ME, Morse DL, Potter ME, et al. 1988. The emergence of Grade A eggs as a major source of Salmonella enteritidis infections. Journal of the American Medical Association 259:2103–7.

605. Drexler M. 2002. Secret Agents: The Menace of Emerging Infections (Washington, DC: Joseph Henry Press, p. 112).

606. Lewis C. 1998. Safety last—the politics of E. coli and other food-borne killers. Statement of the Chairman, Center for Public Integrity, February 26.

607. Mexicans are the leading egg eaters. 2006. Poultry International 45(2):4–6.

608. Swayne DE, Beck JR. 2004. Heat inactivation of avian influenza and Newcastle disease viruses in egg products. Avian Pathology 33:512–8.

609. 2006. No bird flu but don't eat chicken, says health Daily Times, April 29. dailytimes.com.pk/default.asp?page=2006%5C04%5C29%5Cstory_29-4-2006 _pg7_36.

610. 2005. Minister warns public to stay alert to bird flu infection. Antara News Agency, July 21. indonesia-1.com/EN/konten.php?nama=News&op=detail _news&id=134.

611. 2004. Timeline: bird flu crisis unfolds. CNN, February. cnn.com/2004/WORLD /asiapcf/02/01/bird.flu.timeline/index.html.

612. 2005. Rome airport takes precautions against bird flu. Agence France Presse, August 20. news24.com/News24/World/News/0,2-10-1462_1757157,00. html.

613. Minder R. 2005. EU bird flu alert as outbreak spreads to Croatia. Financial Times, October 25.

614. Animal Health and Welfare Panel of the European Food Safety Authority. 2005. Animal health and welfare aspects of avian influenza. European Food Safety Authority Journal 266:1–21.

615. Swayne DE, Akey BL. 2003. Avian influenza control strategies in the United States of America. In: Schrijver RS, Koch G (eds.), Proceedings of the Frontis Workshop on Avian Influenza: Prevention and Control (Wageningen, The Netherlands, pp. 113–30).

616. Swayne DE, Akey BL. 2003. Avian influenza control strategies in the United States of America. In: Schrijver RS, Koch G (eds.), Proceedings of the Frontis Workshop on Avian Influenza: Prevention and Control (Wageningen, The Netherlands, pp. 113–30).

617. Swayne DE. 2003. Transcript of the question and answer session from the Fifth International Symposium on Avian Influenza. Avian Diseases 47:1219–55.

618. Swayne DE, Akey BL. 2003. Avian influenza control strategies in the United States of America. In: Schrijver RS, Koch G (eds.), Proceedings of the Frontis Workshop on Avian Influenza: Prevention and Control (Wageningen, The Netherlands, pp. 113–30).

619. Food and Agriculture Organization of the United Nations, World Organization for Animal Health, and World Health Organization, United Nations. 2004. Technical Consultation on the Control of Avian Influenza: Conclusion and Recommendations. www.oie.int/eng/AVIAN_INFLUENZA/avian_rome _feb04_report.pdf.

620. Food and Agriculture Organization of the United Nations and World Organization for Animal Health, United Nations. 2005. Second FAO/OIE Regional Meeting on Avian Influenza Control on Asia (Ho Chi Minh City, Vietnam), www.oie.int/eng/AVIAN_INFLUENZA/HPAI%20HCMC%20Recommen dations_March%2005.pdf.

621. Simon S. 2002. Outcry over pets in pet food. Los Angeles Times, January 6.

622. Swayne DE, Akey BL. 2003. Avian influenza control strategies in the United States of America. In: Schrijver RS, Koch G (eds.), Proceedings of the Frontis Workshop on Avian Influenza: Prevention and Control (Wageningen, The Netherlands, pp. 113–30).

623. Ross B. 2005. Avian flu: is the government ready for an epidemic? Virus poses risk of massive casualties around the world. ABC News Primetime, September 15. abcnews.go.com/Primetime/Investigation/story?id=1130392&page=1.

624. Walsh B, Johnson K. 2005. Emergency measures; avian flu is on the rise in Vietnam and is now endemic in much of Asia. Time International, February 7, p. 22.

625. Alexander DJ, Brown IH. 2000. Recent zoonoses caused by influenza A viruses. Revue Scientifique et Technique 19:197–225.

626. Lee PJ, Krilov LR. 2005. When animal viruses attack: SARS and avian influenza. Pediatric Annals 34(1):43–52.

627. Editorial. 2004. Avian influenza: the threat looms. Lancet 363(9405):257.

628. De Jong MD, Van Cam D, Qui PT, et al. 2005. Fatal avian influenza A (H5N1) in a child presenting with diarrhea followed by coma. New England Journal of Medicine 352:686–91.

629. Chutinimitkul S, Bhattarakosol P, Srisuratanon S, et al. 2006. H5N1 influenza A virus and infected human plasma. Emerging Infectious Diseases 12(6). www.cdc.gov/ncidod/EID/vol12no06/06-0227.htm.

630. Iwasaki T, Itamura S, Nishimura H, et al. 2004. Productive infection in the murine central nervous system with avian influenza virus A (H5N1) after intranasal inoculation. Acta Neuropathologica 108:485–92.

631. Drexler M. 2002. Secret Agents: The Menace of Emerging Infections (Washington, DC: Joseph Henry Press) p 165.

632. Berger S. 2005. I felt as if I was in hell, says bird flu survivor. Daily Telegraph, October 22.

633. 2005. Avian influenza virus: are we prepared? Canadian Medical Association Journal 172:965.

634. Berger S. 2005. I felt as if I was in hell, says bird flu survivor. Daily Telegraph, October 22.

635. Reynolds G. 2004. The flu hunters. New York Times, November 7. tinyurl.com/mqy5u.

636. Mackay N. 2005. Warning: this bird could kill. Sunday Herald, August 28. www.sundayherald.com/51482.

637. Editorial. 2005. Bird flu outbreak could kill 1.5 billion. New Scientist, February 5. www.newscientist.com/channel/health/bird-flu/mg18524853.100.

638. Obama B, Luger R. 2005. Grounding a pandemic. New York Times, June 6.

639. Nelson B. 2005. Bird flu outbreak; global threat; experts say deadly virus presents grave risk if we don't "get our act together." Newsday, March 6, p. A03.

640. World Health Organization. 2005. Avian influenza: assessing the pandemic threat, January 1. www.who.int/csr/disease/influenza/H5N1-9reduit.pdf.

641. Katz JM, Lim W, Bridges CB, et al. 1999. Antibody response in individuals infected with avian influenza A (H5N1) viruses and detection of anti-H5 antibody among household and social contacts. Journal of Infectious Diseases 180:1763–70.

642. Reeth KV. 2000. Cytokines in the pathogenesis of influenza. Veterinary Microbiology 74:109–16.

643. Fox M. 2005. U.S. children's hospital on frontline in bird flu war. Reuters, September 16. tinyurl.com/ma8s8.

644. Frist B. 2005. Floor statement—remarks as prepared for delivery, September 28. frist.senate.gov/index.cfm?FuseAction=Speeches.Detail&Speech _id=291&Month=9&Year=2005.

645. Walsh B. 2005. A wing and a prayer. Times Asia, September 19. www.time .com/time/europe/magazine/printout/0,13155,901051017-1115613,00.html.

646. Loft K. 2005. Bird of prey. Tampa Tribune, March 7.

647. American Experience Transcript. 1918 influenza people and events: Victor Vaughan. Public Broadcasting System. www.pbs.org/wgbh/amex/influenza /peopleevents/pandeAMEX90.html.

648. Public Broadcasting System. American Experience Transcript. 1918 Influenza. pbs.org/wgbh/amex/influenza/filmmore/transcript/transcript1.html.

649. Osterholm M, Colwell R, Garrett L, Fauci AS. 2005. The Council on Foreign Relations meeting: the threat of global pandemics. Federal News Service, June 16. www.cfr.org/publication/8198/threat_of_global_pandemics .html.

650. Antigua KJC, Choi WS, Baek YH, Song MS. 2019. The emergence and decennary distribution of clade 2.3 4.4 HPAI H5Nx. Microorganisms. 7(6):e156. https://doi.org/10.3390/microorganisms7060156.

651. Weekly Epidemiological Record. 2005. H5N1 avian influenza: first steps towards development of a human vaccine. Weekly Epidemiological Record 80:277–8.

652. Walsh B. 2005. A wing and a prayer. Times Asia, September 19. www.time .com/time/asia/magazine/printout/0,13675,501050926-1106457,00.html.

653. Frist B. 2005. Floor statement—remarks as prepared for delivery, September 28. frist.senate.gov/index.cfm?FuseAction=Speeches.Detail&Speech_ id=291&Month=9&Year=2005.

654. Osterholm MT. 2005. Preparing for the next pandemic. Foreign Affairs 84(4). www.foreignaffairs.org/20050701faessay84402/michael-t-osterholm/preparing -for-the-next-pandemic.html.

655. World Health Organization, Department of Communicable Disease Surveillance and Response, Global Influenza Programme. 2004. Vaccines for pandemic influenza: informal meeting of WHO, influenza vaccine manufacturers,

656. Centers for Disease Control and Prevention. 2006. Update: influenza vaccine supply and recommendations for prioritization during the 1009–05 influenza season. Morbidity and Mortality Weekly Reports 54(34):850.

657. Trust for America's Health. 2005. A killer flu? healthyamericans.org/reports /flu/Flu2005.pdf.

658. Caplan A. 2006. What's really scary about bird flu. MSNBC, April 21. msnbc .msn.com/id/12411469/.

659. Lederberg J, Shope RE, Oaks SC. 1992. Emerging Infections: Microbial Threats to Health in the United States (Washington, DC: National Academies Press).

660. Osterholm M, Colwell R, Garrett L, Fauci AS. 2005. The Council on Foreign Relations meeting: the threat of global pandemics. Federal News Service, June 16. www.cfr.org/publication/8198/threat_of_global_pandemics.html.

661. Garrett L. 2005. The next pandemic? Probable cause. Foreign Affairs 84(4). www.foreignaffairs.org/20050701faessay84401/laurie-Garrett/the-next-pan demic.html.

662. Lurie N, Saville M, Hatchett R, Halton J. 2020. Developing Covid-19 vaccines at pandemic speed. N Engl J Med. [Epub ahead of print 2020 Mar 30; accessed 2020 Apr 8]. https://doi.org/10.1056/NEJMp2005630.

663. Shute N, Querna E, Bainbridge B, Brink S, Ramachandran N. 2005. Of birds and men. U.S. News and World Report 138(12):40–9.

664. Woodrow Wilson International Center for Scholars. 2005. Emerging pandemic: costs and consequences of an avian influenza outbreak. September 19. wilsoncenter.org/index.cfm?topic_id=116811&fuseaction=topics.event _summary&event_id=142787.

665. Kennedy M. 2005. Parallels with the 1918 Spanish flu outbreak. National Post, March 9.

666. Garrett L. 2005. The next pandemic? Probable cause. Foreign Affairs 84(4). www.foreignaffairs.org/20050701faessay84401/laurie-Garrett/the-next-pan demic.html.

667. Osterholm M, Colwell R, Garrett L, Fauci AS. 2005. The Council on Foreign Relations meeting: the threat of global pandemics. Federal News Service, June 16. www.cfr.org/publication/8198/threat_of_global_pandemics.html.

668. Guan Y, Chen H. 2005. Resistance to anti-influenza agents. Lancet 366: 1139–40.

669. Centers for Disease Control and Prevention. 1997. Isolation of avian influenza A(H5N1) viruses from humans—Hong Kong, May–December 1997. Morbidity and Mortality Weekly Report 46:1204–7.

670. Sipress A. 2005. Bird flu drug rendered useless; Chinese chickens given medication made for humans. Washington Post, June 18. www.washingtonpost.com /wp-dyn/content/article/2005/06/17/AR2005061701214.html.

671. Guan Y, Poon LLM, Cheung CY, et al. 2004. H5N1 influenza: a protean pandemic threat. Proceedings of the National Academy of Sciences 101:8156–61.

672. Hayden F. 2004. Pandemic influenza: is an antiviral response realistic? Pediatric Infectious Disease Journal 23:S262–9.

673. Webster RG, Kawaoka Y, Bean WJ, Beard CW, Brugh M. 1985. Chemotherapy and vaccination: a possible strategy for the control of highly virulent influenza virus. Journal of Virology 55:173–6.

674. Webster RG, Kawaoka Y, Bean WJ, Beard CW, Brugh M. 1985. Chemotherapy and vaccination: a possible strategy for the control of highly virulent influenza virus. Journal of Virology 55:173–6.

675. U.S. Food and Drug Administration. 2019 Dec 10. 2018 summary report on antimicrobials sold or distributed for use in food-producing animals. FDA; [accessed 2020 Apr 6]. https://www.fda.gov/media/133411/download.

676. Cassell GH, Mekalanos J. 2001. Development of antimicrobial agents in the era of new and reemerging infectious diseases and increasing antibiotic resistance. Journal of the American Medical Association 285:601–5.

677. Nierenberg D. 2005. Happier Meals: Rethinking the Global Meat Industry. Worldwatch Paper 171, September. www.worldwatch.org/pubs/paper/171/.

678. Nature Web. 2005. Web Focus—avian flu timeline. Nature. www.nature.com /nature/focus/avianflu/timeline.html.

679. Kaiser L, Wat C, Mills T, Mahoney P, Ward P, Hayden F. 2003. Impact of os-eltamivir treatment on influenza-related lower respiratory tract complications and hospitalizations. Arch Intern Med. 163(14):1667–1672. https://doi.org/10 .1001/archinte.163.14.1667.

680. Dyer O. 2020. What did we learn from Tamiflu? BMJ. 368:m626. https://doi .org/10.1136/bmj.m626.

681. Abbasi K. 2014. The missing data that cost $20bn. BMJ. 348:g2695. https:// doi.org/10.1136/bmj.g2695.

682. Gupta YK, Meenu M, Mohan P. 2015. The Tamiflu fiasco and lessons learnt. Indian J Pharmacol. 47(1):11–16. https://dx.doi.org/10.4103/0253-7613.150308.

683. Normile D, Enserink M. 2005. Infectious diseases: lapses worry bird flu experts. Science 308:1849–51.

684. Scholtissek C, Webster RG. 1998. Long-term stability of the anti-influenza A compounds—amantadine and rimantadine. Antiviral Research 38:213–5.

685. Scholtissek C, Webster RG. 1998. Long-term stability of the anti-influenza A compounds—amantadine and rimantadine. Antiviral Research 38:213–5.

686. Sipress A. 2005. Bird flu drug rendered useless; Chinese chickens given medication made for humans. Washington Post, June 18. www.washingtonpost.com /wp-dyn/content/article/2005/06/17/AR2005061701214.html.

687. Abbott A. 2005. Avian flu special: what's in the medicine cabinet? Nature 435:407–9. nature.com/news/2005/050523/full/435407a.html.

688. Tooley P. 2002. Drug resistance and influenza pandemics. Lancet 360:1703–4.

689. Harbrecht L. 2005. Doctoral student's research brings lessons, insight to a looming pandemic. AScribe Newswire, October 25.

690. Bor J. 2005. A versatile virus: an expert in infectious diseases explains why avian flu could trigger the next pandemic. Baltimore Sun, July 1. baltimore sun.com/news/health/bal-hs.flu01jul01,1,3742451.story?coll=bal-health -storyutil.

691. Ho S. 2005. Health experts sound alarm over avian flu. Voice of America News, September 20. www.voanews.com/english/archive/2005-09/2005-09 -20-voa45.cfm?CFID=10139428&CFTOKEN=91980581.

692. Kennedy M. 2005. Bird flu could kill millions: global pandemic warning from WHO. Gazette (Montreal), March 9, p. A1.

693. Healy B. 2005. Unprepared for bird flu. U.S. News and World Report, October 24. www.usnews.com/usnews/health/articles/051024/24healy.htm.

694. Rubinson L, Vaughn F, Nelson S, Giordano S, Kallstrom T, Buckley T, Burney T, Hupert N, Mutter R, Handrigan M, et al. 2010. Mechanical ventilators in US acute care hospitals. Disaster Med Public Health Prep. 4(3):199–206. https://doi.org/10.1001/dmp.2010.18.

695. Osterholm M, Colwell R, Garrett L, Fauci AS. 2005. The Council on Foreign Relations meeting: the threat of global pandemics. Federal News Service, June 16. www.cfr.org/publication/8198/threat_of_global_pandemics.html.

696. McNeil DG. 2006. Hospitals short on ventilators if bird flu hits. New York Times, March 12. nytimes.com/2006/03/12/national/12vent.html.?ex=11431 76400&en=2854ac45ce09a66f&ei=5070.

697. Osterholm MT. 2005. Preparing for the next pandemic. Foreign Affairs 84(4). www.foreignaffairs.org/20050701faessay84402/michael-t-osterholm/preparing -for-the-next-pandemic.html.

698. Santora M. 2005. When a bug becomes a monster; city and state prepare an overburdened system for the threat of avian flu. New York Times, August 21.

699. Institute of Medicine. A Shared Destiny: Community Effects of Uninsurance (Washington, DC: National Academies Press). fermat.nap.edu/ books/0309087260/html./R1.html.

700. Hockberger R. 2003. Even without a flu epidemic, ERs are in crisis. Los Angeles Times, December 27.

701. Reynolds G. 2004. The flu hunters. New York Times, November 7. tinyurl .com/mqy5u.

702. Hockberger R. 2003. Even without a flu epidemic, ERs are in crisis. Los Angeles Times, December 27.

703. Lauerman J. 2006. Bird-flu pandemic, even mild one, will overwhelm U.S. hospitals. Bloomberg, March 31. bloomberg.com/apps/news?pid=10000103&s id=a4LQlizkeMqo&refer=us.

704. Augustine JJ. 2019 Oct 20. The latest emergency department utilization numbers are in. ACEP Now. 38(10).

705. American Hospital Association. 2018. Trendwatch chartbook 2018. Appendix 3. Table 3.3. Washington(DC): AHA; [accessed 2020 Apr 6]. https://www .aha.org/system/files/2018-07/2018-chartbook-table-3-3.pdf.

706. Goldstein J. 2005. The next flu pandemic: Are we ready? Miami Herald, September 20, p. 10E.

707. Reynolds G. 2004. The flu hunters. New York Times, November 7. tinyurl .com/mqy5u.

708. Hayden F. 2004. Pandemic influenza: Is an antiviral response realistic? Pediatric Infectious Disease Journal 23:S262–9.

709. Democracy Now. 2005. Transcript—Mike Davis on The Monster at Our Door: The Global Threat of Avian Flu. Democracy Now. October 19. democ racynow.org/article.pl?sid=05/10/19/1332209.

710. Davis M. 2005. Avian flu: a state of unreadiness. The Nation, July 18–25, pp. 27–30.

711. Schoch-Spana M. 2001. "Hospital's full-up": the 1918 influenza pandemic. Public Health Reports 116:S32–3.

712. Fehr-Snyder K. 2005. Arizona, world may not be ready for flu outbreak. Arizona Republic, October 4. www.azcentral.com/health/news/articles /1004birdflu04.html.

713. Woodrow Wilson International Center for Scholars. 2005. Emerging pandemic: costs and consequences of an avian influenza outbreak. September 19. wilsoncenter.org/index.cfm?topic_id=116811&fuseaction=topics.event _summary&event_id=142787.

714. Balicer RD, Omer SB, Barnett DJ, Everly Jr GS. 2006. Local public health workers' perceptions toward responding to an influenza pandemic. BMC Public Health 6:99.

715. Upshur REG, et al. 2006. Stand on Guard for Thee: Ethical Considerations. In: Preparedness Planning for Pandemic Influenza (Toronto: University of Toronto Joint Centre for Bioethics Pandemic Influenza Working Group, p. 11). utoronto.ca/jcb/home/documents/pandemic.pdf.

716. Choo K. 2005. The avian flu time bomb. American Bar Association Journal, November, pp. 36–41.

717. Shute N, Querna E, Bainbridge B, Brink S, Ramachandran N. 2005. Of birds and men. U.S. News and World Report 138(12):40–9.

718. Cooper S, Coxe D. 2005. An investor's guide to Avian Flu. BMO Nesbit Burns Research, August. bmonesbittburns.com/economics/reports/20050812/avian _flu.pdf.

719. Grammaticas D. 2005. Bird flu. Is it the new BSE? Independent, August 28.

720. McMichael T. 2001. Transitions in human health: surviving this millennium by learning from the past one hundred millennia. Global Change and Human Health 2:76–7.

721. Kaneda T, Haub C. 2020 Jan 23. How many people have ever lived on earth? Washington(DC): Population Reference Bureau; [accessed 2020 Apr 7]. https://www.prb.org/howmanypeoplehaveeverlivedonearth/.

722. Garrett L. 2004. How dangerous is the bird flu? YaleGlobal, February 6. yale-global.yale.edu/display.article?id=3278.

723. Kennedy M. 2005. Flu pandemic would kill millions: warning signal clear that world set to be hit by deadly mutation: Expert. Ottawa Citizen, January 25, p. A7.

724. Hoeling AA. 1961. The Great Epidemic (Boston, MA: Little, Brown and Company).

725. Crosby AW. 2003. America's Forgotten Pandemic: The Influenza of 1918 (Cambridge, UK: Cambridge University Press).

726. Johnson RT. 2003. Emerging viral infections of the nervous system. Journal of NeuroVirology 9:140–7.

727. Lashley FR. 2004. Emerging infectious diseases: vulnerabilities, contributing factors and approaches. Expert Review of Anti-infective Therapy 2(2):299–316.

728. Wilson ME. 1995. Travel and the emergence of infectious diseases. Epidemiology and Infection 1(2):39–46.

729. Milbank D. 2005. Capitol Hill flu briefing was no trick, and no treat. Washington Post, October 13, p. A02. www.washingtonpost.com/wp-dyn/content /article/2005/10/12/AR2005101202250.html.

730. 2004. Russian expert says flu epidemic may kill over one billion this year. Moscow News, October 28. www.mosnews.com/news/2004/10/28/pandemic .shtml.

731. Humphrey HH. 2005. Stave off flu pandemic with concerted action. TwinCities .com Pioneer Press, August 11. www.twincities.com/mld/twincities/news /editorial/12351138.htm.

732. Taubenberger JK, Reid AH, Lourens RM, Wang R, Jin G, Fanning TG. Taubenberger et al. Reply. Nature 440:E9–10.

733. Frist B. 2005. Manhattan project for the 21st century. Harvard Medical School Health Care Policy Seidman Lecture, June 1. frist.senate.gov/_files /060105manhattan.pdf.

734. Branswell H. 2005. World as we know it may be at stake: UN pandemic czar. Canadian Press, October 2. cnews.canoe.ca/CNEWS/ Canada/2005/10/02/1245355-cp.html.

735. Vieth W. 2005. The health secretary is leading a drive to boost federal efforts, and funding, to prepare for a global outbreak if avian flu mutates. Los Angeles Times, October 3, p. A9.

736. Mydans S. 2005. Preparations for bird flu are urgent, Asia is warned. International Herald Tribune, October 11. www.iht.com/articles/2005/10/10/news /flu.php.

737. Specter M. 2005. Nature's bioterrorist. New Yorker, February 28, pp. 52–61.

738. Carr-Brown J. 2005. Britain prepares for bird flu death toll of thousands. The Sunday Times, August 7. timesonline.co.uk/article/0,2087 -1724318,00.html.

739. Knox N. 2005. Europe braces for avian flu. USA Today, October 9. www .usatoday.com/news/health/2005-10-09-europe-avian-flu_x.htm.

740. MacKenzie D. 2005. U.S scientists resurrect 1918 flu, study deadliness. New Scientist, October 5. www.newscientist.com/article.ns?id=dn8103.

741. Arieff I. 2005. Flu pandemic could kill 150 million, UN warns. Reuters, September 30.

742. Armstrong RE, Prior SD. 2005. Flu year's eve. Center for Technology and National Security Policy. October. www.ndu.edu/ctnsp/life_sci/FluOpEd.pdf.

743. 2005. Flu pandemic could kill half million in U.S. Report: America not prepared for large outbreak of disease. Reuters, June 24.

744. World Health Organization. 2004. World is ill-prepared for "inevitable" flu pandemic. Bulletin of the World Health Organization 82(4). who.int/bulletin /volumes/82/4/who%20news.pdf.

745. Institute of Medicine. 2005. Microbial Threats to Health: The Threat of Pandemic Influenza (Washington, DC: National Academies Press). darwin.nap.edu /books/0309097177/html./R1.html.

746. Bor J. 2005. A versatile virus: an expert in infectious diseases explains why avian flu could trigger the next pandemic. Baltimore Sun, July 1. baltimoresun.com/news/health/bal-hs.flu01jul01,1,3742451.story?coll=bal -health-storyutil.

747. Stöhr K. 2005. Interview with WHO bird flu expert: a ticking time bomb in your backyard. Spiegel, March 7. service.spiegel.de/cache/international /0,1518,345165,00.html.

748. Macmahon E. 2005. Preface. Journal of Antimicrobial Chemotherapy 55:i1.

749. Parry J. 2003. Hong Kong under WHO spotlight after flu outbreak. British Medical Journal 327:308.

750. Snowbeck C. 2005. Officials gather today in New York to discuss how to stave off a potential pandemic flu threatening millions. Worse than hurricanes? Pittsburgh Post-Gazette, September 23.

751. Ward A, Turner M. 2005. World "unprepared" for flu pandemic. Financial Times, September 19.

752. Nakashima E. 2005. Officials urge farm overhauls to avert bird flu pandemic. Washington Post, February 26, p. A16. www.washingtonpost.com/wp-dyn /articles/A54542-2005Feb25.html.

753. Honigsbaum M. 2005. On a wing and a prayer. Observer, March 20, p. 26. observer.guardian.co.uk/magazine/story/0,11913,1440214,00.html.

754. FAOSTAT. 2019. Live animals data. Food and Agriculture Organization of the United Nations; [updated 2020 Mar 4; accessed 2020 Apr 7]. http://www.fao .org/faostat/en/#data/QA.

755. Delgado C, Rosegrant M, Steinfeld H, Ehui S, Courbois C. 1999. Livestock to 2020: the next food revolution. Food, Agriculture, and the Environment Discussion Paper 28. For the International Food Policy Research Institute, the Food and Agriculture Organization of the United Nations and the International Livestock Research Institute. ifpri.org/2020/dp/dp28.pdf.

756. Fox M. 2005. Experts call for creating U.S. bird flu czar. Reuters, October 12.

757. Kazmin A. 2005. UN targets farming habits to beat bird flu. Financial Times, July 7, p. 11.

758. Food and Agriculture Organization of the United Nations News Release. 2005. Enemy at the gate: saving farms and people from bird flu. April 11. www .fao.org/newsroom/en/focus/2005/100356/.

759. 2004. Flu scientists fear massive outbreak; millions could die; Asian virus eyed. Ottawa Sun, November 18, p. 17. canoe.ca/NewsStand/OttawaSun/News /2004/11/18/719222.html.

760. Sydney Morning Herald. 2005. Tackle bird flu at its source, vet urges. Fairfax Digital, October 17. www.smh.com.au/news/health/tackle-bird-flu-at-its -source-vet-urges/2005/10/16/1129401145763.html.

761. Wire services. 2004. Flu pandemic plan might shut schools, ration drugs. St. Petersburg Times, August 26, p. 7A.

762. Nelson B. 2005. Bird flu outbreak; global threat; experts say deadly virus presents grave risk if we don't "get our act together." Newsday, March 6, p. A03.

763. 2005. Next flu pandemic due "any time," could kill 150 million. Associated Press, September 29. tinyurl.com/mucjp.

764. 2005. Human-to-human bird flu pandemic expected "in very near future." BBC Monitoring Former Soviet Union, August 3.

765. Underwood A, Adler J, Rosenberg D, Seno A. 2004. Scary strains. Newsweek 114(18):46–9.

766. Doshi P. 2006. Selling "pandemic flu" through a language of fear. Christian Science Monitor, March 21.

767. Shortridge K. 2006. H5N1 "bird flu"—some insight. New Zealand Pharmacy, April, pp. 23–7.

768. Ross E. 2004. Asia is the traditional cradle of influenza, although disease can originate anywhere. Biotech Week, February 25, p. 628.

769. Fox M. 2005. Bird flu poses "ominous" threat. Toronto Star, February 22, p. A01.

770. Potter CW. 2001. A history of influenza. Journal of Applied Microbiology 91:572–9.

771. New Zealand Ministry of Health. 2005. Influenza, avian influenza, pandemic influenza FAQ. Scoop Independent News, September 15. www.scoop.co.nz/stories /GE0509/S00077.htm.

772. Potter CW. 1998. Chronicle of influenza pandemics. In: Nicholson KG, Webster RG, Hay AJ (eds.), Textbook of Influenza (Oxford: Blackwell Science, pp. 3–18).

773. Shortridge KF. 1992. Pandemic influenza: a zoonosis? Seminars in Respiratory Infections 7:11–25.

774. Walsh B, Johnson K. 2005. Emergency measures; avian flu is on the rise in Vietnam and is now endemic in much of Asia. Can heightened vigilance keep it at bay? Time International, February 7, p. 22.

775. Chen S, Yang J, Yang W, Wang C, Bärnighausen T. 2020. COVID-19 control in China during mass population movements at New Year. Lancet 395(10226):764–766. https://doi.org/10.1016/S0140-6736(20)30421-9.

776. Mittelstadt M. 2005. Experts: Bird flu plan needs work. The Dallas Morning News, October 5. dallasnews.com/sharedcontent/dws/news/washington/mmit telstadt/stories/100605dnnatbirdflu.17794709.html.

777. Marx PA, Apetrei C, Drucker E. 2004. AIDS as a zoonosis? Confusion over the origin of the virus and the origin of the epidemics. Journal of Medical Primatology 33:220–6.

778. Enserink M. 2004. Tiptoeing around Pandora's box. Science 306:594–5.

779. Enserink M. 2004. Tiptoeing around Pandora's box. Science 306:594–5.

780. Enserink M. 2004. Tiptoeing around Pandora's box. Science 306:594–5.

781. Branswell H. 2005. Entry controls won't stop spread of pandemic flu or SARS, study shows. Canadian Press, September 24.

782. Sample I. 2005. How much notice will we get of a flu pandemic? Guardian, January 27, Science Pages, p. 3.

783. Ross B. 2005. Avian flu: is the government ready for an epidemic? Virus poses risk of massive casualties around the world. ABC News Primetime, September 15. abcnews.go.com/Primetime/Investigation/story?id =1130392&page=1.

784. 2005. Scientists stockpile bird flu drugs. The Age, September 23. theage .com.au/news/National/Scientists-stockpile-bird-flu-drugs/2005/09/23 /1126982206794.html.

785. McKie R, Revill J, Aglionby J, Watts J. 2004. Warning as bird flu crossover

danger escalates. Observer, December 12. observer.guardian.co.uk/international /story/0,6903,1371917,00.html.

786. Goetz T. 2006. The battle to stop bird flu. Wired, January, p. 111–5.

787. Phillips H, Killingray D. 2003. Introduction. In: Phillips H, Killingray D (eds.), The Spanish Influenza Pandemic of 1918–19: New Perspectives (London, UK: Routledge, pp. 1–26).

788. Drexler M. 2002. Secret Agents: The Menace of Emerging Infections (Washington, DC: Joseph Henry Press).

789. World Health Organization. 2020 Mar 31. Coronavirus disease 2019 (COVID-19) situation report—71. Geneva: WHO; [accessed 2020 Apr 6]. https://www .who.int/docs/default-source/coronaviruse/situation-reports/20200331-sitrep -71-covid-19.pdf.

790. Kennedy M. 2005. No way of knowing effectiveness of pandemic plan until outbreak hits. Vancouver Sun, March 11, p. A4.

791. Reid AH, Taubenberger JK, Fanning TG. 2001. The 1918 Spanish influenza: Integrating history and biology. Microbes and Infection 3:81–87.

792. Lee PJ, Krilov LR. 2005. When animal viruses attack: SARS and avian influenza. Pediatric Annals 34(1):43–52.

793. Lee PJ, Krilov LR. 2005. When animal viruses attack: SARS and avian influenza. Pediatric Annals 34(1):43–52.

794. Osterholm MT. 2005. Preparing for the next pandemic. Foreign Affairs 84(4). www.foreignaffairs.org/20050701faessay84402/michael-t-osterholm/preparing -for-the-next-pandemic.html.

795. MacKenzie JS, Drury P, Ellis A., et al. 2004. The WHO Response to SARS and preparations for the future. In: Knobler S, Mahmoud A, Lemon S, Mack A, Sivitz L, Oberholtzer K (eds.), Learning from SARS, Preparing for the Next Disease Outbreak, Workshop Summary (Washington, DC: National Academies Press, pp. 42–9).

796. Osterholm MT. 2005. Preparing for the next pandemic. Foreign Affairs 84(4). www.foreignaffairs.org/20050701faessay84402/michael-t-osterholm/preparing -for-the-next-pandemic.html.

797. Oxford JS. 2005. Preparing for the first influenza pandemic of the 21st century. Lancet Infectious Diseases 5:129–31.

798. 2005. Massive flu outbreak could happen at any moment, WHO warns. Today online, July 23. todayonline.com/articles/62928.asp.

799. Garrett L. 2005. The next pandemic? Probable cause. Foreign Affairs 84(4). www.foreignaffairs.org/20050701faessay84401/laurie-Garrett/the-next -pandemic.html.

800. Ross B. 2005. Avian flu: is the government ready for an epidemic? Virus poses risk of massive casualties around the world. ABC News Primetime, September 15. abcnews.go.com/Primetime/Investigation/story?id=1130392&page=1.

801. World Health Organization. 2005. WHO global influenza preparedness plan. The role of WHO and recommendations for national measures before and during pandemics. www.who.int/csr/resources/publications/influenza/GIP _2005_5Eweb.pdf.

802. Sternberg S. 2005. Imagine what would happen if a Category 5 viral storm hit every state. USA Today, November 10, p. 1A. www.usatoday.com/printedition /news/20051011/1a_cover11.art.htm.

803. Mena K. 2020 Mar 28. Cuomo on possible New York quarantine: 'I don't think it's legal' and it would be a 'federal declaration of war.' CNN. [accessed 2020 Apr 12]. https://www.cnn.com/2020/03/28/politics/cuomo-ny-quarantine -cnntv/index.html.

804. Emerson. 1917 Some practical considerations. American Journal of Medical Sciences 153: 170 as cited in Fee E, Fox DM (eds.), 1988. AIDS: The Burdens of History (Berkeley: University of California Press) ark.cdlib.org/ark:/13030 /ft7t1nb59n/.

805. Risse GB. 1988. Epidemics and history: ecological perspectives and social responses. In: Fee E, Fox DM (eds.), AIDS: The Burdens of History (Berkeley, CA: University of California Press, pp. 33–66).

806. Sternberg S. 2005. Imagine what would happen if a Category 5 viral storm hit every state. USA Today, November 10, p. 1A. www.usatoday.com/printedition /news/20051011/1a_cover11.art.htm.

807. CBC News. 2005. Bush wants military to keep order in bird flu pandemic scenario. October 4. cbc.ca/story/world/national/2005/10/04/Bush-Pandemic 1004.html.

808. Orent W. 2005. The fear contagion: a flu quarantine? No, sir. Washington Post, October 16, p. B01. washingtonpost.com/wp-dyn/content/article/2005/10/15 /AR2005101500102_pf.html.

809. Laver WG, Garman E. 2001. The origin and control of pandemic influenza. Science 293:1776–7.

810. Orent W. 2005. The fear contagion: a flu quarantine? No, sir. Washington Post, October 16, p. B01. washingtonpost.com/wp-dyn/content/article/2005 /10/15/AR2005101500102_pf.html.

811. Fox M. 2005. Experts call for creating U.S. bird flu czar. Boston Globe. October 12. tinyurl.com/roy8g.

812. Orent W. 2005. The fear contagion: a flu quarantine? No, sir. Washington Post, October 16, p. B01. washingtonpost.com/wp-dyn/content/article/2005 /10/15/AR2005101500102_pf.html.

813. Reynolds J. 2005. Bird flu: 20% of globe may be hit. Scotsman, May 26, p. 31. news.scotsman.com/international.cfm?id=573902005.

814. Garrett L. 2005. The next pandemic? Probable cause. Foreign Affairs 84(4). www.foreignaffairs.org/20050701faessay84401/laurie-Garrett/the-next -pandemic.html.

815. Oxford J, Balasingam S, Lambkin R. 2004. A new millennium conundrum: How to use a powerful class of influenza anti-neuraminidase drugs (NAIs) in the community. Journal of Antimicrobial Chemotherapy 53:133–6.

816. Bhattacharya S. 2003. Airports scan for SARS victims' flushed faces. New Scientists, April 24. www.newscientist.com/article/dn3656.html.

817. Bridges CB, Kuehnert MJ, Hall CB. Transmission of influenza: implications for control in health care settings. Clinical Infectious Diseases 37:1094–101.

818. De Gennaro N. 2005. Avian flu pandemic real threat, says national expert. Daily News Journal, October 8. dnj.midsouthnews.com/apps/pbcs.dll/article? AID=/20051008/LIFESTYLE/510080316/1024.

819. Bridges CB, Kuehnert MJ, Hall CB. Transmission of influenza: implications for control in health care settings. Clinical Infectious Diseases 37:1094–101.

820. 2006. Bird flu: the untold story. Oprah Winfrey Show, January 24.

821. Goldmann DA. 2001. Epidemiology and prevention of pediatric viral respiratory infections in health-care institutions. Emerging Infectious Diseases 7:249–53.

822. Hammond GW, Raddatz RL, Gelskey DE. 1989. Impact of atmospheric dispersion and transport of viral aerosols on the epidemiology of influenza. Reviews of Infectious Diseases 11:494–7.

823. Annas GJ. 2005. Bush's risky flu pandemic plan. Boston Globe, October 8. boston.com/news/globe/editorial_opinion/oped/articles/2005/10/08/bushs _risky_flu_pandemic_plan/.

824. Lederberg J, Shope RE, Oaks SC. 1992. Emerging Infections: Microbial Threats to Health in the United States (Washington, DC: National Academies Press).

825. Loven J. 2005. Bush considers military role in flu fight. Associated Press, October 4.

826. Cowen T. 2005. Avian flu: what should be done. Mercatus Center at George Mason University: Working Paper Series, November 11.

827. 2005. Bush: military may have to help if bird flu breaks out. CNN, October 5. cnn.com/2005/POLITICS/10/04/bush.avianflu/index.html.

828. 2005. Bush military bird flu role slammed. CNN, October 5. edition.cnn.com /2005/POLITICS/10/05/bush.reax/.

829. 2005. They knew what to expect. Reuters, September 2.

830. Editorial. 2005. What will happen if the flu comes to a bird near you? USA Today, November 1. www.usatoday.com/news/opinion/editorials/2005-11-01 -bird-flu-edit_x.htm.

831. Arnst C. 2005. A hot zone in the heartland. Little could be done to contain a deadly avian flu outbreak. Business Week, September 19. businessweek.com /magazine/content/05_38/b3951008.htm.

832. Milbank D. 2005. Colonel finally saw whites of their eyes. Washington Post, October 20, p. A04. washingtonpost.com/wp-dyn/content/article/2005/10/19 /AR2005101902246.html.

833. Najera JA. 1989. Malaria and the work of the WHO. Bulletin of the World Health Organization 67:229–43.

834. Crawford D. 2000. The Invisible Enemy: A Natural History of Viruses (New York, NY: Oxford University Press).

835. Davis RJ, Lederberg J (eds.), 2001. Emerging Infectious Diseases from the Global to the Local Perspective: A Summary of a Workshop of the Forum of Emerging Infections (Washington, DC: National Academies Press). darwin.nap .edu/books/0309071844/html./.

836. Selgelid MJ. 2005. Ethics and infectious disease. Bioethics 19(3):272–89. www .blackwell-synergy.com/doi/abs/10.1111/j.1467-8519.2005.00441.x.

837. Burnet M, White DO. 1962. Natural History of Infectious Disease, 4th Edition (Cambridge, UK: Cambridge University Press).

838. Davis RJ, Lederberg J (eds.), 2001. Emerging Infectious Diseases from the Global to the Local Perspective: A Summary of a Workshop of the Forum of Emerging Infections (Washington, DC: National Academies Press). darwin. nap.edu/books/0309071844/html./.

839. Davis RJ, Lederberg J (eds.), 2001. Emerging Infectious Diseases from the Global to the Local Perspective: A Summary of a Workshop of the Forum of Emerging Infections (Washington, DC: National Academies Press). darwin .nap.edu/books/0309071844/html./.

840. Selgelid MJ. 2005. Ethics and infectious disease. Bioethics 19(3):272–89. www .blackwell-synergy.com/doi/abs/10.1111/j.1467-8519.2005.00441.x.

841. Davis RJ, Lederberg J (eds.), 2001. Emerging Infectious Diseases from the Global to the Local Perspective: A Summary of a Workshop of the Forum of Emerging Infections (Washington, DC: National Academies Press). darwin. nap.edu/books/0309071844/html./.

842. World Health Organization. 1996. The World Health Report 1996: Fighting disease, Fostering development (Geneva, Switzerland: WHO). www.who.int/ whr/1996/en/.

843. Liu L, Oza S, Hogan D, Chu Y, Perin J, Zhu J, Lawn JE, Cousens S, Mathers C, Black RE. 2016. Global, regional, and national causes of under-5 mortality in 2000–15: an updated systematic analysis with implications for the Sustainable Development Goals. Lancet. 388(10063):3027–3035. https://doi.org/10 .1016/S0140-6736(16)31593-8.

844. Laurance J. 2004. New diseases pose threat to world health. Independent, January 14. www.findarticles.com/p/articles/mi_qn4158/is_20040114/ai _n9687521.

845. Cookson C. 1993. Bugs that come to plague us: the renewed war against disease. Financial Times (London, UK), August 21.

846. Gill JM, Rechtschaffen JA, Rubenstein LR. 2000. Expect the unexpected: the West Nile virus wake up call. Report of the Minority Staff, Senate Governmental Affairs Committee, July 24. www.senate.gov/~gov_affairs/wnvfinalreport.pdf.

847. Cohen FL, Larson E. 1996. Emerging infectious diseases: nursing responses. Nursing Outlook 44:164–8.

848. Crosby AW. 2003. America's Forgotten Pandemic: The Influenza of 1918 (Cambridge, UK: Cambridge University Press).

849. Hayes R. 1992. The modern plagues. Palm Beach Post, October 23, p. 1D.

850. Brown C. 2000. Emerging infectious diseases of animals: an overview. In: Brown C, Bolin C (eds.), Emerging Diseases of Animals (Washington, DC: ASM Press, pp. 1–12).

851. Pubmed keyword search for Communicable Diseases, Emerging/ limited to prior to 2012 compared to 2012–2020. Accessed April 1, 2020.

852. Brown C. 2000. Emerging infectious diseases of animals: an overview. In: Brown C, Bolin C (eds.), Emerging Diseases of Animals (Washington, DC: ASM Press, pp. 1–12)

853. National Agricultural Research, Extension, Education, and Economics. 2004. Protecting Our Food System from Current and Emerging Animal and Plant Diseases and Pathogens: Implications for Research, Education, Extension, and Economics. NAREEE Advisory Board Meeting and Focus Session, Washington Court Hotel, 525 New Jersey Ave., N.W., Washington, DC, October 27–29.

854. Epstein PR, Chivian E, Frith K. 2003. Emerging diseases threaten conservation. Environmental Health Perspectives 111(10):A506.

855. Woolhouse MEJ. 2002. Population biology of emerging and re-emerging pathogens. Trends in Microbiology 10:S3–7.

856. Murphy FA. 1999. Emerging zoonoses. Emerging Infectious Diseases 4(3):429–35.

857. Wain-Hobson S, Meyerhans A. 1999. On viral epidemics, zoonoses and memory. Trends in Microbiology 7:389–91.

858. Mantovani A. 2001. Notes on the development of the concept of zoonoses. WHO Mediterranean Zoonoses Control Centre Information Circular 51. www.mzcp-zoonoses.gr/pdf.en/circ_51.pdf.

859. Taylor LH, Latham SM, Woolhouse MEJ. 2001. Risk factors for human disease emergence. Philosophical Transactions of the Royal Society of London, Series B 356:983–9.

860. Wolfe DN, Eitel MN, Gockowski J, et al. 2000. Deforestation, hunting and the ecology of microbial emergence. Global Change and Human Health 1:10–25.

861. Clough JD. 2004. Birds, viruses, and history: the current "genuine adventure." Cleveland Clinical Journal of Medicine 71:270.

862. Mayo Clinic staff. 2005. Bird flu (avian influenza). Infectious Disease Center, August 10. ads.mayoclinic.com/health/bird-flu/DS00566/DSECTION=7.

863. Torrey EF, Yolken RH. 2005. Their bugs are worse than their bite. Washington Post, April 3, p. B01.

864. Editorial. 2004. Avian influenza: the threat looms. Lancet 363(9405):257.

865. 2005. Frequently Asked Questions about Med-Vet-Net. Network for the Prevention and Control of Zoonoses, March 23. edvetnet.org/cms/templates/doc .php?id=18.

866. McKenna MAJ. 2004. Animal diseases threaten humans. Cox News Service, March 2.

867. Lederberg J, Shope RE, Oaks SC. 1992. Emerging Infections: Microbial Threats to Health in the United States (Washington, DC: National Academies Press).

868. World Health Organization, Food and Agricultural Organization of the United Nations, and World Organization for Animal Health. 2004. Report of the WHO/FAO/OIE joint consultation on emerging zoonotic diseases. At whqlibdoc .who.int/hq/2004/WHO_CDS_CPE_ZFK_2004.9.pdf.

869. Morse SS. 1997. The public health threat of emerging viral disease. Journal of Nutrition 127:951S-56S.

870. Voigt K. 2005. What ails Asia. Wall Street Journal, April 22.

871. Beran GW, Steele JH. 1994. Handbook of Zoonoses (London, UK: CRC Press).

872. Calvert S, Kohn D. 2005. Out of Africa: a baffling variety of diseases. Baltimore Sun, May 15, p. 4A.

873. Calvert S, Kohn D. 2005. Out of Africa: a baffling variety of diseases. Baltimore Sun, May 15, p. 4A.

874. Benenson AS (ed.), 1990. Control of Communicable Diseases in Man, 15th Edition (Washington, DC: American Public Health Association).

875. Torrey EF, Yolken RH. 2005. Beasts of the Earth: Animals, Humans, and Disease (New Brunswick, NJ: Rutgers University Press).

876. Fox N. 1997. Spoiled: The Dangerous Truth about a Food Chain Gone Haywire (New York, NY: Basic Books).

877. Lubroth J. 2005. Regional and global challenges of the avian influenza outbreaks in Asia and FAO's prospective. World's Poultry Science Journal 61:55–6.

878. Torrey EF, Yolken RH. 2005. Beasts of the Earth: Animals, Humans, and Disease (New Brunswick, NJ: Rutgers University Press).

879. Weber DJ, Rutala WA. 1999. Zoonotic infections. Occupational Medicine: State of the Art Reviews 14(2):247–84.

880. Epstein PR, Chivian E, Frith K. 2003. Emerging diseases threaten conservation. Environmental Health Perspectives 111(10):A506–7.

881. Ritvo H. 2004. Animal planet. Environmental History 9(2):204. www.history cooperative.org/journals/eh/9.2/index.html.

882. Torrey EF, Yolken RH. 2005. Their bugs are worse than their bite. Washington Post, April 3, p. B01.

883. Dubos R, Dubos J. 1952. The White Plague: Tuberculosis, Man and Society (Boston, MA: Little, Brown, p. 8).

884. Espinosa de los Monteros LE, Galán JC, Gutierrez M, et al. 1998. Allele-specific PCR method based on pncA and oxyR sequences for distinguishing Mycobacterium bovis from Mycobacterium tuberculosis: Intraspecific M. bovis pncA sequence polymorphism. Journal of Clinical Microbiology 36:239–42.

885. Torrey EF, Yolken RH. 2005. Their bugs are worse than their bite. Washington Post, April 3, p. B01.

886. World Health Organization. 2019. Global Health Observatory data. How many TB cases and deaths are there? Geneva: WHO; [accessed 2020 Apr 6]. https://www.who.int/gho/tb/epidemic/cases_deaths/en/.

887. World Health Organization. 2000. Tuberculosis, fact sheet 104, April. www.who.int/mediacentre/factsheets/fs104/en/.

888. Waddington K. 2002. Safe meat and healthy animals: BSE and bovine TB. History and Policy, Cambridge University. www.historyandpolicy.org/archive/policy-paper-04.html.

889. Collins CH. 2000. The bovine tubercle bacillus. British Journal of Biomedical Science 57:234–40.

890. Scott C, Cavanaugh JS, Pratt R, Silk BJ, LoBue P, Moonan PK. 2016. Human tuberculosis caused by Mycobacterium bovis in the United States, 2006–2013. Clin Infect Dis. 63(5):594–601. https://doi.org/10.1093/cid/ciw371.

891. Dankner WM, Davis CE. 2000. Mycobacterium bovis as a significant cause of

tuberculosis in children residing along the United States–Mexico border in the Baja California region. Pediatrics 105:E79–83.

892. Weiss RA. 2001. The Leeuwenhoek Lecture 2001. Animal origins of human infectious disease. Philos Trans R Soc Lond B Biol Sci. 356(1410):957–977. https://dx.doi.org/10.1098%2Frstb.2001.0838.

893. Daszak P, Cunningham AA. 2002. Emerging infectious diseases: a key role for conservation medicine. In: Aguirre AA, Ostfeld RS, Tabor GM, House C, Pearl MC (eds.), Conservation Medicine: Ecological Health in Practice (New York, NY: Oxford University Press, pp. 40–61).

894. Torrey EF, Yolken RH. 2005. Their bugs are worse than their bite. Washington Post, April 3, p. B01.

895. Diamond J. 1992. The arrow of disease. Discover, October 13(10):64–73.

896. Gubser C, Hué S, Kellam P, Smith GL. 2004. Poxvirus genomes: a phylogenetic analysis. J Gen Virol. 85(Pt 1):105–117. https://doi.org/10.1099/vir.0.19565-0.

897. Torrey EF, Yolken RH. 2005 Apr 3. Their bugs are worse than their bite. Washington Post. p. B01.

898. Shortridge KF. 2003. Severe acute respiratory syndrome and influenza: virus incursions from southern China. Am J Respir Crit Care Med. 168(12):1416–1420. https://doi.org/10.1164/rccm.2310005.

899. McMichael T. 2001. Human Frontiers, Environments and Disease (Cambridge, UK: Cambridge University Press).

900. McMichael T. 2001. Human Frontiers, Environments and Disease (Cambridge, UK: Cambridge University Press).

901. Rodrigo MJ, Dopazo J. 1995. Evolutionary analysis of the Picornavirus family. Journal of Molecular Evolution 40:362–71 as cited in Torrey EF, Yolken RH. 2005. Beasts of the Earth: Animals, Humans, and Disease (New Brunswick, NJ: Rutgers University Press, p. 50).

902. McMichael T. 2001. Human Frontiers, Environments and Disease (Cambridge, UK: Cambridge University Press).

903. De Groote D, Ducatelle R, Haesebrouck F. 2000. Helicobacters of possible zoonotic origin: a review. Acta Gastro-Enterologica Belgica 63:380–7.

904. Suerbaum S, Michetti P. 2002. Helicobacter pylori infection. New England Journal of Medicine 347:1175–86 as cited in Torrey EF, Yolken RH. 2005. Beasts of the Earth: Animals, Humans, and Disease (New Brunswick, NJ: Rutgers University Press, p. 40).

905. Centers for Disease Control and Prevention National Center for Infectious Diseases/Division of Bacterial and Mycotic Diseases. 2005.Helicobacter pylori Infections (H. pylori). October 12. www.cdc.gov/ncidod/dbmd/diseaseinfo/hpylori_t.htm.

906. Dore MP, Sepulveda AR, El-Zimaity H., et al. 2001. Isolation of Helicobacter pylori from sheep-implications for transmission to humans. American Journal of Gastroenterology 96(5):1396–401.

907. American Heritage Dictionaries (ed.), 2004. The American Heritage Dictionary of the English Language, 4th Edition (Boston, MA: Houghton Mifflin).

908. De Groote D, Ducatelle R, Haesebrouck F. 2000. Helicobacters of possible zoonotic origin: a review. Acta Gastro-Enterologica Belgica 63:380–7.

909. Yoo D, Willson P, Pei Y, et al. 2001. Prevalence of hepatitis E virus antibodies in Canadian swine herds and identification of a novel variant of swine hepatitis E virus. Clinical and Diagnostic Laboratory Immunology 8:1213–9.

910. Sooryanarain H, Heffron CL, Hill DE, Fredericks J, Rosenthal BM, Werre SR, Opriessnig T, Meng XJ. 2020. Hepatitis E virus in pigs from slaughterhouses, United States, 2017–2019. Emerg Infect Dis. 26(2):354–357. https://doi.org /10.3201/eid2602.191348.

911. Tei S, Kitajima N, Takahashi K, Mishiro S. 2003. Zoonotic transmission of hepatitis E virus from deer to human beings. Lancet 362:371–3.

912. Yoo D, Willson P, Pei Y, et al. 2001. Prevalence of hepatitis E virus antibodies in Canadian swine herds and identification of a novel variant of swine hepatitis E virus. Clinical and Diagnostic Laboratory Immunology 8:1213–9.

913. Darwin C. 1839. Chapter XIX: Australia. The Voyage of the Beagle. darwin .thefreelibrary.com/The-Voyage-of-the-Beagle/19-1.

914. Diamond J. 1997. Guns, Germs and Steel: The Fates of Human Societies (New York, NY: Norton and Company).

915. Diamond J. 1997. Guns, Germs and Steel: The Fates of Human Societies (New York, NY: Norton and Company).

916. Diamond J. 1992. The arrow of disease. Discover, October 13(10):64–73.

917. Armelagos GJ, Barnes KC, Lin J. 1996. Disease in human evolution: the re-emergence of infectious disease in the third epidemiological transition. National Museum of Natural History Bulletin for Teachers 18(3).

918. National Agricultural Research, Extension, Education, and Economics. 2004. Protecting Our Food System from Current and Emerging Animal and Plant Diseases and Pathogens: Implications for Research, Education, Extension, and Economics. NAREEE Advisory Board Meeting and Focus Session, Washington Court Hotel, 525 New Jersey Ave., N.W., Washington, DC, October 27–29.

919. Centers for Disease Control and Prevention. 2006. National Center for Chronic Disease Prevention and Health Promotion. Chronic disease prevention. March 17. www.cdc.gov/nccdphp/.

920. World Health Organization. Facts related to chronic diseases. who.int/dietphysi calactivity/publications/facts/chronic/en/index.html.

921. World Health Organization. 2003. Diet, Nutrition and The Prevention of Chronic Diseases (Geneva: World Health Organization). www.who.int/hpr/NPH /docs/who_fao_expert_report.pdf.

922. Armelagos GJ, Barnes KC, Lin J. 1996. Disease in human evolution: the re-emergence of infectious disease in the third epidemiological transition. National Museum of Natural History Bulletin for Teachers 18(3).

923. Glasser RJ. 2004. We are not immune: influenza, SARS, and the collapse of public health. Harper's Magazine, July. www.harpers.org/WeAreNotImmune .html.

924. Weinhold B. 2004. Infectious disease: the human costs of our environmental errors Environmental Health Perspectives 112(1).

925. 2004. Animal diseases "threaten humans." BBC News, January 13.

926. Walters MJ. 2003. Six Modern Plagues and How We are Causing Them (Washington, DC: Island Press).

927. Kelly W. 1987. Pogo: We Have Met the Enemy and He Is Us (New York, NY: Simon & Schuster).

928. McMichael AJ. 2004. Environmental and social influences on emerging infectious diseases: past, present, and future. Philosophical Transactions of the Royal Society of London 359:1049–58.

929. Drexler M. 2002. Secret Agents: The Menace of Emerging Infections (Washington, DC: Joseph Henry Press).

930. Cooper S. 2006 (How to stop) The next killer flu. Seed Magazine, February–March.

931. Fleck F. 2004. Experts urge action to stop animal diseases infecting humans. British Medical Journal 328(7449):1158.

932. World Health Organization Department of Communicable Disease Surveillance. 1999. Future trends in veterinary public health. Weekly Epidemiological Record 74(19):154–6. www.who.int/docstore/wer/pdf./1999/wer7419.pdf.

933. Rohr JR, Barrett CB, Civitello DJ, Craft ME, Delius B, DeLeo GA, Hudson PJ, Jouanard N, Nguyen KH, Ostfeld RS, et al. 2019. Emerging human infectious diseases and the links to global food production. Nat Sustain. 2(6):445–456. https://doi.org/10.1038/s41893-019-0293-3.

934. Schrag S, Wiener P. 1995. Emerging infectious disease: What are the relative roles of ecology and evolution? Trends in Ecology and Evolution 10(8):319–324.

935. Aldo Leopold Nature Center. Who was Aldo Leopold. naturenet.com/alnc/aldo.html.

936. Friend M, McLean RG, Dein FJ. 2001. Disease emergence in birds: Challenges for the twenty-first century. The Auk 118:290–303.

937. Pimm SL, Ayres M, Balmford A, et al. 2001. Can we defy nature's end? Science 293(5538):2207–8. www.sciencemag.org/cgi/content/summary/293/5538/2207?ck=nck.

938. FAO Newsroom. 2005. Cattle ranching is encroaching on forests in Latin America. Food and Agriculture Organization of the United Nations. June 8. fao.org/newsroom/en/news/2005/102924/.

939. World Resources Institute. 1998–99. Land conversion. Environmental Change and Human Health. population.wri.org/pubs_content_text.cfm?ContentID=1322.

940. Patz JA, Wolfe ND. 2002. Global ecological change and human health. In: Aguirre AA, Ostfeld RS, Tabor GM, House C, Pearl MC (eds.), Conservation Medicine: Ecological Health in Practice (New York, NY: Oxford University Press, pp. 167–181).

941. Arzt J, White WR, Thomsen BV, Brown CC. 2010. Agricultural diseases on the move early in the third millennium. Vet Pathol. 47(1):15–27. https://doi.org/10.1177/0300985809354350.

942. Taylor D. 1997. Seeing the forests for more than the trees. Environ Health Perspect. 105(11):1186–1191.

943. Chakraborty S, Andrade FCD, Ghosh S, Uelmen J, Ruiz MO. 2019. Historical expansion of Kyasanur forest disease in India from 1957 to 2017: a retrospective analysis. GeoHealth. 3(2):44–55. https://doi.org/10.1029/2018GH000164.

944. Hoff B, Smith C III. 2000. Mapping Epidemics: a Historical Atlas of Disease (New York, NY: Grolier Publishing).

945. Wattam R. 2004. Junin virus. Pathogen Portal Web Project. May 11. pathport.vbi.vt.edu/pathinfo/pathogens/Junin_virus.html.

946. Guenno BL. 1997. Haemorrhagic fevers and ecological perturbations. Archives of Virology 13:A191–9.

947. Cohen FL, Larson E. 1996. Emerging infectious diseases: nursing responses. Nursing Outlook 44:164–8.

948. Guenno BL. 1997. Haemorrhagic fevers and ecological perturbations. Archives of Virology 13:A191–9.

949. Cullington BJ. 1990. Emerging viruses, emerging threat. Science 247:279–80.

950. Cullington BJ. 1990. Emerging viruses, emerging threat. Science 247:279–80.

951. 2005. Dryden's Grant Information. Washington and Jefferson College. Tick-borne disease research. www.washjeff.edu/tickresearch/.

952. National Institute of Allergy and Infectious Diseases. 2000. Lyme disease vaccine: preventing an emerging disease January 13. niaid.nih.gov/publications/discovery/lyme.htm.

953. Cowley G, Underwood A. 2003. How progress makes us sick. Newsweek, May 5, p. 33.

954. Walters MJ. 2003. Six Modern Plagues and How We Are Causing Them (Washington, DC: Island Press).

955. Avasthi A. 2004. Bush-meat trade breeds new HIV. New Scientist, August. www.newscientist.com/article.ns?id=dn6239.

956. Rose AL. 1996. The African great ape bushmeat crisis. Pan Africa News 3(2):1–6.

957. Rose, AL. 1998. Growing commerce in bushmeat destroys great apes and threatens humanity. African Primates 3:6–10.

958. Walsh PD, Abernethy KA, Bermejo M, et al. 2003. Catastrophic ape decline in western equatorial Africa. Nature 422:611–614.

959. Fox M. 2000. The killer out of Africa. Hobart Mercury (Australia), February 9.

960. Karpowicz P, Cohen CB, van der Kooy D. 2004. Is it ethical to transplant human stem cells into nonhuman embryos? Nature Medicine 10(4):331–5.

961. Gunter C, Dhand R. 2005. The chimpanzee genome. Nature 437(7055):47.

962. Lovgren S. 2005. Chimps, humans 96 percent the same, gene study finds. National Geographic News, August 31. news.nationalgeographic.com/news/2005/08/0831_050831_chimp_genes.html.

963. Karesh WB, Cook RA, Bennett EL, Newcomb J. 2005. Wildlife trade and global disease emergence. Emerging Infectious Diseases 11(7). cdc.gov/ncidod/EID/vol11no07/05-0194.htm.

964. Drexler M. 2002. Secret Agents: The Menace of Emerging Infections (Washington, DC: Joseph Henry Press).

965. National AIDS Trust. 2005. Global statistics. Fact sheet. www.worldaidsday .org/files/stats_global_2005.doc.

966. Hahn BH, Shaw GM, De Cock KM, Sharp PM. 2000. AIDS as a zoonosis: scientific and public health implications. Science 287:607–14.

967. Laurance J. 2004. New diseases pose threat to world health. Independent, January 14. www.findarticles.com/p/articles/mi_qn4158/is_20040114/ai _n9687521.

968. World Health Organization. 2020. Global Health Observatory (GHO) data. Geneva: WHO; [accessed 2020 Apr 7]. https://www.who.int/gho/hiv/en/.

969. Wolfe ND, Switzer WM, Carr JK, et al. 2004. Naturally acquired simian retrovirus infections in central African hunters. Lancet 363(9413):932–7.

970. Hawkes N. 2004. Monkey virus found in man "may lead to new epidemic." Times Online, March 19. www.timesonline.co.uk/article/0,8122-1043946,00.html.

971. Wolfe ND, Switzer WM, Carr JK, et al. 2004. Naturally acquired simian ret- rovirus infections in central African hunters. Lancet 363(9413):932–7. jhsph .edu/cameroon/documents/Papers/Wolfe2.pdf.

972. Peeters M. 2004. Cross-species transmissions of simian retroviruses in Africa and risk for human health. Lancet 363(9413):9111–2.

973. Meslin FX, Stöhr K, Heymann D. 2000. Public health implications of emerg- ing zoonoses. Revue Scientifique et Technique Office International des Epizo- oties 19(1):310–7.

974. Preston R. 1994. The Hot Zone: A Terrifying True Story (New York, NY: Random House).

975. 2004. The American Heritage Dictionary of the English Language, 4th Edition (Boston, MA: Houghton Mifflin).

976. Van Loon J. 2000. Parasite politics: on the significance of symbiosis and as- semblage in theorizing community formations. In: Pierson C, Tormey S (eds.), Politics at the Edge (London, UK: Political Studies Association).

977. Ryan F. 1997. Virus X: Tracking the New Killer Plagues—Out of the Present and and Into the Future (Boston, MA: Little, Brown and Company).

978. Ryan F. 1997. Virus X: Tracking the New Killer Plagues—Out of the Present and and Into the Future (Boston, MA: Little, Brown and Company).

979. Villarreal LP, Defilippis VR, Gottlieb KA. 2000. Acute and persistent viral life strategies and their relationship to emerging diseases. Virology 272:1–6.

980. Merriam-Webster Inc. 2006. Simian. Merriam-Webster Online Dictionary. www.m-w.com/dictionary/simian.

981. Peeters M, Courgnaud V, Abela B, et al. 2002. Risk to human health from a plethora of simian immunodeficiency viruses in primate bushmeat. Emerging Infectious Diseases 8(5) cdc.gov/ncidod/eid/vol8no5/01-0522.htm.

982. O'Rourke LG. 2000. Xenotransplantation. In: Brown C, Bolin C (eds.), Emerging Diseases of Animals (Washington, DC: ASM Press, pp. 59–84).

983. Hahn BH, Shaw GM, De Cock KM, Sharp PM. 2000. AIDS as a zoonosis: scientific and public health implications. Science 287:607–14.

984. Kida H. Hokkaido University Research Center for Zoonosis Control. Director's Message. hokudai.ac.jp/czc/message/index-e.html.

985. Fa JE, Peres CA, Meeuwig JJ. 2002. Bushmeat exploitation in tropical forests: an intercontinental comparison. Conserv Biol. 16(1):232–237.

986. Karesh W, Cook RA. 2005. The human-animal link. Foreign Affairs 84(4):38–50.

987. Bell D, Roberton S, Hunter PR. 2004. Animal origins of SARS coronavirus: Possible links with the international trade in small carnivores. Philosophical Transactions of the Royal Society of London. Series B: Biological Sciences 359(1447):1107–14.

988. Chen H, Deng G, Li Z, et al. 2004. The evolution of H5N1 influenza viruses in ducks in southern China. Proceedings of the National Academy of Sciences of the United States of America 101(28):10452–7.

989. Jun Y. 2004. Are wild animals safe? China Daily, November 12. www.china .org.cn/english/environment/111979.htm.

990. Bray M. 2005. Unhealthy mix of animals, humans. CNN.com International. May 9. edition.cnn.com/2005/WORLD/asiapcf/05/03/eyeonchina.virus/.

991. Lynch DJ. 2003. Wild animal markets in China may be breeding SARS. USA Today, October 28.

992. Lawrie M. 2004. Animal welfare gains from avian influenza? Australian Veterinary Journal 82:135.

993. Brummitt C. 2004. Indonesians enjoy civet-dropping coffee. USA Today, January 20. www.usatoday.com/news/offbeat/2004-01-20-civet-coffee_x.htm.

994. Bell D, Roberton S, Hunter PR. 2004. Animal origins of SARS coronavirus: possible links with the international trade in small carnivores. Philosophical Transactions of the Royal Society of London. Series B: Biological Sciences 359(1447):1107–14.

995. Kasper LR. A recipe for shower flower cake. Scripps Howard News Service. www .diynetwork.com/diy/lc_beverages/article/0,2041,DIY_13997_2278719,00 .html.

996. Marshall S. 1999. Coffee that satisfies a discerning civet cat is excellent indeed. Wall Street Journal, March 17.

997. William J. 2003 The story of civet. The Pharmaceutical Journal 271(7280): 859–861.

998. Lee PJ, Krilov LR. 2005. When animal viruses attack: SARS and avian influenza. Pediatric Annals 34(1):43–52.

999. Mack TM. 2005. The ghost of pandemics past. Lancet 365(9468):1370–2.

1000. Davis M. 2005. The Monster at Our Door: The Global Threat of Avian Flu (New York, NY: The New Press).

1001. Ming Z. 2004. Humans should shoulder blame for SARS. China Daily, October 14. english.people.com.cn/200410/12/eng20041012_159879.html.

1002. Bell D, Roberton S, Hunter PR. 2004. Animal origins of SARS coronavirus: possible links with the international trade in small carnivores. Philosophical Transactions of the Royal Society of London. Series B: Biological Sciences 359(1447):1107–14.

1003. Karesh WB, Cook RA, Bennett EL, Newcomb J. 2005. Wildlife trade and global disease. Emerging Infectious Diseases 11(7). www.cdc.gov/ncidod/EID /vol11no07/05-0194.htm.

1004. Gilbert M, Wint W, Slingenbergh J. 2004. The ecology of highly pathogenic avian influenza in East and South-east Asia: outbreaks distribution, risk factors and policy implications. Consultancy report for the Animal Health Service of the Animal Production and Health Division of the Food and Agriculture Organization of the United Nations, Rome, Italy, August.

1005. Nuwer R. 2020 Feb 19. To prevent next coronavirus, stop the wildlife trade, conservationists say. New York Times. [accessed 2020 Apr 18]; https://www.nytimes.com/2020/02/19/health/coronavirus-animals-markets.html.

1006. Cook RA. 2005. Emerging diseases at the interface of people, domestic animals, and wildlife. The role of wildlife in our understanding of highly pathogenic avian influenza. Yale J Biol Med. 78(5):339–349.

1007. Brown C. 2004. Emerging zoonoses and pathogens of public health significance—an overview. Revue Scientifique et Technique 23:435–42.

1008. Lee PJ, Krilov LR. 2005. When animal viruses attack: SARS and avian influenza. Pediatric Annals 34(1):43–52.

1009. Shields DA, Mathews KH Jr. 2003. Interstate livestock movements. USDA Economic Research Service: Electronic Outlook Report from the Economic Research Service, June. usda.mannlib.cornell.edu/reports/erssor/livestock/ldp-mbb/2003/ldp-m108-01.pdf.

1010. Wilson TM, Gregg DA, King DJ, et al. 2001. Agroterrorism, biological crimes, and biowarfare targeting animal agriculture: the clinical, pathological, diagnostic, and epidemiologic features of some important animal diseases. Clinics in Laboratory Medicine 21:549–91.

1011. Transport of Livestock. 2001. In: Chambers PG, Grandin T, Guidelines for Humane Handling, Transport and Slaughter of Livestock (Bangkok, Thailand: Food and Agriculture Organization of the United Nations). www.fao.org/DOCREP/003/X6909E/x6909e08.htm.

1012. Scientific Committee on Animal Health and Animal Welfare. 2004. The welfare of animals during transport (details for horses, pigs, sheep and cattle). For the European Commission. europa.eu.int/comm/food/fs/sc/scah/out71_en.pdf.

1013. Storz J, Lin X, Purdy CW, et al. 2000. Coronavirus and pasteurella infections in bovine shipping fever pneumonia and Evans' criteria for causation. Journal of Clinical Microbiology 38(9):3291–8. jcm.asm.org/cgi/content/full/38/9/3291.

1014. Pfizer, Inc. 2004. Bovine respiratory disease. Pharmacia Animal Health, Beef Health Management. www.excenel.com/Health.asp?country=UK&lang=EN&species=BF&drug=EP&index=601&view=print.

1015. Scientific Committee on Animal Health and Animal Welfare. 2004. The welfare of animals during transport (details for horses, pigs, sheep and cattle). For the European Commission. seuropa.eu.int/comm/food/fs/sc/scah/out71_en.pdf.

1016. Scientific Committee on Animal Health and Animal Welfare. 2004. The welfare of animals during transport (details for horses, pigs, sheep and cattle). For the European Commission. seuropa.eu.int/comm/food/fs/sc/scah/out71_en.pdf.

1017. Barham AR, Barham BL, Johnson AK, Allen DM, Blanton JR, Miller MF. 2002. Effects of the transportation of beef cattle from the feedyard to the packing plant on prevalence levels of Escherichia coli O157 and Salmonella ssp. Journal of Food Protection 65:280–3.

1018. Marg H, Scholz HC, Arnold T, Rosler U, Hensel A. 2001. Influence of long-time transportation stress on reactivation of Salmonella typhimurium DT104 in experimentally infected pigs. Berliner und Munchener tierarztliche Wochenschrift 114(9–10):385–8.

1019. European Commission Health and Consumer Protection Directorate General. 2002. The Welfare of Animals During Transport, 14–19 (adopted March 11).

1020. Marg H, Scholz HC, Arnold T, Rosler U, Hensel A. 2001. Influence of long-time transportation stress on reactivation of Salmonella Typhimurium DT 104 in experimentally infected pigs. Berliner und Münchener tierärztliche Wochenschrift. 114:385–8.

1021. Food and Agriculture Organization of the United Nations. 1998. Europe vulnerable to livestock epidemics, warning delivered at FAO press conference. FAO News and Highlights, February 17. www.fao.org/news/1998/980204-e .htm.

1022. U.S. Department of Agriculture, Animal and Plant Health Inspection Service Centers for Epidemiology and Animal Health. 1994. Foot and Mouth Disease: sources of outbreaks and hazard categorization of modes of virus transmission. December.

1023. World Organization for Animal Health. 2001. OIE/FAO International Scientific Conference on foot and mouth disease. April 17–18. www.oie.int/eng/press /a_010418.htm.

1024. Food and Agriculture Organization of the United Nations. 2002. Improved animal health for poverty reduction and sustainable livelihoods. FAO Animal Production and Health Paper. www.fao.org/documents/show_cdr.asp?url _file=/DOCREP/005/Y3542E/Y3542E00.HTM.

1025. Federation of Veterinarians of Europe. 2001. Transport of live animals: FVE Position Paper. May 18. www.fve.org/papers/pdf./aw/position_papers/01 _043.pdf.

1026. Kohnen A. 2000. Responding to the threat of agroterrorism: specific recommendations for the U.S. Department of Agriculture. BCSIA Discussion Paper 2000-29, ESDP Discussion Paper ESDP-2000-04 (John F. Kennedy School of Government, Harvard University).

1027. United States Government Accountability Office. 2005. Homeland Security: Much is being done to protect agriculture from a terrorist attack, but important challenges remain. Report to Congressional Requesters. March. www.gao .gov/new.items/d05214.pdf.

1028. Chalk P. 2004. Hitting America's soft underbelly: the potential threat of deliberate biological attacks against the U.S. agricultural and food industry. Prepared for the Office of the Secretary of Defense. National Defense Research Institute, RAND Corporation. www.rand.org/pubs/monographs/2004/RAND _MG135.pdf.

1029. Ishmael W. 2003. A soft underbelly. Beef, July 1, p. 11. beef-mag.com/mag/beef_soft_underbelly/index.html.

1030. Chalk P. 2004. Hitting America's soft underbelly: the potential threat of deliberate biological attacks against the U.S. agricultural and food industry. Prepared for the Office of the Secretary of Defense. National Defense Research Institute, RAND Corporation. www.rand.org/pubs/monographs/2004/RAND_MG135.pdf.

1031. National Agricultural Statistics Service, USDA. 2017. Table 18. Cattle and calves—number sold per farm by sales: 2017. 2017 Census of Agriculture—United States Data. [accessed 2020 Apr 6]; https://www.nass.usda.gov/Publications/AgCensus/2017/Full_Report/Volume_1,_Chapter_1_US/st99_1_0017_0019.pdf.

1032. National Agricultural Statistics Service, USDA. 2017. Table 30. Poultry—inventory and number sold: 2017 and 2012. 2017 Census of Agriculture—United States Data. [accessed 2020 Apr 6]; https://www.nass.usda.gov/Publications/AgCensus/2017/Full_Report/Volume_1,_Chapter_1_US/st99_1_0030_0031.pdf.

1033. Chalk P. 2004. Hitting America's soft underbelly: the potential threat of deliberate biological attacks against the U.S. agricultural and food industry. Prepared for the Office of the Secretary of Defense. National Defense Research Institute, RAND Corporation. www.rand.org/pubs/monographs/2004/RAND_MG135.pdf.

1034. Chalk P. 2004. Hitting America's soft underbelly: the potential threat of deliberate biological attacks against the U.S. agricultural and food industry. Prepared for the Office of the Secretary of Defense. National Defense Research Institute, RAND Corporation. www.rand.org/pubs/monographs/2004/RAND_MG135.pdf.

1035. Chalk P. 2004. Hitting America's soft underbelly: the potential threat of deliberate biological attacks against the U.S. agricultural and food industry. Prepared for the Office of the Secretary of Defense. National Defense Research Institute, RAND Corporation. www.rand.org/pubs/monographs/2004/RAND_MG135.pdf.

1036. Watts G. 2005. Harnessing Mother Nature against your fellow humans. British Medical Journal 331:1228.

1037. Avasthi A. 2004. Bush-meat trade breeds new HIV. New Scientist, August. www.newscientist.com/article.ns?id=dn6239.

1038. Wyler LS, Sheikh PA. 2013. International illegal trade in wildlife: threats and U.S. policy. Congressional Research Service. July 23. [accessed 2020 Apr 14]; https://fas.org/sgp/crs/misc/RL34395.pdf.

1039. Weinhold B. 2004. Infectious disease: the human costs of our environmental errors. Environmental Health Perspectives 112(1):A32–9. www.ehponline.org/docs/2004/112-1/focus-abs.html.

1040. Marchione M. 2003. Globetrotting boosts exotic diseases. Milwaukee Journal Sentinel, June 15, p. 1. www.findarticles.com/p/articles/mi_qn4196/is_20030615/ai_n10879847.

1041. Marchione M. 2003. Tighter rules sought on exotic pets after trade, risks increase. Milwaukee Journal Sentinel, August 6.

1042. Marchione M. 2003. Globetrotting boosts exotic diseases. Milwaukee Journal Sentinel, June 15, p. 1. www.findarticles.com/p/articles/mi_qn4196/is _20030615/ai_n10879847.

1043. Lashley FR. 2004. Emerging infectious diseases: vulnerabilities, contributing factors and approaches. Expert Review of Anti-infective Therapy 2(2):299–316.

1044. Marchione M. 2003. Globetrotting boosts exotic diseases. Milwaukee Journal Sentinel, June 15, p. 1. www.findarticles.com/p/articles/mi_qn4196/is _20030615/ai_n10879847.

1045. Avasthi A. 2004. Bush-meat trade breeds new HIV. New Scientist, August. www.newscientist.com/article.ns?id=dn6239.

1046. Marchione M. 2003. Globetrotting boosts exotic diseases. Milwaukee Journal Sentinel, June 15, p. 1. www.findarticles.com/p/articles/mi_qn4196/is _20030615/ai_n10879847.

1047. Centers for Disease Control and Prevention. 2003. What you should know about monkeypox. June 12. cdc.gov/ncidod/monkeypox/factsheet2.htm.

1048. Antia R, Regoes RR, Koella JC, Bergstrom CT. 2003. The role of evolution in the emergence of infectious diseases. Nature 426(6967):658–61.

1049. Centers for Disease Control and Prevention. 2003. Update: multistate outbreak of monkeypox—Illinois, Indiana, Kansas, Missouri, Ohio, and Wisconsin. Morbidity and Mortality Weekly Report 52(27):642–46. cdc.gov/mmwr /preview/mmwrhtml./mm5227a5.htm.

1050. Shoichet CE. 2003. Global travel fans disease. Atlanta Journal and Constitution, July 21, p. 1A.

1051. Fritsch P. 2003. Containing the outbreak: scientists search for human hand behind outbreak of jungle virus. Wall Street Journal, June 19.

1052. Johnson RT. 2003. Emerging viral infections of the nervous system. Journal of NeuroVirology 9:140–7.

1053. McCormack JG. 2005. Hendra and Nipah viruses: New zoonotically-acquired human pathogens. Respiratory Care Clinics of North America 11(1):59–66.

1054. Cowley G, Underwood A. 2003. How progress makes us sick. Newsweek, May 5, p. 33.

1055. Mohd Nor MN, Gan CH, Ong BL. 2000. Nipah virus infection of pigs in peninsular Malaysia. Revue scientifique et technique 19(1):160–5.

1056. Ng FKS. 1999. Hendra-like (NIPAH) virus: Malaysia epidemic. Pighealth.com. pighealth.com/News99/NIPAH.HTM.

1057. Uppal PK. 2000. Emergence of Nipah virus in Malaysia. Annals of the New York Academy of Sciences 916:354–7. www.blackwell-synergy.com/doi/abs/10 .1111/j.1749-6632.2000.tb05312.x.

1058. Uppal PK. 2000. Emergence of Nipah virus in Malaysia. Annals of the New York Academy of Sciences 916:354–7. www.blackwell-synergy.com/doi/abs/10 .1111/j.1749-6632.2000.tb05312.x.

1059. Mohd Nor MN, Gan CH, Ong BL. 2000. Nipah virus infection of pigs in peninsular Malaysia. Revue scientifique et technique 19(1):160–5.

1060. Smith S. 2003. Crossing the species barrier from AIDS to Ebola: Our most deadly diseases have made the leap from animals to humans. Boston Globe, April 29, p. C1.

1061. Specter M. 2005. Nature's bioterrorist. New Yorker, February 28, pp. 52–61.

1062. Central Intelligence Agency. 2006. World Factbook. Malaysia. cia.gov/cia /publications/factbook/geos/my.html.

1063. Smith S. 2003. Crossing the species barrier from AIDS to Ebola: Our most deadly diseases have made the leap from animals to humans. Boston Globe, April 29, p. C1.

1064. Lam S-K. 2003. Nipah virus—a potential agent of bioterrorism? Antiviral Research 57(1–2):113–9.

1065. Fritsch P. 2003. Containing the outbreak: scientists search for human hand behind outbreak of jungle virus. Wall Street Journal, June 19.

1066. Wong KT, Shieh WJ, Zaki SR, Tan CT. 2002. Nipah virus infection, an emerging paramyxoviral zoonosis. Springer Seminars in Immunopathology 24:215–28.

1067. Wong SC, Ooi MH, Wong MNL, Tio PH, Solomon T, Cardosa MJ. 2001. Late presentation of Nipah virus encephalitis and kinetics of the humoral immune response. Journal of Neurology, Neurosurgery and and Psychiatry 71:552–4.

1068. Harcourt BH, Lowe L, Tamin A, et al. 2004. Genetic characterization of Nipah virus, Bangladesh, 2004. Centers for Disease Control and Prevention, Emerging Infectious Diseases 11(10). www.cdc.gov/ncidod/EID/vol11no10/05 -0513.htm.

1069. Fritsch P. 2003. Containing the outbreak: scientists search for human hand behind outbreak of jungle virus. Wall Street Journal, June 19.

1070. Ludwig B, Kraus FB, Allwinn R, Doerr HW, Preiser W. 2003. Viral zoonoses— a threat under control? Intervirology 46:71–8.

1071. U.S. Central Intelligence Agnency. 2006. Malaysia. CIA World Fact Book. March 29. cia.gov/cia/publications/factbook/geos/my.html.

1072. Newman SH, Epstein JH, Schloegel LM. 2005. The nature of emerging zoonotic diseases: Ecology, prediction, and prevention. Medical Laboratory Observer. 37(7):10(9).

1073. Ai SY. 2000. Profile of a virus. Jabatan Perkhidmatan Haiwan, Department of Veterinary Services. agrolink.moa.my/jph/dvs/nipah/star000410/nipah -profile.html.

1074. Nierenberg D. 2005. Happier Meals: Rethinking the Global Meat Industry. Worldwatch Paper 171, September. www.worldwatch.org/pubs/paper/171/.

1075. RaboBank International 2003. China's meat industry overview. Food and Agribusiness Research. May. www.rabobank.com/Images/rabobank_publication _china_meat_2003_tcm25-139.pdf.

1076. Gosline A. 2005. Mysterious disease outbreak in China baffles WHO. Newsci entist.com. July. www.newscientist.com/article.ns?id=dn7740.

1077. Streptococcus suis infection. Merk Veterinary Manual. merckvetmanual.com /mvm/index.jsp?cfile=htm/bc/54302.htm&word=Strep%2csuis.

1078. Huang YT, Teng LJ, Ho SW, Hsueh PR. 2005. Streptococcus suis infection. Journal of Microbiology, Immunology and Infection 38:306–13. jmii.org/con tent/abstracts/v38n5p306.php.

1079. Gosline A. 2005. Mysterious disease outbreak in China baffles WHO. Newsci entist.com. July. www.newscientist.com/article.ns?id=dn7740.

1080. Altman LK. 2005. Pig disease in China worries UN. New York Times, August 5. iht.com/bin/print_ipub.php?file=/articles/2005/08/05/news/pig.php.

1081. Nolan T. 2005. 40 people die from pig-borne bacteria. AM radio transcript. www.abc.net.au/am/content/2005/s1441324.htm.

1082. World Health Organization. 2005. Streptococcus suis fact sheet. www.wpro .who.int/media_centre/fact_sheets/fs_20050802.htm.

1083. U.S. Department of Agriculture, Veterinary Services, Center for Emerging Issues. 2005. Streptococcus suis outbreak, swine and human, China: Emerging disease notice. www.aphis.usda.gov/vs/ceah/cei/taf/emergingdiseasenotice _files/strep_suis_china.htm.

1084. 2005. China drafts, revises laws to safeguard animal welfare. China View, November 4. news.xinhuanet.com/english/2005-11/04/content_3729580.htm.

1085. Du W. 2005. Streptococcus suis, (S. suis) pork production and safety. Ontario Ministry of Agriculture, Food and Rural Affairs. www.omafra.gov.on.ca/english /livestock/swine/news/novdec05a5.htm.

1086. Nierenberg D. 2005. Happier Meals: Rethinking the Global Meat Industry. Worldwatch Paper 171, September. www.worldwatch.org/pubs/paper/171/.

1087. Arends JP, Hartwig N, Rudolphy M, Zanen HC. 1984. Carrier rate of Strep- tococcus suis capsular type 2 in palatine tonsils of slaughtered pigs. Journal of Clinical Microbiology 20(5):945–947.

1088. FAOSTAT Database. 2005. Agricultural data. faostat.fao.org/faostat/collectio ns?version=ext&hasbulk=0&subset=agriculture.

1089. Du W. 2005. Streptococcus suis, (S. suis) pork production and safety. Ontario Ministry of Agriculture, Food and Rural Affairs. www.omafra.gov.on.ca/english /livestock/swine/news/novdec05a5.htm.

1090. Gottschalk M. 2004. Porcine Streptococcus suis strains as potential sources of infections in humans: an underdiagnosed problem in North America? Journal of Swine Health and Production 12(4):197–9.

1091. Cole D, Todd L, Wing S. 2000. Concentrated swine feeding operations and public health: a review of occupational and community health effects. Environ- mental Health Perspectives 108:685–99.

1092. World Health Organization. 2005. Streptococcus suis fact sheet. www.wpro .who.int/media_centre/fact_sheets/fs_20050802.htm.

1093. Du W. 2005. Streptococcus suis, (S. suis) pork production and safety. Ontario Ministry of Agriculture, Food and Rural Affairs. www.omafra.gov.on.ca/english /livestock/swine/news/novdec05a5.htm.

1094. MacKenzie D. 1998. This little piggy fell ill. New Scientist, September 12, p. 1818.

1095. Meredith M. 2004. Zoonotic disease risks—2004 update. American Association of Swine Veterinarians. October 1. www.aasv.org/news/story.php ?id=1221.

1096. McMichael AJ. 2004. Environmental and social influences on emerging infectious diseases: Past, present, and future. Philosophical Transactions of the Royal Society of London 359:1049–58.

1097. World Health Organization, Food and Agricultural Organization of the United Nations, and World Organization for Animal Health. 2004. Report of the WHO/FAO/OIE joint consultation on emerging zoonotic diseases. At whqlib doc.who.int/hq/2004/WHO_CDS_CPE_ZFK_2004.9.pdf.

1098. Pappaioanou M. 2004. Veterinary medicine protecting and promoting the public's health and well-being. Preventive Veterinary Medicine 62:153–63.

1099. Krushinskie EA. 2006. Preparedness for an HPAI outbreak. Avian Influenza: dealing with the challenge. Watt, January 10. bulldogsolutions.net/WattPublishing/WPC01102006/frmEventDescription.aspx.

1100. Photo credit: Compassion Over Killing.

1101. 2005. Top U.S. broiler producing companies mid-2005. Feedstuffs, September 14, p. 5.

1102. United Egg Producers Certified. 2004. Industry history. www.uepcertified .com/industryhistory.html./.

1103. Lymbery P. 2002. Laid Bare: The Case Against Enriched Cages in Europe (Hampshire, UK: Compassion in World Farming Trust). www.ciwf.org.uk /publications/reports/laid_bare_2002.pdf.

1104. United Egg Producers. 2017. Animal husbandry guidelines for U.S. egg-laying flocks. United Egg Producers. [accessed 2020 Apr 14]; https://uepcertified .com/wp-content/uploads/2020/02/Caged-UEP-Guidelines_17.pdf.

1105. Mench JA. 2002. Consumer voices, dollars are changing animal welfare standards. UC Davis Sustainable Agriculture Newsletter 14(2). sarep.ucdavis.edu/newsltr /v14n2/sa-1.htm

1106. Nierenberg D. 2005. Happier Meals: Rethinking the Global Meat Industry. Worldwatch Paper 171, September. www.worldwatch.org/pubs/paper/171/.

1107. Torrey EF, Yolken RH. 2005. Beasts of the Earth: Animals, Humans, and Disease (New Brunswick, NJ: Rutgers University Press).

1108. Brown C. 2000. Emerging infectious diseases of animals: an overview. In: Brown C, Bolin C (eds.), Emerging Diseases of Animals (Washington, DC: ASM Press, pp. 1–12).

1109. Kazmin A. 2004. Greater livestock density blamed for disease rise. Financial Times, January 28, p. 12.

1110. Delgado CL, Narrod CA, Tiongco MM. 2003. Policy, technical, and environmental determinants and implications of the scaling-up of livestock production in four fast-growing developing countries: a synthesis. Submitted to the Food and Agricultural Organization of the United Nations by the International Food Policy Research Institute. July 24. www.fao.org/WAIRDOCS/LEAD/x6170e /x6170e00.htm.

1111. Food and Agriculture Organization of the United Nations. 2006. FAOSTAT data. faostat.fao.org/faostat/collections?version=ext&hasbulk=0&subset=agriculture.

1112. Industry-funded organizations. Sourcewatch.org. www.sourcewatch.org/index .php?title=Industry-funded_organizations.

1113. Council for Agricultural Science and Technology 2005. Global risks of infectious animal diseases. Issue Paper no. 28. www.cvmbs.colostate.edu/aphi /aphiweb/PDF.s/Global%20Risks%20of%20Infectious%20Animal%20Dis eases%20FINAL.pdf.

1114. Tilman D, Cassman KG, Matson PA, Naylor R, Polasky S. 2002. Agricultural sustainability and intensive production practices. Nature 418:671–7.

1115. Delgado CL, Narrod CA. 2003. Policy, technical, and environmental determinants and implications of the scaling-up of livestock production in four fast-growing developing countries: a synthesis. International Food Policy Research Institute report. fao.org/WAIRDOCS/LEAD/X6170E/x6170e00 .htm#Contents.

1116. Ferrari J. 1997. Fierce creatures. The Australian, December 10, p. 19.

1117. Drexler M. 2002. Secret Agents: The Menace of Emerging Infections (Washington, DC: Joseph Henry Press).

1118. Tauxe RV. 2002. Emerging foodborne pathogens. International Journal of Food Microbiology 78:31–41.

1119. Drexler M. 2002. Secret Agents: The Menace of Emerging Infections (Washington, DC: Joseph Henry Press).

1120. Galvin J. 2005. The worst jobs in science—manure inspector. Popular Science, February 27. www.popsci.com/popsci/science/806ffb24a5f27010vgnvc m1000004eecbccdrcrd/9.html.

1121. Purdue Research Foundation. 2001. Beef and dairy cows. Livestock Manure Handling on the Farm. danpatch.ecn.purdue.edu/~epados/farmstead/yards/src /cattle.htm.

1122. Drexler M. 2002. Secret Agents: The Menace of Emerging Infections (Washington, DC: Joseph Henry Press).

1123. Potter ME, Tauxe RV. 1997. Epidemiology of foodborne disease: tools and applications. World Health Organization Mediterranean Zoonoses Control, Information Circular (48):8. www.mzcp-zoonoses.gr/pdf.en/circ_48.pdf.

1124. Ministry of Agriculture, Fisheries, and Food. 1998. A review of antimicrobial resistance in the food chain. A technical report for the UK Ministry of Agriculture, Fisheries, and Food, July.

1125. Muir WM, Aggrey SE. 2003. Introductory editorial: Breeding for disease resistance in its evolutionary context in Poultry Genetics, Breeding and Biotechnology (Oxfordshire, UK: CAB International, pp. ix–xiv).

1126. Riemenschneider CH. 2005. Avian influenza and other transboundary animal diseases. Health in Foreign Policy Forum 2005, Academy Health, Washington, DC, February 4. www.academyhealth.org/NHPC/foreignpolicy/2005/agenda .htm.

1127. Tilman D, Cassman KG, Matson PA, Naylor R, Polasky S. 2002. Agricultural sustainability and intensive production practices. Nature 418:671–7.

1128. Agricultural Research Service. 2002. USDA Stakeholder Workshop for Animal Agriculture. Goal 3: Protect Animal Health (Washington, DC: U.S. Department of Agriculture). www.ars.usda.gov/docs.htm?docid=1083&page=6.

1129. Murphy FA. 1999. Emerging zoonoses. Emerging Infectious Diseases 4(3):429–35.

1130. Franco DA. 2003. Livestock development in developing countries. Render Magazine, December.

1131. Das P. 2002. Interview: Michael Osterholm—medical detective to fighting bioterrorism. Lancet Infectious Diseases 2:502–5.

1132. Delgado CL, Narrod CA, Tiongco MM. 2003. Policy, technical, and environmental determinants and implications of the scaling-up of livestock production in four fast-growing developing countries: a synthesis. Submitted to the Food and Agricultural Organization of the United Nations by the International Food Policy Research Institute. July 24. www.fao.org/WAIRDOCS/LEAD/x6170e/x6170e00.htm.

1133. Agricultural Research Service. 2006. Animal health national action plan (Washington, DC: U.S. Department of Agriculture). February 6. www.ars.usda.gov/research/programs/programs.htm?np_code=103&docid=820.

1134. Peters CJ. 2002. Hurrying toward disaster? Perspectives in Health: Magazine of the Pan American Health Organization 7(1).

1135. Puvadolpirod S, Thaxton JP. 2000. Model of physiological stress in chickens 1. Response parameters. Poultry Science 79:363–9.

1136. Battaglia RA. 2001. Handbook of Livestock Management, 3rd Edition (Weimar, Texas: Culinary and Hospitality Industry Publications Services).

1137. Cameron RDA. 2000. Food and Agricultural Organization of the United Nations, Animal Production and Health Commission for Asia and the Pacific. A review of the industrialization of pig production worldwide with particular reference to the Asian region. May. aphca.org/publications/files/pig_awi_oz/pig_awi_oz.pdf.

1138. Liang AP. 2002. Current state of foodborne illness. Conference for Food Safety Education. Orlando, FL, September 27. fsis.usda.gov/Orlando2002/presentations/aliang/aliang.pdf.

1139. Liang AP. 2002. Current state of foodborne illness. Conference for Food Safety Education. Orlando, FL, September 27. fsis.usda.gov/Orlando2002/presentations/aliang/aliang.pdf.

1140. Cookson C. 1993. Bugs that come to plague us: the renewed war against disease. Financial Times (London, UK), August 21.

1141. Galvin J. 2005. The worst jobs in science—manure inspector. Popular Science, February 27. www.popsci.com/popsci/science/806ffb24a5f27010vgnvcm1000004eecbccdrcrd/9.html.

1142. Cole D, Todd L, Wing S. 2000. Concentrated swine feeding operations and public health: a review of occupational and community health effects. Environmental Health Perspectives 108:685–99.

1143. Boyd W. 2001. Making meat: science, technology, and American poultry production. Technology and Culture 42:631–64.

1144. Glasgow HB, Burkholder JM, Morton SL, Springer J. 2001. A second species of Ichthyotoxic pfiesteria (dinamoebales, dinophyceae). Phycologia 40(3):234–45.

1145. Center for Mathematics and Science Education. 1998. The fuss over pfiesteria. University of North Carolina, Chapel Hill. June 5. unc.edu/depts/cmse/science /pfiesteria.html.

1146. Burkholder JM, Glasgow HB. 1995. Insidious effects of toxic estuarine dinoflagellate on fish survival and human health. Journal of Toxicology and Environmental Health 46(4):501–22.

1147. Mahy BWJ, Brown CC. 2000. Emerging zoonoses: crossing the species barrier. Revue Scientifique et Technique Office International des Epizooties 19(1):33–40.

1148. Goodman PS. 1999. Who pays for what is thrown away? Washington Post, August 3, p.A1. www.washingtonpost.com/wp-srv/local/daily/aug99/chicken3 .htm.

1149. Lederberg J, Shope RE, Oaks SC. 1992. Emerging Infections: Microbial Threats to Health in the United States (Washington, DC: National Academies Press).

1150. Avens JS. 1987. Overview: Salmonella—what's the problem? Third Poultry Symposium Proceedings: Managing for Profit (Fort Collins, CO: Colorado State University, pp. 119–123).

1151. Delgado C, Rosegrant M, Steinfeld H, Ehui S, Courbois C. 1999. Livestock to 2020: the next food revolution. Food, Agriculture, and the Environment Discussion Paper 28. For the International Food Policy Research Institute, the Food and Agriculture Organization of the United Nations and the International Livestock Research Institute. ifpri.org/2020/dp/dp28.pdf.

1152. Adams M, Motarjemi Y. 1999. Basic Food Safety for Health Workers (Geneva, Switzerland: World Health Organization Press).

1153. Tauxe RV. 2002. Emerging foodborne pathogens. International Journal of Food Microbiology 78:31–41.

1154. Waltner-Toews D, Lang T. 2000. A new conceptual base for food and agricultural policy: the emerging model of links between agriculture, food, health, environment and society. Global Change and Human Health 1:116–30.

1155. Division of Environmental Health, State of Alaska. Food Safety and Sanitation Program: Food Myths. dec.state.ak.us/eh/fss/consumers/food_myths.htm.

1156. Centers for Disease Control and Prevention. 2020. Foodborne germs and illnesses. U.S. Department of Health and Human Services; [last reviewed 2020 Mar 18; accessed 2020 Apr 7]. https://www.cdc.gov/foodsafety/foodborne -germs.html.

1157. Tauxe RV. 2002. Emerging foodborne pathogens. International Journal of Food Microbiology 78:31–41.

1158. Bjerklie S. 1999. Starting over. Meat Processing, March, p. 90.

1159. Adak GT, Meakins SM, Yip H, Lopman BA, O'Brien SJ. 2005. Disease risks from foods, England and Wales, 1996–2000. Emerging Infectious Diseases 11(3):365–72.

1160. Adak GT, Meakins SM, Yip H, Lopman BA, O'Brien SJ. 2005. Disease risks from foods, England and Wales, 1996–2000. Emerging Infectious Diseases 11(3):365–72.

1161. Ernst RA. 1995. University of California Cooperative Extension, Poultry fact sheet No. 20, June. animalscience.ucdavis.edu/Avian/pfs20.htm.

1162. United Egg Producers. 2002. Animal Husbandry Guidelines for U.S. Egg Laying Flocks 2002 Edition (Alpharetta, GA: United Egg Producers).

1163. Dawkins MS, Hardie S. 1989. Space needs of laying hens. British Poultry Science 30:413–6.

1164. Fox N. 1997. Spoiled: The Dangerous Truth about a Food Chain Gone Haywire (New York, NY: Basic Books, pp. 196–7).

1165. Kite-Powell H. 2004. Down on the farm. raising fish. Oceanus, September 21. whoi.edu/oceanus/viewArticle.do?id=2468.

1166. Chapman FA. 1992. Farm-raised channel catfish. Circular 1052, Department of Fisheries and Aquatic Sciences, Florida Cooperative Extension Service, Institute of Food and Agricultural Sciences, University of Florida. www.edis.ifas.ufl.edu/FA010.

1167. Smith GL, Irving WL, McCauley JW, Rowlands DJ (eds.) 2001. New Challenges to Health: The Threat of Virus Infection (Cambridge, UK: Cambridge University Press).

1168. Fisheries Department, FAO. 2000. The State of the World Fisheries and Aquaculture (Rome, Italy: Food and Agriculture Organization of the United Nations).

1169. Brown C. 2000. Emerging infectious diseases of animals: an overview. In: Brown C, Bolin C (eds.), Emerging Diseases of Animals (Washington, DC: ASM Press, pp. 1–12).

1170. Massicot P. 2005. Boto (Amazon River dolphin). Animal Info—Information on endangered mammals. November 2. www.animalinfo.org/species/cetacean/iniageof.htm.

1171. Goh SH, Driedger D, Gillett S, et al. 1998. Streptococcus iniae, a human and animal pathogen: Specific identification by the chaperonin 60 gene identification method. Journal of Clinical Microbiology 36(7):2164–66.

1172. Weinstein MR, Litt M, Kertesz DA, et al. Invasive infections due to a fish pathogen, Streptococcus iniae. New England Journal of Medicine 337:589–94.

1173. Weinstein MR, Litt M, Kertesz DA, et al. Invasive infections due to a fish pathogen, Streptococcus iniae. New England Journal of Medicine 337:589–94.

1174. Lederberg J, Shope RE, Oaks SC. 1992. Emerging Infections: Microbial Threats to Health in the United States (Washington, DC: National Academies Press).

1175. Brown C. 2000. Emerging infectious diseases of animals: an overview. In: Brown C, Bolin C (eds.), Emerging Diseases of Animals (Washington, DC: ASM Press, pp. 1–12).

1176. Beers MH, Berkow R (eds.), 2005. Bacterial infections, The Merck Manual, 17th Edition (Rahway, NJ: The Merck Publishing Group). www.merck.com/mrkshared/mmanual/section17/chapter227/227a.jsp.

1177. Centers for Disease Control and Prevention. 2005. Urinary tract infections. National Center for Infectious Diseases/Division of Bacterial and Mycotic Diseases. October 25. www.cdc.gov/ncidod/dbmd/diseaseinfo/urinarytractinfec tions_t.htm.

1178. Meslin FX, Stöhr K, Heymann D. 2000. Public health implications of emerging zoonoses. Revue Scientifique et Technique Office International des Epizooties 19(1):310–7.

1179. National Institutes of Health. 2005. Foodborne diseases. National Institute of Allergy and Infectious Disease fact sheet. February. www.niaid.nih.gov/fact sheets/foodbornedis.htm.

1180. Centers for Disease Control and Prevention. 2005. Escherichia coli O157:H7. National Center for Infectious Diseases/Division of Bacterial and Mycotic Diseases. October 6. www.cdc.gov/ncidod/dbmd/diseaseinfo/escherichiacoli _g.htm.

1181. Phillips ML. 2005. ExPECting the worst. Environmental Health Perspectives 113(6). http://www.ehponline.org/docs/2005/113-6/forum.html.

1182. Schoenl JL, Doyle MP. 1994. Variable colonization of chickens perorally inoculated with Escherichia coli O157:H7 and subsequent contamination of eggs. Applied Environmental Microbiology 60(8):2958–62.

1183. Jones TF, Schaffner W. 2005. Perspectives on the persistent scourge of foodborne disease. Journal of Infectious Disease 205:1029–31.

1184. Liu CM, Stegger M, Aziz M, Johnson TJ, Waits K, Nordstrom L, Gauld L, Weaver B, Rolland D, Statham S, et al. 2018. Escherichia coli ST131-H22 as a foodborne uropathogen. mBio. 9(4):e00470-18. https://doi.org/10.1128/mBio .00470-18.

1185. Brownlee C. 2005. Beef about UTIs. Science News, January 15.

1186. Slifko TR, Smith HV, Rose JB. 2000. Emerging parasite zoonoses associated with water and food. International Journal for Parasitology 30:1379–93.

1187. Mayer JD. 2000. Geography, ecology and emerging infectious diseases. Social Science and Medicine 50:937–52.

1188. Centers for Disease Control and Prevention: Morbidity and Mortality Weekly Report. 2002. Alfalfa sprouts—Arizona, California, Colorado, and New Mexico, February–April 2001. Journal of the American Medical Association 287(5):581–2. jama.ama-assn.org/cgi/content/full/287/5/581.

1189. U.S. Food and Drug Administration, Center for Food Safety and Applied Nutrition. 2005. Public Meeting: 2005 Sprout safety. May 17. www.cfsan.fda.gov /~dms/sprotran.html.

1190. Taormina PJ, Beuchat LR, Slutsker L. Infections associated with eating seed sprouts: an international concern. Emerging Infectious Diseases 5(5). www .cdc.gov/ncidod/eid/vol5no5/taormina.htm.

1191. Taormina PJ, Beuchat LR, Slutsker L. Infections associated with eating seed sprouts: an international concern. Emerging Infectious Diseases 5(5). www .cdc.gov/ncidod/eid/vol5no5/taormina.htm.

1192. Beuchat LR, Ryu J-H. 1997. Produce handling and processing practices. Emerging Infectious Diseases 3(4). www.cdc.gov/ncidod/eid/vol3no4/beuchat.htm.

1193. Centers for Disease Control and Prevention: Morbidity and Mortality Weekly Report. 2002. Alfalfa sprouts—Arizona, California, Colorado, and New Mexico, February–April 2001. Journal of the American Medical Association 287(5):581–2. jama.ama-assn.org/cgi/content/full/287/5/581.

1194. U.S. Food and Drug Administration. 2018. What you need to know about egg safety. Washington(DC): FDA; [last reviewed 2018 Mar 28; accessed 2020 Apr 6]. https://www.fda.gov/food/buy-store-serve-safe-food/what-you-need-know-about-egg-safety.

1195. McDowell RM, McElvaine MD. 1997. Long-term sequelae to foodborne disease. Revue Scientifique et Technique 16(2):337–41.

1196. U.S. Food and Drug Administration. 2017. 2015 NARMS integrated report. FDA, CDC, USDA; [accessed 2020 Apr 8]. https://www.fda.gov/media/108304/download.

1197. McDowell RM, McElvaine MD. 1997. Long-term sequelae to foodborne disease. Revue Scientifique et Technique 16(2):337–41.

1198. Tauxe RV. 2002. Emerging foodborne pathogens. International Journal of Food Microbiology 78:31–41.

1199. Liang AP. 2002. Current state of foodborne illness. Conference for Food Safety Education. Orlando, FL, September 27. fsis.usda.gov/Orlando2002/presentations/aliang/aliang.pdf.

1200. Drexler M. 2002. Secret Agents: The Menace of Emerging Infections (Washington, DC: Joseph Henry Press).

1201. Lecuit M. Abachin R, Martin A, et al. 2004. Immunoproliferative small intestinal disease associated with campylobacter jejuni. New England Journal of Medicine 350:239–48.

1202. U.S. Department of Agriculture. 1991. Campylobacter questions and answers. Food Safety and Inspection Service Background Document. www.fsis.usda.gov/Frame/FrameRedirect.asp?main= www.fsis.usda.gov/OA/background/campy_qa.htm.

1203. Linden J. 2005. Campylobacter gradually reveals its secrets. Poultry International, December.

1204. Hingley A. 1999. Campylobacter: low-profile bug is food poisoning leader. FDA Consumer, September-October. www.fda.gov/fdac/features/1999/599_bug.html.

1205. McNamara TS. 2002. Diagnosis and control of zoonotic infections: pathology and early recognition of zoonotic disease outbreaks. In: The Emergence of Zoonotic Diseases: Understanding the Impact on Animal and Human Health—Workshop Summary (Washington, DC: National Academies Press, p. 126).

1206. Cools I, Uyttendaele M, Cerpentier J, D'Haese E, Nelis HJ, Debevere J. 2005. Persistence of Campylobacter jejuni on surfaces in a processing environment and on cutting boards. Letters in Applied Microbiology 40:418–23.

1207. Frontline. Modern meat: what is HAACP? WGBH Educational Foundation. www.pbs.org/wgbh/pages/frontline/shows/meat/evaluating/haccp.html.

1208. Mattera P. 2004. USDA Inc.: How agribusiness has hijacked regulatory policy at the U.S. Department of Agriculture. Corporate Research Project of Good

Jobs First. July 23. www.agribusinessaccountability.org/pdf.s//289_USDA %20Inc.pdf.

1209. 1998. Industry Forum. Meat and Poultry, March.

1210. Moore T. 2002. Largest meat recall in USDA history: Wampler Foods recall expands to 27 million pounds. Associated Press, October 12.

1211. United States Government Accountability Office. 2004. Food safety: USDA and FDA need to better ensure prompt and complete recalls of potentially unsafe food. Report to Congressional Requesters. www.gao.gov/new.items/d0551 .pdf.

1212. Leonard R. 1999. Food Safety mismanagement puts consumer health at risk. Nutrition Week, April 16, pp. 4–5.

1213. Linden J. 2005. Campylobacter gradually reveals its secrets. Poultry International, December.

1214. Center for Science in the Public interest. 1999. Regulatory Comments and Petitions. Re: Docket No. 97P-076P. April 26. cspinet.org/foodsafety/irradia tion_usda.html.

1215. 1995. Superglue advocated for preventing fecal leakage in poultry. Food Chemical News, April 24, p. 12.

1216. DeWaal CS. 1996. Playing chicken: the human cost of inadequate regulation of the poultry industry. March. cspinet.org/reports/polt.html.

1217. Drummer R. 1995. Pacer backing new use for glue. Inland Valley Daily Bulletin, May 16.

1218. Phua K, Lee LK. 2005. Meeting the challenges of epidemic infectious disease outbreaks: an agenda for research. Journal of Public Health Policy 26:122–32.

1219. Stapp K. 2004. Scientists warn of fast-spreading global viruses. IPS-Inter Press Service, February 23.

1220. Lawrence J, Otto D. 2006. Economic importance of Montana's cattle industry. Cattleman's Beef Board and National Cattleman's Beef Association. www.beef .org/NEWSECONOMICIMPORTANCEOFMONTANASCATTLEINDUS TRY2711.aspx.

1221. Rampton S, Stauber J. 1997. Mad Cow USA (Monroe, ME: Common Courage Press).

1222. Satchell M, Hedges SJ. 1997. The next bad beef scandal? Cattle feed now contains things like manure and dead cats. U.S. News and World Report, September 1.

1223. Animal Industry Foundation. 1989. Animal Agriculture: Myths and Facts (Arlington, VA: Animal Industry Foundation).

1224. Kimberlin RH. 1992. Human spongiform encephalopathies and BSE. Medical Laboratory Sciences 49:216–17.

1225. Ensminger ME. 1990. Feeds and Nutrition. (Clovis, CA: Ensminger Publishing Co.).

1226. Flaherty M. 1993. Mad Cow disease dispute U.W. conference poses frightening questions. Wisconsin State Journal, September 26, p. 1C.

1227. 1990 Mad, bad and dangerous to eat? Economist. February, pp. 89–90.

1228. World Health Organization and Office International des Epizooties. 1999. WHO Consultation on Public Health and Animal Transmissible Spongiform Encephalopathies: Epidemiology, Risk and Research Requirements. December 1–31.

1229. Collee G. 1993. BSE stocktaking 1993. Lancet 342(8874):790–3. www.cyber-dyne.com/~tom/essay_collee.html.

1230. U.S. Department of Agriculture and Animal and Plant Health Inspection Service. 2005. List of USDA-Recognized Animal Health Status of Countries/Areas Regarding Specific Livestock or Poultry Diseases, April, 12. oars.aphis.usda.gov/NCIE/country.html.

1231. Albert D. 2000. EU meat meal industry wants handout to survive ban. Reuters World Report, December 5.

1232. Harrison PJ, Roberts GW. 1992. How now mad cow. British Medical Journal 304(6832):929–30.

1233. Harrison PJ, Roberts GW. 1992. How now mad cow. British Medical Journal 304(6832):929–30.

1234. Brown P, Liberski PP, Wolff A, Gajdusek DC. 1990. Resistance of scrapie infectivity to steam autoclaving after formaldehyde fixation and limited survival after ashing at 360 degrees C: Practical and theoretical implications. Journal of Infectious Diseases 161(3):467–72.

1235. Bentor Y. 2003. Lead. Chemical Element.com. www.chemicalelements.com/elements/pb.html.

1236. Harrison PJ, Roberts GW. 1991. "Life, Jim, but not as we know it": Transmissible dementias and the prion protein. British Journal of Psychiatry 158:457–70.

1237. Glanze WD, Anderson KN, Anderson LE (eds.), 1992. The Mosby Medical Encyclopedia (New York, NY: C.V. Mosby Company).

1238. Dealler SF, Lacey RW. 1990. Transmissible spongiform encephalopathies. Food Microbiology 7:253–79.

1239. Gibbs CJ. 1994. BSE and other spongiform encephalopathies in humans and animals: causative agent, pathogenesis and transmission. Food Science Seminar Series, Department of Food Science, Cornell University, December 1.

1240. Smith PG. 2003. The epidemics of bovine spongiform encephalopathy and variant Creutzfeldt-Jakob Disease: current status and future prospects. Bulletin of the World Health Organization 81(2):123–30. www.who.int/bulletin/volumes/81/2/en/PHR0203.pdf.

1241. Oxford University Press. 1996. Oxford Textbook of Medicine 2:3981.

1242. Ricketts MN. 2004. Public health and the BSE epidemic. Current Topics in Microbiology and Immunology 284:49–119.

1243. Brown P, Preece M, Brandel JP, et al. 2000. Iatrogenic Creutzfeldt-Jakob disease at the millennium. Neurology 55(8):1075.

1244. Diack AB, Will RG, Manson JC. 2017. Public health risks from subclinical variant CJD. PLoS Pathog. 13(11):e1006642. https://dx.doi.org/10.1371/journal.ppat.1006642.

1245. Pearson J. 1998. CJD is "worst form of death"—Dorrell tells BSE probe. PA News, November 30.

1246. Northoff E. 2004. BSE controls in many countries are still not sufficient. Food and Agriculture Organization of the United Nations, FAO Newsroom, January 12. www.fao.org/english/newsroom/news/2003/26999-en.html.

1247. Department of Health and Human Services, Food and Drug Administration. 2005. Substances Prohibited from Use in Animal Food or Feed. Proposed Rules, Federal Register 70(193):58570–58601, October 6.

1248. Public Citizen. 2001. Letter to the FDA and USDA RE: BSE. April 21. www.citizen.org/print_article.cfm?ID=1562.

1249. Mississippi State University Cooperative Extension Service. 1998. Broiler litter as a feed or fertilizer in livestock operations. msstate.edu/dept/poultry/pub1998.htm.

1250. Food and Drug Administration Sec. 685.100 Recycled Animal Waste (CPG 7126.34). www.fda.gov/ora/compliance_ref/cpg/cpgvet/cpg685-100.html.

1251. Tilman D, Cassman KG, Matson PA, Naylor R, Polasky S. 2002. Agricultural sustainability and intensive production practices. Nature 418:671–7.

1252. Fontenot JP, Webb KE Jr., Harmon BW, Tucker RE, Moore WEC. 1971. Studies of processing, nutritional value and palatability of broiler litter for ruminants. In: Proceedings of the International Symposium on Livestock Wastes (St. Joseph, Michigan: American Society of Agricultural Engineers, pp. 271–301).

1253. Satchell M, Hedges SJ. 1997. The next bad beef scandal? Cattle feed now contains things like manure and dead cats. U.S. News and World Report, September 1.

1254. Fontenot JP. 2001. Utilization of poultry litter as feed for beef cattle. Food and Drug Administration Public Hearing on Animal Feeding Regulation, October 30. www.fda.gov/ohrms/dockets/dailys/01/Nov01/110501/ts00014.doc.

1255. Fontenot JP. 1996. Feeding poultry wastes to cattle. Department of Animal and Poultry Sciences. Virginia Polytechnic Institute. September 18. www.rem.sfu.ca/FRAP/9809.pdf.

1256. McKinley B, Broome M, Oldham L. 2000. Poultry nutrient management through livestock feedstuffs. Mississippi State University Extension Service. msucares.com/pubs/misc/m1146.htm.

1257. Fontenot JP. 1996. Feeding poultry wastes to cattle. Department of Animal and Poultry Sciences. Virginia Polytechnic Institute. September 18. www.rem.sfu.ca/FRAP/9809.pdf.

1258. Fontenot JP, Webb KE Jr., Harmon BW, Tucker RE, Moore WEC. 1971. Studies of processing, nutritional value and palatability of broiler litter for ruminants. In: Proceedings of the International Symposium on Livestock Wastes (St. Joseph, Michigan: American Society of Agricultural Engineers, pp. 271–301).

1259. Kunkle WE, Jacob JP, Tervola RS, Miles RD, Mather FB. 1997. Broiler litter, part 2: feeding to ruminants. Dairy and Poultry Sciences Department, University of Florida Cooperative Extension, fact sheet PS-14. edis.ifas.ufl.edu/pdffiles/ps/ps00200.pdf.

1260. Fontenot JP. 1996. Feeding poultry wastes to cattle. Department of Animal and Poultry Sciences. Virginia Polytechnic Institute. September 18. www.rem.sfu.ca/FRAP/9809.pdf.

1261. University of Missouri Agriculture Extension. 2001. Feeding poultry litter to beef cattle. Publication G2077, February 15.

1262. University of Missouri Agriculture Extension. 2001. Feeding poultry litter to beef cattle. Publication G2077, February 15.

1263. Mississippi State University Cooperative Extension Service. 1998. Broiler litter as a feed or fertilizer in livestock operations. msstate.edu/dept/poultry/pub 1998.htm.

1264. Alabama Cooperative Extension Service. 2001. U.S. policy of feeding "broiler litter" (chicken sh**) to beef cattle. February 19.

1265. Mills B. 1998. Alabama cries "foul." Beef, January 1. beef-mag.com/mag/beef _alabama_cries_foul/index.html.

1266. Roybal J. 1997. The public sees it as "manure." Beef, December 1. beef-mag.com /mag/beef_litter_feeding_isnt/index.html.

1267. Price DP. 1998. More on poultry litter. Beef, March 1. beef-mag.com/mag/beef _poultry_litter/.

1268. Mills B. 1998. Alabama cries "foul." Beef, January 1. beef-mag.com/mag/beef _alabama_cries_foul/index.html.

1269. European Commission. Chronological list of Community legislation. europa .eu.int/comm/food/fs/bse/legislation_en.html.

1270. Evans E. 1996. Agency to ban some feeds to block mad-cow disease. Reuters World Report, May 13.

1271. 1994. AVMA casts doubt on spread of BSE through sheep offal. Food Chemical News, November 28, pp. 42–45.

1272. 1993. BSE/scrapie group share research, debate feed bans. Food Chemical News, July 5 July, pp. 57–59.

1273. Rampton S, Stauber J. 1997. Mad Cow USA (Monroe, ME: Common Courage Press).

1274. 1996. Dangerous food. Burrelle's Information Services, Oprah Winfrey Show, April 16.

1275. 1996. Dangerous food. Burrelle's Information Services, Oprah Winfrey Show, April 16.

1276. U.S. Department of Agriculture, Animal and Plant Health Inspection Service, and Veterinary Services. 1993. Dairy herd management practices focusing on preweaned heifers: April 1991–July 1992. National Dairy Heifer Evaluation Project. nahms.aphis.usda.gov/dairy/ndhep/dr91des1.pdf.

1277. U.S. Department of Agriculture, Animal and Plant Health Inspection Service, and Veterinary Services. 1993. Dairy herd management practices focusing on preweaned heifers: April 1991–July 1992. National Dairy Heifer Evaluation Project. nahms.aphis.usda.gov/dairy/ndhep/dr91des1.pdf.

1278. U.S. Department of Agriculture, Animal and Plant Health Inspection Service, and Veterinary Services. 1993. Dairy herd management practices focusing on preweaned heifers: April 1991–July 1992. National Dairy Heifer Evaluation Project. nahms.aphis.usda.gov/dairy/ndhep/dr91des1.pdf.

1279. Quigley J. 2001. Red blood cell protein in calf milk replacers. Calf Notes 49. calfnotes.com/pdf.files/CN049.pdf.

1280. Quigley J. 2001. Red blood cell protein in calf milk replacers. Calf Notes 49. calfnotes.com/pdf.files/CN049.pdf.

1281. Schlosser E. 2004. The cow jumped over the USDA. New York Times, January 2. organicconsumers.org/madcow/usda1204.cfm.

1282. European Commission Health and Consumer Protection Directorate. 2002. General scientific steering committee opinion on the implications of the recent papers on transmission of BSE by blood. European Commission, September 13. europa.eu.int/comm/food/fs/bse/scientificadvice08en.html.

1283. European Commission Health and Consumer Protection Directorate. 2002. General scientific steering committee opinion on the implications of the recent papers on transmission of BSE by blood. European Commission, September 13. europa.eu.int/comm/food/fs/bse/scientificadvice08en.html.

1284. European Commission Health and Consumer Protection Directorate. 2002. General scientific steering committee opinion on the implications of the recent papers on transmission of BSE by blood. European Commission, September 13. europa.eu.int/comm/food/fs/bse/scientificadvice08en.html.

1285. Milk replacer is up to 15 percent red blood cell protein (Quigley J. Red blood cell protein in calf milk replacers. calfnotes.com/pdf.files/CN049.pdf) and calves drink up to five quarts per day (U.S. Department of Agriculture. 1993. Dairy Herd Management Practices Focusing on Preweaned Heifers, N129.0793. July). cofcs66.aphis.usda.gov/vs/ceah/cahm/DairyCattle/ndhep /dr91des1.pdf.

1286. American Protein Corporation, Inc. 2002. Overview. functionalproteins.com /overview/index.html.

1287. American Protein Corporation, Inc. The basic science behind spray-dried plasma and serum proteins. Series on Plasma and Serum Proteins, Discoveries. www.functionalproteins.com/functional_prots/images/thebasicscience.pdf.

1288. American Protein Corporation, Inc. The basic science behind spray-dried plasma and serum proteins. Series on Plasma and Serum Proteins, Discoveries. www.functionalproteins.com/functional_prots/images/thebasicscience.pdf.

1289. National Renderers Association. Rendered animal products for swine. www .renderers.org/links/swine.htm.

1290. Nobel Foundation. 1976. The 1976 Nobel Prize in Physiology or Medicine. News release, October 14. nobelprize.org/medicine/laureates/1976/press.html.

1291. Gajdusek DC. 1997. NBC Dateline, March 14.

1292. Pearce F. 1996. BSE may lurk in pigs and chickens. New Scientist, April 6, p. 5. www.newscientist.com/article/mg15020240.300.html.

1293. Centers for Epidemiology and Animal Health, USDA: APHIS Based on average 7.9 week weaning period USDA Dairy Herd Management Practices Focusing on Preweaned Heifers N129.0793. July 1993. nahms.aphis.usda.gov/dairy/ndhep /dr91des1.pdf.

1294. American Feed Industry Association. 2001. Testimony of Richard Sellers. In: Government and Industry Programs to Prevent BSE from Entering the U.S. U.S. Senate Subcommittee on Consumer Affairs, April 4. commerce.senate.gov /hearings/0404sel.PDF.

1295. Piper E. 2000. Stop factory farming and end BSE, UK scientists say. Reuters, December 4.

1296. National Cattlemen's Beef Association. 2005. NCBA statement regarding today's USDA announcement. Member eUpdate, June 10. beefusa.org/NEWSMembere Update-June10200522511.aspx.

1297. Drury A. 2003 Critics say U.S. needs to do more to protect against mad cow. Journal News (New York), May 29. tinyurl.com/pclw2.

1298. Coiro A. 2003. Mad cow disease in Canada. Forum. KQED, May 23. www .kqed.org/programs/programarchive.jsp?progID=RD19&ResultStart=1& ResultCount=10&type=radio.

1299. World Health Organization, Food and Agricultural Organization of the United Nations, and World Organization for Animal Health. 2001. Joint WHO/FAO /OIE Technical Consultation on BSE: Public health, animal health and trade. oie.int/eng/publicat/rapports/en_BSE%20WHO-FAO-OIE.htm.

1300. Murphy D. 2003. FDA changes in feed restriction won't reduce BSE risk, industry groups say. Meatingplace.com, January 15.

1301. Matravers P, Bridgeman J, Ferguson-Smith M. 2000. Report of the BSE Inquiry. www.bseinquiry.gov.uk/report/volume1/execsum2.htm.

1302. Waltner-Toews D. 2002. Veterinary public health. In: Breslow L (ed.), Encyclopedia of Public Health (New York, NY: Macmillan Reference, New York). www.idmed.slu.se/VPH/VPH-Waltner-Toews.pdf.

1303. Murphy D. 2003. FDA changes in feed restriction won't reduce BSE risk, industry groups say. Meatingplace.com, January 15.

1304. Walters MJ. 2003. Six Modern Plagues and How We Are Causing Them (Washington, DC: Island Press).

1305. Meslin FX, Stöhr K, Heymann D. 2000. Public health implications of emerging zoonoses. Revue Scientifique et Technique Office International des Epizooties 19(1):310–7.

1306. Drexler M. 2002. Secret Agents: The Menace of Emerging Infections (Washington, DC: Joseph Henry Press).

1307. Eisnitz G. 1997. Slaughterhouse (New York, NY: Prometheus).

1308. Eisnitz G. 1997. Slaughterhouse (New York, NY: Prometheus).

1309. Bjerklie S. 1995. Who really has the world's safest meat supply? Meat and Poultry, August.

1310. Bjerklie S. 1995. Who really has the world's safest meat supply? Meat and Poultry, August.

1311. U.S. Food and Drug Administration. [date unknown]. What you need to know about egg safety. Washington (DC): FDA; [last reviewed 2018 Mar 28; accessed 2020 Apr 6]. https://www.fda.gov/food/buy-store-serve-safe-food/what-you -need-know-about-egg-safety.

1312. Drexler M. 2002. Secret Agents: The Menace of Emerging Infections (Washington, DC: Joseph Henry Press).

1313. Nestle M. 2003. Safe Food: Bacteria, Biotechnology, and Bioterrorism (Berkeley and Los Angeles, California: University of California Press, p. 1).

1314. U.S. Food and Drug Administration. 2017. 2015 NARMS integrated report.

FDA, CDC, USDA; [accessed 2020 Apr 8]. https://www.fda.gov/media/108304/download.

1315. Burrows M. 2006. More Salmonella is reported in chickens. New York Times, March 8. nytimes.com/2006/03/08/dining/08well.html.

1316. Bjerklie S. 1995. Who really has the world's safest meat supply? Meat and Poultry, August.

1317. Food and Nutrition Board, Institute of Medicine, and Board on Agriculture, National Research Council. 1988. Ensuring Safe Food: From Production to Consumption (Washington, DC: National Academies Press).

1318. United States Government Accountability Office. 2001. Weaknesses in meat and poultry inspection pilot should be addressed before implementation. Report to the Committee on Agriculture, Nutrition, and Forestry, U.S. Senate. December. www.gao.gov/cgi-bin/getrpt?GAO-02-59.

1319. Food and Nutrition Board, Institute of Medicine, and Board on Agriculture, National Research Council. 1988. Ensuring Safe Food: From Production to Consumption (Washington, DC: National Academies Press).

1320. Food Marketing Institute Board of Directors. 1988. Long-Range Priorities for Food Safety (Washington, DC: Food Marketing Institute).

1321. Nestle M. 2003. Safe Food: Bacteria, Biotechnology, and Bioterrorism (Berkeley and Los Angeles, California: University of California Press).

1322. Food Safety and Inspection Service. 2002. Colorado firm recalls beef trim and ground beef products for possible E. coli O157:H7. Recall Release: FSIS-RC-055-2002, July 19. www.fsis.usda.gov/OA/recalls/prelease/pr055-2002.htm.

1323. Carman D. 2002. Just cook the crud out of it. Denver Post, July 25.

1324. Nestle M. 2003. Safe Food: Bacteria, Biotechnology, and Bioterrorism (Berkeley and Los Angeles, California: University of California Press).

1325. Fox N. 1997. Spoiled: The Dangerous Truth about a Food Chain Gone Haywire (New York, NY: Basic Books, p. 344).

1326. Crump JA, Sulka AC, Langer AJ, et al. 2002. An outbreak of Escherichia coli O157:H7 infections among visitors to a dairy farm. New England Journal of Medicine 347:555–60.

1327. Torrey EF, Yolken RH. 2005. Their bugs are worse than their bite. Washington Post, April 3, p. B01.

1328. Raloff J. 1998. Hay! What a way to fight E. coli. Science News Online, September 19. www.sciencenews.org/pages/sn_arc98/9_19_98/food.htm.

1329. Nou X, Rivera-Betancourt M, Bosilevac JM, et al. 2003. Effect of chemical dehairing on the prevalence of Escherichia coli O157:H7 and the levels of aerobic bacteria and Enterobacteriaceae on carcasses in a commercial beef processing plant. Journal of Food Protection 66(11):2005–9. www.ingentaconnect.com/content/iafp/jfp/2003/00000066/00000011/art00006.

1330. Boyd W. 2001. Making meat: science, technology, and American poultry production. Technology and Culture 42:631–64.

1331. Boyd W. 2001. Making meat: science, technology, and American poultry production. Technology and Culture 42:631–64.

1332. Office of Technology Assessment. 1979. Drugs in livestock feed: Volume 1

Technical Report (Washington, DC: U.S. Government Printing Office). www
.govinfo.library.unt.edu/ota/Ota_5/DATA/1979/7905.PDF.

1333. Office of Technology Assessment. 1979. Drugs in livestock feed: Volume 1
Technical Report (Washington, DC: U.S. Government Printing Office). www
.govinfo.library.unt.edu/ota/Ota_5/DATA/1979/7905.PDF.

1334. Cole D, Todd L, Wing S. 2000. Concentrated swine feeding operations and
public health: a review of occupational and community health effects. Environmental Health Perspectives 108:685–99.

1335. Boyd W. 2001. Making meat: science, technology, and American poultry production. Technology and Culture 42:631–64.

1336. Wallner-Pendleton E, Dunn P. 2004. Sulfonamide toxicity in poultry. In: 76th
Northeastern Conference on Avian Diseases: June 9–11 (State College, Penn-
sylvania: Department of Veterinary Science, College of Agricultural Sciences,
Pennsylvania State University, p. 38). www.vetsci.psu.edu/NECAD/NECAD
Proceedings.pdf.

1337. Anderson AD, McClellan J, Rossiter S, Angulo FJ. 2003. Public health consequences of use of antimicrobial agents in agriculture. In: The Resistance Phenomenon in Microbes and Infectious Disease Vectors: Implications for Human
Health and Strategies for Containment: Workshop Summary (Washington,
DC: National Academies Press, pp. 231–43).

1338. Tilman D, Cassman KG, Matson PA, Naylor R, Polasky S. 2002. Agricultural
sustainability and intensive production practices. Nature 418:671–7.

1339. Lees W. 2004. Section 5: Disease control actions taken. In: Comprehensive
report on the 2004 outbreak of high pathogenicity avian influenza (H7N3) in
the Fraser Valley of British Columbia, Canada, June 30 (Canadian Food Inspection Agency). www.inspection.gc.ca/english/anima/heasan/disemala/avflu
/2004rep/5e.shtml.

1340. Tilman D, Cassman KG, Matson PA, Naylor R, Polasky S. 2002. Agricultural
sustainability and intensive production practices. Nature 418:671–7.

1341. Anderson AD, McClellan J, Rossiter S, Angulo FJ. 2003. Public health consequences of use of antimicrobial agents in agriculture. In: The Resistance Phenomenon in Microbes and Infectious Disease Vectors: Implications for Human
Health and Strategies for Containment: Workshop Summary (Washington,
DC: National Academies Press, pp. 231–43).

1342. Mellon MG, Benbrook C, Benbrook KL. 2001. Hogging It! Estimates of Antimicrobial Abuse in Livestock (Cambridge, MA: Union of Concerned Scientists).

1343. U.S. Food and Drug Administration. 2016 Dec. 2015 summary report on
antimicrobials sold or distributed for use in food-producing animals. FDA; [ac-
cessed 2020 Apr 6]. https://www.fda.gov/files/about fda/published/2015-Su
mmary-Report-on-Antimicrobials-Sold-or-Distributed-for-Use-in-Food-Produ
cing-Animals.pdf.

1344. U.S. Food and Drug Administration. 2019 Nov 22. NARMS now: integrated
data. Rockville(MD): U.S. Department of Health and Human Services; [ac-
cessed 2020 Apr 9]. https://www-aws.fda.gov/animal-veterinary/national
-antimicrobial-resistance-monitoring-system/narms-now-integrated-data.

1345. U.S. Food and Drug Administration. 2017. 2015 NARMS integrated report. FDA, CDC, USDA; [accessed 2020 Apr 8]. https://www.fda.gov/media/108304/download.

1346. Thaxton YV. 2006 Mar 16. Chicken industry needs the power of positive PR. Meatingplace.com. meatingplace.com/MembersOnly/webNews/details.aspx?item=15666.

1347. Aitken SL, Dilworth TJ, Heil EL, Nailor MD. 2016. Agricultural applications for antimicrobials. A danger to human health: an official position statement of the Society of Infectious Diseases Pharmacists. Pharmacotherapy. 36(4):422–432. https://doi.org/10.1002/phar.1737.

1348. U.S. Food and Drug Administration. 2016 Dec. 2015 summary report on antimicrobials sold or distributed for use in food-producing animals. FDA; [accessed 2020 Apr 6]. https://www.fda.gov/files/about fda/published/2015-Summary-Report-on-Antimicrobials-Sold-or-Distributed-for-Use-in-Food-Producing-Animals.pdf.

1349. Cima G. 2015. Antimicrobial sales outpace meat production: regulators, industry caution that sales may differ from use. JAVMA. 246(12):1279–1280.

1350. Watkins RR, Smith TC, Bonomo RA. 2016. On the path to untreatable infections: colistin use in agriculture and the end of 'last resort' antibiotics. Expert Rev Anti Infect Ther. 14(9):785–788. https://doi.org/10.1080/14787210.2016.1216314.

1351. 1968. A bitter reckoning. New Scientist, January 4, pp. 14–5.

1352. Alanis AJ. 2005. Resistance to antibiotics: Are we in the post-antibiotic era? Archives of Medical Research 36:697–705.

1353. 1998. EU bans farm antibiotics. BBC News, December 14. news.bbc.co.uk/2/hi/europe/234566.stm.

1354. World Health Organization. 2006. Zoonoses and veterinary public health. www.who.int/emc/diseases/zoo/zoo97_4.html.

1355. American Medical Association House of Delegates Annual Meeting. 2001. Resolution 508: Antimicrobial use and resistance. www.keepantibioticsworking.com/new/resources_library.cfm?refID=36325.

1356. American Public Health Association. 2003. Precautionary Moratorium on new concentrated animal feed operations. apha.org/legislative/policy/policysearch/index.cfm?fuseaction=view&id=1243.

1357. Animal Health Institute. 2004. Does the use of antibiotics in food animals pose a risk to human health? A critical review of published data. ahi.org/antibiotics Debate/documents/Factsheet-JAC1-15.pdf.

1358. United States Government Accountability Office. 2004. Antibiotic resistance: Federal agencies need to better focus efforts to address risk to humans from antibiotic use in animals. Report to Congressional Requesters. www.gao.gov/new/.items/d04490.pdf.

1359. National Research Council. 1999. Costs of eliminating subtherapeutic use of antibiotics, chapter 7. In: Committee on Drug Use in Food Animals, Panel on Animal Health, Food Safety, and Public Health, Board on Agriculture, and National Research Council, The Use of Drugs in Food Animals: Benefits and

Risk (Washington, DC: National Academies Press, p. 179). newton.nap. edu/html./foodanim/.

1360. American College of Physicians. Facts and figures. Emerging antibiotic resistance. acponline.org/ear/factsfigs.htm.

1361. Office of Communications and Public Liaison. 2004. The problem of antibiotic resistance. National Institute of Allergy and Infectious Diseases, National Institutes of Health fact sheet, April. www.niaid.nih.gov/factsheets/antimicro.htm.

1362. Jukes TH. 1973. Public health significance of feeding low levels of antibiotics to animals. Advances in Applied Microbiology 16:1–29.

1363. Jukes TH. 1973. Public health significance of feeding low levels of antibiotics to animals. Advances in Applied Microbiology 16:1–29.

1364. Public Broadcasting Service. 2002. Antibiotic debate overview. Is your meat safe? Modern meat. Frontline. pbs.org/wgbh/pages/frontline/shows/meat/safe /overview.html.

1365. Anderson AD, McClellan J, Rossiter S, Angulo FJ. 2003. Public health consequences of use of antimicrobial agents in agriculture. In: The Resistance Phenomenon in Microbes and Infectious Disease Vectors: Implications for Human Health and Strategies for Containment: Workshop Summary (Washington, DC: National Academies Press, pp. 231–43).

1366. Keep Antibiotics Working. 2005. Bayer commended for ending 5-year opposition to FDA ban on use of Cipro-like antibiotics in poultry. News Release, September 7. www.keepantibioticsworking.com/new/resources_library.cfm ?refID=76541.

1367. Price LB, Johnson E, Vailes R, Silbergeld E. 2005. Fluoroquinolone-resistant Campylobacter isolates from conventional and antibiotic-free chicken products. Environmental Health Perspectives 113(5):557–60. www.ehponline.org/members /2005/7647/7647.html.

1368. Anderson AD, McClellan J, Rossiter S, Angulo FJ. 2003. Public health consequences of use of antimicrobial agents in agriculture. In: The Resistance Phenomenon in Microbes and Infectious Disease Vectors: Implications for Human Health and Strategies for Containment: Workshop Summary (Washington, DC: National Academies Press, pp. 231–43). fermat.nap.edu/openbook /0309088542/html./231.html.

1369. Helms M, Simonsen J, Olsen KE, Molbak K. 2005. Adverse health events associated with antimicrobial drug resistance in Campylobacter species: a registry -based cohort study. Journal of Infectious Disease 191:1051.

1370. Palmer E. 2002. Bayer urged to eliminate animal version of Cipro. Kansas City Star, February 20. keepantibioticsworking.com/news/news.cfm?News _ID=176.

1371. 2005. Bayer pulls Baytril. Journal of the American Veterinary Medical Association News, October 15. avma.org/onlnews/javma/oct05/051015e.asp.

1372. Price LB, Johnson E, Vailes R, Silbergeld E. 2005. Fluoroquinolone-resistant Campylobacter isolates from conventional and antibiotic-free chicken products. Environmental Health Perspectives 113(5):557–60. www.ehponline.org/mem bers/2005/7647/7647.html.

1373. Henig RM. 1997. The People's Health: A Memoir of Public Health and Its Evolution at Harvard (Washington, DC: Joseph Henry Press, p. 88).

1374. Epstein S. 1989. U.S. policy turns blind side to dangers of meat additives. Austin American-Statesman, March 8, p. A15.

1375. Dutton D. 1988. Worse Than the Disease: The Pitfalls of Medical Progress, (Cambridge, UK: Cambridge University Press).

1376. Lerner S. 2001. Risky chickens. Village Voice, November 28–December 4. villagevoice.com/news/0148,lerner,30287,1.html.

1377. Kestin SC, Knowles TG, Tinch AE, Gregory NG. 1992. Prevalence of leg weakness in broiler chickens and its relationship with genotype. Veterinary Record 131 (9):190–4. veterinaryrecord.bvapublications.com/cgi/content /abstract/131/9/190.

1378. Martin D. 1997. Researcher studying growth-induced diseases in broilers. Feedstuffs, May 26.

1379. Office of Technology Assessment. 1979. Drugs in livestock feed: Volume 1 Technical Report (Washington, DC: U.S. Government Printing Office). www .govinfo.library.unt.edu/ota/Ota_5/DATA/1979/7905.PDF.

1380. Varma JK, Greene KD, Ovitt J, Barrett TJ, Medalla F, Angulo FJ. 2005. Hospitalization and antimicrobial resistance in Salmonella outbreaks, United States, 1984–2002. Emerging Infectious Diseases 11(6):943–6. www.cdc.gov /ncidod/EID/vol11no06/pdf.s/04-1231.pdf.

1381. Drexler M. 2002. Secret Agents: The Menace of Emerging Infections (Washington, DC: Joseph Henry Press).

1382. Angulo F. 1999. Use of antimicrobial agents in aquaculture: potential for public health impact. Centers for Disease Control Memo to the Record, National Aquaculture Association Release, October 18. www.nationalaquaculture.org /pdf./CDC%20Memo%20to%20the%20Record.pdf.

1383. Centers for Disease Control and Prevention. Outbreak of multidrug-resistant Salmonella Newport—United States, January–April 2002. Morbidity and Mortality Weekly Report 51(25):545–8. cdc.gov/mmwr/preview/mmwrhtml ./mm5125a1.htm.

1384. Schroeder CM, Naugle AL, Schlosser WD, et al. 2005. Estimate of illnesses from Salmonella enteritidis in eggs, United States, 2000. Emerging Infectious Diseases 11(1):113–5. www.cdc.gov/foodnet/pub/publications/2005/040401 _schroeder.pdf.

1385. Burrows M. 2006. More Salmonella is reported in chickens. New York Times, March 8. nytimes.com/2006/03/08/dining/08well.html.

1386. World Health Organization. 2000. Drug resistance threatens to reverse medical progress. Press Release, June 12.

1387. Drexler M. 2002. Secret Agents: The Menace of Emerging Infections (Washington, DC: Joseph Henry Press).

1388. Drexler M. 2002. Secret Agents: The Menace of Emerging Infections (Washington, DC: Joseph Henry Press).

1389. Drexler M. 2002. Secret Agents: The Menace of Emerging Infections (Washington, DC: Joseph Henry Press).

1390. National Cattlemen's Beef Association. 2006. Antibiotic resistant bacteria found in U.S. poultry. Food Safety and Health. www.beefusa.org/NEWSAnti bioticResistantBacteriaFoundinUSPoultry14111.aspx.

1391. Boyd W. 2001. Making meat: science, technology, and American poultry production. Technology and Culture 42:631–64.

1392. Worldwatch Institute. 2004. Meat: now, it's not personal! But like it or not, meat-eating is becoming a problem for everyone on the planet. World Watch magazine, July/August, pp. 12–20.

1393. Torres-Vélez F, Brown C. 2004. Emerging infections in animals—potential new zoonoses. Clinics in Laboratory Medicine 24:825–38.

1394. Kaplan MM, Webster RG. 1977. The epidemiology of influenza. Scientific American 237:88–106.

1395. Silverstein AM. 1981. Pure Politics and Impure Science, the Swine Flu Affair (Baltimore, Maryland: Johns Hopkins University Press, pp. 129–31).

1396. Davies P. 1999. The plague in waiting. Guardian, August 7. www.guardian.co .uk/birdflu/story/0,14207,1131477,00.html.

1397. Davis M. 2005. Has time run out? Commentary: on The Monster at Our Door—the coming flu pandemic. Mother Jones, August 17. motherjones.com /commentary/columns/2005/08/has_time_run_out.html.

1398. Taylor M. 2005. Is there a plague on the way? Farm Journal, March 10. www .agweb.com/get_article.asp?pageid=116037.

1399. Lee M. 2005. Panel: plan for flu crisis now; world isn't prepared to combat pandemic, health experts say. Star Tribune (Minneapolis, MN) June 17, p. 8A.

1400. Drexler M. 2002. Secret Agents: The Menace of Emerging Infections (Washington, DC: Joseph Henry Press).

1401. Laver G. 2002. Influenza virus surface glycoproteins, haemagglutinin and neuraminidase: a personal account. Perspectives in Medical Virology 7:31.

1402. Kaplan MM. 1982. The epidemiology of influenza as a zoonosis. Veterinary Record 110:395–9.

1403. Webby RJ, Webster RG. 2001. Emergence of influenza A viruses. Philosophical Transactions of the Royal Society of London 356:1817–28.

1404. 2001. The virus hunters. South China Morning Post, May 25, p. 15.

1405. World Health Organization. 2005. H5N1 avian influenza: Timeline. October 28. www.who.int/csr/disease/avian_influenza/Timeline_28_10a.pdf.

1406. Gadsby P. 1999. Fear of flu—pandemic influenza outbreaks. Discover, January.

1407. Webster RG. 1997. Influenza virus: Transmission between species and relevance to emergence of the next human pandemic. Archives of Virology 13:S105–13.

1408. Naegel LCA. 1990. A review of public health problems associated with the integration of animal husbandry and aquaculture, with a special emphasis on Southeast Asia. Biological Wastes 31:69–83.

1409. Torrey EF, Yolken RH. 2005. Beasts of the Earth: Animals, Humans, and Disease (New Brunswick, NJ: Rutgers University Press).

1410. Matsui S. 2005. Protecting human and ecological health under viral threats in Asia. Water Science and Technology 51(8):91–7.

1411. Normile D. 2004. Asia struggles to keep humans and chickens apart. Science 306:399.

1412. Scholtissek C, Naylor E. 1988. Fish farming and influenza pandemics. Nature 331:215.

1413. Scholtissek C, Naylor E. 1988. Fish farming and influenza pandemics. Nature 331:215.

1414. Matsui S. 2005. Protecting human and ecological health under viral threats in Asia. Water Science and Technology 51(8):91–7.

1415. United States Food and Drug Administration. 1992. Vibrio cholerae Serogroup Non-O1. Foodborne pathogenic microorganisms and natural toxins handbook. www.cfsan.fda.gov/~mow/chap8.html.

1416. Lederberg J, Shope RE, Oaks SC. 1992. Emerging Infections: Microbial Threats to Health in the United States (Washington, DC: National Academies Press).

1417. Bondad-Reantaso MG, Subasinghe RP, Arthur JR. 2005. Disease and health management in Asian aquaculture. Veterinary Parasitology 132(3–4):249–72.

1418. Naegel LCA. 1990. A review of public health problems associated with the integration of animal husbandry and aquaculture, with a special emphasis on Southeast Asia. Biological Wastes 31:69–83.

1419. Naylor E, Scholtissek C. 1989. A potential human health hazard in integrated aquaculture-agriculture systems which include both pigs and poultry. Pig News and Information, March 1989, Volume 10, No. 1, pp. 17–8.

1420. Nelson B. 2005. Bird flu outbreak; global threat; experts say deadly virus presents grave risk if we don't "get our act together." Newsday, March 6, p. A03.

1421. Osterholm M, Colwell R, Garrett L, Fauci AS. 2005. The Council on Foreign Relations meeting: the threat of global pandemics. Federal News Service, June 16. www.cfr.org/publication/8198/threat_of_global_pandemics.html.

1422. McDonald H. 2003. China's unsafe farming practices may be breeding more than pigs, Sydney Morning Herald, April 7.

1423. Webster RG. 1997. Influenza virus: transmission between species and relevance to emergence of the next human pandemic. Archives of Virology 13:S105–13.

1424. Buras N, Duek L, Niv S, Hepher B, Sandbank E. 1987. Microbiological aspects of fish grown in treated wastewater. Water Research 21(1):1–10.

1425. Scholtissek C. 1992. Cultivating a killer virus. Natural History 1(92):2–6.

1426. Torrey EF, Yolken RH. 2005. Beasts of the Earth: Animals, Humans, and Disease (New Brunswick, NJ: Rutgers University Press).

1427. Mathias, JA. 1995. Aquaculture: The Blue Revolution. Canadian Business and Current Affairs Ecodecision, September, pp. 66–70.

1428. Bailey C, Jentoft S, Sinclair P. 1996. Aquaculture Development: Social Dimensions of an Emerging Industry (Boulder, CO: Westview Press).

1429. Edwards P. 1991. Fish-fowl-pig farming uncommon. World Aquaculture 22(3):2–3.

1430. Osterholm MT. 2005. Preparing for the next pandemic. Foreign Affairs 84(4). www.foreignaffairs.org/20050701faessay84402/michael-t-osterholm/preparing-for-the-next-pandemic.html.

1431. Manci WE. 1991. Let's promote discussion. World Aquaculture 22(3):6.

1432. Torrey EF, Yolken RH. 2005. Beasts of the Earth: Animals, Humans, and Disease (New Brunswick, NJ: Rutgers University Press).

1433. Cullington BJ. 1990. Emerging viruses, emerging threat. Science 247: 279–80.

1434. Naeve CW, Hinshaw VS, Webster RG. 1984. Mutations in the hemagglutinin receptor-binding site can change the biological properties of an influenza virus. Journal of Virology 51:567–9.

1435. Osterhaus ADME, de Jong JC, Rimmelzwaan GF, Class ECJ. 2002. H5N1 influenza in Hong Kong: virus characterizations. Vaccine 20:S82–3.

1436. Davies P. 2000. The Devil's Flu (New York, NY: Henry Holt and Company).

1437. Taubenberger JK, Kash JC, Morens DM. 2019. The 1918 influenza pandemic: 100 years of questions answered and unanswered. Sci Transl Med. 11(502):eaau5485. https://doi.org/10.1126/scitranslmed.aau5485.

1438. Smith GJ, Bahl J, Vijaykrishna D, Zhang J, Poon LL, Chen H, Webster RG, Peiris JS, Guan Y. 2009. Dating the emergence of pandemic influenza viruses. Proc Natl Acad Sci U S A. 106(28):11709–11712. https://doi.org/10.1073/pnas.0904991106.

1439. Zhou NN, Senne DA, Landgraf JS, Swenson SL, Erickson G, Rossow K, Liu L, Yoon Kj, Krauss S, Webster RG. 1999. Genetic reassortment of avian, swine, and human influenza A viruses in American pigs. J Virol. 73(10):8851–8856.

1440. dos Reis M, Hay AJ, Goldstein RA. 2009. Using non-homogeneous models of nucleotide substitution to identify host shift events: application to the origin of the 1918 'Spanish' influenza pandemic virus. J Mol Evol. 69(4):333–345. https://doi.org/10.1007/s00239-009-9282-x.

1441. Guan Y, Vijaykrishna D, Bahl J, Zhu H, Wang J, Smith GJ. 2010. The emergence of pandemic influenza viruses. Protein Cell. 1(1):9–13. https://doi.org/10.1007/s13238-010-0008-z.

1442. Guan Y, Vijaykrishna D, Bahl J, Zhu H, Wang J, Smith GJ. 2010. The emergence of pandemic influenza viruses. Protein Cell. 1(1):9–13. https://doi.org/10.1007/s13238-010-0008-z.

1443. Brockwell-Staats C, Webster RG, Webby RJ. Diversity of influenza viruses in swine and the emergence of a novel human pandemic influenza A (H1N1). Influenza Other Respir Viruses. 3(5):207–213. https://doi.org/10.1111/j.1750-2659.2009.00096.x.

1444. Wuethrich B. 2003. Infectious disease. Chasing the fickle swine flu. Science. 299(5612):1502–1505. https://doi.org/10.1126/science.299.5612.1502.

1445. Sturgis S. 2009 May 5. Swine flu genes traced to North Carolina factory farm. Durham: Facing South; [accessed 2020 Apr 18]. https://www.facingsouth.org/2009/05/swine-flu-genes-traced-to-north-carolina-hog-farm.html.

1446. Zhou NN, Senne DA, Landgraf JS, et al. 1999. Genetic reassortment of avian, swine, and human influenza A viruses in American pigs. Journal of Virology 73:8851–6.

1447. Webby RJ, Swenson SL, Krauss SL, Gerrish PJ, Goyal SM, Webster RG. 2000. Evolution of swine H3N2 influenza viruses in the United States. Journal of Virology 74:8243–51.

1448. Wuethrich B. 2003. Infectious disease. Chasing the fickle swine flu. Science. 299(5612):1502–1505. https://doi.org/10.1126/science.299.5612.1502.

1449. Wilson TM, Logan-Henfrey L, Weller R, Kellman B. 2000. Agroterrorism, biological crimes, and biological warfare targeting animal agriculture. In: Brown C, Bolin C, editors. Emerging diseases of animals. Washington (DC): ASM Press. p. 23–57. https://doi.org/10.1128/9781555818050.ch3.

1450. Shields DA, Mathews KH. 2003. Interstate livestock movements. USDA Economic Research Service. Report No.: LDP-M-108-01; [updated 2003 June 5; accessed 2020 Apr 2]. https://www.ers.usda.gov/webdocs/publications/37685/15376_ldpm10801_1_.pdf.

1451. Burrell A. 2002. Animal disease epidemics: implications for production, policy and trade. Outlook Agric. 31(3):151–160. https://doi.org/10.5367/000000002101294001.

1452. Strelioff CC, Vijaykrishna D, Riley S, Guan Y, Peiris JSM, Lloyd-Smith JO. 2013. Inferring patterns of influenza transmission in swine from multiple streams of surveillance data. Proc Biol Sci. 280(1762):20130872. https://dx.doi.org/10.1098/rspb.2013.0872.

1453. Wallace RG. 2009. Breeding influenza: the political virology of offshore farming. Antipode. 41(5):916–951.

1454. Mena I, Nelson MI, Quezada-Monroy F, Dutta J, Cortes-Fernández R, Lara-Puente JH, Castro-Peralta F, Cunha LF, Trovão NS, Lozano-Dubernard B, et al. 2016. Origins of the 2009 H1N1 influenza pandemic in swine in Mexico. eLife. 5:e16777. https://dx.doi.org/10.7554/eLife.16777.

1455. Suriya R, Hassan L, Omar AR, Aini I, Tan CG, Lim YS, Kamaruddin MI. 2008. Seroprevalence and risk factors for influenza A viruses in pigs in Peninsular Malaysia. Zoonoses Public Health. 55(7):342–351. https://doi.org/10.1111/j.1863-2378.2008.01138.x.

1456. Beltran-Alcrudo D, Falco JR, Raizman E, Dietze K. 2019. Transboundary spread of pig diseases: the role of international trade and travel. BMC Vet Res. 15(1):64. https://doi.org/10.1186/s12917-019-1800-5.

1457. Webby RJ, Swenson SL, Krauss SL, Gerrish PJ, Goyal SM, Webster RG. 2000. Evolution of swine H3N2 influenza viruses in the United States. J Virol. 74(18):8243–8251. https://doi.org/10.1128/jvi.74.18.8243-8251.2000.

1458. Environmental Defense. 2000 Nov. Factory hog farming: the big picture. New York: Environmental Defense Fund; [accessed 2020 Apr 9]. https://web.archive.org/web/20081102210913/http://www.edf.org/documents/2563_FactoryHogFarmingBigPicture.pdf.

1459. Center on Globalization, Governance & Competitiveness. 2006. Hog farming: overview. Durham(NC): Duke University; [updated 2006 Feb 23; accessed 2020 Apr 9]. https://web.archive.org/web/20061013165542/http://www.soc.duke.edu/NC_GlobalEconomy/hog/overview.php.

1460. North Carolina Department of Agriculture and Consumer Services. 2001. North Carolina agriculture overview: livestock. [updated 2001 Feb 23; accessed 2020 Apr 9]. https://web.archive.org/web/20040810163842/http://www.ncagr.com:80/stats/general/livestoc.htm.

1461. Byerly CR. 2005. Fever of war: the influenza epidemic in the U.S. Army during World War I. New York: New York University Press. p. 160.

1462. Maes D, Deluyker H, Verdonck M, Castryck F, Miry C, Vrijens B, de Kruif A. 2000. Herd factors associated with the seroprevalences of four major respiratory pathogens in slaughter pigs from farrow-to-finish pig herds. Vet Res. 31(3):313–327. https://doi.org/10.1051/vetres:2000122.

1463. Madec F, Rose N. 2003. How husbandry practices may contribute to the course of infectious diseases in pigs. In: 4th International Symposium on Emerging and Re-emerging Pig Diseases; 2003 June 29–July 2; Rome. Ploufragan (France): French Agency for Food Safety. p. 9–18.

1464. Enøe C, Mousing J, Schirmer AL, Willeberg P. 2002. Infectious and rearing-system related risk factors for chronic pleuritis in slaughter pigs. Prev Vet Med. 54(4):337–349. https://doi.org/10.1016/S0167-5877(02)00029-6.

1465. Maes D, Deluyker H, Verdonck M, Castryck F, Miry C, Vrijens B, de Kruif A. 2000. Herd factors associated with the seroprevalences of four major respiratory pathogens in slaughter pigs from farrow-to-finish pig herds. Vet Res. 31(3):313–327. https://doi.org/10.1051/vetres:2000122.

1466. Poljak Z, Carman S, McEwen B. Assessment of seasonality of influenza in swine using field submissions to a diagnostic laboratory in Ontario between 2007 and 2012. Influenza Other Respir Viruses. 8(4):482–492.

1467. Crawford D. 2000. The invisible enemy: a natural history of viruses. Oxford: Oxford University Press.

1468. Baudon E, Peyre M, Peiris M, Cowling BJ. 2017. Epidemiological features of influenza circulation in swine populations: a systematic review and meta-analysis. PLoS ONE. 12(6):e0179044. https://doi.org/10.1371/journal.pone.0179044.

1469. Takemae N, Shobugawa Y, Nguyen PT, Nguyen T, Nguyen TN, To TL, Thai PD, Nguyen TD, Nguyen DT, Nguyen DK, et al. 2016. Effect of herd size on subclinical infection of swine in Vietnam with influenza A viruses. BMC Vet Res. 12(1):227. https://doi.org/10.1186/s12917-016-0844-z.

1470. Poljak Z, Dewey CE, Martin SW, Christensen J, Carman S, Friendship RM. 2008. Prevalence of and risk factors for influenza in southern Ontario swine herds in 2001 and 2003. Can J Vet Res. 72(1):7–17.

1471. Maes D, Deluyker H, Verdonck M, Castryck F, Miry C, Vrijens B, de Kruif A. 2000. Herd factors associated with the seroprevalences of four major respiratory pathogens in slaughter pigs from farrow-to-finish pig herds. Vet Res. 31(3):313–327. https://doi.org/10.1051/vetres:2000122.

1472. de Souza Almeida HM, Storino GY, Pereira DA, Gatto IRH, Mathias LA, Montassier HJ, de Oliveira LG. 2017. A cross-sectional study of swine influenza in intensive and extensive farms in the northeastern region of the state of São Paulo, Brazil. Trop Anim Health Prod. 49(1):25–30. https://doi.org/10.1007/s11250-016-1153-z.

1473. Wuethrich B. 2003. Infectious disease. Chasing the fickle swine flu. Science. 299(5612):1502–1505. https://doi.org/10.1126/science.299.5612.1502.

1474. 1993. Overcrowding pigs pays—if it's managed properly. National Hog Farmer, November 15.

1475. Wuethrich B. 2003. Infectious disease. Chasing the fickle swine flu. Science. 299(5612):1502–1505. https://doi.org/10.1126/science.299.5612.1502.

1476. Yan JZ, Morrison B, Meyer T, Deen J. 2003. Inside China. Pig Progress. 19(1):9–14. [updated 2006 Aug 17; accessed 2020 Apr 3]. https://www.pig progress.net/Home/General/2003/1/Inside-China-PP005236W/.

1477. Gardner IA, Willeberg P, Mousing J. 2002. Empirical and theoretical evidence for herd size as a risk factor for swine diseases. Anim Health Res Rev. 3(1):43–55.

1478. Ludwig S, Stitz L, Planz O, Van H, Fitch WM, Scholtissek C. 1995. European swine virus as a possible source for the next influenza pandemic? Virology 212:555–61.

1479. SmithField Foods. 2005. Thirty years of progress 1975–2005. smithfieldfoods .com/Investor/Pdf./AnnualReports/SmithfieldFoods_05AR_LoRes.pdf.

1480. Kettlewell J. 2004. Polish factory farms cause a stink. BBC News, November 24. news.bbc.co.uk/2/hi/science/nature/4035081.stm.

1481. MacKenzie D. 1998. This little piggy fell ill. New Scientist, September 12.

1482. Webster RG, Sharp GB, Claas CJ. 1995. Interspecies transmission of influenza viruses. Americal Journal of Respiratory and Critical Care Medicine 152:525–30.

1483. Agriculture and Agri-Food Canada. 1997. The hog and pork industries of Denmark and the Netherlands: a competitiveness analysis. March. agr.gc.ca:8081 /spb/rad-dra/publications/hognprk/hognprk_e.pdf.

1484. 2003. Too many, too smelly. Economist, August 7. economist.com/displayStory .cfm?story_id=1979752.

1485. Decision News Media SAS 2004. Danish pork industry on the rise. October 24. foodproductiondaily.com/news/ng.asp?id=49755-danish-pork-industry.

1486. MacKenzie D. 1998. This little piggy fell ill. New Scientist, September 12.

1487. MacKenzie D. 1998. This little piggy fell ill. New Scientist, September 12.

1488. Delgado C, Rosegrant M, Steinfeld H, Ehui S, Courbois C. 1999. Livestock to 2020: the next food revolution. Food, Agriculture, and the Environment Discussion Paper 28. For the International Food Policy Research Institute, the Food and Agriculture Organization of the United Nations and the International Livestock Research Institute. ifpri.org/2020/dp/dp28.pdf.

1489. MacKenzie D. 1998. This little piggy fell ill. New Scientist, September 12, p. 1818.

1490. MacKenzie D. 1998. This little piggy fell ill. New Scientist, September 12, p. 1818.

1491. Choi YK, Lee JH, Erickson G, et al. 2004. H3N2 influenza virus transmission from swine to turkeys, United States. Emerging Infectious Diseases. 10:2156–60.

1492. Webster RG, Hulse DJ. 2004. Microbial adaptation and change: avian influenza. Rev Sci Tech. 23(2):453–465. https://doi.org/10.20506/rst.23.2.1493.

1493. U.S. Department of Agriculture. 2009 Feb 25. Poultry slaughter 2008 annual summary. Ithaca: USDA Economics, Statistics and Market Information System; [accessed 2020 Apr 2]. https://downloads.usda.library.cornell.edu/usda-esmis /files/pg15bd88s/kd17cw364/qn59q6557/PoulSlauSu-02-25-2009.pdf.

1494. U.S. Department of Agriculture. 2009 Feb 26. Chickens and eggs 2008 summary. Ithaca: USDA Economics, Statistics and Market Information System;

[accessed 2020 Apr 2]. https://downloads.usda.library.cornell.edu/usda-esmis/files/1v53jw96n/7h149s210/p5547v38d/ChickEgg-02-26-2009.pdf.

1495. Graham JP, Leibler JH, Price LB, Otte JM, Pfeiffer DU, Tiensin T, Silbergeld EK. 2008. The animal-human interface and infectious disease in industrial food animal production: rethinking biosecurity and biocontainment. Public Health Rep. 123(3):282–299. https://doi.org/10.1177/003335490812300309.

1496. Dawood FS, Iuliano AD, Reed C, Meltzer MI, Shay DK, Cheng P-Y, Bandaranayake D, Breiman RF, Brooks WA, Buchy P, et al. 2012. Estimated global mortality associated with the first 12 months of 2009 pandemic influenza A H1N1 virus circulation: a modelling study. Lancet Infect Dis. 12(9):687–695. https://doi.org/10.1016/S1473-3099(12)70121-4.

1497. Myers KP, Olsen CW, Gray GC. 2007. Cases of swine influenza in humans: a review of the literature. Clin Infect Dis. 44(8):1084–1088. https://doi.org/10.1086/512813.

1498. Wells DL, Hopfensperger DJ, Arden NH, et al. 1991. Swine influenza virus infections: transmission from ill pigs to humans at a Wisconsin agricultural fair and subsequent probable person-to-person transmission. Journal of the American Medical Association 265(4):478–81.

1499. Claas ECJ, de Jong JC, van Beek R, Rimmelzwaan GF, Osterhaus ADME. 1998. Human influenza virus A/HongKong/156/97 (H5N1) infection. Vaccine 16:977–8.

1500. Matrosovich MN, Matrosovich TY, Gray T, Roberts NA, Klenk HD. 2004. Human and avian influenza viruses target different cell types in cultures of human airway epithelium. Proceedings of the National Academy of Sciences of the United States of America 101(13):4620–4.

1501. Arnst C. 2005. A hot zone in the heartland. Little could be done to contain a deadly avian flu outbreak. Business Week, September 19. businessweek.com/magazine/content/05_38/b3951008.htm.

1502. Taubenberger JK, Morens DM. 2006. 1918 influenza: the mother of all pandemics. Emerging Infectious Diseases 12(1):15–22.

1503. Shortridge KF, Gao P, Guan Y, et al. 2000. Interspecies transmission of influenza viruses: H5N1 virus and a Hong Kong SAR perspective. Veterinary Microbiology 74:141–7.

1504. Arnst C. 2005. A hot zone in the heartland. Little could be done to contain a deadly avian flu outbreak. Business Week, September 19. businessweek.com/magazine/content/05_38/b3951008.htm.

1505. Gargan EA. 1997. As avian flu spreads, China is seen as its epicenter. New York Times, December 21, p. 10. query.nytimes.com/gst/fullpage.html.?res=9803E6DF173EF932A15751C1A961958260&sec=health&pagewanted=print.

1506. Food and Agriculture Organization of the United Nations. 2020. Sources of meat. Rome: FAO; [updated 2014 Nov 25; accessed 2020 Apr 8].

1507. Environmental Defense. 2000. Factory hog farming: the big picture. November. environmentaldefense.org/documents/2563_FactoryHogFarmingBigPicture.pdf.

1508. Iowa Egg Council. 2002. Production. iowaegg.org/allabouteggs/production.html.

1509. Food and Agriculture Organization of the United Nations. 2006. FAO-STAT database. Livestock primary, January 24. faostat.fao.org/faostat/collec tions?subset=agriculture.

1510. Webby RJ, Swenson SL, Krauss SL, Gerrish PJ, Goyal SM, Webster RG. 2000. Evolution of swine H3N2 influenza viruses in the United States. J Virol. 74(18):8243–8251. https://doi.org/10.1128/jvi.74.18.8243-8251.2000.

1511. Karasin AI, Carman S, Olsen CW. 2006. Identification of human H1N2 and human-swine reassortant H1N2 and H1N1 influenza A viruses among pigs in Ontario, Canada (2003 to 2005). J Clin Microbiol. 44(3):1123–1126. https://doi.org/10.1128/JCM.44.3.1123-1126.2006.

1512. Fleites MÁ, Buenfil JCR, Carrasco AC, Guzmán LR, Tavera GA, Correa JCS. 2004. Serological profile of porcine influenza virus, Mycoplasma hyopneumoniae and Actinobacillus pleuropneumoniae, in farms of Yucatan, Mexico. Vet Méx. 35(4):295–305.

1513. Lee CS, Kang BK, Kim HK, Park SJ, Park BK, Jung K, Song DS. 2008. Phylogenetic analysis of swine influenza viruses recently isolated in Korea. Virus Genes. 37(2):168–176. https://doi.org/10.1007/s11262-008-0251-z.

1514. Smith GJ, Vijaykrishna D, Bahl J, Lycett SJ, Worobey M, Pybus OG, Ma SK, Cheung CL, Raghwani J, Bhatt S, et al. 2009. Origins and evolutionary genomics of the 2009 swine-origin H1N1 influenza A epidemic. Nature. 459(7250):1122–1125. https://doi.org/10.1038/nature08182.

1515. Trovão NS, Nelson MI. 2020. When pigs fly: pandemic influenza enters the 21st century. PLoS Pathog. 16(3):e1008259. https://doi.org/10.1371/journal.ppat .1008259.

1516. Ma W, Liu Q, Qiao C, del Real G, García-Sastre A, Webby RJ, Richt JA. 2014. North American triple reassortant and Eurasian H1N1 swine influenza viruses do not readily reassort to generate a 2009 pandemic H1N1-like virus. mBio. 5(2):e00919–13. https://dx.doi.org/10.1128/mBio.00919-13.

1517. Drew TW. 2011. The emergence and evolution of swine viral diseases: to what extent have husbandry systems and global trade contributed to their distribution and diversity? Rev Sci Tech. 30(1):95–106. https://doi.org/10.20506/rst .30.1.2020.

1518. Rajao DS, Anderson TK, Kitikoon P, Stratton J, Lewis NS, Vincent AL. 2018. Antigenic and genetic evolution of contemporary swine H1 influenza viruses in the United States. Virology. 518:45–54. https://doi.org/10.1016/j.virol.2018 .02.006.

1519. Fabrizio TP, Sun Y, Yoon SW, Jeevan T, Dlugolenski D, Tripp RA, Tang L, Webby RJ. 2016. Virologic differences do not fully explain the diversification of swine influenza viruses in the United States. J Virol. 90(22):10074–10082. https://doi.org/10.1128/JVI.01218-16.

1520. Hari J. 2009 May 1. Life-threatening disease is the price we pay for cheap meat. Independent (London, United Kingdom). [accessed 2020 Apr 2]; https://www.independent.co.uk/voices/commentators/johann-hari/johann -hari-life-threatening-disease-is-the-price-we-pay-for-cheap-meat-1677067 .html.

1521. Fablet C, Simon G, Dorenlor V, Eono F, Eveno E, Gorin S, Quéguiner S, Madec F, Rose N. 2013. Different herd level factors associated with H1N1 or H1N2 influenza virus infections in fattening pigs. Prev Vet Med. 112(3-4): 257–265. https://doi.org/10.1016/j.prevetmed.2013.07.006.

1522. Lawrence AB, Petherick JC, McLean KA, Deans LA, Chirnside J, Gaughan A, Clutton E, Terlouw EMC. 1994. The effect of environment on behaviour, plasma cortisol and prolactin in parturient sows. Appl Anim Behav Sci. 39 (3-4):313–330. https://doi.org/10.1016/0168-1591(94)90165-1.

1523. Siegel HS. 1983. Effects of intensive production methods on livestock health. Agro—Ecosystems. 8(3-4):215–230. https://doi.org/10.1016/0304 -3746(83)90005-7.

1524. André F, Tuyttens M. 2005. The importance of straw for pig and cattle welfare: a review. Appl Anim Behav Sci. 92(3):261–282. https://doi.org/10.1016/j .applanim.2005.05.007.

1525. Ewald C, Heer A, Havenith U. 1994. Factors associated with the occurrence of influenza A virus infections in fattening swine. Berl Munch Tierarztl Wochenschr. 107(8):256–262.

1526. Crowding pigs pays—if it's managed properly. National Hog Farmer. November 15, 1993;62.

1527. Kennedy RF Jr. 1999. I don't like green eggs and ham! Newsweek, April 26.

1528. Corzo CA, Culhane M, Dee S, Morrison RB, Torremorell M. 2013. Airborne detection and quantification of swine influenza A virus in air samples collected inside, outside and downwind from swine barns. PLoS ONE. 8(8):e71444. https://doi.org/10.1371/journal.pone.0071444.

1529. Torremorell M, Alonso C, Davies PR, Raynor PC, Patnayak D, Torchetti M, McCluskey B. 2016. Investigation into the airborne dissemination of H5N2 highly pathogenic avian influenza virus during the 2015 spring outbreaks in the Midwestern United States. Avian Dis. 60(3):637–643. https://doi.org/10.1637 /11395-021816-Reg.1.

1530. Zhao Y, Richardson B, Takle E, Chai L, Schmitt D, Xin H. 2019. Airborne transmission may have played a role in the spread of 2015 highly pathogenic avian influenza outbreaks in the United States. Sci Rep. 9(1):11755. https://doi .org/10.1038/s41598-019-47788-z.

1531. Graham JP, Leibler JH, Price LB, Otte JM, Pfeiffer DU, Tiensin T, Silbergeld EK. 2008. The animal-human interface and infectious disease in industrial food animal production: rethinking biosecurity and biocontainment. Public Health Rep. 123(3):282–299. https://doi.org/10.1177/003335490812300309.

1532. Saenz RA, Hethcote HW, Gray GC. 2006. Confined animal feeding operations as amplifiers of influenza. Vector Borne Zoonotic Dis. 6(4):338–346. https://doi.org/10.1089/vbz.2006.6.338.

1533. Fragaszy E, Ishola DA, Brown IH, Enstone J, Nguyen-Van-Tam JS, Simons R, Tucker AW, Wieland B, Williamson SM, Hayward AC, et al. 2016. Increased risk of A(H1N1)pdm09 influenza infection in UK pig industry workers compared to a general population cohort. Influenza Other Respir Viruses. 10(4):291–300. https://dx.doi.org/10.1111/irv.12364.

1534. Lantos PM, Hoffman K, Höhle M, Anderson B, Gray GC. 2016. Are people living near modern swine production facilities at increased risk of influenza virus infection? Clin Infect Dis. 63(12):1558–1563. https://doi.org/10.1093/cid/ciw646.

1535. Koçer ZA, Obenauer J, Zaraket H, Zhang J, Rehg JE, Russell CJ, Webster RG. 2013. Fecal influenza in mammals: selection of novel variants. J Virol. 87(21):11476–11486. https://dx.doi.org/10.1128/JVI.01544-13.

1536. Haas B, Ahl R, Böhm R, Strauch D. 1995. Inactivation of viruses in liquid manure. Rev Sci Tech. 14(2):435–445. https://doi.org/10.20506/rst.14.2.844.

1537. Michiels A, Piepers S, Ulens T, Van Ransbeeck N, Del Pozo Sacristán R, Sierens A, Haesebrouck F, Demeyer P, Maes D. 2015. Impact of particulate matter and ammonia on average daily weight gain, mortality and lung lesions in pigs. Prev Vet Med. 121(1-2):99–107. https://doi.org/10.1016/j.prevetmed.2015.06.011.

1538. Desrosiers R, Boutin R, Broes A. 2004. Persistence of antibodies after natural infection with swine influenza virus and epidemiology of the infection in a herd previously considered influenza-negative. J Swine Health Prod. 12(2):78–81.

1539. Sawabe K, Hoshino K, Isawa H, Sasaki T, Hayashi T, Tsuda Y, Kurahashi H, Tanabayashi K, Hotta A, Saito T, et al. 2006. Detection and isolation of highly pathogenic H5N1 avian influenza A viruses from blow flies collected in the vicinity of an infected poultry farm in Kyoto, Japan, 2004. Am J Trop Med Hyg. 75(2):327–332.

1540. Centers for Disease Control and Prevention. [date unknown]. 2009 H1N1 pandemic. U.S. Department of Health and Human Services; [last reviewed 2019 June 11; accessed 2020 Apr 2]. https://www.cdc.gov/flu/pandemic-resources/2009-h1n1-pandemic.html.

1541. Centers for Disease Control and Prevention. 2009. Outbreak of swine-origin influenza A (H1N1) virus infection—Mexico, March–April 2009. U.S. Department of Health and Human Services. MMWR. 58(Dispatch):1-3; [last reviewed 2009 Apr 30; accessed 2020 Apr 2]. https://www.cdc.gov/mmwr/preview/mmwrhtml/mm58d0430a2.htm.

1542. Shapiro P. 2020 Mar 24. One root cause of pandemics few people think about. Sci Am. [accessed 2020 Apr 6]. https://blogs.scientificamerican.com/observations/one-root-cause-of-pandemics-few-people-think-about/.

1543. Maillard P. 2006. Adaptation rapide du virus influenza aviaire H5N1 au mammifère: la pandémie de grippe aviaire tiendrait-elle à un acide aminé? Virologie. 10(6):458–460.

1544. Wertheim HFL, Nghia HDT, Taylor W, Schultsz C. 2009. Streptococcus suis: an emerging human pathogen. Clin Infect Dis. 48(5):617–625. https://doi.org/10.1086/596763.

1545. U.S. Department of Agriculture. 2005 Aug. Streptococcus suis outbreak, swine and human, China. Riverdale(MD): USDA, APHIS; [accessed 2020 Apr 9]. https://web.archive.org/web/20090815051837/http://www.aphis.usda.gov/vs/ceah/cei/taf/emergingdiseasenotice_files/strep_suis_china.htm.

1546. World Health Organization Regional Office for the Western Pacific. 2005 Aug 2. Streptococcus suis. Manila(Philippines): WPRO; [accessed 2020 Apr 9]. https://web.archive.org/web/20091210033358/http://www.wpro.who.int/media_centre/fact_sheets/fs_20050802.htm.

1547. Pulliam JR, Epstein JH, Dushoff J, Rahman SA, Bunning M, Jamaluddin AA, Hyatt AD, Field HE, Dobson AP, Daszak P, et al. 2012. Agricultural intensification, priming for persistence and the emergence of Nipah virus: a lethal bat-borne zoonosis. J R Soc Interface. 9(66):89–101. https://doi.org/10.1098/rsif.2011.0223.

1548. Benfield C. 2009 Mar 24. Antibiotics in livestock 'threatens humans.' Yorkshire Post.

1549. Pew Commission on Industrial Farm Animal Production. 2008. Expert panel highlights serious public health threats from industrial animal agriculture. Press release issued April 11. www.pewtrusts.org/news_room_detail.aspx?id=37968. Accessed August 26, 2008.

1550. Pew Commission on Industrial Farm Animal Production. 2008 Apr 29. Putting meat on the table: industrial farm animal production in America. Executive summary. Philadelphia: PEW Charitable Trusts. p. 13. http://www.pewtrusts.org/~/media/Assets/2008/PCIFAP_Exec-Summary.pdf.

1551. American Public Health Association. 2019 Nov 5. Precautionary moratorium on new and expanding concentrated animal feeding operations. Washington: APHA; [accessed 2020 Apr 2]. https://www.apha.org/policies-and-advocacy/public-health-policy-statements/policy-database/2020/01/13/precautionary-moratorium-on-new-and-expanding-concentrated-animal-feeding-operations.

1552. Arizona State Legislature. 2007. 13–2910.07. Cruel and inhumane confinement of a pig during pregnancy or of a calf raised for veal. State of Arizona; [accessed 2020 Apr 9]. https://web.archive.org/web/20090321091854/https://www.azleg.gov/FormatDocument.asp?inDoc=/ars/13/02910-07.htm&Title=13&DocType=ARS.

1553. California Legislative Information. 2008. Chapter 13.8. Farm animal cruelty. 25991. Definitions. State of California; [amended 2018 Nov 6; accessed 2020 Apr 6]. https://leginfo.legislature.ca.gov/faces/codes_displaySection.xhtml?lawCode=HSC&sectionNum=25991.

1554. Colorado General Assembly. 2008 May 14. Chapter 228. Agriculture. An act concerning requirements for confinement of specified livestock. State of Colorado; [accessed 2020 Apr 6]. https://leg.colorado.gov/sites/default/files/images/olls/2008a_sl_228.pdf.

1555. Florida Legislature. [date unknown]. Article X. Section 21. Limiting cruel and inhumane confinement of pigs during pregnancy. State of Florida; [accessed 2020 Apr 6]. http://www.leg.state.fl.us/Statutes/index.cfm?Mode=Constitution&Submenu=3&Tab=statutes#A10S21.

1556. Maine Legislature. 2020. Section 4020. Cruel confinement of calves raised for veal and sows during gestation. State of Maine; [accessed 2020 Apr 6]. http://www.mainelegislature.org/legis/statutes/7/title7sec4020.html.

1557. Ballotpedia. 2016. Massachusetts minimum size requirements for farm animal containment, question 3 (2016). Ballotpedia; [accessed 2020 Apr 6]. https://ballotpedia.org/Massachusetts_Minimum_Size_Requirements_for_Farm_Animal_Containment,_Question_3_(2016).

1558. Michigan Legislature. 2020. Enrolled senate bill no. 174. Animal industry act. State of Michigan; [accessed 2020 Apr 6]. www.legislature.mi.gov/documents/2019-2020/publicact/pdf/2019-PA-0132.pdf.

1559. LAWriter. 2016. Ohio administrative code. Chapter 901:12-8 swine. Lawriter LLC; [accessed 2020 Apr 6]. http://codes.ohio.gov/oac/901:12-8.

1560. OregonLaws.org. 2017. ORS 600.150 Prohibition against restrictive confinement. Public Technology Ltd; [accessed 2020 Apr 6]. https://www.oregonlaws.org/ors/600.150.

1561. Rhode Island General Assembly. [date unknown]. Section 4-1.1-3. Unlawful confinement. State of Rhode Island; [accessed 2020 Apr 6]. http://webserver.rilin.state.ri.us/Statutes/TITLE4/4-1.1/4-1.1-3.HTM.

1562. Wuethrich B. 2003. Infectious disease. Chasing the fickle swine flu. Science. 299(5612):1502–1505. https://doi.org/10.1126/science.299.5612.1502.

1563. Webby RJ, Rossow K, Erickson G, Sims Y, Webster R. 2004. Multiple lineages of antigenically and genetically diverse influenza A virus co-circulate in the United States swine population. Virus Res. 103(1-2):67–73. https://doi.org/10.1016/j.virusres.2004.02.015.

1564. Chen H, Cheung CL, Tai H, Zhao P, Chan JFW, Cheng VCC, Chan KH, Yuen KY. 2009. Oseltamivir-resistant influenza A pandemic (H1N1) 2009 virus, Hong Kong, China. Emerg infect Dis. 15(12):1970–1972. https://dx.doi.org/10.3201/eid1512.091057.

1565. Wei K, Sun H, Sun Z, Sun Y, Kong W, Pu J, Ma G, Yin Y, Yang H, Guo X, et al. 2014. Influenza A virus acquires enhanced pathogenicity and transmissibility after serial passages in swine. J Virol. 88(20):11981–11994. https://doi.org/10.1128/JVI.01679-14.

1566. Taubenberger JK, Morens DM. 2013. Influenza viruses: breaking all the rules. mBio. 4(4):e00365-13. https://doi.org/10.1128/mBio.00365-13.

1567. Keim B. 2009 May 1. Swine flu ancestor born on U.S. factory farms. Wired.com; [accessed 2020 Apr 9]. https://web.archive.org/web/20140706145323/http://www.wired.com/2009/05/swineflufarm/.

1568. Wuethrich B. 2003. Infectious disease. Chasing the fickle swine flu. Science. 299(5612):1502–1505. https://doi.org/10.1126/science.299.5612.1502.

1569. De Jong JC, de Ronde-Verloop JM, Bangma PJ, Van Kregten E, Kerckhaert J, Paccaud MF, Wicki F, Wunderli W. 1986. Isolation of swine-influenza-like A (H1N1) viruses from man in Europe, 1986. Lancet. 328(8519):1329–1330. https://doi.org/10.1016/S0140-6736(86)91450-9.

1570. De Jong JC, de Ronde-Verloop JM, Bangma PJ, Van Kregten E, Kerckhaert J, Paccaud MF, Wicki F, Wunderli W. 1986. Isolation of swine-influenza-like A (H1N1) viruses from man in Europe, 1986. Lancet. 328(8519):1329–1330. https://doi.org/10.1016/S0140-6736(86)91450-9.

1571. Wiley S. 2020. The 2009 influenza pandemic: 10 years later. Nursing2020.

50(1):17–20. https://journals.lww.com/nursing/Fulltext/2020/01000/The_2009_influenza_pandemic__10_years_later.6.aspx.

1572. Wong JY, Kelly H, Ip DKM, Wu JT, Leung GM, Cowling BJ. 2013 Nov. Case fatality risk of influenza A (H1N1pdm09): a systematic review. Epidemiology. 24(6). https://dx.doi.org/10.1097/EDE.0b013e3182a67448.

1573. Dawood FS, Iuliano AD, Reed C, Meltzer MI, Shay DK, Cheng P-Y, Bandaranayake D, Breiman RF, Brooks WA, Buchy P, et al. 2012. Estimated global mortality associated with the first 12 months of 2009 pandemic influenza A H1N1 virus circulation: a modelling study. Lancet Infect Dis. 12(9):687–695. https://doi.org/10.1016/S1473-3099(12)70121-4.

1574. 2001. The virus hunters. South China Morning Post, May 25, p. 15.

1575. Shortridge KF. 1992. Pandemic influenza: a zoonosis? Seminars in Respiratory Infections 7:11–25.

1576. Shortridge KF. 1982. Avian influenza A viruses of southern China and Hong Kong: ecological aspects and implications for man. Bulletin of the World Health Organization 60:129–35.

1577. Elegant S. 2003. The breeding grounds: what other bugs are out there? Time, April 7. time.com/time/asia/magazine/printout/0,13675,501030407-438944,00.html./.

1578. Shortridge KF. 2003. Severe Acute Respiratory Syndrome and influenza virus incursions from Southern China. American Journal of Respiratory and Critical Care Medicine 168:1416–20.

1579. U.S. State Department Bureau of East Asian and Pacific Affairs. 2006. Hong Kong Special Administrative Region. January. state.gov/r/pa/ei/bgn/2747.htm.

1580. Travelsmart.com. Hong Kong. Population and people. travelsmart.net/hk/hotels/.

1581. Fielding R, Lam WW, Ho EY, Lam TH, Hedley AJ, Leung GM. 2005. Avian influenza risk perception, Hong Kong. Emerging Infectious Diseases 11(5):677–82.

1582. FAO/OIE/WHO. 2005. Consultation on avian influenza and human health: risk reduction measures in producing, marketing, and living with animals in Asia. Renaissance Hotel, Kuala Lumpur, Malaysia 4–6 July.

1583. Ellis MT, Bousfield RB, Bissett LA, et al. 2004. Investigation of outbreaks of highly pathogenic H5N1 avian influenza in waterfowl and wild birds in Hong Kong in late 2002. Avian Pathology 33:492–505.

1584. Sims LD, Ellis TM, Liu KK, et al. 2003. Avian influenza in Hong Kong 1997–2002. Avian Diseases 47:832–8.

1585. Marwick C. 1998. Could virulent virus be harbinger of "new flu"? Journal of the American Medical Association 279:259–60.

1586. Shortridge KF, Peiris JS, Guan Y. 2003. The next influenza pandemic: lessons from Hong Kong Journal of Applied Microbiology 94(1):70.

1587. Fielding R, Lam WT, Ho EYY, Lam TH, Hedley AJ, Leung GM. 2005. Avian influenza risk perception, Hong Kong. Emerging Infectious Diseases 11(5):677–82.

1588. Parry J. 2003. Hong Kong under WHO spotlight after flu outbreak. British Medical Journal 327:308.

1589. Fong J. 2004. Beating "bird flu" against the odds. Greatreporter.com, March 3. greatreporter.com/mambo/content/view/227/2/.

1590. Macan-Markar M. 2005. Bird flu pandemic may hang on for years. Inter Press Service, February 26.

1591. Dronamraju K (ed.), 2004. Infectious Disease and Host-Pathogen Evolution (Cambridge, UK: Cambridge University Press).

1592. Fielding R, Lam WT, Ho EYY, Lam TH, Hedley AJ, Leung GM. 2005. Avian influenza risk perception, Hong Kong. Emerging Infectious Diseases 11(5):677–82.

1593. Hedley AJ, Leung GM, Fielding R, Lam TH. 2004. The prevention of avian influenza in Hong Kong: observations on the HKSAR government's consultation document. Department of Community Medicine and Unit for Behavioural Sciences, School of Public Health, The University of Hong Kong. legco.gov.hk /yr03-04/english/panels/fseh/papers/fe0604cb2-2583-03-e.pdf.

1594. Choi MJ, Torremorell M, Bender JB, Smith K, Boxrud D, Ertl JR, Yang M, Suwannakarn K, Her D, Nguyen J, et al. 2015. Live animal markets in Minnesota: a potential source for emergence of novel influenza A viruses and interspecies transmission. Clin Infect Dis. 61(9):1355–1362. https://doi.org /10.1093/cid/civ618.

1595. Wu Y, Shi W, Lin J, Wang M, Chen X, Liu K, Xie Y, Luo L, Anderson BD, Lednicky JA, et al. 2017. Aerosolized avian influenza A (H5N6) virus isolated from a live poultry market, China. J Infect. 74(1):89–91. https://doi.org/10 .1016/j.jinf.2016.08.002.

1596. Bertran K, Balzli C, Kwon Y-K, Tumpey TM, Clark A, Swayne DE. 2017. Airborne transmission of highly pathogenic influenza virus during processing of infected poultry. Emerg Infect Dis. 23(11):1806–1814. https://doi.org/10 .3201/eid2311.170672.

1597. Chen H, Deng G, Li Z, et al. 2004. The evolution of H5N1 influenza viruses in ducks in southern China. Proceedings of the National Academy of Sciences of the United States of America 101(28):10452–7.

1598. Appenzeller T. 2005. Tracking the next killer flu. National Geographic, October. www7.nationalgeographic.com/ngm/0510/feature1/.

1599. Webster RG, Hulse DJ. 2004. Microbial adaptation and change: avian influenza. Revue Scientifique et Technique 23(2):453–65.

1600. Hedley AJ, Leung GM, Fielding R, Lam TH. 2004. The prevention of avian influenza in Hong Kong: observations on the HKSAR government's consultation document. Department of Community Medicine and Unit for Behavioural Sciences, School of Public Health, The University of Hong Kong. legco.gov.hk /yr03-04/english/panels/fseh/papers/fe0604cb2-2583-03-e.pdf.

1601. FAO/WHO global forum of food safety regulators in Marrekech, Morocco, January 28–30. www.fao.org/DOCREP/MEETING/004/AB427E.HTM.

1602. Webster RG, Hulse DJ. 2004. Microbial adaptation and change: avian influenza. Revue Scientifique et Technique 23(2):453–65.

1603. Lam A. 2004. China's dangerous wild tastes. Pacific News Service, January 1.

1604. Fielding R, Lam WT, Ho EYY, Lam TH, Hedley AJ, Leung GM. 2005. Avian influenza risk perception, Hong Kong. Emerging Infectious Diseases 11(5):677–82.

1605. 2006. Live birds back on sale despite ban. Shanghai Daily News, March 2. english.eastday.com/eastday/englishedition/node20665/node20669/node22813/node95960/node95963/node95964/node95966/userobject1ai1885583.html.

1606. Hoo S. 2005. China closes all Beijing poultry markets. Associated Press, November 7. katv.com/news/stories/1105/275446.html.

1607. 2006. Hong Kong to ban live poultry sales in three years. Agence France Presse. news.yahoo.com/s/afp/healthfluhongkong;_ylt=Ak6dh2DxZxiPZHN HKChGjwiTvyIi;_ylu=X3oDMTBiMW04NW9mBHNlYwMlJVRPUCUl.

1608. Webby RJ, Webster RG. 2001. Emergence of influenza A viruses. Philosophical Transactions of the Royal Society of London 356:1817–28.

1609. Perez DR, Nazarian SH, McFadden G, Gilmore MS. 2005. Miscellaneous threats: Highly pathogenic avian influenza, and novel bio-engineered organisms. In: Bronze MS, Greenfield RA (eds.), Biodefense: Principles and Pathogens (Norfolk, UK: Horizon Bioscience).

1610. Brown C. 1999. Economic considerations of agricultural diseases. Annals New York Academy of Sciences 894:92–94.

1611. Alexander DJ. 2000. A review of avian influenza in different bird species. Veterinary Microbiology 74:3–13.

1612. Stubbs EL. 1925. Fowl pest. Sixty-Second Annual Meeting of the American Veterinary Medical Association, Portland, Oregon, July 21–24.

1613. Linares JA, Gayle L, Sneed L, Wigle W. 2004. H5N2 avian influenza outbreak in Texas. In: 76th Northeastern Conference on Avian Diseases: June 9–11 (State College, Pennsylvania: Department of Veterinary Science, College of Agricultural Sciences, Pennsylvania State University, p. 14). www.vetsci.psu.edu/NECAD/NECADProceedings.pdf.

1614. Suarez DL, Spackman E, Senne DA. 2003. Update on molecular epidemiology of H1, H5, and H7 influenza virus infections in poultry in North America. Avian Diseases 47:888–97.

1615. Shane S. 2004. Live-bird markets are under the microscope: as the United States battles new outbreaks of bird flu, the role and necessity of live-bird markets must be examined. National Provisioner 218(4):38. www.findarticles.com/p/articles/mi_hb314/is_200404/ai_hibm1G1117180028.

1616. Suarez DL, Spackman E, Senne DA. 2003. Update on molecular epidemiology of H1, H5, and H7 influenza virus infections in poultry in North America. Avian Diseases 47:888–97.

1617. Senne DA, Pederson JC, Panigrahy B. 2003. Live-bird markets in the Northeastern United States: a source of avian influenza in commercial poultry. In: Schrijver RS, Koch G (eds.), Proceedings of the Frontis Workshop on Avian Influenza: Prevention and Control (Wageningen, The Netherlands, pp. 19–24).

1618. Kingsbury K. 2004. Animal markets are alive with controversy. Columbia News Service. February 16. www.jrn.columbia.edu/studentwork/cns/2004-02-16/455.asp.

1619. Choi YK, Seo SH, Kim JA, Webby RJ, Webster RG. 2005. Avian influenza viruses in Korean live poultry markets and their pathogenic potential. Virology 332:529–537.

1620. Lashley FR. 2004. Emerging infectious diseases: vulnerabilities, contributing factors and approaches. Expert Review of Anti-infective Therapy 2(2):299–316.

1621. Shane S. 2004. Live-bird markets are under the microscope: as the United States battles new outbreaks of bird flu, the role and necessity of live-bird markets must be examined. National Provisioner 218(4):38. findarticles .com/p/articles/mi_hb314/is_200404/ai_hibm1G1117180028.

1622. Shane S. 2004. Live-bird markets are under the microscope: as the United States battles new outbreaks of bird flu, the role and necessity of live-bird markets must be examined. National Provisioner 218(4):38. findarticles .com/p/articles/mi_hb314/is_200404/ai_hibm1G1117180028.

1623. Suarez DL, Spackman E, Senne DA. 2003. Update on molecular epidemiology of H1, H5, and H7 influenza virus infections in poultry in North America. Avian Diseases 47:888–97.

1624. Suarez DL, Spackman E, Senne DA. 2003. Update on molecular epidemiology of H1, H5, and H7 influenza virus infections in poultry in North America. Avian Diseases 47:888–97.

1625. Shane S. 2004. Live-bird markets are under the microscope: as the United States battles new outbreaks of bird flu, the role and necessity of live-bird markets must be examined. National Provisioner 218(4):38. findarticles .com/p/articles/mi_hb314/is_200404/ai_hibm1G1117180028.

1626. Webster RG. 2004. Wet markets—a continuing source of severe acute respiratory syndrome and influenza? Lancet 363:234–6.

1627. Swayne DE. 2003. Transcript of the question and answer session from the Fifth International Symposium on Avian Influenza. Avian Diseases 47:1219–55.

1628. Suarez DL, Spackman E, Senne DA. 2003. Update on molecular epidemiology of H1, H5, and H7 influenza virus infections in poultry in North America. Avian Diseases 47:888–97.

1629. Mullaney R. 2003. Live-bird market closure activities in the northeastern United States. Avian Diseases 47:1096–8.

1630. 2004. Bird flu found at four New Jersey live chicken markets. USA Today, February 12. usatoday.com/news/nation/2004-02-12-bird-flu_x.htm.

1631. Kingsbury K. 2004. Animal markets are alive with controversy. Columbia News Service. February 16. www.jrn.columbia.edu/studentwork/cns/2004 -02-16/455.asp.

1632. Shane S. 2004. Live-bird markets are under the microscope: as the United States battles new outbreaks of bird flu, the role and necessity of live-bird markets must be examined. National Provisioner 218(4):38. findarticles .com/p/articles/mi_hb314/is_200404/ai_hibm1G1117180028.

1633. Bulaga LL, Garber L, Senne D, et al. 2003. Descriptive and surveillance studies of suppliers to New York and New Jersey retail live-bird markets. Avian Diseases 47:1169–76.

1634. U.S. Department of Agriculture. Agriculture Research Service. 2005. Science Hall of Fame. December 16. www.ars.usda.gov/careers/hof/browse.htm.

1635. Thacker C. 2006. Live markets: a risk for entry of bird flu into US. Dow Jones Newswires, March 31. cattlenetwork.com/content.asp?contentid=26782.

1636. U.S. Department of Agriculture Food Safety Inspection Service. 2005. Guidance for determining whether a poultry slaughter or processing operation is exempt from inspection requirements of the Poultry Products Inspection Act. June. www.fsis.usda.gov/OPPDE/rdad/FSISNotices/Poultry_Slaughter _Exemption_0605.pdf.

1637. Iowa Department of Agriculture and Land Stewardship Meat and Poultry Inspection Bureau. Slaughter-processing-labeling-marketing: the basics. www .agriculture.state.ia.us/thebasics.htm.

1638. Shane S. 2004. Live-bird markets are under the microscope: as the United States battles new outbreaks of bird flu, the role and necessity of live-bird markets must be examined. National Provisioner 218(4):38. www.findarticles.com /p/articles/mi_hb314/is_200404/ai_hibm1G1117180028.

1639. Hedley AJ, Leung GM, Fielding R, Lam TH. 2004. The prevention of avian influenza in Hong Kong: observations on the HKSAR government's consultation document. Department of Community Medicine and Unit for Behavioural Sciences, School of Public Health, The University of Hong Kong. legco.gov.hk /yr03-04/english/panels/fseh/papers/fe0604cb2-2583-03-e.pdf.

1640. Webby RJ, Webster RG. 2001. Emergence of influenza A viruses. Philosophical Transactions of the Royal Society of London 356:1817–28.

1641. Food and Agriculture Organization of the United Nations. Technical Task Force on Avian Influenza. 2005. Update on the avian influenza situation. Avian Influenza Disease Emergency News, issue 28. www.fao.org/ag/againfo/subjects /documents/ai/AVIbull028.pdf.

1642. BirdLife International. 2005. Waterbird culls and wetland drainage could worsen spread of Avian Influenza, BirdLife warns. News release, October 20. birdlife.org/news/pr/2005/10/bird_flu_measures.html.

1643. Boon D. 2006. Wild birds, poultry, and avian influenza. Lancet Infectious Diseases 6:262.

1644. Melville DS, Shortridge KF. 2004. Influenza: time to come to grips with the avian dimension. Lancet Infectious Diseases 4:261–2.

1645. Food and Agriculture Organization of the United Nations. 2005. Army of volunteers helps detect flu early. fao.org/newsroom/en/focus/2005/100356 /article_100556en.html.

1646. 2004. Bird flu death toll rises to 18 in Asia. Associated Press, February 5.

1647. Sipress A. 2005. Bird flu adds new danger to bloody game; cockfighting among Asian customs that put humans at risk. Washington Post, April 14.

1648. Reynolds G. 2004. Our lives in their hands; they scour the earth for clues that could prevent millions of deaths. Independent, November 15. findarticles .com/p/articles/mi_qn4158/is_20041115/ai_n12822423.

1649. 2004. Cock-fighters the culprits. September 16. e.sinchew-i.com/content.pht ml.?sec=2&artid=200409160005.

1650. Taipei Times. 2005. Cockfighting to resume in Thailand. December 6. taipei times.com/News/world/archives/2005/12/06/2003283202.

1651. 2004. Fighting cocks fan Thai flu fears. The Australian, February 4.

1652. Food and Agriculture Organization of the United Nations. Army of volunteers helps detect flu early. 2005. fao.org/newsroom/en/focus/2005/100356 /article_100556en.html.

1653. Gilbert M, Chaitaweesub P, Parakamawongsa T, et al. 2006. Free-grazing ducks and highly pathogenic avian influenza, Thailand. Emerging Infectious Diseases 12(2):227–34.

1654. Delgado CL, Narrod CA, Tiongco MM. 2003. Policy, Technical, and Environmental Determinants and Implications of the Scaling-Up of Livestock Production in Four Fast-Growing Developing Countries: A Synthesis. Submitted to the Food and Agricultural Organization of the United Nations by the International Food Policy Research Institute. July 24. www.fao.org/WAIRDOCS/ LEAD/x6170e/x6170e00.htm.

1655. Shane S. 2004. The Asian AI outbreak and what it means to the U.S. poultry industry. Meating Place, February, 2.

1656. 2005. Fatal flu. The NewsHour with Jim Lehrer transcript #8201. April 7.

1657. Sipress A. 2005. Bird flu adds new danger to bloody game; cockfighting among Asian customs that put humans at risk. Washington Post, April 14. washing tonpost.com/wp-dyn/articles/A51593-2005Apr13.html.

1658. Clifton M. 2004. Cockfighters spread Asian killer flu. Animal People, March.

1659. Piller C. 2005. Squawking at bird flu warning. Los Angeles Times, September 1. latimes.com/news/science/la-sci-cockfighting1sep01,0,1160398 .story?coll=la-home-science.

1660. Griffin J. 2014 Jan. Cockfighting laws. Washington(DC): National Conference of State Legislatures; [accessed 2020 Apr 18]. https://www.ncsl.org/research /agriculture-and-rural-development/cockfighting-laws.aspx.

1661. Pagan G. 2005. SB 156 bill analysis. January 28. info.sen.ca.gov/pub/bill/sen /sb_0151-0200/sb_156_cfa_20060109_123745_asm_comm.html.

1662. Veneman AM. 2004. Letter from U.S. Department of Agriculture Secretary to U.S. Senator Robert Bennet. May 24.

1663. Frabotta D. 2005. Bird flu's U.S. flyby? DVM Newsmagazine, December 1. www.dvmnewsmagazine.com/dvm/article/articleDetail.jsp?id=274373.

1664. Gallegly E. 2005. Smuggling cockfighting roosters a conduit to bird flu. Santa Barbara News-Press, December 11. tinyurl.com/m4369.

1665. Blumenauer E. 2003. USDA needs funding to fight animal abuse. Agriculture and Animal Welfare. Floor Speeches, July 14. www.blumenauer.house.gov/issues /FloorSpeechSummary.aspx?NewsID=71&IssueID=3.

1666. Estrada RT. 2003. Fighting roosters spreading disease? Modesto Bee, February 9. modbee.com/local/story/6130728p-7083314c.html.

1667. Estrada RT. 2003. Fighting roosters spreading disease? Modesto Bee, February 9. modbee.com/local/story/6130728p-7083314c.html.

1668. U.S. Department of Transportation. 1998. USDA, APHIS, PPQ—Agricultural quarantine inspections database; the potential for international travelers to transmit foreign animal diseases to U.S. livestock or poultry. August, as cited in U.S. Department of Agriculture APHIS. Newcastle Disease in Luxembourg, December 1999 Impact Worksheet. www.aphis.usda.gov/vs/ceah/cei /taf/iw_1999_files/foreign/newcastle_lux1.htm.

1669. Aviagen. Welcome to Aviagen. www.aviagen.com/output.aspx?sec=10& con=334&siteId=1.

1670. Fernández-Gutiérrez A. Controlling highly pathogenic avian influenza. ThePoultrySite. thepoultrysite.com/FeaturedArticle/FAType. asp?AREA=game&Display=414.

1671. Carolina on the West Coast. 2005. Avian flu and our game birds. The Gamecock, December, p. 96.

1672. Gallegly E. 2005. Smuggling cockfighting roosters a conduit to bird flu. Santa Barbara News-Press, December 11. tinyurl.com/m4369.

1673. Blumenauer E. 2003. Cockfighting. U.S. Department of Agriculture Animal Welfare Information Center. March 31. www.nal.usda.gov/awic/cockfighting .htm.

1674. Public Health-Disease Control Programs, Department of Health Services, County of Los Angeles. 2003. Veterinary public health and rabies control: Cockfighting. www.lapublichealth.org/vet/docs/cockfight.pdf.

1675. Piller C. 2005. A virus stalks the henhouse. Los Angeles Times, December 13. www.latimes.com/news/printedition/front/la-sci-poultry13dec13,1,6174614 ,full.story?coll=la-headlines-frontpage.

1676. Estrada RT. 2003. Fighting roosters spreading disease? Modesto Bee, February 9. modbee.com/local/story/6130728p-7083314c.html.

1677. Frommer FJ. 2001. Senate passes anti-cockfighting bill. Associated Press, July 31. speakout.com/activism/apstories/10005-1.html.

1678. 2003. Project pork. ABC 7, May 13. abclocal.go.com/kgo/news/ iteam/051303_iteam_project_pork_chickens.html.#.

1679. Saville A (ed.), 2006. The American Game Fowl Standards (Belton, SC: The American Game Fowl Society).

1680. Slasherfowl. 2006. World Slasher Derby 2006. January 18, 2:05 AM. Game Rooster Public Forums Gamefowl Board. Accessed January 18, 2006. www .gamerooster.com.

1681. Murillo MAS. 2004. Weekender. Business World (Philippines) Financial Times Information Limited—Asia Intelligence Wire, January 30.

1682. Gay L. 2005. With threat of avian flu, bird smuggling becomes issue. Scripps Howard News Service, October 26. www.knoxstudio.com/shns/story.cfm ?pk=AVIANFLU-10-26-05&cat=AN.

1683. National Chicken Council. 2004. NCC backs increased penalties for cockfighting. April 12. www.poultryandeggnews.com/poultrytimes/news/April2004 /210283.html.

1684. Powelson R. 2005. Should the feds regulate cock fighting? Capitol Hill Blue, August 23. www.capitolhillblue.com/artman/publish/article_7259.shtml.

1685. Hearn J. 2004. Chicken lobby: curb cockfights. The Hill, April 7. www.hill news.com/business/040704_chicken.aspx.

1686. Food and Agriculture Organization of the United Nations. 2004. Animal health special report: avian influenza questions and answers. www.fao.org/ag /againfo/subjects/en/health/diseases-cards/avian_qa.html.

1687. Chen H. 2009. Avian influenza vaccination: the experience in China. Rev Sci Tech. 28(1):267–274. https://doi.org/10.20506/rst.28.1.1860.

1688. Specter M. 2005. Nature's bioterrorist. New Yorker, February 28, pp. 52–61.

1689. Rosenthal E. 2006. A scientific puzzle: some Turks have bird flu virus but aren't sick. New York Times, January 11, p. A10.nytimes.com/2006/01/11 /international/europe/11flu.html.?ex=1294635600&en=7a724fa647544955& ei=5090&partner=rssuserland&emc=rss.

1690. Gilbert M, Wint W, Slingenbergh J. 2004. The ecology of highly pathogenic avian influenza in East and South-east Asia: outbreaks distribution, risk factors and policy implications. Consultancy report for the Animal Health Service of the Animal Production and Health Division of the Food and Agriculture Organization of the United Nations, Rome, Italy, August.

1691. 2005. Bird Shippers of America Answers HSUS Charges. November 5.bird shippers.org/archives/2005/11/bird_shippers_o_1.html.

1692. Clifton M. 2005. Flu threat spreads opposition to cockfighting. Animal People, September, p. 1.

1693. Who's Who in the Egg and Poultry Industries in the USA and Canada—2005 /2006 (Mt. Morris, IL: Watt Publishing Company).

1694. Clifton M. 2005. Flu threat spreads opposition to cockfighting. Animal People, September, p. 1.

1695. Webster A. 1993. Thermal stress on chickens in transit. British Poultry Science 34(2):267–77.

1696. Whyte P, Collins JD, McGill K, Monahan C, O'Mahony H. 2001. The effect of transportation stress on excretion rates of campylobacters in market-age broilers. Poultry Science 80(6):817–20.

1697. Wildlife Conservation Society. 2004. Avian flu: Wildlife experts say that clos- ing overseas wild bird markets would help prevent spread of disease. Science Daily, February 4. www.sciencedaily.com/releases/2004/02/040203225930 .htm.

1698. Weinhold B. 2004. Infectious disease: the human costs of our environmental errors. Environmental Health Perspectives 112(1):A32–9. ehponline.org/mem bers/2004/112-1/EHP112pa32PDF.PDF.

1699. Weinhold B. 2004. Infectious disease: the human costs of our environmental errors. Environmental Health Perspectives 112(1):A32–9. ehponline.org/mem bers/2004/112-1/EHP112pa32PDF.PDF.

1700. Gerberding JL. Order of the Centers for Disease Control and Prevention, Department of Health and Human Services, March 10. www.cdc.gov/flu/avian /pdf./malaysia.pdf.

1701. Gay L. 2005. With threat of avian flu, bird smuggling becomes issue. Scripps Howard News Service, October 26. www.knoxstudio.com/shns/story.cfm ?pk=AVIANFLU-10-26-05&cat=AN.

1702. Wildlife Conservation Society. 2004. Avian flu: wildlife experts say that closing overseas wild bird markets would help prevent spread of disease. Science Daily, February 4. www.sciencedaily.com/releases/2004/02/040203225930.htm.

1703. Chong J. 2006. Bird flu defies control efforts. Los Angeles Times, March 27. latimes.com/news/printedition/la-sci-birdflu27mar27,0,2708107,full .story?coll=la-home-headlines.

1704. Gay L. 2005. With threat of avian flu, bird smuggling becomes issue. Scripps Howard News Service, October 26. www.knoxstudio.com/shns/story.cfm ?pk=AVIANFLU-10-26-05&cat=AN.

1705. U.S. Department of State. 2005. United States announces global coalition against wildlife trafficking. September 23. state.gov/r/pa/prs/ps/2005/53926.htm.

1706. Gay L. 2005. With threat of avian flu, bird smuggling becomes issue. Scripps Howard News Service, October 26. www.knoxstudio.com/shns/story.cfm ?pk=AVIANFLU-10-26-05&cat=AN.

1707. Gay L. 2005. With threat of avian flu, bird smuggling becomes issue. Scripps Howard News Service, October 26. www.knoxstudio.com/shns/story.cfm ?pk=AVIANFLU-10-26-05&cat=AN.

1708. MacKenzie D. 2004. Europe has close call with deadly bird flu. New Scientist, October 26. www.newscientist.com/article.ns?id=dn6575.

1709. Borm S, Thomas I, Hanquet G, et al. 2005. Highly pathogenic H5N1 influenza virus in smuggled Thai eagles, Belgium. Emerging Infectious Diseases 11(5):702–5. www.cdc.gov/ncidod/eid/vol11no05/05-0211.htm.

1710. Borm S, Thomas I, Hanquet G, et al. 2005. Highly pathogenic H5N1 influenza virus in smuggled Thai eagles, Belgium. Emerging Infectious Diseases 11(5):702–5. www.cdc.gov/ncidod/eid/vol11no05/05-0211.htm.

1711. MacKenzie D. 2004. Europe has close call with deadly bird flu. New Scientist, October 26. www.newscientist.com/article.ns?id=dn6575.

1712. Johnson RT. 2003. Emerging viral infections of the nervous system. Journal of NeuroVirology 9:140–7.

1713. Stapp K. 2004. Scientists warn of fast-spreading global viruses. IPS-Inter Press Service, February 23.

1714. Ronca SE, Murray KO, Nolan MS. 2019. Cumulative incidence of West Nile virus infection, continental United States, 1999–2016. Emerg Infect Dis. 25(2):325–327. https://doi.org/10.3201/eid2502.180765.

1715. Ludwig B, Kraus FB, Allwinn R, Doerr HW, Preiser W. 2003. Viral zoonoses— a threat under control? Intervirology 46:71–8.

1716. Food and Agriculture Organization of the United Nations. Technical Task Force on Avian Influenza. 2005. Update on the avian influenza situation. Avian Influenza Disease Emergency News, issue 28. www.fao.org/ag/againfo/subjects /documents/ai/AVIbull028.pdf.

1717. Gardiner B. 2005. Global bird trade raises bird flu concerns. Associated Press, October 24. abcnews.go.com/Business/print?id=1247482.

1718. ProMED-mail. 2004. Avian influenza, human—East Asia. January 29. www .promedmail.org/pls/promed/f?p=2400:1202:11412984429089452986::N

O::F2400_P1202_CHECK_DISPLAY,F2400_P1202_PUB_MAIL_ID:X
,24295.

1719. Office of Communications, U.S. Department of Agriculture. 2005. Transcript of technical briefing regarding avian influenza, October 26. Transcript
Release No. 0461.05. www.usda.gov/wps/portal/!ut/p/_s.7_0_A/7_0_1OB
?contentidonly=tru%C2%AD&contentid=2005/10/0461.xml.

1720. Department for Environment, Food and Rural Affairs. 2005. Epidemiology report published on H5N1 in Essex quarantine. DEFRA News Release, November 15. www.defra.gov.uk/news/2005/051115b.htm.

1721. Bureau of Animal and Plant Health Inspection and Quarantine Council of
COA, Executive Yuan. H5N1 Avian influenza virus detected in smuggled
birds from China. Government Information Office, Republic of China
(Taiwan), October 26. english.www.gov.tw/e-Gov/index.jsp?categid=217&
recordid=87565.

1722. Department for Environment, Food and Rural Affairs. 2005. Epidemiology report published on H5N1 in Essex quarantine. DEFRA News Release, November
15. www.defra.gov.uk/news/2005/051115b.htm.

1723. Schmit J. 2005. Pet bird buyers asking sellers about avian flu. USA Today,
November 11. www.usatoday.com/money/industries/health/2005-11-27-bird
-questions-usat_x.htm?csp=N009.

1724. Watts G. 2006. An old problem finds a new role. Watt PoultryUSA 7:82–3.

1725. Europa Press Release. 2005. Avian influenza: EU bans imports of captive live
birds from third countries. October 26. europa.eu.int/rapid/pressReleases
Action.do?reference=IP/05/1351&format=HTML.&aged=0&language=EN&g
uiLanguage=en.

1726. Centers for Disease Control and Prevention. 2006. Embargoed African rodents
and monkeypox virus. January 26. www.cdc.gov/ncidod/monkeypox/animals
.htm.

1727. Centers for Disease Control and Prevention. 2003. Update: multistate outbreak of monkeypox—Illinois, Indiana, Kansas, Missouri, Ohio, and Wisconsin. Morbidity and Mortality Weekly Report 52(27):642–46. cdc.gov/mmwr
/preview/mmwrhtml./mm5227a5.htm.

1728. McKenna MAJ. 2004. Smuggled birds may harbor avian flu; AMA to hear
experts warn how Southeast Asian virus could become a global threat. Atlanta
Journal-Constitution, December 6, p. 1A. www.cste.org/PS/2003pdf.s/03
-ID-13%20-%20FINAL.pdf.

1729. Gay L. 2005. With threat of avian flu, bird smuggling becomes issue. Scripps
Howard News Service, October 26. www.knoxstudio.com/shns/story.cfm
?pk=AVIANFLU-10-26-05&cat=AN.

1730. Frabotta D. 2005. Bird flu's U.S. flyby? DVM Newsmagazine, December 1.
www.dvmnewsmagazine.com/dvm/article/articleDetail.jsp?id=274373.

1731. McKenna MAJ. 2004. Smuggled birds may harbor avian flu; AMA to hear
experts warn how Southeast Asian virus could become a global threat. Atlanta
Journal-Constitution, December 6, p. 1A. wildaid.org/index.asp?CID=8&PID
=331&SUBID=&TERID=86.

1732. McKenna MAJ. 2004. Smuggled birds may harbor avian flu; AMA to hear experts warn how Southeast Asian virus could become a global threat. Atlanta Journal-Constitution, December 6, p. 1A. wildaid.org/index.asp?CID=8&PID=331&SUBID=&TERID=86.

1733. American Bird Conservancy, Defenders of Wildlife, Eurogroup for Animal Welfare, et al. An NGO call to halt wild bird imports into the European Union. European Union Wild Bird Declaration. birdsareforwatching.org/WB DecFinal.pdf.

1734. Gay L. 2005. With threat of avian flu, bird smuggling becomes issue. Scripps Howard News Service, October 26. www.knoxstudio.com/shns/story.cfm ?pk=AVIANFLU-10-26-05&cat=AN.

1735. Bradshaw B. 2006. United Kingdom Parliament House of Commons. Wild birds. April 25. www.publications.parliament.uk/pa/cm200506/cmhansrd /cm060425/text/60425w05.htm.

1736. Wright TF, Toft CA, Enkerlin-Hoeflich E, et al. 2001. Nest poaching in neo-tropical parrots. Conservation Biology 15(3):710–20.

1737. Born Free Foundation. Groups urge EU to end wild bird imports. bornfree .org.uk/birds.shtml.

1738. Editorial. 2003. Trade in wild animals: a disaster ignored Lancet Infectious Diseases 2(7):391.

1739. Bhattacharya S. 2005. Bird flu outbreaks expected in more countries. New Scientist, October 17. www.newscientist.com/article.ns?id=dn8140.

1740. 2005. Scientists say migratory birds may carry H5N1 avian flu virus to U.S. next year. People's Daily Online, October 29. english.people.com.cn/200510/29/eng 20051029_217622.html.

1741. Shortridge KF. 1999. Influenza—a continuing detective story. Lancet 354:siv29.

1742. Webster RG, Bean WJ, Gorman OT, Chambers TM, Kawaoka Y. 1992. Evolu-tion and ecology of influenza A viruses. Microbiological Reviews 56(1):152–79.

1743. Webster RG. 1997. Influenza virus: transmission between species and relevance to emergence of the next human pandemic. Archives of Virology 13:S105–13.

1744. Webster RG, Bean WJ, Gorman OT, Chambers TM, Kawaoka Y. 1992. Evolu-tion and ecology of influenza A viruses. Microbiol Rev. 56(1):152–179.

1745. Drexler M. 2002. Secret Agents: The Menace of Emerging Infections (Wash-ington, DC: Joseph Henry Press).

1746. Webster RG, Bean WJ, Gorman OT, Chambers TM, Kawaoka Y. 1992. Evolu-tion and ecology of influenza A viruses. Microbiological Reviews 56(1):152–79.

1747. Webster RG, Bean WJ, Gorman OT, Chambers TM, Kawaoka Y. 1992. Evolu-tion and ecology of influenza A viruses. Microbiological Reviews 56(1):152–79.

1748. Laver WG, Bischofberger N, Webster RG. 2000. The origin and control of pandemic influenza. Perspectives in Biology and Medicine 43(2):173–92.

1749. Wobeser GA. 1997. Diseases of Wild Waterfowl (New York, NY: Plenum Press).

1750. Webster RG, Shortridge KF, Kawaoka Y. 1997. Influenza: Interspecies trans-mission and emergence of new pandemics. Federation of European Microbio-logical Societies Immunology and Medical Microbiology 18:275–9.

1751. Murphy B. 1993. Factors restraining emergence of new influenza viruses. In: Morse SS (ed.), Emerging Viruses (New York, NY: Oxford University Press, pp. 234–40).

1752. Webster RG, Wright SM, Castrucci MR, Bean WJ, Kawaoka Y. 1993. Influenza—a model of an emerging virus disease. Intervirology 35:16–25.

1753. Shortridge KF. 1992. Pandemic influenza: a zoonosis? Seminars in Respiratory Infections 7:11–25.

1754. Webster RG, Bean WJ, Gorman OT, Chambers TM, Kawaoka Y. 1992. Evolution and ecology of influenza A viruses. Microbiological Reviews 56(1):152–79.

1755. Webby RJ, Webster RG. 2001. Emergence of influenza A viruses. Philosophical Transactions of the Royal Society of London 356:1817–28.

1756. Webster RG, Bean WJ, Gorman OT, Chambers TM, Kawaoka Y. 1992. Evolution and ecology of influenza A viruses. Microbiological Reviews 56(1):152–79.

1757. Handwerk B. 2002. Sharks falling prey to humans' appetites. National Geographic News, June 3. news.nationalgeographic.com/news/2002 /06/0603_020603_shark1.html.

1758. Sharp GB, Kawaoka Y, Jones DJ, et al. 1997. Coinfection of wild ducks by influenza A viruses: distribution patterns and biological significance. Journal of Virology 71:6128–35. jvi.asm.org/cgi/reprint/71/8/6128.pdf.

1759. Kurtz J, Manvell RJ, Banks J. 1996. Avian influenza virus isolated from a woman with conjunctivitis. Lancet. 348(9031):901–2.

1760. Webster RG, Geraci J, Petursson G, Skirnisson K. 1981. Conjunctivitis in human beings caused by influenza A virus of seals. New England Journal of Medicine 304(15):911.

1761. Davis M. 2005. The Monster at Our Door: The Global Threat of Avian Flu (New York, NY: The New Press).

1762. Horimoto T, Kawaoka Y. 2001. Pandemic threat posed by Avian Influenza A viruses. Clinical Microbiology Reviews 14:129–49.

1763. Subbarao K, Katz J. 2000. Avian influenza viruses infecting humans. Cellular and Molecular Life Sciences 57:1770–84.

1764. Webby RJ, Webster RG. 2001. Emergence of influenza A viruses. Philosophical Transactions of the Royal Society of London 356:1817–28.

1765. Whitney D. 2005. Bird flu battle on horizon: scientists fear the deadly virus is adapting and will hit the U.S. hard. Sacramento Bee, August 13, p. A3.

1766. Honigsbaum M. 2005. Flying Dutchman to the rescue: "virus hunter" sees bird flu as greatest threat. Guardian, June 3, p. 23. www.guardian.co.uk/life/feature /story/0,13026,1491811,00.html.

1767. Torrey EF, Yolken RH. 2005. Beasts of the Earth: Animals, Humans, and Disease (New Brunswick, NJ: Rutgers University Press).

1768. Shortridge KF. 1997. Is China an influenza epicentre? Chinese Medical Journal 110(8):637–41.

1769. Shortridge KF. 1992. Pandemic influenza: a zoonosis? Seminars in Respiratory Infections 7:11–25.

1770. Steneroden K, Roth R, Ramirez A, Spickler AR. Avian influenza (highly pathogenic): fowl plague, fowl pest, Brunswick bird plague, fowl disease, fowl or bird grippe. www.cfsph.iastate.edu/DiseaseInfo/notes/AvianInfluenza.pdf.

1771. Daszak P, Cunningham AA. 2002. Emerging infectious diseases: a key role for conservation medicine. In: Aguirre AA, Ostfeld RS, Tabor GM, House C, Pearl MC (eds.), Conservation Medicine: Ecological Health in Practice (New York, NY: Oxford University Press, pp. 40–61).

1772. Suarez DL, Garcia M, Latimer J, Senne D, Perdue M. 1999. Phylogenetic analysis of H7 avian influenza viruses isolated from the live bird markets of the northeastern United States. Journal of Virology 73:3567–73.

1773. Dronamraju K (ed.), 2004. Infectious Disease and Host-Pathogen Evolution (Cambridge, UK: Cambridge University Press).

1774. Hollenbeck JE. 2005. An avian connection as a catalyst to the 1918–1919 influenza pandemic. International Journal of Medical Sciences 2(2):87–90. pubmedcentral.nih.gov/articlerender.fcgi?artid=1145139.

1775. Webster RG. 1998. Influenza: an emerging microbial pathogen. In: Emerging Infections (San Diego, CA: Academic Press, pp. 275–300).

1776. Suarez DL, Perdue ML, Cox N, et al. 1998. Comparisons of highly virulent H5N1 influenza A viruses isolated from humans and chickens from Hong Kong. Journal of Virology 72:6678–88.

1777. Shortridge KF. 1992. Pandemic influenza: a zoonosis? Seminars in Respiratory Infections 7:11–25.

1778. Suarez DL. 2000. Evolution of avian influenza viruses. Veterinary Microbiology 74:15–27.

1779. Capua I, Alexander DJ. 2004. Avian influenza: recent developments. Avian Pathology 33:393–404.

1780. Sturm-Ramirez KM, Hulse-Post DJ, Govorkova EA. 2005. Are ducks contributing to the endemicity of highly pathogenic H5N1 influenza virus in Asia?

1781. Marwick C. 1998. Investigators present latest findings on Hong Kong "bird flu" to the FDA. Journal of the American Medical Association 279(9):643–44.

1782. Van Blerkom LM. 2003. Role of viruses in human evolution. Yearbook of Physical Anthropology 46:14–46. tinyurl.com/ksh92.

1783. Hayden D. 2003. Pox: Genius, Madness, and the Mysteries of Syphilis (New York, NY: Basic Books).

1784. Knell RJ. 2004. Syphilis in Renaissance Europe: rapid evolution of an introduced sexually transmitted disease? Proceedings of the Royal Society of London. Series B: Biological Sciences 7:271(Suppl 4):S174–6. www.ncbi.nlm.nih.gov/entrez/query.fcgi?cmd=Retrieve&db=pubmed&dopt=Abstract&list_uids=15252975&itool=iconabstr&query_hl=12&itool=pubmed_docsum.

1785. Flint SJ, Enquist LW, Racaniello VR, Skalka AM. 2004. Principles of Virology: Molecular Biology, Pathogenesis and Control of Animal Viruses (Washington, DC: American Society of Microbiology Press).

1786. Ryan F. 1997. Virus X: Tracking the New Killer Plagues—Out of the Present and Into the Future (Boston, MA: Little, Brown and Company).

1787. Dieckmann U, Metz JAJ, Sabelis MW, Sigmund K. 2002. Adaptive dynamics of infectious diseases: In: Pursuit of Virulence Management (Cambridge, UK: Cambridge University Press).

1788. Diamond J. 1992. The arrow of disease. Discover, October 13(10):64–73.

1789. Truyen U, Parrish CR, Harder TC, Kaaden O. 1995. There is nothing permanent except change. The emergence of new virus diseases. Veterinary Microbiology 43:103–22.

1790. Dimmock NJ, Easton A, Leppard K. 2001. Introduction to Modern Virology (Blackwell Publishing).

1791. Davis M. 2005. The Monster at Our Door: The Global Threat of Avian Flu (New York, NY: The New Press).

1792. Suarez DL. 2000. Evolution of avian influenza viruses. Veterinary Microbiology 74:15–27.

1793. Torrey EF, Yolken RH. 2005. Beasts of the Earth: Animals, Humans, and Disease (New Brunswick, NJ: Rutgers University Press).

1794. World Health Organization. 2005. Avian influenza: assessing the pandemic threat, January 1. www.who.int/csr/disease/influenza/H5N1-9reduit.pdf.

1795. Ito T, Goto H, Yamamoto E, et al. Generation of a highly pathogenic avian influenza A virus from an avirulent field isolate by passaging in chickens. Journal of Virology 75(9):4439–43. pubmedcentral.com/articlerender.fcgi?artid=114193.

1796. Capua I, Marangon S. 2003. The use of vaccination as an option for the control of avian influenza. In: 71st General Session International Committee of the World Organization for Animal Health (Paris, France, May 18–23).

1797. Morris RS, Jackson R. 2005. Epidemiology of H5N1 avian influenza in Asia and implications for regional control. Food and Agriculture Organization of the United Nations. January–February 11. thepoultrysite.com/FeaturedArticle/FAType.asp?AREA=turkeys&Display=121.

1798. Suarez DL, Spackman E, Senne DA. 2003. Update on molecular epidemiology of H1, H5, and H7 influenza virus infections in poultry in North America. Avian Diseases 47:888–97.

1799. U.S. Department of Agriculture, Agriculture Research Service. 2006. People and places. www.ars.usda.gov/pandp/people/people.htm?personid=5507.

1800. Ito T, Goto H, Yamamoto E, et al. Generation of a highly pathogenic avian influenza A virus from an avirulent field isolate by passaging in chickens. Journal of Virology 75(9):4439–43. pubmedcentral.com/articlerender.fcgi?artid=114193.

1801. Becker WB. 1966. The isolation and classification of tern virus: influenza A/tern/South Africa/1961. Journal of Hygiene 64(3):309–20.

1802. Sabirovic M. 2004. Qualitative risk analysis: HPAI in ostriches in South Africa. United Kingdom Department of Environment, Food and Rural Affairs. www.defra.gov.uk%A0///animalh/diseases/monitoring/pdf./hpai_safrica.pdf.

1803. Alexander DJ. 1986. Avian influenza—historical aspects. Proceedings of the Second International Symposium on Avian Influenza (University of Wisconsin: U.S. Animal Health Association, pp. 4–13).

1804. Dhingra MS, Artois J, Dellicour S, Lemey P, Dauphin G, Von Dobschuetz S, Van Boeckel TP, Castellan DM, Morzaria S, Gilbert M. 2018. Geographical and historical patterns in the emergences of novel highly pathogenic avian influenza (HPAI) H5 and H7 viruses in poultry. Front Vet Sci. 5:84. https://doi.org/10.3389/fvets.2018.00084.

1805. Stegeman A (Chairman). 2003. Workshop 1: Introduction and spread of avian influenza. In: Schrijver RS, Koch G (eds.), Proceedings of the Frontis Workshop on Avian Influenza: Prevention and Control. library.wur.nl/frontis/avian_influenza/workshop1.pdf.

1806. Brown EG, Liu H, Kit LC, Baird S, Nesrallah M. 2001. Pattern of mutation in the genome of influenza A virus on adaptation to increased virulence in the mouse lung: identification of functional themes. Proceedings of the National Academy of Sciences of the United States of America 98(12):6883–8.

1807. Brown EG, Liu H, Kit LC, Baird S, Nesrallah M. 2001. Pattern of mutation in the genome of influenza A virus on adaptation to increased virulence in the mouse lung: identification of functional themes. Proceedings of the National Academy of Sciences of the United States of America 98(12):6883–8.

1808. Domingo E, Menendez-Arias L, Holland JJ. 1997. RNA virus fitness. Reviews in Medical Virology 7:87–96.

1809. Brown E. 2006. Personal communication. May 4.

1810. Horimoto T, Kawaoka Y. 2001. Pandemic threat posed by Avian Influenza A viruses. Clinical Microbiology Reviews 14:129–49.

1811. Rhorer AR. 2005. Controlling avian flu: the case for a low-path control program. Watt PoultryUSA, July, pp. 28–35.

1812. Hall C. 2004. Impact of avian influenza on U.S. poultry trade relations—2002: H5 or H7 low pathogenic avian influenza. Annals of the New York Academy of Science 1026:47–53. www.blackwell-synergy.com/doi/abs/10.1196/annals.1307.006.

1813. Rhorer AR. 2005. Controlling avian flu: the case for a low-path control program. Watt PoultryUSA, July, pp. 28–35.

1814. Rojas H, Moreira R, Avalos P, Capua I, Marangon S. 2002. Avian influenza in poultry in Chile. Vet Rec. 151:188.

1815. Naeem K, Siddique N, Ayaz M, Jalalee MA. 2007. Avian influenza in Pakistan: outbreaks of low- and high-pathogenicity avian influenza in Pakistan during 2003–2006. Avian Dis. 51:189–193.

1816. Centers for Disease Control and Prevention. 2006. Guidance and recommendations. Interim guidance for protection of persons involved in U.S. avian influenza outbreak disease control and eradication activities. January 14. www.cdc.gov/flu/avian/professional/protect-guid.htm.

1817. Pringle CR. 2005. Avian influenza, human—East Asia (121): migratory birds. ProMED-mail, September 1. promedmail.org/pls/promed/f?p=2400:1001:::NO::F2400_P1001_BACK_PAGE,F2400_P1001_PUB_MAIL_ID:1000%2C30265.

1818. Tam JS. 2002. Influenza A (H5N1) in Hong Kong: an overview. Vaccine 20:S77–81.

1819. Kristensson K. 2006. Avian influenza and the brain—comments on the occasion of resurrection of the Spanish flu virus. Brain Research Bulletin 68:406–13.

1820. Shortridge KF. 1999. Influenza—a continuing detective story. Lancet 354:siv29.

1821. Webby RJ, Webster RG. 2001. Emergence of Influenza A Viruses. Philosophical Transactions of the Royal Society of London 356:1817–28.

1822. Campitelli L, Mogavero E, Alessandra M, et al. 2004. Interspecies transmission of an H7N3 influenza virus from wild birds to intensively reared domestic poultry in Italy. Virology 323:24–36.

1823. Reid AH, Taubenberger JK, Fanning TG. 2001. The 1918 Spanish influenza: integrating history and biology. Microbes and Infection 3:81–87.

1824. Gambaryan A, Webster R, Matrosovich M. 2002. Differences between influenza virus receptors on target cells of duck and chicken. Archives of Virology 147:1197–208.

1825. Matrosovich MN, Krauss S, Webster RG. 2001. Rapid communication: H9N2 influenza A viruses from poultry in Asia have human virus-like receptor specificity. Virology 281:156–62.

1826. Gambaryan A, Webster R, Matrosovich M. 2002. Differences between influenza virus receptors on target cells of duck and chicken. Archives of Virology 147:1197–208.

1827. Gambaryan A, Webster R, Matrosovich M. 2002. Differences between influenza virus receptors on target cells of duck and chicken. Archives of Virology 147:1197–208.

1828. Gambaryan A, Yamnikova S, Lvov D, et al. 2005. Receptor specificity of influenza viruses from birds and mammals: new data on involvement of the inner fragments of the carbohydrate chain. Virology 334(2):276–83.

1829. Olofsson S, Kumlin U, Dimock K, Amberg N. 2005. Avian influenza and sialic acid receptors: more than meets the eye. Lancet Infectious Diseases 5:184–8.

1830. Wolfe DN, Eitel MN, Gockowski J, et al. 2000. Deforestation, hunting and the ecology of microbial emergence. Global Change and Human Health 1:10–25.

1831. Garrett L. 1994. The Coming Plague: Newly Emerging Diseases in a World Out of Balance (New York, NY: Farrar, Straus, Giroux).

1832. Campitelli L, Mogavero E, Alessandra M, et al. 2004. Interspecies transmission of an H7N3 influenza virus from wild birds to intensively reared domestic poultry in Italy. Virology 323:24–36.

1833. Perez DR, Lim W, Seiler JP, et al. 2003. Role of quail in the interspecies transmission of H9 influenza A viruses: molecular changes on HA that correspond to adaptations from ducks to chickens. Journal of Virology 77:3148–56. jvi.asm.org/cgi/content/full/77/5/3148?view=full&pmid=12584339.

1834. University of Georgia Southeastern Cooperative Wildlife Disease Study. 1986. July. Avian influenza in live poultry markets. SCWDS Briefs, July.

1835. Centers for Disease Control and Prevention. 2005. Transmission of influenza A viruses between animals and people. October 17. www.cdc.gov/flu/avian/gen-info/transmission.htm.

1836. Orent W. 2005. Playing with viruses. Washington Post, April 17, p. B01. www.washingtonpost.com/wp-dyn/articles/A58300-2005Apr16.html.

1837. Oxford JS, Sefton A, Jackson R, Innes W, Daniels RS, Johnson NPAS. 2002. World War I may have allowed the emergence of "Spanish" influenza. Lancet Infectious Diseases 2:111–4.

1838. Phillips H, Killingray D. 2003. Introduction. In: Phillips H, Killingray D (eds.), The Spanish Influenza Pandemic of 1918–19: New Perspectives (London, UK: Routledge, pp. 1–26).

1839. Byerly CR. 2005. Fever of War: The Influenza Epidemic in the U.S. Army during World War I (New York, NY: New York University Press, p. 94).

1840. McGirk T, Adiga A, Glacier S. 2005. Will the next pandemic rival 1918? Times Asia, July 4. time.com/time/asia/magazine/printout/0,13675,501050711-107 9528,00.html.

1841. Barry JM. 2004. The site of origin of the 1918 influenza pandemic and its public health implications. Journal of Translational Medicine 2:3–7.

1842. Kolata G. 1999. Flu: The Story of the Great Influenza Pandemic (New York, NY: Simon & Schuster, Inc.).

1843. Elegant S. 2003. The breeding grounds: what other bugs are out there? Time, April 7. time.com/time/asia/magazine/printout/0,13675,501030407-438 944,00.html.

1844. Drexler M. 2002. Secret Agents: The Menace of Emerging Infections (Washington, DC: Joseph Henry Press).

1845. Shortridge KF. 1999. The 1918 "Spanish" flu: pearls from swine? Nature Medicine 5:384–5.

1846. Oxford JS. 2001. The so-called Great Spanish Influenza Pandemic of 1918 may have originated in France in 1916. Philosophical Transactions of the Royal Society of London 356:1857–9.

1847. Webster RG. 2001. A molecular whodunit. Science 293:1773–5.

1848. Oxford JS, Novelli P, Sefton A, Lambkin R. 2002. New millennium antivirals against pandemic and epidemic influenza: the neuraminidase inhibitors. Antiviral Chemistry and Chemotherapy 13:205–17.

1849. Ross E. 2004. Asia is the traditional cradle of influenza, although disease can originate anywhere. Biotech Week, February 25, p. 628.

1850. Oxford JS. 2001. The so-called Great Spanish Influenza Pandemic of 1918 may have originated in France in 1916. Philosophical Transactions of the Royal Society of London 356:1857–9.

1851. Jordan E. 1927. Epidemic Influenza, 1st Edition (Chicago, Illinois: American Medical Association).

1852. Hollenbeck JE. 2005. An avian connection as a catalyst to the 1918–9 influenza pandemic. International Journal of Medical Sciences 2(2):87–90. medsci .org/v02p0087.htm.

1853. Gladwell M. 1997. The dead zone. New Yorker, July 28. gladwell .com/1997/1997_09_29_a_flu.htm.

1854. Hollenbeck JE. 2005. An avian connection as a catalyst to the 1918–9 influenza pandemic. International Journal of Medical Sciences 2(2):87–90. medsci.org /v02p0087.htm.

1855. Hollenbeck JE. 2005. An avian connection as a catalyst to the 1918–9 influenza pandemic. International Journal of Medical Sciences 2(2):87–90. medsci .org/v02p0087.htm.

1856. Barry JM. 2004. The site of origin of the 1918 influenza pandemic and its public health implications. Journal of Translational Medicine 2:3–7.

1857. Thomson D, Thomson R. 1934. Influenza: Annals of the Pickett-Thomson Research Laboratory, 1st Edition (Baltimore, MD: Williams and Wilkens).

1858. Burnet FM, Clark E. 1942. Influenza: a survey of the last fifty years (Melbourne, Australia: Macmillan Co).

1859. Gladwell M. 1997. The dead zone. New Yorker, July 28. gladwell.com/1997 /1997_09_29_a_flu.htm.

1860. Ewald P.1994. Evolution of Infectious Disease (Oxford: Oxford University Press, p. 117).

1861. Rennie J. 2005. Bird reaper, pt. III: Paul Ewald replies. SciAm Observations, November 2. blog.sciam.com/index.php?title=bird_reaper_pt_iii_paul_ewald _replies&more=1&c=1&tb=1&pb=1.

1862. Rennie J. 2005. Bird reaper, pt. III: Paul Ewald replies. SciAm Observations, November 2. blog.sciam.com/index.php?title=bird_reaper_pt_iii_paul_ewald _replies&more=1&c=1&tb=1&pb=1.

1863. Rennie J. 2005. Bird reaper, pt. III: Paul Ewald replies. SciAm Observations, November 2. blog.sciam.com/index.php?title=bird_reaper_pt_iii_paul_ewald _replies&more=1&c=1&tb=1&pb=1.

1864. Orent W. 2005. Playing with viruses. Washington Post, April 17, p. B01. washingtonpost.com/wp-dyn/articles/A58300-2005Apr16.html.

1865. Normile D. 2005. Avian Influenza: pandemic skeptics warn against crying wolf. Science 310(5751):1112–3.

1866. Ewald PW. 1996. Guarding against the most dangerous emerging pathogens: Insights from evolutionary biology. Emerging Infectious Diseases 2(4). www .cdc.gov/ncidod/eid/vol2no4/ewald.htm.

1867. Wilson WO. 1966. Poultry production. Scientific American 215(1):56–64.

1868. Boyd W, Watts M. 1997. Agro-industrial just-in-time: the chicken industry and postwar American capitalism. In: Goodman D, Watts M (eds.), Globalising Food: Agrarian Questions and Global Restructuring (London, UK: Routledge, pp. 192–224).

1869. Tracy M. 1982. Agriculture in Western Europe—Challenge and Response 1880–1980 (London, UK: Granada).

1870. National Chicken Council. [date unknown]. Per capita consumption of poultry and livestock, 1960 to forecast 2020, in pounds. Washington: NCC [updated 2020 Mar; accessed 2020 Apr 8]. https://www.nationalchickencouncil.org/about -the-industry/statistics/per-capita-consumption-of-poultry-and-livestock-1965 -to-estimated-2012-in-pounds.

1871. Smil V. Worldwide transformation of diets, burdens of meat production and opportunities for novel food proteins. Enzyme and Medical Technology 30 (2002) 305–11.

1872. Boyd W, Watts M. 1997. Agro-industrial just-in-time: the chicken industry and postwar American capitalism. In: Goodman D, Watts M (eds.), Globalising Food: Agrarian Questions and Global Restructuring (London, UK: Routledge, pp. 192–224).

1873. Boyd W, Watts M. 1997. Agro-industrial just-in-time: the chicken industry and postwar American capitalism. In: Goodman D, Watts M (eds.), Globalising Food: Agrarian Questions and Global Restructuring (London, UK: Routledge, pp. 192–224).

1874. Dekich MA. 1998. Broiler industry strategies for control of respiratory and enteric diseases. Poultry Science 77:1176–80.

1875. Dekich MA. 1998. Broiler industry strategies for control of respiratory and enteric diseases. Poultry Science 77:1176–80.

1876. Boyd W, Watts M. 1997. Agro-industrial just-in-time: the chicken industry and postwar American capitalism. In: Goodman D, Watts M (eds.), Globalising Food: Agrarian Questions and Global Restructuring (London, UK: Routledge, pp. 192–224).

1877. Bellis M. The history of the vitamins. Vitamins—production methods. Inventors. About.com. inventors.about.com/library/inventors/bl_vitamins.htm.

1878. Novus International Incorporated. Alimet® and Novus tradition of excellence vision of the future. novusint.com/Public/About/HistoryComplete.asp.

1879. Jacob JP, Mather FB. 1998. The home broiler chicken flock. University of Florida, Institute of Food and Agricultural Sciences. edis.ifas.ufl.edu/PS035.

1880. Cheng HH. 2003. Industrial selection for disease resistance: molecular genetic techniques. In: Muir WM, Aggrey SE (eds.), Poultry Genetics, Breeding and Biotechnology (Wallingford, UK: CABI Publishing, pp. 385–98).

1881. Boyd W. 2001. Making meat: science, technology, and American poultry production. Technology and Culture 42:631–64.

1882. Wilson WO. 1966. Poulrty production. Scientific American 215(1):56–64.

1883. Drexler M. 2002. Secret Agents: The Menace of Emerging Infections (Washington, DC: Joseph Henry Press).

1884. Walters MJ. 2003. Six Modern Plagues and How We Are Causing Them (Washington, DC: Island Press).

1885. Boyd W. 2001. Making meat: science, technology, and American poultry production. Technology and Culture 42:631–64.

1886. Boyd W. 2001. Making meat: science, technology, and American poultry production. Technology and Culture 42:631–64.

1887. Boyd W. 2001. Making meat: science, technology, and American poultry production. Technology and Culture 42:631–64.

1888. U.S. Department of Agriculture Animal and Plant Health Inspection Service. 1995. APHIS history: a chronology of significant events, milestones and accomplishments of APHIS and its predecessor organizations. Sept. 13. permanent.access.gpo.gov/lps3025/history.html.

1889. Boyd W. 2001. Making meat: science, technology, and American poultry production. Technol Cult. 42(4):631–664.

1890. Ramos SE, MacLachlan M, Melton A. 2017. Impacts of the 2014–2015 highly pathogenic avian influenza outbreak on the U.S. poultry sector. A report from the Economic Research Service. U.S. Department of Agriculture. Report No.: LDPM-282-02. [updated 2017 Dec 20; accessed 2020 Apr 7]. https://www.ers.usda.gov/publications/pub-details/?pubid=86281.

1891. Hafez HM. 2003. Emerging and re-emerging diseases in poultry. World Poultry 19(7):23–7.

1892. Price LB, Johnson E, Vailes R, Silbergeld E. 2005. Fluoroquinolone-resistant Campylobacter isolates from conventional and antibiotic-free chicken products. Environmental Health Perspectives 113(5):557–60. www.ehponline.org/members/2005/7647/7647.html.

1893. Shane SM. 2003. Disease continues to impact the world's poultry industries. World Poultry 19(7):22–7.

1894. GRAIN. 2006. Fowl play: the poultry industry's central role in the bird flu crisis. grain.org/briefings/?id=194.

1895. ProMed-mail. 1998. Newcastle disease virus, mutation—Australia. December 11. promedmail.org/pls/promed/f?p=2400:1202:11447257451621287002::NO::F2400_P1202_CHECK_DISPLAY,F2400_P1202_PUB_MAIL_ID:X,4299.

1896. Tasmania Department of Primary Industries, Water and Environment. Newcastle Disease in poultry. www.dpiwe.tas.gov.au/inter.nsf/Attachments/CART-6FQ8LZ/$FILE/backyarders.pdf.

1897. Shane SM. 2003. Disease continues to impact the world's poultry industries. World Poultry 19(7):22–7.

1898. Madec F, Rose N. 2003. How husbandry practices may contribute to the course of infectious diseases in pigs. In: 4th International Symposium on Emerging and Re-emerging Pig Diseases, June 29—July 2 (Rome, Italy). unipr.it/arpa/facvet/dip/dipsa/ric/prrs2003/9-18.pdf.

1899. Ritchie BW. 1995. Avian Viruses: Function and Control (Lake Worth, FL: Wingers Publishing).

1900. Bueckert D. 2004. Avian flu outbreak raises concerns about factory farms. Daily Herald-Tribune (Grande Prairie, Alberta), April 8, p. 6. cp.org/english/online/full/agriculture/040407/a040730A.html.

1901. Boyd W. 2001. Making meat: science, technology, and American poultry production. Technology and Culture 42:631–64.

1902. Davis M. 2005. Has time run out? Commentary: On the Monster at Our Door—the coming flu pandemic. Mother Jones, August 17.

1903. Girard D. 2004. Coping with the flu virus. Toronto Star, April 10, p. F1.

1904. Brady M. 2004. The comeback kids: Just when you thought it was safe to go back outside, along comes another pestilence from the past. Ottawa Citizen, May 23.

1905. Manavalan T. 2004. From fowl to pigs to humans? New Straits Times, February 8.

1906. Mackenzie D. 2004. Review 2004: Bird flu threatens the world. New Scientist issue 2479, December 25.

1907. Stöhr K, Meslin FX. 1997. The role of veterinary public health in the prevention of zoonoses. Archives Virology 13:S207–18.

1908. Pheasant B. 2004. A virus of our hatching. The Financial Review (Australia), January 30.

1909. Capua I, Marangon S. 2003. The use of vaccination as an option for the control of avian influenza. World Organization for Animal Health 71st General Session in Paris, France, May 18–23. www.oie.int/eng/AVIAN_INFLUENZA/A_71%20SG_12_CS3E.pdf.

1910. Vidal J. 2006. Flying in the face of nature. Guardian, February 22. society.guardian.co.uk/health/story/0,1714703,00.html.

1911. Zhihong H, Shuyi Z, Zhu C. 2005. Zoonoses: the deadly diseases that animals pass on to us. Global Agenda: Magazine of World Economic Forum Annual Meeting. globalagendamagazine.com/2005/huzhihongzhangshuyichenzhu.asp.

1912. Pheasant B. 2004. A virus of our hatching. The Financial Review (Australia), January 30.

1913. Chastel C. 2004. Emergence of new viruses in Asia: is climate change involved? Médecine et maladies infectieuses 34:499–505.

1914. Prowse S. 2005. Biosecurity and emerging infectious diseases. Australia Academy of Technological Sciences and Engineering Focus No 136, March/April.

1915. Boyd W. 2001. Making meat: science, technology, and American poultry production. Technology and Culture 42:631–64.

1916. United Nations. 2005. UN task forces battle misconceptions of avian flu, mount Indonesian campaign. UN News Centre, October 24. un.org/apps/news/story.asp?NewsID=16342&Cr=bird&Cr1=flu.

1917. United Nations. 2005. UN task forces battle misconceptions of avian flu, mount Indonesian campaign. UN News Centre, October 24. un.org/apps/news/story.asp?NewsID=16342&Cr=bird&Cr1=flu.

1918. 2005. Preeminent vaccinologist led eradication of world's deadliest childhood diseases, saving and protecting millions. American Association of Immunologists Newsletter, June/July, p. 8. aai.org/newsletter/PDF.s/2005/JunJul PDF.pdf.

1919. Prince Mahidol Award Foundation. 1998. Professor Kennedy F Shortridge, PhD. kanchanapisek.or.th/kp10/awardees/bio.en.html.?type=ind&id=2005-12-26%2008:58:08.

1920. 2004. Avian influenza researcher to receive UQ honorary doctorate. University of Queensland. September 8. uq.edu.au/news/?article=5877uq.edu.au/news/?article=5877.

1921. Cooper S. 2006 (How to stop) The next killer flu. Seed Magazine, February–March.

1922. Vidal J. 2006. Flying in the face of nature. Guardian, February 22. society.guardian.co.uk/health/story/0,1714703,00.html.

1923. Ritchie BW. 1995. Avian Viruses: Function and Control (Lake Worth, FL: Wingers Publishing).

1924. Delgado C, Rosegrant M, Steinfeld H, Ehui S, Courbois C. 1999. Livestock to 2020: the next food revolution. Food, Agriculture, and the Environment Discussion Paper 28. For the International Food Policy Research Institute, the Food and Agriculture Organization of the United Nations and the International Livestock Research Institute. ifpri.org/2020/dp/dp28.pdf.

1925. Hafez HM. 2003. Emerging and re-emerging diseases in poultry. World Poultry 19(7):23–7.

1926. Tsukamoto K, Imada T, Tanimura N, Okamatsu M, Mase M, Mizuhara T, Swayne D, Yamaguchi S. 2007. Impact of different husbandry conditions on contact and airborne transmission of H5N1 highly pathogenic avian influenza virus to chickens. Avian Dis. 51(1):129–132.

1927. Narayan O, Lang G, Rouse BT. 1969. A new influenza A virus infection in turkeys. IV. Experimental susceptibility of domestic birds to virus strain turkey/Ontario 7732/1966. Archiv Gesamte Virusforsch. 26:149–165. https://doi.org/10.1007/BF01241184.

1928. Hugh-Jones ME, Hubbert WT, Hagsad HV. 1995. Zoonoses: Recognition, Control, and Prevention (Ames, IA: Iowa State University Press).

1929. North MO, Bell DD. 1990. Commercial Chicken Production Manual, 4th Edition (New York, NY: Van Nostrand Reinhold).

1930. Edwards K. 1996. Short, but not sweet: the life of the meat chicken. Animals Today, February–April, pp. 29–31.

1931. Hugh-Jones ME, Hubbert WT, Hagsad HV. 1995. Zoonoses: Recognition, Control, and Prevention (Ames, IA: Iowa State University Press).

1932. United Egg Producers Certified. 2004. Industry history. United Egg Producers. uepcertified.com/industryhistory.html.

1933. United Egg Producers. 2002. Animal Husbandry Guidelines for U.S. Egg Laying Flocks 2002 Edition (Alpharetta, GA: United Egg Producers).

1934. Dawkins MS, Hardie S. 1989. Space needs of laying hens. British Poultry Science 30:413–6.

1935. United Egg Producers. 2005. United Egg Producers Animal Husbandry Guidelines for U.S. Egg Laying Flocks (Alpharetta, GA: United Egg Producers). www.animalcarecertified.com/docs/2005_UEPanimal_welfare_guidelines.pdf.

1936. University of California, Davis. 1998. Egg-type Layer Flock Care Practices. www.vetmed.ucdavis.edu/vetext/INF-PO_EggCarePrax.pdf.

1937. Royal Geographical Society. 2004. Bird flu across Asia. Geography in the News, February 23. www.geographyinthenews.rgs.org/news/article/?id=270.

1938. European Commission. [date unknown]. Broilers. Belgium: European Commission; [accessed 2020 Apr 18]. https://ec.europa.eu/food/animals/welfare/practice/farm/broilers_en.

1939. Fanatico A. 2002. Sustainable poultry: production overview—Part II. National Center for Appropriate Technology. thepoultrysite.com/FeaturedArticle/FATopic.asp?AREA=ProductionMgmt&Display=113.

1940. 1999. Battery hen cages to be outlawed. BBC News, June 15. news.bbc.co.uk/1/hi/world/europe/369555.stm.

1941. Photo credit: Compassion Over Killing.

1942. California Legislative Information. 2008. Chapter 13.8. Farm animal cruelty. 25991. Definitions. State of California; [amended 2018 Nov 6; accessed 2020 Apr 6]. https://leginfo.legislature.ca.gov/faces/codes_displaySection.xhtml?lawCode=HSC&sectionNum=25991.

1943. Ballotpedia. 2016. Massachusetts minimum size requirements for farm animal containment, question 3 (2016). Ballotpedia; [accessed 2020 Apr 6]. https://ballotpedia.org/Massachusetts_Minimum_Size_Requirements_for_Farm _Animal_Containment,_Question_3_(2016).

1944. Michigan Legislature. 2020. Enrolled senate bill no. 174. Animal industry act. State of Michigan; [accessed 2020 Apr 6]. www.legislature.mi.gov/documents /2019-2020/publicact/pdf/2019-PA-0132.pdf.

1945. Oregon Legislative Assembly. 2019. Enrolled Senate Bill 1019. State of Oregon; [accessed 2020 Apr 7]. https://olis.leg.state.or.us/liz/2019R1/Downloads /MeasureDocument/SB1019/Enrolled.

1946. Rhode Island General Assembly. 2018. H 7456 Substitute A. An act relating to animals and animal husbandry—unlawful confinement of a covered animal. State of Rhode Island; [accessed 2020 Apr 7]. http://webserver.rilin.state.ri.us /BillText/BillText18/HouseText18/H7456A.pdf.

1947. Washington State Legislature. 2019. HB 2049-2019-20. Concerning commercial egg layer operations. State of Washington; [accessed 2020 Apr 7]. https://app.leg.wa.gov/billsummary/?billNumber=2049&year=2019& initiative=False.

1948. LAWriter. 2016. Ohio administrative code. Chapter 901:12-9 poultry layers. Lawriter LLC; [accessed 2020 Apr 7]. http://codes.ohio.gov/oac /901:12-9.

1949. World Health Organization, Food and Agricultural Organization of the United Nations, and World Organization for Animal Health. 2004. Report of the WHO/FAO/OIE joint consultation on emerging zoonotic diseases. At whqlibdoc.who.int/hq/2004/WHO_CDS_CPE_ZFK_2004.9.pdf.

1950. European Commission Scientific Committee on Animal Health and Animal Welfare. 2000. The Welfare of Chickens Kept for Meat Production (Broilers). March 21. europa.eu.int/comm/food/fs/sc/scah/out39_en.pdf.

1951. Sanchez M. 2005. Influenza pandemic, could something have been done? Washington Post, October 6. washingtonpost.com/wp-dyn/content/article /2005/10/06/AR2005100601186_pf.html.

1952. Moore JE, et al. 1996. Erythromycin-resistant thermophilic Campylobacter species isolated from pigs. Veterinary Record 138:306–7.

1953. Orent W. 2005. Chicken flu is no big peril: fear sick people, not poultry. Los Angeles Times, February 28, p. 9.

1954. Bulloch W. 1979. The History of Bacteriology (New York, NY: Oxford University Press).

1955. Lim TT, Heber AJ, Ni J-Q. 2005. Air quality measurements at a laying hen house: ammonia concentrations and emissions. Purdue Agricultural Air Quality Laboratory.

1956. Scientific Panel on Animal Health and Welfare. 2005. Scientific report on the animal health and welfare aspects of avian influenza. Annex to European Food Safety Authority Journal 266:1–21. 64.233.179.104/search? q=cache:bShJ5Q424WgJ:www.offlu.net/LinkClick.aspx%3Flink%3Dpdf. %252Fahaw_op_ej266_Avian%2BInfluenza_annex_en.pdf.%26tabid%3D54 %26mid%3D426+survival+influenza+virus+wet+manure&hl=en&gl=us& ct=clnk&cd=17&lr=lang_en.

1957. Webster RG, Sharp GB, Claas CJ. 1995. Interspecies transmission of influenza viruses. American Journal of Respiratory and Critical Care Medicine 152:525–30.

1958. Food and Agriculture Organization of the United Nations. 2004. Emergency prevention system transboundary animal diseases, Bulletin No. 25 January-June. ftp://ftp.fao.org/docrep/fao/007/y5537e/y5537e00.pdf.

1959. Perry M. 2005. Asia must change age-old farming to stop disease. Reuters, September 22.

1960. Villarreal LP, Defilippis VR, Gottlieb KA. 2000. Acute and persistent viral life strategies and their relationship to emerging diseases. Virology 272:1–6.

1961. Shortridge KF. 1992. Pandemic influenza: a zoonosis? Seminars in Respiratory Infections 7:11–25.

1962. Afelt A, Frutos R, Devaux C. 2018. Bats, coronaviruses, and deforestation: toward the emergence of novel infectious diseases? Front Microbiol. 9:702. https://dx.doi.org/10.3389/fmicb.2018.00702.

1963. Webster RG, Sharp GB, Claas CJ. 1995. Interspecies transmission of influenza viruses. American Journal of Respiratory and Critical Care Medicine 152:525–30.

1964. Webster RG. 1998. Influenza: an emerging microbial pathogen. In: Emerging Infections (San Diego, CA: Academic Press, pp. 275–300).

1965. Laver WG, Garman E. 2001. The origin and control of pandemic influenza. Science 293:1776–7.

1966. Frederick MA. 1999. The threat posed by the global emergence of livestock, food-borne, and zoonotic pathogens. Annals of the New York Academy of Sciences 894:20–7.

1967. André F, Tuyttens M. 2005. The importance of straw for pig and cattle welfare: a review. Applied Animal Behavior Science, 92(3)261.

1968. Maes D, Deluyker H, Verdonck M, et al. 2000. Herd factors associated with the seroprevalences of four major respiratory pathogens in slaughter pigs from farrow-to-finish pig herds. Veterinary Research 31:313–27.

1969. Quattro JD. 1999. Three scientists introduced into ARS hall of fame. ARS /USDA News and Events, September 17. ars.usda.gov/is/pr/1999/990917. htm.

1970. Witter RL. 1998. Control strategies for Marek's Disease: a perspective for the future. Poultry Science 77:1197–203.

1971. El-Lethey H, Huber-Eicher B, Jungi TW. 2003. Exploration of stress-induced immunosuppression in chickens reveals both stress-resistant and stress-susceptible antigen responses. Veterinary Immunology and Immunopathology 95:91–101.

1972. Siegel HS. 1983. Effects of intensive production methods on livestock health. Agro-Ecosystems 8:215–30.

1973. André F, Tuyttens M. 2005. The importance of straw for pig and cattle welfare: a review. Applied Animal Behavior Science, 92(3)261.

1974. Puvadolpirod S, Thaxton JP. 2000. Model of physiological stress in chickens. 1. Response parameters. Poultry Science 79:363–9.

1975. European Commission. Scientific Veterinary Committee. 1996. Report on the Welfare of Laying Hens (Brussels, Belgium: Scientific Veterinary Committee).

1976. Grandin T. 2001. Corporations can be agents of great improvements in animal welfare and food safety and the need for minimum decent standards. National Institute of Animal Agriculture, April 4. grandin.com/welfare/corporation. agents.html.

1977. MacArthur M. 2002. Analyst says poultry growers oblivious to poor conditions. Western Producer, December 12.

1978. Dawkins MS, Hardie S. 1989. Space needs of laying hens. British Poultry Science 30:413–6.

1979. Craig JV. 1978. Aggressive behavior of chickens: some effects of social and physical environments. 27th Annual National Breeder's Roundtable; 1978 May 11; Kansas City. Department of Animal Sciences and Industry, Kansas State University. www.poultryscience.org/pba/1952-2003/1978/1978%20Craig .pdf.

1980. Siegel HS. 1983. Effects of intensive production methods on livestock health. Agro-Ecosystems 8:215–30.

1981. Urrutia S. 1997. Broilers for next decade: what hurdles must commercial broiler breeders overcome? World Poultry 13(7):28–30.

1982. J. Byrnes. 1976. Raising pigs by the calendar at Maplewood Farms. Hog Farm Management, September, p. 30.

1983. Siegel HS. 1983. Effects of intensive production methods on livestock health. Agro-Ecosystems 8:215–30.

1984. André F, Tuyttens M. 2005. The importance of straw for pig and cattle welfare: a review. Applied Animal Behavior Science, 92(3)261.

1985. Ewald C, Heer A, Havenith U. 1994. Factors associated with the occurrence of influenza A virus infections in fattening swine. Berliner und Munchener Tierarztliche Wochenschrift. 107:256–62.

1986. European Commission Scientific Committee on Animal Health and Animal Welfare. 2000. The Welfare of Chickens Kept for Meat Production (Broilers). March 21. europa.eu.int/comm/food/fs/sc/scah/out39_en.pdf.

1987. Webster B. 2002. American Meat Institute Stunning Conference, Feb. 21–22 as cited in Davis K. The need for legislation and elimination of electrical immobilization. United Poultry Concerns. www.upc-online.org/slaughter/report .html.

1988. Duncan IJH. 2001. Animal welfare issues in the poultry industry: is there a lesson to be learned? Journal Applied Animal Welfare Science 4(3):207–21.

1989. Duncan IJH. 2001. Animal welfare issues in the poultry industry: is there a lesson to be learned? Journal Applied Animal Welfare Science 4(3):207–21.

1990. Mench JA. 1992. The welfare of poultry in modern production systems. Poultry Science 4:108–9.

1991. Duncan IJ. 2003. Letter to Nancy Halpern, New Jersey Department of Agriculture. June 25.

1992. Fraser D, Mench J, Millman S. 2001. Farm Animals and Their Welfare in 2000: State of the Animals (Washington, DC: Humane Society Press, p. 90).

1993. Parker HS. 2002. Agricultural Bioterrorism: A Federal Strategy to Meet the Threat. McNair Paper 65 (Washington, DC: National Defense University Institute for National Strategic Studies).

1994. Duncan IJH. 2001. Welfare problems of meat-type chickens. Farmed Animal Well-Being Conference at the University of California-Davis, June 28–29.

1995. Donaldson, WE. 1995. Early poult mortality: the role of stressors and diet. Turkey World, January–February, p. 27.

1996. O'Keefe T. 2005. Starting on the farm. Watt PoultryUSA, June, pp. 12–16.

1997. Kuhlein U, Aggrey SE, Zadworny A. 2003. Progress and prospects in resistance to disease. In: Muir WM, Aggrey SE (eds.), Poultry Genetics, Breeding and Biotechnology (Oxfordshire, UK: CAB International).

1998. Thorp BH, Luiting E. 2000. Breeding for resistance to production diseases in poultry. In: Axford RFE, Bishop SC, Nicholas FW, Owen JB (eds.), Breeding for Disease Resistance in Farm Animals (Wallingford, UK: CABI Publishing, pp. 357–77).

1999. North MO, Bell DD. 1990. Commercial Chicken Production Manual, 4th Edition (New York, NY: Van Nostrand Reinhold).

2000. U.S. Department of Agriculture, APHIS. 2004. Highly pathogenic avian influenza: a threat to U.S. poultry. Program Aid No. 1704. March.

2001. Wilson WO. 1966. Poulrty production. Scientific American 215(1):56–64.

2002. Shacklesford AD. 1988. Modifications of processing methods to control Salmonella in poultry. Poultry Science 67:933–5.

2003. Weeks CA, Danbury TD, Davies HC, Hunt P, Kestin SC. 2000. The behaviour of broiler chickens and its modification by lameness. Applied Animal Behavior Science 67:111–25.

2004. Grandin T, Johnson C. 2005. Animals in Translation (New York, NY: Scribner, p. 270).

2005. Shacklesford AD. 1988. Modifications of processing methods to control Salmonella in poultry. Poultry Science 67:933–5.

2006. Gregory E, Barnhart H, Dreesen DW, Stern NJ, Corn JL. 1997. Epidemiological study of Campylobacter spp. In: Broilers: source, time of colonization, and prevalence. Avian Diseases 41:890–8.

2007. Horowitz R. 2006. Putting Meat on the American Table: Taste, Technology and Transformation (Baltimore, MD: Johns Hopkins University Press, p. 125).

2008. Cole DJ, Hill VR, Humenik FJ, Sobsey MD. 1999. Health, safety, and environmental concerns of farm animal waste. Occupational Medicine: State of the Art Reviews 14(2):423–48.

2009. North MO, Bell DD. 1990. Commercial Chicken Production Manual, 4th Edition (New York, NY: Van Nostrand Reinhold).

2010. European Commission Scientific Committee on Animal Health and Animal Welfare. 2000. The Welfare of Chickens Kept for Meat Production (Broilers). March 21. europa.eu.int/comm/food/fs/sc/scah/out39_en.pdf.

2011. Madec F, Rose N. 2003. How husbandry practices may contribute to the course of infectious diseases in pigs. In: 4th International Symposium on Emerging and Re-emerging Pig Diseases (Rome, Italy June 29–July 2, pp. 9–18).

2012. Cooper GL, Venables LM, Lever MS. 1996. Airborne challenge of chickens vaccinated orally with the genetically-defined Salmonella enteritidis aroA strain CVL30. Veterinary Record 139(18):447–8.

2013. Van der Sluis W. 2005. Housing conditions affect broiler welfare more than stocking density. World Poultry 21(8):22–3.

2014. Van der Sluis W. 2005. Housing conditions affect broiler welfare more than stocking density. World Poultry. 21:22–23.

2015. National Turkey Federation. Meat bird production/growout. Food safety best management practices for the production of turkeys, Dec. 1995.

2016. Sims LD, Ellis TM, Liu KK, et al. 2003. Avian Influenza in Hong Kong 1997–2002. Avian Diseases 47:832–8.

2017. Hafez HM. 2000. Factors influencing turkey diseases. World Poultry Turkey Health Special, pp. 6–8.

2018. European Commission Scientific Committee on Animal Health and Animal Welfare. 2000. The Welfare of Chickens Kept for Meat Production (Broilers). March 21. europa.eu.int/comm/food/fs/sc/scah/out39_en.pdf.

2019. Cole DJ, Hill VR, Humenik FJ, Sobsey MD. 1999. Health, safety, and environmental concerns of farm animal waste. Occupational Medicine: State of the Art Reviews 14(2):423–48.

2020. Cole DJ, Hill VR, Humenik FJ, Sobsey MD. 1999. Health, safety, and environmental concerns of farm animal waste. Occupational Medicine: State of the Art Reviews 14(2):423–48.

2021. Madelin TM, Wathes CM. 1989. Air hygiene in a broiler house: Comparison of deep litter with raised netting floors. British Poultry Science 30:23–37.

2022. Collins JD, Wall PG. 2004. Food safety and animal production systems: controlling zoonoses at farm level. Revue Scientifique et Technique Office International des Epizooties 23(2):680–700. oie.int/eng/publicat/rt/2302/PDF ./685-700collins.pdf.

2023. Zavala G. 1998. An overview of myeloid leukosis in meat-type chickens. Technical News, Special Technical Bulletin, January 1998:S1–4.

2024. Gregory EH, Dreesen DW, Stern NJ, Corn JL. 1997. Epidemiological study of Campylobacter spp. In: Broilers: source, time of colonation, and prevalence. Avian Diseases 41:890–8.

2025. Advisory Committee on the Microbiological Safety of Food. 1996. Report on Poultry Meat (London, UK: HSMO, p 92).

2026. Linden J. 2005. Campylobacter gradually reveals its secrets. Poultry International, December.

2027. Vaillancourt JP. 2002. Biosecurity now. Poultry International. 411:12–8.

2028. Vaillancourt JP. 2002. Biosecurity now. Poultry International. 411:12–8.

2029. Fontenot JP. 2001. Utilization of poultry litter as feed for beef cattle. Food and Drug Administration Public Hearing on Animal Feeding Regulation, October 30. www.fda.gov/ohrms/dockets/dailys/01/Nov01/110501/ts00014.doc.

2030. Cole DJ, Hill VR, Humenik FJ, Sobsey MD. 1999. Health, safety, and environmental concerns of farm animal waste. Occupational Medicine: State of the Art Reviews 14(2):423–48.

2031. 2000. Humidity and litter moisture important factors in Salmonella and E.coli multiplication. World Poultry 16(10).

2032. Shane SM. 1997. Campylobacteriosis. In: Calnek BW (ed.), Diseases of Poultry, 10th Edition (Ames, IA: Iowa State University Press, pp. 235–245).

2033. Shortridge KF, Zhou NN, Guan Y, et al. 1998. Characterization of avian H5N1 influenza viruses from poultry in Hong Kong. Virology 252:331–42.

2034. Delgado CL, Narrod CA 2002. Impact of the changing market forces and policies on structural change in the livestock industries of selected fast-growing developing countries. Final Research Report of Phase I, International Food Policy Research Institute.

2035. Food and Agriculture Organization of the United Nations. Technical Task Force on Avian Influenza. 2005. Update on the avian influenza situation. Avian Influenza Disease Emergency News, issue 28. www.fao.org/ag/againfo/subjects/documents/ai/AVIbull028.pdf.

2036. Taubenberger JK, Morens DM. 2006. 1918 influenza: the mother of all pandemics. Emerging Infectious Diseases 12(1):15–22.

2037. Halvorson DA, Kelleher CJ, Senne DA. 1985. Epizootiology of avian influenza: effect of seasonal incidence in sentinel ducks and domestic turkey in Minnesota. Applied and Environmental Microbiology 49:914–9.

2038. Ritchie BW. 1995. Avian Viruses: Function and Control (Lake Worth, FL: Wingers Publishing).

2039. Drexler M. 2002. Secret Agents: The Menace of Emerging Infections (Washington, DC: Joseph Henry Press).

2040. Bridges CB, Kuehnert MJ, Hall CB. 2003. Transmission of influenza: implications for control in health care settings. Clinical Infectious Diseases 37:1094–101.

2041. Collier R. 1974. The Plague of the Spanish Lady: The Influenza Pandemic of 1918–1919 (New York, NY: Atheneum).

2042. Naylor MF, Farmer KC. Sun damage and prevention. health.howstuffworks.com/framed.htm?parent=sunscreen.htm&url= www.telemedicine.org/sundam2.4.1.html.

2043. Bridges CB, Kuehnert MJ, Hall CB. 2003. Transmission of influenza: implications for control in health care settings. Clinical Infectious Diseases 37:1094–101.

2044. Food and Agriculture Organization of the United Nations. 2004. FAO recommendations on the prevention, control and eradication of highly pathogenic avian influenza (HPAI) in Asia. www.fao.org/ag/againfo/subjects/en/health/diseases-cards/27septrecomm.pdf.

2045. Russell SM, Fairchild BD. 2005. Poultry production China's way. Watt Poultry USA, February, Volume 6, No. 2, pp. 26–30.

2046. Mason J, Singer P. 1990. Animal Factories (New York, NY: Crown Publishers).

2047. Maegraith D. 2004. When fear takes flight. Weekend Australian, January 31, p. C13.

2048. Arthur JA, Albers GAA. 2003. Industrial perspective on problems and issues associated with poultry breeding. In: Muir WM, Aggrey SE (eds.), Poultry Genetics, Breeding and Biotechnology (Wallingford, UK: CABI Publishing, pp. 1–12).

2049. Arthur JA, Albers GAA. 2003. Industrial perspective on problems and issues associated with poultry breeding. In: Muir WM, Aggrey SE (eds.), Poultry Genetics, Breeding and Biotechnology (Wallingford, UK: CABI Publishing, pp. 1–12).

2050. Boyd W. 2001. Making meat: science, technology, and American poultry production. Technology and Culture 42:631–64.

2051. Arthur JA, Albers GAA. 2003. Industrial perspective on problems and issues associated with poultry breeding. In: Muir WM, Aggrey SE (eds.), Poultry Genetics, Breeding and Biotechnology (Wallingford, UK: CABI Publishing, pp. 1–12).

2052. Fraser D, Mench J, Millman S. 2001. Farm Animals and Their Welfare in 2000: State of the Animals (Washington, DC: Humane Society Press, p. 90).

2053. MacArthur M. 2002. Analyst says poultry growers oblivious to poor conditions. Western Producer, December 12; and Fraser D, Mench J, Millman S. 2001. Farm Animals and Their Welfare in 2000: State of the Animals (Washington, DC: Humane Society Press, p. 90).

2054. Arthur JA, Albers GAA. 2003. Industrial perspective on problems and issues associated with poultry breeding. In: Muir WM, Aggrey SE (eds.), Poultry Genetics, Breeding and Biotechnology (Wallingford, UK: CABI Publishing, pp. 1–12).

2055. Boyd W. 2001. Making meat: science, technology, and American poultry production. Technology and Culture 42:631–64.

2056. Arshad M. 1999. An ecological study of red junglefowl (Gallus gallus spadiceus) in agricultural areas. Universiti Putri Malasia.

2057. Canadian Egg Marketing Agency. 2002. Egg facts. eggs.ca/eggfacts/egg down.asp.

2058. Clubb S. 2001. Stop the practice of starving birds for egg production. Association of Avian Veterinarians Newsletter, June-August.

2059. Parkinson G. 1993. Osteoporosis and bone fractures in the laying hen. Progress Report of Work at the Victorian Institute of Animal Science, Attwood.

2060. Dekich MA. 1998. Broiler industry strategies for control of respiratory and enteric diseases. Poultry Science 77:1176–80.

2061. Hafez HM. 2000. Enteric diseases. World Poultry (Elsevier Special 2000) p. 6.

2062. McCarthy M. 2001. Animal welfare: the growing pains of a selectively bred chicken; a plan to accelerate further the unnatural growth rate of broiler birds is condemned by campaign groups. Independent, December 10, p. 7.

2063. Duncan IJH. 2001. Welfare problems of meat-type chickens. Farmed Animal Well-Being Conference at the University of California-Davis, June 28–29.

2064. University of Arkansas Division of Agriculture Cooperative Extension Service. kidsarus.org/kids_go4it/growit/raiseit/chickens.htm.

2065. Boyd W. 2001. Making meat: science, technology, and American poultry production. Technology and Culture 42:631–64.

2066. Warren DC. 1958. A half century of advances in the genetics and breeding improvement of poultry. Poultry Science 37:5–6.

2067. Davenport CB. 1910. Eugenics, a subject for investigation rather than instruction. American Breeders Magazine 1:68.

2068. Quigley M. 1995. The roots of the I.Q. debate: eugenics and social control. The Public Eye, March. publiceye.org/magazine/v09n1/eugenics.html.

2069. Boyd W. 2001. Making meat: science, technology, and American poultry production. Technology and Culture 42:631–64.

2070. Davenport CB. 1907. Inheritance in pedigree breeding of poultry. In: Proceedings of the American Breeders' Association, volume 3 (Washington, DC).

2071. Patterson C. 2005. Animals, slavery, and the holocaust. Logos 4(2). logosjournal.com/issue_4.2/patterson.htm.

2072. Lindhe B, Philipsson J. 1998. Conventional breeding programmes and genetic resistance to animal diseases. International Office of Epizootics 17(1):291–301.

2073. Thornton G. 1996. High yielding broiler production: the big trade-off. Broiler Industry 59:18–22.

2074. European Commission Scientific Committee on Animal Health and Animal Welfare. 2000. The Welfare of Chickens Kept for Meat Production (Broilers). March 21. europa.eu.int/comm/food/fs/sc/scah/out39_en.pdf.

2075. European Commission Scientific Committee on Animal Health and Animal Welfare. 2000. The Welfare of Chickens Kept for Meat Production (Broilers). March 21. europa.eu.int/comm/food/fs/sc/scah/out39_en.pdf.

2076. Martin D. 1997. Researcher studying growth-induced diseases in broilers. Feedstuffs, May 26.

2077. European Commission Scientific Committee on Animal Health and Animal Welfare. 2000. The Welfare of Chickens Kept for Meat Production (Broilers). March 21. europa.eu.int/comm/food/fs/sc/scah/out39_en.pdf.

2078. U.S. Department of Agriculture National Agricultural Statistics Service. 2005. Poultry Slaughter: 2004 Annual Summary. usda.mannlib.cornell.edu/reports/nassr/poultry/ppy-bban/pslaan05.txt.

2079. European Commission Scientific Committee on Animal Health and Animal Welfare. 2000. The Welfare of Chickens Kept for Meat Production (Broilers). March 21. europa.eu.int/comm/food/fs/sc/scah/out39_en.pdf.

2080. Rauw WM, Kanis E, Noordhuizen-Stassen EN, Grommers FJ. 1998. Undesirable side effects of selection for high production efficiency in farm animals: a review. Livestock Production Science 56:15–33.

2081. Yunis R, Ben-David A, Heller ED, Cahaner A. 2000. Immunocompetence and viability under commercial conditions of broiler groups differing in growth rates and in antibody response to Escherichia coli vaccine. Poultry Science 79:810–6.

2082. Han PFS, Smyth JR. 1972. The influence of growth rate on the development of Marek's Disease in chickens. Poultry Science 51:975–85.

2083. Nestor KE, Saif YM, Zhu J, Noble DO. 1996. Influence of growth selection in turkeys on resistance to Pasteurella multocida. Poultry Science 75(10):1161–3.

2084. Yunis R, Ben-David A, Heller ED, Cahaner A. 2002. Antibody responses and morbidity following infection with infectious bronchitis virus and challenge with Escherichia coli, in lines divergently selected on antibody response. Poultry Science 81:149–59.

2085. Johnson AL. 2005. Avian influenza: Complicated issue with a simple message. Watt PoultryUSA, December, p. 16–7.

2086. Hawken RJ, Beattie CW, Schook LB. 1998. Resolving the genetics of resistance to infectious diseases. International Office of Epizootics Scientific and Technical Review 17(1):17–25.

2087. Huff GR, Huff WE, Balog JM, Rath NC, Anthony NB, Nestor KE. 2005. Stress response differences and disease susceptibility reflected by heterophil ratio in turkeys selected for increased body weight. Poultry Science 84:709–17.

2088. Bayyari GR, Huff WE, Rath NC, et al. 1997. Effect of the genetic selection of turkeys for increased body weight and egg production on immune and physiological responses. Poultry Science 76:289–96.

2089. Tsai HJ, Saif YM, Nestor KE, Emmerson DA, Patterson RA. 1992. Genetic Variation in Resistance of Turkeys to Experimental Infection with Newcastle Disease Virus. Avian Diseases 36:561–5.

2090. Saif YM, Nestor KE, Dearth RN, Renner PA. 1984. Case report: Possible genetic variation in resistance of turkeys to Erysipelas and fowl cholera. Avian Diseases 28:770–3.

2091. Kowalski, A, Mormede P, Jakubowski K, Jedlinska-Krakowska M. 2002. Comparison of susceptibility to stress in two genetic lines of turkey broilers BUT-9 and Big-6. Polish Journal of Veterinary Science 5:145–150.

2092. Huff GR, Huff WE, Balog JM, Rath NC, Anthony NB, Nestor KE. 2005. Stress response differences and disease susceptibility reflected by heterophil ratio in turkeys selected for increased body weight. Poultry Science 84:709–17.

2093. Rauw WM, Kanis E, Noordhuizen-Stassen EN, Grommers FJ. 1998. Undesirable side effects of selection for high production efficiency in farm animals: a review. Livestock Production Science 56:15–33.

2094. Rauw WM, Kanis E, Noordhuizen-Stassen EN, Grommers FJ. 1998. Undesirable side effects of selection for high production efficiency in farm animals: a review. Livestock Production Science 56:15–33.

2095. Rauw WM, Kanis E, Noordhuizen-Stassen EN, Grommers FJ. 1998. Undesirable side effects of selection for high production efficiency in farm animals: a review. Livestock Production Science 56:15–33.

2096. Smith R. 1991. Cutting edge poultry researchers doing what birds tell them to do. Feedstuffs. September 9, p. 22.

2097. Wise D, Jennings A. 1972. Dyschondroplasia in domestic poultry. Veterinary Record. 91:285–6.

2098. Kamyab A. 2001. Enlarged sternal bursa and focal ulcerative dermatitis in male turkeys. World's Poultry Science Journal 57:5–12.

2099. Ekstrand C, Algers B. 1997 Rearing conditions and foot-pad dermatitis in Swedish turkey poults. Acta-Veterinaria-Scandinavica 38(2):167–174.

2100. Bayyari GR, Huff WE, Rath NC, et al. 1997. Effect of the genetic selection of turkeys for increased body weight and egg production on immune and physiological responses. Poultry Science 76:289–96.

2101. Beaumont C, Dambrine G, Chaussé AM, Flock D. 2003. Selection for disease resistance: conventional breeding for resistance to bacteria and viruses. In: Muir WM, Aggrey SE (eds.), Poultry Genetics, Breeding and Biotechnology (Wallingford, UK: CABI Publishing, pp. 357–84).

2102. Beaumont C, Dambrine G, Chaussé AM, Flock D. 2003. Selection for disease resistance: conventional breeding for resistance to bacteria and viruses. In: Muir WM, Aggrey SE (eds.), Poultry Genetics, Breeding and Biotechnology (Wallingford, UK: CABI Publishing, pp. 357–84).

2103. Beaumont C, Dambrine G, Chaussé AM, Flock D. 2003. Selection for disease resistance: conventional breeding for resistance to bacteria and viruses. In: Muir WM, Aggrey SE (eds.), Poultry Genetics, Breeding and Biotechnology (Wallingford, UK: CABI Publishing, pp. 357–84).

2104. Knap PW, Bishop SC. 2000. Relationships between genetic change and infectious disease in domestic livestock. In: Hill WG, Bishop SC, McGuirk B, McKay JC, Simm G, Webb AJ (eds.), The challenge of genetic change in animal production, Proceedings of an Occasional Meeting Organized by the British Society of Animal Science (Edinburgh, Scotland: BSAS Occasional Publication, pp. 65–80).

2105. Boa-Amponsem K, Dunnington EA, Baker KS, Siegel PB. 1999. Diet and immunological memory of lines of white leghorn chickens divergently selected for antibody response to sheep red blood cells. Poultry Science 78:165–70.

2106. Van der Zijpp AJ. 1983. Breeding for immune responsiveness and disease resistance. World's Poultry Science Journal 39(2):118–31.

2107. Huff GR, Huff WE, Balog JM, Rath NC, Anthony NB, Nestor KE. 2005. Stress response differences and disease susceptibility reflected by heterophil ratio in turkeys selected for increased body weight. Poultry Science 84:709–17.

2108. Hawken RJ, Beattie CW, Schook LB. 1998. Resolving the genetics of resistance to infectious diseases. International Office of Epizootics Scientific and Technical Review 17(1):17–25.

2109. Mangel M, Stamps J. 2001. Trade-offs between growth and mortality and the maintenance of individual variation in growth. Evolutionary Ecology Research 3:583–93.

2110. Lindhe B, Philipsson J. 1998. Conventional breeding programmes and genetic resistance to animal diseases. International Office of Epizootics 17(1):291–301.

2111. Sinclair MC, Nielsen BL, Oldham JD, Reid HW. 1999. Consequences for immune function of metabolic adaptations to load. In: Oldham JD, Simm G, Groen AF, Nielsen BL, Pryce JF, Lawrence TLJ (eds.), Metabolic Stress in Dairy Cows (Edinburgh: British Society of Animal Science, pp. 113–118).

2112. Lindhe B, Philipsson J. 1998. Conventional breeding programmes and genetic resistance to animal diseases. International Office of Epizootics 17(1):291–301.

2113. Sinclair MC, Nielsen BL, Oldham JD, Reid HW. 1999. Consequences for immune function of metabolic adaptations to load. In: Oldham JD, Simm G, Groen AF, Nielsen BL, Pryce JF, Lawrence TLJ (eds.), Metabolic Stress in Dairy Cows (Edinburgh: British Society of Animal Science, pp. 113–118).

2114. Norris K, Evans MR. 2000. Ecological immunology: life history trade-offs and immune defense in birds. Behavioral Ecology 11:19–26.

2115. Cheema MA, Qureshi MA, Havenstein GB. 2003. A comparison of the immune response of a 2001 commercial broiler with a 1957 randombred broiler strain when fed representative 1957 and 2001 broiler diets. Poultry Science 82:1519–29.

2116. Koenen ME, Boonstra-Blom AG, Jeurissen SHM. 2002. Immunological differences between layer- and broiler-type chickens. Veterinary Immunology and Immunopathology 89:47–56.

2117. Cheema MA, Qureshi MA, Havenstein GB. 2003. A comparison of the immune response of a 2001 commercial broiler with a 1957 randombred broiler strain when fed representative 1957 and 2001 broiler diets. Poultry Science 82:1519–29.

2118. Madden RH. 1994. Microbial hazards in animal products. Proceedings of the Nutrition Society 53:209–16.

2119. Riddell C, Springer R. 1984. An epizootiological study of acute death syndrome and leg weakness in broiler chickens in western Canada. Avian Diseases 29:90–102.

2120. European Commission Scientific Committee on Animal Health and Animal Welfare. 2000. The Welfare of Chickens Kept for Meat Production (Broilers). March 21. europa.eu.int/comm/food/fs/sc/scah/out39_en.pdf.

2121. Mangel M, Stamps J. 2001. Trade-offs between growth and mortality and the maintenance of individual variation in growth. Evolutionary Ecology Research 3:583–93.

2122. Lochmiller RL, Deerenberg C. 2000. Trade-offs in evolutionary immunology: just what is the cost of immunity? Oikos 88:87–98.

2123. Gross WB, Siegel PB. 1988. Environment-genetic influences on immunocompetence. Journal of Animal Science 66:2091–2094.

2124. Klasing KC, Laurin DE, Peng RK, Fry DM. 1987. Immunologically mediated growth depression in chicks: influence of feed intake, Corticosterone and Interleukin-1. Journal of Nutrition 117(9):1629–37.

2125. Mangel M, Stamps J. 2001. Trade-offs between growth and mortality and the maintenance of individual variation in growth. Evolutionary Ecology Research 3:583–93.

2126. Klasing KC, Laurin DE, Peng RK, Fry DM. 1987. Immunologically mediated growth depression in chicks: influence of feed intake, corticosterone and
interleukin-1. Journal of Nutrition 117(9):1629–37.

2127. Freeman BM, Manning ACC, Harrison GF, Coates ME. 1975. Dietary
aureomycin and the response of the fowl to stressors. British Poultry Science
16:395–404.

2128. Johnson RW. 1999. Stress and disease: resetting the biological machinery of
growth. Illini PorkNet, October 21. www.traill.uiuc.edu/porknet/paperDisplay
.cfm?Type=paper&ContentID=83.

2129. Lochmiller RL, Deerenberg C. 2000. Trade-offs in evolutionary immunology:
just what is the cost of immunity? Oikos 88:87–98.

2130. Lochmiller RL, Deerenberg C. 2000. Trade-offs in evolutionary immunology:
just what is the cost of immunity? Oikos 88:87–98.

2131. Thorp BH, Luiting E. 2000. Breeding for resistance to production diseases in
poultry. In: Axford RFE, Bishop SC, Nicholas FW, Owen JB (eds.), Breeding
for Disease Resistance in Farm Animals (Wallingford, UK: CABI Publishing,
pp. 357–77).

2132. Gavora JS. 1990. Disease genetics. In: Crawford RD (ed.), Poultry Breeding and
Genetics (Amsterdam, The Netherlands: Elsevier Publishing Co., pp. 805–46).

2133. Boa-Amponsem K, O'Sullivan NP, Gross WB, Dunnington EA, Siegel PB.
1991. Genotype, feeding regimen, and diet interactions in meat chickens.
Poultry Science 70:697–701.

2134. Kolok A, Oris JT. 1995. The relationship between specific growth rate and
swimming performance in male fathead minnows (Pimephales promelas).
Canadian Journal of Zoology 73:2165–7.

2135. Gregory TR, Wood CM. 1998. Individual variation and interrelationships
between swimming performance, growth rate, and feeding in juvenile rainbow
trout (Oncorhynchus mykiss). Canadian Journal of Fisheries and Aquatic Sciences 55:1583–90.

2136. Farrell AP, Bennett W, Devlin RH. 1997. Growth-enhanced transgenic
salmon can be inferior swimmers. Canadian Journal of Zoology 75:335–7.

2137. Boyd W. 2001. Making meat: science, technology, and American poultry production. Technology and Culture 42:631–64.

2138. Huff GR, Huff WE, Balog JM, Rath NC, Anthony NB, Nestor KE. 2005.
Stress response differences and disease susceptibility reflected by heterophil ratio in turkeys selected for increased body weight. Poultry Science 84:709–17.

2139. Van der Zijpp AJ. 1983. Breeding for immune responsiveness and disease resistance. World's Poultry Science Journal 39(2):118–31.

2140. Boyd W. 2001. Making meat: science, technology, and American poultry production. Technology and Culture 42:631–64.

2141. Thornton G. 1996. High yielding broiler production: the big trade-off. Broiler
Industry 59:18–22.

2142. Carson R. 1962. Silent Spring (New York, NY: Mariner Books), chap. 15.

2143. Boyd W. 2001. Making meat: science, technology, and American poultry production. Technology and Culture 42:631–64.

2144. Urrutia S. 1997. Broilers for next decade: what hurdles must commercial broiler breeders overcome? World Poultry 13(7):28–30.

2145. Baskin C. 1978. Confessions of a chicken farmer. Country Journal, April, p. 38.

2146. Albers GAA. 1993. Breeding for disease resistance: fact and fiction. Archiv für Geflügelkunde 57(2):56–8.

2147. Arthur JA, Albers GAA. 2003. Industrial perspective on problems and issues associated with poultry breeding. In: Muir WM, Aggrey SE (eds.), Poultry Genetics, Breeding and Biotechnology (Wallingford, UK: CABI Publishing, pp. 1–12).

2148. Thorp BH, Luiting E. 2000. Breeding for resistance to production diseases in poultry. In: Axford RFE, Bishop SC, Nicholas FW, Owen JB (eds.), Breeding for Disease Resistance in Farm Animals (Wallingford, UK: CABI Publishing, pp. 357–77).

2149. Tabler GT, Mendenhall AM. 2003. Broiler nutrition, feed intake and grower economics. Avian Advice 5(4):8–10.

2150. Bayyari GR, Huff WE, Rath NC, et al. 1997. Effect of the genetic selection of turkeys for increased body weight and egg production on immune and physiological responses. Poultry Science 76:289–96.

2151. Thorp BH, Luiting E. 2000. Breeding for resistance to production diseases in poultry. In: Axford RFE, Bishop SC, Nicholas FW, Owen JB (eds.), Breeding for Disease Resistance in Farm Animals (Wallingford, UK: CABI Publishing, pp. 357–77).

2152. U.S. Food and Drug Administration. 2017. 2015 NARMS integrated report. FDA, CDC, USDA; [accessed 2020 Apr 8]. https://www.fda.gov/media/108304/download.

2153. Schroeder CM, Naugle AL, Schlosser WD, et al. 2005. Estimate of illnesses from Salmonella enteritidis in eggs, United States, 2000. Emerging Infectious Diseases 11(1):113–5. www.cdc.gov/foodnet/pub/publications/2005/040401_schroeder.pdf.

2154. European Commission Scientific Committee on Animal Health and Animal Welfare. 2000. The Welfare of Chickens Kept for Meat Production (Broilers). March 21. europa.eu.int/comm/food/fs/sc/scah/out39_en.pdf.

2155. Walker A, MacLeod M. 2004. Limits to the performance of poultry. In: Wiseman J, Sylvester-Bradley R. 2005. Yields of Farmed Species: Constraints and Opportunities in the 21st Century (Nottingham: Nottingham University Press).

2156. Urrutia S. 1997. Broilers for next decade: what hurdles must commercial broiler breeders overcome? World Poultry 13(7):28–30.

2157. Boyd W. 2001. Making meat: science, technology, and American poultry production. Technology and Culture 42:631–64.

2158. Koenen ME, Boonstra-Blom AG, Jeurissen SHM. 2002. Immunological differences between layer- and broiler-type chickens. Veterinary Immunology and Immunopathology 89:47–56.

2159. Thorp BH, Luiting E. 2000. Breeding for resistance to production diseases in poultry. In: Axford RFE, Bishop SC, Nicholas FW, Owen JB (eds.), Breeding for Disease Resistance in Farm Animals (Wallingford, UK: CABI Publishing, pp. 357–77).

2160. Decuypere E, Bruggeman V, Barbato GF, Buyse J. 2003. Growth and reproductive problems associated with selection for increased broiler meat production. In: Muir WM, Aggrey SE (eds.), Poultry Genetics, Breeding and Biotechnology (Wallingford, UK: CABI Publishing, pp. 13–28).

2161. Thorp BH, Luiting E. 2000. Breeding for resistance to production diseases in poultry. In: Axford RFE, Bishop SC, Nicholas FW, Owen JB (eds.), Breeding for Disease Resistance in Farm Animals (Wallingford, UK: CABI Publishing, pp. 357–77).

2162. Thorp BH, Luiting E. 2000. Breeding for resistance to production diseases in poultry. In: Axford RFE, Bishop SC, Nicholas FW, Owen JB (eds.), Breeding for Disease Resistance in Farm Animals (Wallingford, UK: CABI Publishing, pp. 357–77).

2163. Parker HS. 2002. Agricultural Bioterrorism: A Federal Strategy to Meet the Threat. McNair Paper 65 (Washington, DC: National Defense University Institute for National Strategic Studies).

2164. Food and Agriculture Organization of the United Nations. 2004. Loss of domestic animal breeds alarming. Press release, March 31.

2165. 2001. Biodiversity shrinks as farm breeds die out, Reuters, September 18. lists .iatp.org/listarchive/archive.cfm?id=36947.

2166. Food and Agriculture Organization of the United Nations. 2004. Loss of domestic animal breeds alarming. Press release, March 31.

2167. Meredith M. 2004. Zoonotic disease risks—2004 update. American Association of Swine Veterinarians. aasv.org/news/story.php?id=1221&lang=en.

2168. Schrag S, Wiener P. 1995. Emerging infectious disease: what are the relative roles of ecology and evolution? Trends in Ecology and Evolution 10(8):319–324.

2169. Huff GR, Huff WE, Balog JM, Rath NC, Anthony NB, Nestor KE. 2005. Stress response differences and disease susceptibility reflected by heterophil ratio in turkeys selected for increased body weight. Poultry Science 84:709–17.

2170. Holland F. 1998. Search for the superchicken. South China Morning Post, February 25, p. 17.

2171. 2000. R&D agreement to develop disease resistant poultry. World Poultry 16(3):50.

2172. Van Blerkom LM. 2003. Role of viruses in human evolution. Yearbook of Physical Anthropology 46:14–46.

2173. Simianer H. 2005. Decision making in livestock conservation. Ecological Economics 53:559–572.

2174. 2005. Bird flu and bird farms. Effect Measure, February 5. effectmeasure. blogspot.com/2005/02/bird-flu-and-bird-farms.html.

2175. Wong M. 2004. Virus hitting chicken immunity may be cause of bird flu. Associated Press, January 28. thepoultrysite.com/LatestNews/Default.asp?AREA=LatestNews&Display=6223.

2176. Cereno TN. Infectious bursal disease: causative agent, diagnosis and prevention. Canadian Poultry Consultants. canadianpoultry.ca/new_page_2.htm.

2177. 2006. Adaptive immunity. Microbiology and Bacteriology, March 5. www
.bact.wisc.edu/Microtextbook/index.php?name=Sections&req=viewarticle&
artid=292&page=1.

2178. Schat KA, Davies CJ. 2000. Viral diseases. In: (eds.) Axford RFE, Bishop SC,
Nicholas FW, Owen JB. Breeding for Disease Resistance in Farm Animals
(Wallingford: CAB International, pp. 271–300).

2179. Bumstead N. 2003. Genetic resistance and transmission of avian bacteria and
viruses. In: Muir WM, Aggrey SE (eds.), Poultry Genetics, Breeding and
Biotechnology (Oxfordshire, UK: CAB International, pp. 311–28).

2180. European Commission Scientific Committee on Animal Health and Animal
Welfare. 2000. The Welfare of Chickens Kept for Meat Production (Broilers).
March 21. europa.eu.int/comm/food/fs/sc/scah/out39_en.pdf.

2181. Saif YM. 1998. Infectious bursal disease and hemorrhagic enteritis. Poultry
Science 77:1186–9.

2182. Saif YM. 1998. Infectious bursal disease and hemorrhagic enteritis. Poultry
Science 77:1186–9.

2183. Cereno TN. Infectious bursal disease: causative agent, diagnosis and prevention. Canadian Poultry Consultants. canadianpoultry.ca/new_page_2.htm.

2184. Silbergeld E. 2006. Avian influenza risks and the animal-human interface.
Avian Flu: The Pandemic Threat and the Global Strategy at the Johns Hopkins
Bloomberg School of Public Health, January 30. commprojects.jhsph.edu/_media
/009_avian_flu.ram.

2185. Fussell L. 1998. Poultry industry strategies for control of immunosuppressive
diseases. Poultry Science 77:1193–6.

2186. Shane SM. 2005. Global disease update—AI overshadowing erosive diseases.
World Poultry 21(7):22–3.

2187. Shane SM. 2003. Disease continues to impact the world's poultry industries.
World Poultry 19(7):22–7.

2188. Daszak P, Cunningham AA, Hyatt AD. 2000. Emerging infectious diseases of
wildlife—threats to biodiversity and human health. Science 287:443–9.

2189. Marek J. 1907. Multiple nervenentzundung (polyneuritis) bei Hubern. Deut-
che Tierarztliche Wochenschrift 15:417–21.

2190. Boyd W. 2001. Making meat: science, technology, and American poultry production. Technology and Culture 42:631–64.

2191. Schat KA, Davies CJ. 2000. Viral diseases. In: Axford RFE, Bishop SC, Nicholas FW, Owen JB. (eds.), Breeding for Disease Resistance in Farm Animals
(Wallingford: CAB International, pp. 271–300).

2192. Nair V. 2005. Evolution of Marek's disease—a paradigm for incessant race
between the pathogen and the host. Veterinary Journal 170:175–83.

2193. Nair V. 2005. Evolution of Marek's disease—a paradigm for incessant race
between the pathogen and the host. Veterinary Journal 170:175–83.

2194. Saif YM. 1998. Infectious bursal disease and hemorrhagic enteritis. Poultry
Science 77:1186–9.

2195. Rosenberger JK and Cloud SS. 1998. Chicken anemia virus. Poultry Science
77:1190–2.

2196. Rosenberger JK and Cloud SS. 1998. Chicken anemia virus. Poultry Science 77:1190–2.

2197. Schat KA. 2005. Chicken infectious anemia virus infection: it is a serious problem. In: Proceedings of the 77th Northeastern Conference on Avian Diseases, June 15–17 (Cornell, NY, pp. 4–6). diaglab.vet.cornell.edu/avian /Proc77NECAD.pdf.

2198. Miller MM, Schat KA. 2004. Chicken infectious anemia virus: an example of the ultimate host-parasite relationship. Avian Diseases 48(4):734–45.

2199. Rosenberger JK, Cloud SS. 1998. Chicken anemia virus. Poultry Science 77:1190–2.

2200. Rosenberger JK, Cloud SS. 1998. Chicken anemia virus. Poultry Science 77:1190–2.

2201. Fussell L. 1998. Poultry industry strategies for control of immunosuppressive diseases. Poultry Science 77:1193–6.

2202. Nair V. 2005. Evolution of Marek's disease—a paradigm for incessant race between the pathogen and the host. Veterinary Journal 170:175–83.

2203. Cereno TN. Infectious bursal disease: causative agent, diagnosis and prevention. Canadian Poultry Consultants. canadianpoultry.ca/new_page_2.htm.

2204. Fussell L. 1998. Poultry industry strategies for control of immunosuppressive diseases. Poultry Science 77:1193–6.

2205. Nair V. 2005. Evolution of Marek's disease—a paradigm for incessant race between the pathogen and the host. Veterinary Journal 170:175–83.

2206. Pond J, Pond W. 2000. Introduction to Animal Science (New York, NY: John Wiley and Sons, Inc.).

2207. Democracy Now. 2005. Transcript—Mike Davis on The Monster at Our Door: The Global Threat of Avian Flu. Democracy Now. October 19. democ racynow.org/article.pl?sid=05/10/19/1332209

2208. Food and Agriculture Organization of the United Nations. 2004. Questions and answers on avian influenza; briefing paper prepared by AI Task Force, Internal FAO Document, January 30. animal-health-online.de/drms/faoinfluenza.pdf.

2209. Lindlaw S. 2006. "Biosecurity" is buzzword vs. bird flu. Associated Press, April 22. seattlepi.nwsource.com/business/1310AP_Bird_Flu_Poultry.html.

2210. Jack A, Cookson C, Kazmin A. 2005. Preparing for a pandemic. Financial Times, March 1, p. 19. sci.tech-archive.net/pdf./Archive/sci.med/2005-03 /0134.pdf.

2211. Wuethrich B. 2003. Chasing the fickle swine flu. Science 299:1502–5.

2212. Webster RG. 1997. Influenza virus: transmission between species and relevance to emergence of the next human pandemic. Archives of Virology 13:S105–13.

2213. Horn R. 2004. Families under fire: Chearavanont. Time Asia, February 23. time.com/time/asia/covers/501040223/chearavanont.html.

2214. Neuykhiew N. 2004. Bird-flu aftermath: loans, free land for chicken farms. The Nation, March 15. tinyurl.com/nwuz5.

2215. Delforge I. 2004. The flu that made agribusiness stronger. Focus on the Global South, July 5. focusweb.org/content/view/363/28/.

2216. Delforge I. 2004. The flu. Vietnam News, February 4 as cited in Davis M. 2005. The Monster at Our Door: The Global Threat of Avian Flu (New York, NY: The New Press, pp. 108–9).

2217. Moore M. 2006. Flu fears are sidelining French poultry. Washington Post, March 2, p. A14. washingtonpost.com/wp-dyn/content/article/2006/03/01/AR2006030102150.html.

2218. Food and Agriculture Organization of the United Nations. 2006. Update on the avian influenza situation. Avian Influenza Disease Emergency News, issue 39.

2219. 2006. France confirms bird flu on poultry farm. Associated Press, February 25. www.guardian.co.uk/print/0,329420997-112338,00.html.

2220. Butler D. 2006. Doubts hang over source of bird flu spread. Nature 439:772.

2221. Delforge I. 2004. Thailand: the world's kitchen. Le Monde Diplomatique, July. mondediplo.com/2004/07/05thailand.

2222. United Nations Food and Agriculture Organization Technical Task Force on Avian Influenza. 2004. Update on the avian influenza situation. Avian Influenza Disease Emergency News, issue 13.

2223. U.S. Department of Agriculture Global Agriculture Information Network. 2005. Laos: poultry and products; avian influenza. GAIN Report, March 16. 2005.www.fas.usda.gov/gainfiles/200503/146119131.pdf.

2224. Steckle MP. 2005. From a management crisis, to becoming better crisis managers: the 2004 avian influenza outbreak in British Columbia. Report of the Standing Committee on Agriculture and Agri-Food. April. parl.gc.ca/committee/CommitteePublication.aspx?SourceId=111249.

2225. Davis M. 2005. The Monster at Our Door: The Global Threat of Avian Flu (New York, NY: The New Press).

2226. Tweed SA, Skowronski DM, David ST, et al. 2004. Human illness from avian influenza H7N3, British Columbia. Emerging Infectious Diseases 10(12):2196–9. cdc.gov/ncidod/EID/vol10no12/pdf.s/04-0961.pdf.

2227. Bhattacharya S. 2004. Bird flu prompts mass cull in Canada. New Scientist, April, p. 22.

2228. 2004. Canadian Broadcasting Corporation, November 8 as cited in Davis M. 2005. The Monster at Our Door: The Global Threat of Avian Flu (New York, NY: The New Press).

2229. Tweed SA, Skowronski DM, David ST, et al. Human illness from avian influenza H7N3, British Columbia. Emerging Infectious Diseases 10(12):2196–9. www.cdc.gov/ncidod/EID/vol10no12/04-0961.htm.

2230. Steckle MP. 2005. From a management crisis, to becoming better crisis managers: the 2004 avian influenza outbreak in British Columbia. Report of the Standing Committee on Agriculture and Agri-Food. April. parl.gc.ca/committee/CommitteePublication.aspx?SourceId=111249.

2231. Bueckert D. 2004. Avian flu outbreak raises concerns about factory farms. Daily Herald-Tribune (Grande Prairie, Alberta), April 8, p. 6. cp.org/english/online/full/agriculture/040407/a040730A.html.

2232. Bueckert D. 2004. Avian flu outbreak raises concerns about factory farms.

Daily Herald-Tribune (Grande Prairie, Alberta), April 8, p. 6. cp.org/english /online/full/agriculture/040407/a040730A.html.

2233. Mench JA. 1992. The welfare of poultry in modern production systems. Poultry Science 4:108–9.

2234. Broom DM. 2000. Does present legislation help animal welfare? Sustainable Animal Production: Workshops, Discussion, Online Resources. June–October. agriculture.de/acms1/conf6/ws5alegisl.htm.

2235. Vaillancourt JP. 2002. Biosecurity now. Poultry International. 411:12–8.

2236. Shane SM. 2005. Global disease update—AI overshadowing erosive diseases. World Poultry 21(7):22–3.

2237. Mabbett T. 2005. People, poultry and avian influenza. Poultry International, Volume 44, Number 9 pp.34–39.

2238. Bueckert D. 2004. Avian flu outbreak raises concerns about factory farms. Daily Herald-Tribune (Grande Prairie, Alberta), April 8, p. 6. cp.org/english /online/full/agriculture/040407/a040730A.html.

2239. Leahy S. 2004. Bird flu defeated—at high cost. IPS-Inter Press Service, August 27. ipsnews.net/interna.asp?idnews=25254.

2240. Bueckert D. 2004. Avian flu outbreak raises concerns about factory farms. Daily Herald-Tribune (Grande Prairie, Alberta), April 8, p. 6. cp.org/english /online/full/agriculture/040407/a040730A.html.

2241. CBC News. 2004. Scientist probe mystery surrounding avian flu. March 26. cbc.ca/bc/story/mar26avianmystery226032004.html.

2242. 2005. A few facts about avian influenza. www.avian-influenza.com. January. thepoultrysite.com/FeaturedArticle/FAType.asp?AREA=broilers&Display=275.

2243. 2005. A few facts about avian influenza. www.avian-influenza.com. January. thepoultrysite.com/FeaturedArticle/FAType.asp?AREA=broilers&Display=275.

2244. Lees W. 2004. Overview: the avian influenza outbreak in BC. Presentation to the Canadian Poultry Industry Forum, Animal Disease Surveillance Unit, CFIA. bcac.bc.ca/documents/C%20CFIA%20Overview%20-%20Dr.%20 Wayne%20Lees.pdf.

2245. Johnson E. 2004. The ducks in the henhouse: wild birds are being blamed for the death of 19 million chickens. Yet factory farms are the real problem. The Tyee, April 13. thetyee.ca/Views/2004/04/13/The_Ducks_in_the_Henhouse/.

2246. Capua I, Alexander DJ. 2004. Avian influenza: recent developments. Avian Pathol. 33:393–404.

2247. Bosman A, Meijer A, Koopmans M. 2005. Final analysis of Netherlands avian influenza outbreaks reveals much higher levels of transmission to humans than previously thought. Eurosurveill. 10:E050106.2.

2248. World Health Organization. 2003. Avian influenza in the Netherlands: disease outbreak reported. Epidemic and Pandemic Alert and Response. April 24. www.who.int/csr/don/2003_04_24/en/.

2249. de Jong MCM, Stegeman A, van der Goot J, Koch G. 2009. Intra- and inter-species transmission of H7N7 highly pathogenic avian influenza virus during the avian influenza epidemic in the Netherlands in 2003. Rev Sci Tech. 28(1): 333–340. https://doi.org/10.20506/rst.28.1.1859.

2250. Lawrence F. 2004. Why factory farms and mass trade make for a world where disease travels far and fast. Experts fear flu virus may spread to other countries and mutate, threatening a human pandemic. Guardian, January 24. www .guardian.co.uk/food/Story/0,2763,1130271,00.html.

2251. de Jong MCM, Stegeman A, van der Goot J, Koch G. 2009. Intra- and interspecies transmission of H7N7 highly pathogenic avian influenza virus during the avian influenza epidemic in the Netherlands in 2003. Rev Sci Tech. 28(1): 333–340. https://doi.org/10.20506/rst.28.1.1859.

2252. Kuiken T, Fouchier R, Rimmelzwaan G, Osterhaus A. 2003. Emerging viral infections in a rapidly changing world. Current Opinion in Biotechnology 14:641–6.

2253. Thomas ME, Bouma A, Ekker HM, Fonken AJM, Stegeman JA, Nielen M. 2005. Risk factors for the introduction of high pathogenicity avian influenza virus into poultry farms during the epidemic in the Netherlands in 2003. Preventive Veterinary Medicine 69:1–11.

2254. Meredith M. 2004. Bird flu epidemics—what more can be done. World Poultry 20(2):28–9.

2255. de Wit E, Munster VJ, van Riel D, Beyer WE, Rimmelzwaan GF, Kuiken T, Osterhaus AD, Fouchier RA. 2010. Molecular determinants of adaptation of highly pathogenic avian influenza H7N7 viruses to efficient replication in the human host. J Virol. 84(3):1597–1606. https://doi.org/10.1128/JVI.01783-09.

2256. Ward P, Small I, Smith J, Suter P, Dutkowski R. 2005. Oseltamivir (Tamiflu) and its potential for use in the event of an influenza pandemic. Journal of Antimicrobial Chemotherapy 55(S1):i5–i21.

2257. Shortridge KF, Peiris JSM, Guan Y. 2003. The next influenza pandemic: lessons from Hong Kong. Journal of Applied Microbiology 94:70–9.

2258. Suarez DL, Senne DA, Banks J, et al. 2004. Recombination resulting in virulence shift in avian influenza outbreak, Chile. Emerging Infectious Diseases 10:693–99.

2259. Capua I, Mutinelli F, Marangon S, Alexander DJ. 2000. H7N1 avian influenza in Italy (1999 to 2000) in intensively reared chickens and turkeys. Avian Pathology 29:537–43.

2260. Webster RG, Shortridge KF, Kawaoka Y. 1997. Influenza: interspecies transmission and emergence of new pandemics. Federation of European Microbiological Societies Immunology and Medical Microbiology 18:275–9.

2261. Infectious Disease Society of America. 2006. Avian influenza (bird flu): agricultural and wildlife considerations. April 4. www.cidrap.umn.edu/idsa/influenza /avianflu/biofacts/avflu.html.

2262. Webster RG, Shortridge KF, Kawaoka Y. 1997. Influenza: interspecies transmission and emergence of new pandemics. Federation of European Microbiological Societies Immunology and Medical Microbiology 18:275–9.

2263. Webster RG. 1997. Predictions for future human influenza pandemics. The Journal of Infectious Diseases 176:S14–9.

2264. Webster RG. 1998. Influenza: an emerging microbial pathogen. In: Emerging Infections (San Diego, CA: Academic Press, pp. 275–300).

2265. Capua I, Marangon S, Selli L, et al. 1999. Outbreaks of highly pathogenic avian influenza (H5N2) in Italy during October 1997 to January 1998. Avian Pathology 28:455–60.

2266. Capua I, Marangon S. 2000. The avian influenza epidemic in Italy, 1999–2000: a review. Avian Pathology 29:289–94.

2267. Capua I, Marangon S. 2000. The avian influenza epidemic in Italy, 1999–2000: a review. Avian Pathology 29:289–94.

2268. Capua I, Mutinelli F, Marangon S, Alexander DJ. 2000. H7N1 avian influenza in Italy (1999 to 2000) in intensively reared chickens and turkeys. Avian Pathology 29:537–43.

2269. Shortridge KF, Zhou NN, Guan Y, et al. 1998. Characterization of avian H5N1 influenza viruses from poultry in Hong Kong. Virology 252:331–42.

2270. Gladwell M. 1997. The dead zone. New Yorker, July 28. gladwell .com/1997/1997_09_29_a_flu.htm.

2271. Straight Dope Science Advisory Board. 2001. How high can birds and bees fly? The Straight Dope, December 11. straightdope.com/mailbag/mbirdbees.html.

2272. Webster RG, Yakhno M, Hinshaw VS, Bean WJ, Murti KG. 1978. Intestinal influenza: replication and characterization of influenza viruses in ducks. Virology 84:268–78.

2273. Hinshaw VS, Webster RG, Turner B. 1980. The perpetuation of orthomyxoviruses and paramyxoviruses in Canadian waterfowl. Canadian Journal of Microbiology 26:622–9.

2274. Pharo HJ. 2003. The impact of new epidemiological information on a risk analysis for the introduction of avian influenza viruses in imported poultry meat. Avian Diseases 47:988–95.

2275. Marshall B. 2006. You call this a wetland? Field and Stream, March 30. fieldandstream.com/fieldstream/columnists/conservation/article/0,13199, 1179434,00.html.

2276. Gumuchian M. 2006. Restoring wetlands key to curbing bird flu—report. Reuters, April 11.

2277. Brown C. 2000. Emerging infectious diseases of animals: an overview. In: Brown C, Bolin C (eds.), Emerging Diseases of Animals (Washington, DC: ASM Press, pp. 1–12).

2278. Alexander DJ. 2000. A review of avian influenza in different bird species. Veterinary Microbiology 74:3–13.

2279. Drexler M. 2002. Secret Agents: The Menace of Emerging Infections (Washington, DC: Joseph Henry Press).

2280. Hafez HM. 2000. Factors influencing turkey diseases. World Poultry Turkey Health Special, pp. 6–8.

2281. Surgeoner GA. 1996. Rodent control in livestock facilities. Ontario Ministry of Agriculture, Food and Rural Affairs. September. www.omafra.gov.on.ca /english/livestock/dairy/facts/86-036.htm.

2282. Shortridge KF, Zhou NN, Guan Y, et al. 1998. Characterization of avian H5N1 influenza viruses from poultry in Hong Kong. Virology 252:331–42.

2283. Nestorowicz A, Kawaoka Y, Bean WJ, Webster RG. 1987. Molecular analysis of the hemagglutinin genes of Australian H7N7 influenza viruses: role of passerine birds in maintenance or transmission? Virology 160:411–18.

2284. Halvorson DA, Kelleher CJ, Senne DA. 1985. Epizootiology of avian influenza: effect of seasonal incidence in sentinel ducks and domestic turkey in Minnesota. Applied and Environmental Microbiology 49:914–9.

2285. Petersen L, Nielsen EM, Engberg J, On SL, Dietz HH. 2001. Comparison of genotypes and serotypes of Campylobacter jejuni isolated from Danish wild mammals and birds and from broiler flocks and humans. Applied and Environmental Microbiology 67(7):3115–21.

2286. Silbergeld E. 2006. Avian influenza risks and the animal-human Interface. Avian flu: the pandemic threat and the global strategy at the Johns Hopkins Bloomberg School of Public Health, January 30. commprojects.jhsph.edu/_media /009_avian_flu.ram.

2287. Axtell RC, Arends JJ. 1990. Ecology and management of arthropod pests of poultry. Annual Review of Entomology 35:101–126.

2288. Rosef O, Kapperud G. 1983. House flies (Musca domestica) as possible vectors of Campylobacter fetus subsp. Applied and Environmental Microbiology 45(2):3811–3.

2289. Iowa State University Center for Food Security and Public Health. 2005. Avian influenza (highly pathogenic). October. www.cfsph.iastate.edu/DiseaseInfo /notes/AvianInfluenza.pdf.

2290. Ito T, Kawaoka Y. 1998. Avian influenza. In: Nicholson KG, Webster RG, Hay AJ (eds.), Textbook of Influenza (Oxford: Blackwell Science, pp. 126–36).

2291. Halvorson DA, Kelleher CJ, Senne DA. 1985. Epizootiology of avian influenza: effect of seasonal incidence in sentinel ducks and domestic turkey in Minnesota. Applied and Environmental Microbiology 49:914–9.

2292. Vaillancourt JP. 2002. Biosecurity now. Poultry International. 411:12–8.

2293. Capua I, Marangon S. 2003. The use of vaccination as an option for the control of avian influenza. In: 71st General Session International Committee of the World Organization for Animal Health (Paris, France, May 18–23).

2294. Capua I, Marangon S. 2003. The use of vaccination as an option for the control of avian influenza. In: 71st General Session International Committee of the World Organization for Animal Health (Paris, France, May 18–23).

2295. Capua I, Marangon S. 2003. Currently available tools and strategies for emergency vaccination in case of avian influenza. In: Schrijver RS, Koch G (eds.), Proceedings of the Frontis Workshop on Avian Influenza: Prevention and Control (Wageningen, The Netherlands, pp. 59–74).

2296. Perdue ML, Suarez DL, Swayne DE. 2000. Avian influenza in the 1990s. Avian and Poultry Biology Reviews 11:11–20.

2297. Krushinskie EA. 2006. U.S. poultry industry preparedness for an HPAI outbreak. Avian influenza: Dealing with the challenge. bulldogsolutions.net/Watt Publishing/WPC01102006/frmEventDescription.aspx.

2298. Cutler GJ. 1986. The nature and impact of layer industry changes. United States Animal Health Association. Second International Symposia on Avian Influenza, pp. 423–6.

2299. Alexander DJ. 1993. Orthomyxovirus infection. In: McFerran JB, McNulty MS (eds.), Virus Infections of Birds (Amsterdam, The Netherlands: Elsevier Science Publishers, pp. 287–316).

2300. U.S. Department of Agriculture APHIS. Backyard biosecurity: practices to keep your birds healthy. September 2004

2301. Canning K. 2005. A matter of pride. www.refrigeratedfrozenfood.com/content.php?s=RF/2005/12&p=8.

2302. Schmit J. 2005. Poultry farm tactics may thwart bird flu. USA Today, November 14. usatoday.com/news/nation/2005-11-13-farmers-birdflu_x.htm?csp=N009.

2303. Tablante NL, San Myint M, Johnson YJ, Rhodes K, Colby M, Hohenhaus G. 2002. A survey of biosecurity practices as risk factors affecting broiler performance on the Delmarva Peninsula. Avian Diseases 46:730–4.

2304. Beard CW. 2003. Minimizing the vulnerability of poultry production chains for avian influenza. In: Schrijver RS, Koch G (eds.), Proceedings of the Frontis Workshop on Avian Influenza: Prevention and Control (Wageningen, The Netherlands, pp. 133–7).

2305. 2003. Dirty money: corporate criminal donations to the two major parties. Corporate Crime Reporter, July 3. www.corporatecrimereporter.com/ccrreport.pdf.

2306. Tyson Foods. 2005. Tyson provides $26 million to fuel family farmers: supplemental energy allowance addresses rising fuel costs. Tyson Press Room. October 3. tysonfoodsinc.com/PressRoom/ViewArticle.aspx?id=1925.

2307. 2005. IBP, Inc. v. Alvarez (03-1238); Tum v. Barber Foods, Inc (04-66) Supreme Court collection. www.law.cornell.edu/supct/cert/03-1238.html.

2308. Schmit J. 2005. Poultry farm tactics may thwart bird flu. USA Today, November 14. usatoday.com/news/nation/2005-11-13-farmers-birdflu_x.htm?csp=N009.

2309. Animal Health and Welfare Panel of the European Food Safety Authority. 2005. Animal health and welfare aspects of avian influenza. European Food Safety Authority Journal 266:1–21.

2310. Beard CW. 2003. Minimizing the vulnerability of poultry production chains for avian influenza. In: Schrijver RS, Koch G (eds.), Proceedings of the Frontis Workshop on Avian Influenza: Prevention and Control (Wageningen, The Netherlands, pp. 133–7).

2311. Stegeman A (Chairman). 2003. Workshop 1: Introduction and spread of avian influenza. In: Schrijver RS, Koch G (eds.), Proceedings of the Frontis Workshop on Avian Influenza: Prevention and Control. library.wur.nl/frontis/avian_influenza/workshop1.pdf.

2312. Shane SM. 2003. Disease continues to impact the world's poultry industries. World Poultry 19(7):22–7.

2313. Rudd K. 1995. Poultry reality check needed. Poultry Digest, December 1995, pp. 12–20.

2314. Rudd K. 1995. Poultry reality check needed. Poultry Digest, December 1995, pp. 12–20.

2315. Anderson I. 2002. Foot and Mouth Disease 2001: Lessons to Be Learned Inquiry Report (London, UK: The Stationery Office). archive.cabinetoffice.gov .uk/fmd/fmd_report/report/.

2316. Shane SM. 2003. Disease continues to impact the world's poultry industries. World Poultry 19(7):22–7.

2317. Pluimers F (Chairman). 2003. Workshop 4: Control measures and legislation. In: Schrijver RS, Koch G (eds.), Proceedings of the Frontis Workshop on Avian Influenza: Prevention and Control (Wageningen, The Netherlands) at library .wur.nl/frontis/avian_influenza/workshop4.pdf.

2318. Halvorson D. 2005. Overview of avian influenza. University of Minnesota University of Minnesota Extension Service. December 9. www.cvm.umn.edu /ai/home.html.

2319. Olsen SJ, Rooney JA, Blanton L, Rolfes MA, Nelson DI, Gomez TM, Karli SA, Trock SC, Fry AM. 2019. Estimating risk to responders exposed to avian influenza A H5 and H7 viruses in poultry, United States, 2014–2017. Emerg Infect Dis. 25(5):1011–1014. https://dx.doi.org/10.3201/eid2505.181253.

2320. Bevins SN, Dusek RJ, White CL, Gidlewski T, Bodenstein B, Mansfield KG, DeBruyn P, Kraege D, Rowan E, Gillin C, et al. 2016. Widespread detection of highly pathogenic H5 influenza viruses in wild birds from the Pacific Flyway of the United States. Sci Rep. 6(1):28980. https://dx.doi.org/10.1038/srep28980.

2321. Lee DH, Bertran K, Kwon JH, Swayne DE. 2017. Evolution, global spread, and pathogenicity of highly pathogenic avian influenza H5Nx clade 2.3.4.4. J Vet Sci. 18(S1):269–280. https://doi.org/10.4142/jvs.2017.18.S1.269.

2322. Lee DH, Bahl J, Torchetti MK, Killian ML, Ip HS, DeLiberto TJ, Swayne DE. 2016. Highly pathogenic avian influenza viruses and generation of novel reassortants, United States, 2014–2015. Emerg Infect Dis. 22(7):1283–1285. https://doi.org/10.3201/eid2207.160048.

2323. U.S. Government Accountability Office. 2017 Apr 13. Avian influenza: USDA has taken actions to reduce risks but needs a plan to evaluate its efforts. Washington: GAO. Report No.: GAO-17-360. [accessed 2020 Apr 7]. https://www .gao.gov/assets/690/684086.pdf.

2324. U.S. Department of Agriculture. 2015 Dec. High pathogenicity avian influenza control in commercial poultry operations—a national approach. USDA. [accessed 2020 Apr 18]. https://www.aphis.usda.gov/stakeholders/downloads /2015/hpai_ea.pdf.

2325. Humane Society of the United States v. U.S. Department of Agriculture, Animal & Plant Health Inspection Service, Veterinary Services, Kevin Shea, Burke Healy, Mark Davidson. 2020 Apr 8. Case 2:20-cv-03258.

2326. Swayne DE, Akey BL. 2003. Avian influenza control strategies in the United States of America. In: Schrijver RS, Koch G (eds.), Proceedings of the Frontis Workshop on Avian Influenza: Prevention and Control (Wageningen, The Netherlands, pp. 113–30).

2327. Gladwell M. 1995. The plague year. New Republic, July 24.

2328. Brown C. 1999. Economic considerations of agricultural diseases. Annals of the New York Academy of Sciences 894:92–94.

2329. Greene JL. 2015 Jul 20. Update on the highly-pathogenic avian influenza outbreak of 2014–2015. Congressional Research Service; [accessed 2020 Apr 7]. https://fas.org/sgp/crs/misc/R44114.pdf.

2330. Senne DA, Pearson JE, Panigrahy B. 1997. Live poultry markets: a missing link in the epidemiology of avian influenza. In: Proceedings of the 3rd International Symposium on Avian Influenza May 27–29 (University of Wisconsin, Madison, pp. 50–8).

2331. Gladwell M. 1995. The plague year. New Republic, July 24.

2332. Laver WG, Bischofberger N, Webster RG. 2000. The origin and control of pandemic influenza. Perspectives in Biology and Medicine 43(2):173–92.

2333. Gladwell M. 1997. The dead zone. New Yorker, July 28. gladwell .com/1997/1997_09_29_a_flu.htm.

2334. Branden C, John T. 1991. Introduction to Protein Structure (New York, NY: Garland Publishing, Inc., pp. 72–75). www.chem.uwec.edu/Chem406/Web pages97/heidi/INTRO.HTM.

2335. Kawaoka Y, Webster RG. 1988. Molecular mechanism of acquisition of virulence in influenza virus in nature. Microbial Pathogenesis 5:311–18.

2336. Laver WG, Bischofberger N, Webster RG. 2000. The origin and control of pandemic influenza. Perspectives in Biology and Medicine 43(2):173–92.

2337. Dierauf L. Avian influenza in wild birds. U.S. Department of the Interior, U.S. Geological Survey. Wildlife Health Bulletin 04-01. www.nwhc.usgs.gov/publi cations/wildlife_health_bulletins/WHB_04_01.jsp.

2338. Dierauf L. Avian influenza in wild birds. U.S. Department of the Interior, U.S. Geological Survey. Wildlife Health Bulletin 04-01. www.nwhc.usgs.gov/publica tions/wildlife_health_bulletins/WHB_04_01.jsp.

2339. Senne DA, Pearson JE, Panigrahy B. 1997. Live poultry markets: a missing link in the epidemiology of avian influenza. In: Proceedings of the 3rd International Symposium on Avian Influenza May 27–29 (University of Wisconsin, Madison, pp. 50–8).

2340. Senne DA, Pearson JE, Panigrahy B. 1997. Live poultry markets: a missing link in the epidemiology of avian influenza. In: Proceedings of the 3rd International Symposium on Avian Influenza May 27–29 (University of Wisconsin, Madison, pp. 50–8).

2341. Perez DR, Nazarian SH, McFadden G, Gilmore MS. 2005. Miscellaneous threats: highly pathogenic avian influenza, and novel bio-engineered organisms. In: Bronze MS, Greenfield RA (eds.), Biodefense: Principles and Pathogens (Norfolk, UK: Horizon Bioscience).

2342. Lee C, Senne DA, Linares JA, et al. 2004. Characterization of recent H5 subtype avian influenza viruses from U.S. poultry. Avian Pathology 33:288–97.

2343. 2004. USDA confirms highly pathogenic Avian Influenza in Texas. West Texas County Courier, February 26. www.wtccourier.com/flats_pdf./2004/02-26 -04.pdf.

2344. Stubbs EL. 1948. Fowl pest. In: Biester HE, Schwarte LH (eds.), Diseases of Poultry, 2nd ed (Ames, IA: Iowa State University Press, pp. 603–614).

2345. Perez DR, Nazarian SH, McFadden G, Gilmore MS. 2005. Miscellaneous threats: highly pathogenic avian influenza, and novel bio-engineered organisms. In: Bronze MS, Greenfield RA (eds.), Biodefense: Principles and Pathogens (Norfolk, UK: Horizon Bioscience).

2346. Senne DA, Pearson JE, Panigrahy B. 1997. Live poultry markets: a missing link in the epidemiology of avian influenza. In: Proceedings of the 3rd International Symposium on Avian Influenza May 27–29 (University of Wisconsin, Madison, pp. 50–8).

2347. Senne DA, Holt TJ, Akey BL. 2003. An overview of the 2002 outbreak of low-pathogenic H7N2 avian influenza in Virginia, West Virginia and North Carolina. In: Schrijver RS, Koch G (eds.), Proceedings of the Frontis Workshop on Avian Influenza: Prevention and Control (Wageningen, The Netherlands, pp. 41–7).

2348. Centers for Disease Control and Prevention. 2005. Outbreaks in North America with transmission to humans. tinyurl.com/n7eu2.

2349. Spackman E, Suarez DL. 2003. Evaluation of molecular markers for pathogenicity in recent H7N2 avian influenza isolates from the northeastern United States. In: Proceedings of the 52nd Western Poultry Disease Conference, pp. 21–3. Sacramento, CA, USA.

2350. Centers for Disease Control and Prevention. 2005. Outbreaks in North America with transmission to humans. tinyurl.com/n7eu2.

2351. Swayne DE, Akey BL. 2003. Avian influenza control strategies in the United States of America. In: Schrijver RS, Koch G (eds.), Proceedings of the Frontis Workshop on Avian Influenza: Prevention and Control (Wageningen, The Netherlands, pp. 113–30).

2352. Shane SM. 2003. Disease continues to impact the world's poultry industries. World Poultry 19(7):22–7.

2353. Swayne DE. 2003. Transcript of the question and answer session from the Fifth International Symposium on Avian Influenza. Avian Diseases 47:1219–55.

2354. Senne DA, Pederson JC, Panigrahy B. 2003. Live-bird markets in the northeastern United States: a source of avian influenza in commercial poultry. In: Schrijver RS, Koch G (eds.), Proceedings of the Frontis Workshop on Avian Influenza: Prevention and Control (Wageningen, The Netherlands, pp. 19–24).

2355. Spackman E, Senne DA, Davison S, Suarez DL. 2003. Sequence analysis of recent H7 avian influenza viruses associated with three different outbreaks in commercial poultry in the United States. Journal of Virology 77:13399–402.

2356. Swayne DE, Akey BL. 2003. Avian influenza control strategies in the United States of America. In: Schrijver RS, Koch G (eds.), Proceedings of the Frontis Workshop on Avian Influenza: Prevention and Control (Wageningen, The Netherlands, pp. 113–30).

2357. Centers for Disease Control and Prevention. 2005. Outbreaks in North America with transmission to humans. tinyurl.com/n7eu2.

2358. Capua I, Alexander DJ. 2004. Avian influenza: recent developments. Avian Pathology 33:393–404.

2359. Senne DA, Pederson JC, Panigrahy B. 2003. Live-bird markets in the northeastern United States: a source of avian influenza in commercial poultry. In:

Schrijver RS, Koch G (eds.), Proceedings of the Frontis Workshop on Avian Influenza: Prevention and Control (Wageningen, The Netherlands, pp. 19–24).

2360. Swayne DE. 2003. Transcript of the question and answer session from the Fifth International Symposium on Avian Influenza. Avian Diseases 47:1219–55.

2361. University of Georgia Southeastern Cooperative Wildlife Disease Study. 1986. July. Avian influenza in live poultry markets. SCWDS Briefs, July.

2362. Spackman E, Senne DA, Davison S, Suarez DL. 2003. Sequence analysis of recent H7 avian influenza viruses associated with three different outbreaks in commercial poultry in the United States. Journal of Virology 77:13399–402.

2363. Swayne DE, Akey BL. 2003. Avian influenza control strategies in the United States of America. In: Schrijver RS, Koch G (eds.), Proceedings of the Frontis Workshop on Avian Influenza: Prevention and Control (Wageningen, The Netherlands, pp. 113–30).

2364. Mullaney R. 2003. Live-bird market closure activities in the northeastern United States. Avian Diseases 47:1096–8.

2365. Senne DA, Pederson JC, Panigrahy B. 2003. Live-bird markets in the northeastern United States: a source of avian influenza in commercial poultry. In: Schrijver RS, Koch G (eds.), Proceedings of the Frontis Workshop on Avian Influenza: Prevention and Control (Wageningen, The Netherlands, pp. 19–24).

2366. Suarez DL, Garcia M, Latimer J, Senne D, Perdue M. 1999. Phylogenetic analysis of H7 avian influenza viruses isolated from the live bird markets of the northeastern United States. Journal of Virology 73:3567–73.

2367. Trock SC, Huntley JP. 2010. Surveillance and control of avian influenza in the New York live bird markets. Avian Dis. 54(s1):340–344. https://doi.org/10.1637/8728-032409-ResNote.1.

2368. Newbury SP, Cigel F, Killian ML, Leutenegger CM, Seguin MA, Crossley B, Brennen R, Suarez DL, Torchetti M, Toohey-Kurth K. 2017. First detection of avian lineage H7N2 in Felis catus. Genome Announc. 5(23):e00457-17. https://dx.doi.org/10.1128/genomeA.00457-17.

2369. Poirot E, Levine MZ, Russell K, Stewart RJ, Pompey JM, Chiu S, Fry AM, Gross L, Havers FP, Li ZN, et al. 2019. Detection of avian influenza A(H7N2) virus infection among animal shelter workers using a novel serological approach—New York City, 2016–2017. J Infect Dis. 219(11):1688–1696. https://doi.org/10.1093/infdis/jiy595.

2370. Belser JA, Pulit-Penaloza JA, Sun X, Brock N, Pappas C, Creager HM, Zeng H, Tumpey TM, Maines TR. A novel A(H7N2) influenza virus isolated from a veterinarian caring for cats in a New York City animal shelter causes mild disease and transmits poorly in the ferret model. J Virol. 91(15):e00672-17. https://doi.org/10.1128/JVI.00672-17.

2371. Senne DA, Pederson JC, Panigrahy B. 2003. Live-bird markets in the northeastern United States: a source of avian influenza in commercial poultry. In: Schrijver RS, Koch G (eds.), Proceedings of the Frontis Workshop on Avian Influenza: Prevention and Control (Wageningen, The Netherlands, pp. 19–24).

2372. 2005. Cornell checking for avian flu in NYC. Ithaca Journal, October 15.

2373. Belser JA, Blixt O, Chen L-M, Pappas C, Maines TR, Van Hoeven N, Donis R,

Busch J, McBride R, Paulson JC, et al. 2008. Contemporary North American influenza H7 viruses possess human receptor specificity: implications for virus transmissibility. Proc Natl Acad Sci U S A. 105(21)7558–7563. https://doi.org/10.1073/pnas.0801259105.

2374. Chander Y, Jindal N, Sreevatsan S, Stallknecht DE, Goyal SM. 2013. Molecular and phylogenetic analysis of matrix gene of avian influenza viruses isolated from wild birds and live bird markets in the USA. Influenza Other Respir Viruses. 7(4):513–520. https://doi.org/10.1111/irv.12003.

2375. Belser JA, Blixt O, Chen L-M, Pappas C, Maines TR, Van Hoeven N, Donis R, Busch J, McBride R, Paulson JC, et al. 2008. Contemporary North American influenza H7 viruses possess human receptor specificity: implications for virus transmissibility. Proc Natl Acad Sci U S A. 105(21)7558–7563. https://doi.org/10.1073/pnas.0801259105.

2376. Yen HL, Lipatov AS, Ilyushina NA, Govorkova EA, Franks J, Yilmaz N, Douglas A, Hay A, Krauss S, Rehg JE, Hoffmann E, et al. 2007. Inefficient transmission of H5N1 influenza viruses in a ferret contact model. J Virol. 81(13):6890–6898. https://doi.org/10.1128/JVI.00170-07.

2377. U.S. Department of Agriculture, Agricultural Research Service. Action plan. tinyurl.com/k56zb.

2378. Graham JP, Leibler JH, Price LB, Otte JM, Pfeiffer DU, Tiensin T, Silbergeld EK. 2008. The animal-human interface and infectious disease in industrial food animal production: rethinking biosecurity and biocontainment. Public Health Rep. 123(3):282–299. https://doi.org/10.1177/003335490812300309.

2379. Suarez DL, Spackman E, Senne DA. 2003. Update on molecular epidemiology of H1, H5, and H7 influenza virus infections in poultry in North America. Avian Diseases 47:888–97.

2380. Veterinary Services; Surveillance, Preparedness, and Response Services; Animal and Plant Health Inspection Service. 2016. Final report for the 2014–2015 outbreak of highly pathogenic avian influenza (HPAI) in the United States. U.S. Department of Agriculture; [revised 2016 Aug 11; accessed 2020 Apr 7]. https://www.aphis.usda.gov/animal_health/emergency_management/downloads/hpai/2015-hpai-final-report.pdf.

2381. Thaxton YV. 2005. Are you prepared for AI? Poultry, April/May, p. 5.

2382. 2005. Flu "would spread to UK in weeks." BBC News, September 14. news.bbc.co.uk/1/hi/health/4245004.stm.

2383. Specter M. 2005. Nature's bioterrorist. New Yorker, February 28, pp. 52–61.

2384. Ferguson NM, Cummings DA, Cauchemez S, Fraser C, Riley S, Meeyai A, Lamsirithaworn S, Burke DS. 2005. Strategies for containing an emerging influenza pandemic in Southeast Asia. Nature 437(7056):209–14.

2385. Longini IM Jr, Nizam A, Xu S, Ungchusak K, Hanshaoworakul W, Cummings DA, Halloran ME. 2005. Containing pandemic influenza at the source. Science. 309(5737):1083–7.

2386. Ferguson NM, Cummings DA, Cauchemez S, Fraser C, Riley S, Meeyai A, Lamsirithaworn S, Burke DS. 2005. Strategies for containing an emerging influenza pandemic in Southeast Asia. Nature 437(7056):209–14.

2387. Ruef C. 2004. A new influenza pandemic-unprepared for a big threat? Infection 32(6):313–4.

2388. Weiss R. 2005. Bird flu could be stopped—if everything is aligned right. Washington Post, August 4, p. A16. www.washingtonpost.com/wp-dyn/content /article/2005/08/03/AR2005080301806.html.

2389. Center for Infectious Disease and Research Policy. 2005. Roche to give flu drug to WHO to fight pandemic. August 24. cidrap.umn.edu/cidrap/content /influenza/panflu/news/aug2405who.html.

2390. Center for Infectious Disease and Research Policy. 2005. Roche to give flu drug to WHO to fight pandemic. August 24. cidrap.umn.edu/cidrap/content /influenza/panflu/news/aug2405who.html.

2391. New Scientist. 2005. Editorial: bird flu—ready or not? New Scientist, August 6, p. 3.

2392. Fox M. 2005. No quick fix for bird flu, experts caution. Reuters, October 11.

2393. Editorial. 2003. We have been warned. Nature 424(6945):113. www.nature .com/nature/journal/v424/n6945/full/424113a.html.

2394. 2005. Weak-link Laos gets U.S. funds for bird flu fight. Reuters, October 13. signonsandiego.com/news/world/20051013-0824-birdflu-laos.html.

2395. Mason M. 2005. Official: preventing pandemic impossible. ABC News, October 15. abcnews.go.com/Health/wireStory?id=1216962&CMP=OTC-RSSFeeds0312.

2396. Institute of Medicine and National Research Council. 2009 Sep. Report brief: sustaining global surveillance and response to emerging zoonotic diseases. Washington(DC): National Academies Press; [accessed 2020 Apr 9].

2397. Weiss R. 2005. Bird flu could be stopped—if everything is aligned right. Washington Post, August 4, p. A16. www.washingtonpost.com/wp-dyn/ content/article/2005/08/03/AR2005080301806.html.

2398. Levy A, Scott-Clark C. 2005. Flu on the wing. Guardian, October 15. www .guardian.co.uk/birdflu/story/0,14207,1591358,00.html.

2399. Stone R. 2006. Combating the bird flu menace, down on the farm. Science 311:944–46.

2400. Bradsher K. 2005. Gaps in affluence strain worldwide bird flu response. New York Times, October 9.

2401. United Nations Food and Agriculture Organization News Release. 2005. Global strategy to fight bird flu in animals faces serious funding gap. September 26. www.fao.org/newsroom/en/news/2005/107804/.

2402. Oxford JS. 2005. Preparing for the first influenza pandemic of the 21st century. Lancet Infectious Diseases 5:129–31.

2403. United Nations. 2005. Fighting bird flu at origin will help prevent human flu pandemic says UN Food and Agriculture Organization. UN Press Release SAG/334, February 23. www.un.org/News/Press/docs/2005/sag334.doc.htm.

2404. Stapp K. 2004. Scientists warn of fast-spreading global viruses. IPS-Inter Press Service, February 23.

2405. Aglionby J. 2004. The politics of poultry. Guardian, January 29. guardian .co.uk/elsewhere/journalist/story/0,7792,1134341,00.html.

2406. Lawrence F. 2004. Why factory farms and mass trade make for a world where disease travels far and fast. Experts fear flu virus may spread to other countries and mutate, threatening a human pandemic. Guardian, January 24. www.guardian.co.uk/food/Story/0,2763,1130271,00.html.

2407. Hookway J. 2005. In the battle against avian flu, rural Asia is seen as vanguard. Wall Street Journal, October 14.

2408. Delforge I. 2004. Thailand: the world's kitchen. Le Monde Diplomatique, July. mondediplo.com/2004/07/05thailand.

2409. Delgado CL, Narrod CA. 2002. Impact of Changing Market Forces and Policies on Structural Change in the Livestock Industries of Selected Fast-Growing Developing Countries Final Research Report of Phase I—Project on Livestock Industrialization, Trade and Social-Health-Environment Impacts in Developing Countries (Washington, DC: International Food Policy Research Institute). fao.org/WAIRDOCS/LEAD/X6115E/X6115E00.HTM.

2410. Horn R. 2004. The families that own Asia—Chearavanont. Time Asia, February 16. www.time.com/time/asia/covers/501040223/chearavanont.html.

2411. Becker J. 2004. Bird flu panic hits China amid fears of global pandemic. Independent, January 31.

2412. Horn R. 2004. The families that own Asia—Chearavanont. Time Asia, February 16. www.time.com/time/asia/covers/501040223/chearavanont.html.

2413. Davis M. 2005. The Monster at Our Door: The Global Threat of Avian Flu (New York, NY: The New Press, pp. 100–1).

2414. Elegant S. 2004. Gauging the threat: Is a human pandemic next? Time International, February 9, p. 14.

2415. Elegant S. 2004. Gauging the threat: Is a human pandemic next? Time International, February 9, p. 14.

2416. Delforge I. 2004. Thailand: the world's kitchen. Le Monde Diplomatique, July. mondediplo.com/2004/07/05thailand.

2417. Davis M. 2005. The Monster at Our Door: The Global Threat of Avian Flu (New York, NY: The New Press, p. 102).

2418. Hermawan A. 2003. No News Is Bad News. Southeast Asian Press Alliance. www.seapabkk.org/newdesign/fellowshipsdetail.php?No=241.

2419. Davis M. 2005. The Monster at Our Door: The Global Threat of Avian Flu (New York, NY: The New Press, p. 105).

2420. Hermawan A. 2003. No News Is Bad News. Southeast Asian Press Alliance. www.seapabkk.org/newdesign/fellowshipsdetail.php?No=241.

2421. Channel News Asia. 2004. WHO raps Asia over handling of bird flu crisis. February 10. www.channelnewsasia.com/stories/afp_world/view/70444/1/.html.

2422. Watts J. 2004. Asian nations step up action to curb spread of avian influenza. Lancet 363:373.

2423. McCurry J. 2004. Bird flu suicides in Japan. Guardian, March 9.

2424. Editorial. Lapses in halting avian flu. Japan Times, March 3. www.japantimes.co.jp/shukan-st/jteds/ed20040319.htm.

2425. Sipress A. 2005. Indonesia neglected bird flu until too late, experts say. Washington Post, October 20, p. A01. www.washingtonpost.com/wp-dyn/content/article/2005/10/19/AR2005101902147.html.

2426. Aglionby J. 2004. The politics of poultry. Guardian, January 29. guardian.co.uk/elsewhere/journalist/story/0,7792,1134341,00.html.

2427. Chanyapate C, Delforge I. 2004. The politics of bird flu in Thailand. Focus on Trade, April, No.98. focusweb.org/publications/FOT%20pdf./fot98.pdf.

2428. Wongchanglaw S. 2004. Thaksin's cover-up: can we trust our leader? Think Centre (ASIA), February 13. www.thinkcentreasia.org/opinions/Thaksincoverup.html.

2429. Avian Influenza Information Centre. 2004. Chicken eating festival. Thai Government fact sheet, February 8. www.thaigov.go.th/avian/index-e.html.

2430. Watt Poultry USA. 2004. KFC gives away free chicken in Thailand to restore consumer confidence. Watt Poultry USA, Industry News Briefs, February 9. www.wattnet.com/Newsroom/ViewNews.cfm?PG=1&nwsNum=14288.

2431. Anthony T. 2004. Eating poultry in China a political act. Associated Press, February 10.

2432. Warden J. 1998. Beef Was Not Perfectly Safe. British Medical Journal 317:1273.

2433. Khalik A. 2005. Anxious minister alone in facing bird flu threat. Jakarta Post, July 30.

2434. Knobler S, Mahmoud A, Lemon S, Mack A, Sivitz L, Oberholtzer K (eds.), 2001. Learning from SARS: Preparing for the Next Disease Outbreak. Workshop Summary (Washington, DC: National Academies Press).

2435. Lee PJ, Krilov LR. 2005. When animal viruses attack: SARS and avian influenza. Pediatric Annals 34(1):43–52.

2436. Channel News Asia. 2004. WHO raps Asia over handling of bird flu crisis. February 10.

2437. Ma J. 2020 Mar 13. Coronavirus: China's first confirmed Covid-19 case traced back to November 17. South China Morning Post. [accessed 2020 Apr 7]; https://www.scmp.com/news/china/society/article/3074991/coronavirus-chinas-first-confirmed-covid-19-case-traced-back.

2438. Yang DL. 2020 Mar 10. Wuhan officials tried to cover up covid-19—and sent it careening outward. Washington Post. [accessed 2020 Apr 7]; https://www.washingtonpost.com/politics/2020/03/10/wuhan-officials-tried-cover-up-covid-19-sent-it-careening-outward/.

2439. Lai S, Ruktanonchai NW, Zhou L, Prosper O, Luo W, Floyd JR, Wesolowski A, Santillana M, Zhang C, Du X, et al. 2020 Mar 13. Effect of non-pharmaceutical interventions for containing the COVID-19 outbreak in China. medRxiv.org. [accessed 2020 Apr 18]. https://doi.org/10.1101/2020.03.03.20029843.

2440. Wong J. 2003. How it began—in case you missed it. Globe and Mail, April 5.

2441. Cropley E. 2005. Myanmar—the world's bird flu black hole? Reuters, October 9.

2442. Butler D. 2005. Flu researchers slam U.S. agency for hoarding data. Nature 437:458–9.

2443. Carr R. 2005. CDC locks up flu data: critics call policy too restrictive. The Atlanta Journal-Constitution, October 3.

2444. Vaillancourt JP. 2002. Biosecurity now. Poultry International. 411:12–8.

2445. Montgomery J. 2005. Public in dark about avian flu cases on farms. News Journal, October 24. www.delawareonline.com/apps/pbcs.dll/article?AID= /20051024/NEWS/510240344.

2446. Rainsford S. 2005. Resentment grows in bird flu town. BBC News, October 11. news.bbc.co.uk/1/hi/world/europe/4329712.stm.

2447. Nordland R. 2005. To stop a virus. Newsweek, October 14. msnbc.msn.com/id /9698067/site/newsweek/.

2448. 2005. Life as we know it. Effect Measure, October 3. effectmeasure.blogspot. com/2005/10/life-as-we-know-it.html.

2449. 2005. After SARS, health experts ponder the next global epidemic. Terra Daily, January 27. terradaily.com/2005/050127124144.c0rr22pn.html.

2450. Nikiforuk A. 2003. Nature always strikes back in global village. Times Colonist, April 6, p. D7.

2451. Weintraub A. 2005. The "horrific" economics of avian flu. Business Week, September 19. www.businessweek.com/magazine/content/05_38/b3951011 .htm.

2452. Knobler S, Mahmoud A, Lemon S, Mack A, Sivitz L, Oberholtzer K (eds.), 2004. Learning from SARS, Preparing for the Next Disease Outbreak, Workshop Summary (Washington, DC: National Academies Press, p. 123). nap .edu/catalog/10915.html.

2453. 2005. Life as we know it. Effect Measure, October 3. effectmeasure.blogspot .com/2005/10/life-as-we-know-it.html.

2454. Fidler DP. 1997. The role of international law in the control of emerging infectious diseases. Bulletin de l'Institut Pasteur 95:57–72.

2455. Walsh B. 2005. A wing and a prayer. Time Asia, September 19. www.time .com/time/asia/magazine/printout/0,13675,501050926-1106457,00.html.

2456. Knox R. 2005. New strategy for pandemic flu. NPR Health News, January 24. npr.org/templates/story/story.php?storyId=4466883.

2457. Wiseman P. 2005. Quick action may stop global bird flu epidemic. USA Today, June 6, p.1A. www.usatoday.com/news/health/2005-06-05-bird-flu-cover_x .htm.

2458. Donnan S, Hidayat T. 2005. Jakarta bird flu vaccine stockpile still low. Financial Times, September 17.

2459. Nissanka JS. 2005. No drugs now if avian flu breaks out. Sunday Observer, October 30. sundayobserver.lk/2005/10/30/new14.html.

2460. Butler D. 2005. Drugs could head off a flu pandemic—but only if we respond fast enough. Nature 436:614–5.

2461. Editorial. 2005. Avian influenza virus: are we prepared? Canadian Medical Association Journal 172:965. cmaj.ca/cgi/content/full/172/8/965.

2462. Lett D. 2005. WHO's call for international pandemic action unheeded. Canadian Medical Association Journal 172:1429. www.cmaj.ca/cgi/reprint/172 /11/1429.

2463. Vesely R. 2005. State tries to save bird flu drug for those most vulnerable to illness. Oakland Tribune, November 30.

2464. Lett D. 2005. WHO's call for international pandemic action unheeded. Canadian Medical Association Journal 172:1429. www.cmaj.ca/cgi/reprint/172/11/1429.

2465. Specter M. 2005. Nature's bioterrorist. New Yorker, February 28, pp. 52–61.

2466. 2005. On the mirage of stopping bird flu. Effect Measure, August 4. effect measure.blogspot.com/2005/08/on-mirage-of-stopping-bird-flu.html.

2467. Council on Foreign Relations. 2005. Conference on the Global Threat of Pandemic Influenza, Session 2: Containment and Control November 16. cfr.org/publication/9244/council_on_foreign_relations_conference_on_the_global_threat_of_pandemic_influenza_session_2.html.

2468. Fox M. 2005. No quick fix for bird flu, experts caution. Reuters, October 11. www.alertnet.org/thenews/newsdesk/N11489775.htm.

2469. Heiberg M. 2005. Two studies model containment strategies for pandemic flu. CIDRAP News, August 3. www.cidrap.umn.edu/cidrap/content/influenza/panflu/news/aug0305panflu.html.

2470. Lyn TE. 2005. South China: Perfect incubator for bird flu pandemic? The Star, September 13. jphpk.gov.my/English/Sept05%2013a.htm.

2471. Osterholm MT. 2005. Preparing for the next pandemic. New England Journal of Medicine 352(18):1839–42. content.nejm.org/cgi/content/full/352/18/1839.

2472. Editorial. 2005. Avian influenza: Perfect storm now gathering? Lancet 365(9462):820.

2473. Gibbs WW, Soares C. 2005. Preparing for a pandemic. Scientific American, October 24.

2474. Tangwisutijit N, Kwankom A. 2005. Not enough drugs to fight a new pandemic. The Nation (Thailand), August 23.

2475. Council on Foreign Relations. 2005. Q&A with Laurie Garrett. Foreign Affairs, May 25. www.foreignaffairs.org/background/pandemic/Garrett2.

2476. Abbott A. 2005. Avian flu special: what's in the medicine cabinet? Nature 435:407–9. nature.com/news/2005/050523/full/435407a.html.

2477. Tangwisutijit N, Kwankom A. 2005. Not enough drugs to fight a new pandemic. The Nation (Thailand), August 23.

2478. Abbott A. 2005. Avian flu special: what's in the medicine cabinet? Nature 435:407–9. nature.com/news/2005/050523/full/435407a.html.

2479. Nebehay S. 2005. WHO's Chan aims to prepare world for bird flu outbreak. Reuters, September 13. msnbc.msn.com/id/9312931/.

2480. Evans B. 2002. Emergency preparedness: a veterinary and animal health community challenge and obligation. Canadian Veterinary Journal 43:797.

2481. Tangwisutijit N, Kwankom A. 2005. Not enough drugs to fight a new pandemic. The Nation (Thailand), August 23.

2482. Nesmith J. 2005. U.S. "woefully unprepared" for bird flu pandemic. Cox News Service, May 26.

2483. Nesmith J. 2005. Flu outbreak could wreak global havoc; scientists warn against complacency. Atlanta Journal-Constitution, June 17, p. 5C.

2484. 2005. Battling bird flu. NewsHour with Jim Lehrer, November 1.

2485. 2005. Vaccines, drugs offer little help in bird flu fight. Governments should instead focus on controlling pandemic, expert cautions. Reuters, October 10.

2486. Marwick C. 1996. Readiness is all: public health experts draft plan outlining pandemic influenza response. Journal of the American Medical Association 275:179–80.

2487. Davis M. 2005. Avian flu: a state of unreadiness. The Nation, July 18–25, pp. 27–30.

2488. Harris G. 2005. Bush plan shows U.S. not ready for deadly flu. New York Times, October 8.

2489. Kennedy EM. 2005. America's response to avian flu. The Boston Globe, October 16.

2490. Neergaard L. 2005. U.S. could restrict travel to prevent flu. Herald News Daily, November 2. heraldnewsdaily.com/stories/news-0094307.html.

2491. Motavalli J. 2005. Laurie Garrett: are we prepared for avian flu? Interviewed by Jim Motavalli. E Magazine, July/August 2005, www.emagazine.com/view/?2826.

2492. Miller S. 2005. Epidemic proportions. Top Producer, February 11.

2493. U.S. Department of Health and Human Services. 2005. Pandemic Influenza Plan. November, p. B7. hhs.gov/pandemicflu/plan/pdf./HHSPandemicInfluenzaPlan.pdf.

2494. Editorial. 2005. The perplexing pandemic flu plan. New York Times, November 20. nytimes.com/2005/11/20/opinion/20sun1.html.?ex=1143090000&en=8d71a46c25138208&ei=5070.

2495. Harris G. 2006. States welcome flu plan but say they need federal money. New York Times, May 4. select.nytimes.com/gst/abstract.html?res=F50F12FA355B0C778CDDAC0894DE404482.

2496. Garrett L. Betrayal of Trust: The Collapse of Global Public Health (New York, NY: Hyperion; 2000).

2497. Osterholm M, Branswell H. 2005. Emerging pandemic: costs and consequences of an avian influenza outbreak (webcast). Woodrow Wilson International Center for Scholars, September 19. www.wilsoncenter.org/index.cfm?topic_id=116811&fuseaction=topics.event_summary&event_id=142787.

2498. Isikoff M, Hosenball M. 2005. Bio-Katrina. Newsweek Web Exclusive, October 12. msnbc.msn.com/id/9675585/site/newsweek/.

2499. Naughton P 2005. Don't panic over bird flu, say EU ministers. Times Online, October 18. timesonline.co.uk/article/0,13509-1831022,00.html.

2500. 2005. "Don't panic." Effect Measure, October 18. effectmeasure.blogspot.com/2005/10/dont-panic.html.

2501. Institute of Medicine Board of Health. The Threat of Pandemic Influenza: Are We Ready? (Washington, DC: National Academies Press).

2502. Barry JM. 2004. The Great Influenza: The Epic Story of the Deadliest Plague in History (New York, NY: Penguin Books).

2503. Colihan K. 2005. Witness to 1918 flu: "Death was there all the time." CNN, November 14. cnn.com/2005/HEALTH/conditions/10/07/1918.flu.witness/index.html.

2504. Public Broadcasting System. American Experience Transcript. 1918 Influenza. pbs.org/wgbh/amex/influenza/filmmore/transcript/transcript1.html.

2505. Davies P. 2000. The Devil's Flu (New York, NY: Henry Holt and Company).

2506. Davies P. 2000. The Devil's Flu (New York, NY: Henry Holt and Company).

2507. Public Broadcasting System. American Experience Transcript. 1918 Influenza Timeline. pbs.org/wgbh/amex/influenza/timeline/index.html.

2508. Colihan K. 2005. Witness to 1918 flu: "Death was there all the time." CNN, November 14. cnn.com/2005/HEALTH/conditions/10/07/1918.flu.witness/index.html.

2509. Torrey EF, Yolken RH. 2005. Beasts of the Earth: Animals, Humans, and Disease (New Brunswick, NJ: Rutgers University Press).

2510. Silverstein AM. 1981. Pure Politics and Impure Science: The Swine Flu Affair (Baltimore, Maryland: Johns Hopkins University Press, pp. 129–31).

2511. Schonberger LB, Bregman DJ, Sullivan-Bolyai JZ, et al. 1979. Guillain-Barré syndrome following vaccination in the national influenza immunization program, United States, 1976–1977. American Journal of Epidemiology 110(2):105–23.

2512. Hilleman M. 1996. Cooperation between government and industry in combating a perceived emerging pandemic: the 1967 swine influenza vaccination program. Journal of the American Medical Association 275:241–3.

2513. Bollet AJ. 2004. Plagues and Poxes: The Impact of Human History on Epidemic Disease (New York, NY: Demos).

2514. Bollet AJ. 2004. Plagues and Poxes: The Impact of Human History on Epidemic Disease (New York, NY: Demos).

2515. Nesmith J. 2005. Experts fret over flu pandemic; U.S. plan for avian threat incomplete. Atlanta Journal-Constitution, May 27, p. 10A. tinyurl.com/joods.

2516. Kennedy M. 2005. Bird flu could kill millions: global pandemic warning from WHO. Gazette (Montreal), March 9, p. A1.

2517. Branswell H. 2006. Health officials worry over flu risk. Canadian Press, March 19. cnews.canoe.ca/CNEWS/Canada/2006/03/19/1495802-cp.html.

2518. Pan American Health Organization. Influenza Pandemic a Brewing Storm, WHO Director-General Says. PAHO news release, September 27. paho.org/English/DD/PIN/pr050927.htm.

2519. Manning A. Big screen horror. USA Today, September 18, p. 6D. usatoday.com/life/2003-09-17-microbes_x.htm.

2520. Peter D. Hart Research Associates. 2006 Apr 26. Gauging the threat: media coverage of pandemic and avian flu. http://healthyamericans.org/reports/flumedia/GaugingReport.pdf

2521. Editorial. 2006 Nov 5. Shrugging at a pandemic. Boston Globe.

2522. Southwell BG, Hwang Y, Torres A. 2006. Avian influenza and US TV news. Emerg Infect Dis. 12(11):1797–1798. http://www.cdc.gov/ncidod/EID/vol12no11/06-0672.htm.

2523. Peter D. Hart Research Associates. 2006 Apr 26. Gauging the threat: media coverage of pandemic and avian flu. http://healthyamericans.org/reports/flumedia/GaugingReport.pdf

2524. 2005. World Reassurance Organization (aka WHO). Effect Measure, September 22. effectmeasure.blogspot.com/2005/09/world-reassurance-organization-aka-who.html.

2525. Nowak G. 2004. Planning for the 2004–05 influenza vaccination season: a communication situation analysis. Centers for Disease Control and Prevention National Immunization Program. urban-renaissance.org/urbanren/images/2004_flu_nowak.pdf.

2526. Sandman PM, Lanard J. 2005. Bird flu: communicating the risks. Perspectives in Health 10(2):2–9.

2527. 2005. Outbreak of bird flu in Asia hits 3 nations. International Herald Tribune, November 4. iht.com/articles/2005/11/04/news/flu.php.

2528. 2005. French ignorant about bird flu but unworried—poll. Reuters, October 15.

2529. 2005. French ignorant about bird flu but unworried—poll. Reuters, October 15.

2530. Sandman PM, Lanard J. 2005. Bird flu: communicating the risks. Perspectives in Health 10(2):2–9.

2531. 2005. Vaccines, drugs offer little help in bird flu fight. Governments should instead focus on controlling pandemic, expert cautions. Reuters, October 10.

2532. 2005. In depth bird flu: the next pandemic? CBC News Online, July 27. cbc.ca/news/background/avianflu/.

2533. Collier R. 1974. The Plague of the Spanish Lady: The Influenza Pandemic of 1918–1919 (New York, NY: Atheneum).

2534. Osterholm M, Branswell H. 2005. Emerging pandemic: costs and consequences of an avian influenza outbreak (webcast). Woodrow Wilson International Center for Scholars, September 19. www.wilsoncenter.org/index.cfm?topic_id=116811&fuseaction=topics.event_summary&event_id=142787.

2535. Editorial. 2005. Avian flu: the U.S. must be more prepared. Philadelphia Inquirer August 14. www.philly.com/mld/inquirer/news/editorial/12376798.htm.

2536. Schwartz R, Bicks M, Chapman S, et al. 2005. Avian flu: is the government ready for an epidemic? ABC News. www.wirednewyork.com/forum/archive/index.php/t-7324.html.

2537. 2005. No local threat from avian flu. KDKA Pittsburg, October 12.

2538. Dillon A. 2005. October 4. Bird flu not expected to affect Arkansas. Daily Citizen thedailycitizen.com/articles/2005/10/05/news/local_news/news02.prt.

2539. Johnson T. Inaction in Indonesia stirs fears it may become pandemic's cradle. Mercury News, October 13.

2540. Kazmin A. 2005. UN targets farming habits to beat bird flu. Financial Times, July 7, p. 11.

2541. Walsh B. 2005. A wing and a prayer. Times Asia, September 19. www.time.com/time/asia/magazine/printout/0,13675,501050926-1106457,00.html.

2542. Branswell. H. 2004. Looming pandemic that could kill tens of millions causing sleepless nights. Canadian Press, November 20. cp.org/awards/view_story.asp?ID=117.

2543. Branswell H. 2006. Health officials worry over flu risk. Canadian Press, March 19. cnews.canoe.ca/CNEWS/Canada/2006/03/19/1495802-cp.html.

2544. Uhlman M. 2005. U.S. unprepared for new flu. Norther Iowan, October 7. fp.uni.edu/northia/archives3.asp?ID=3878.

2545. Lueck S, Mathews AW. 2005. Bush proposes $7.1 billion outlay to fight pandemic-flu threat. Wall Street Journal, November 2, p. A6.

2546. Milbank D. 2005. Capitol Hill flu briefing was no trick, and no treat. Washington Post, October 13, p. A02. www.washingtonpost.com/wp-dyn/content/article/2005/10/12/AR2005101202250.html.

2547. Editorial. 2004. Fowl flu fuels fears. Nature Medicine 10:211–211.

2548. Clayton J. 2003. Looming flu pandemic has experts crying fowl, Nature Medicine 9(4):375. nature.com/nm/journal/v9/n4/full/nm0403-275.html.

2549. Stein R. 2005. Vaccine appears to ward off bird flu. Washington Post, August 7, p. A01. washingtonpost.com/wp-dyn/content/article/2005/08/06/AR2005080600849.html.

2550. 2005. The Karl Rove bird flu strategy. Effect Measure, August 9. effectmeasure.blogspot.com/2005/08/karl-rove-bird-flu-strategy.html.

2551. Altman LK, Bradsher K. 2005. A successful vaccine alone is not enough to prevent avian flu epidemic. New York Times, August 8.

2552. Heinen PP, Rijsewijk FA, de Boer-Luijtze EA, Bianchi AT. 2002. Vaccination of pigs with a DNA construct expressing an influenza virus M2-nucleoprotein fusion protein exacerbates disease after challenge with influenza A virus. Journal of General Virology 83(Pt 8):1851–9.

2553. Branswell H. Bird flu vaccine requires huge doses; stretching strategies critical: experts. Canadian Press, August 9. www.freerepublic.com/focus/f-news/1459633/posts.

2554. Branswell H. Bird flu vaccine requires huge doses; stretching strategies critical: experts. Canadian Press, August 9. www.freerepublic.com/focus/f-news/1459633/posts.

2555. Perry S. 2006. Bird flu: "This thing just continues to march." City Pages, March 22. citypages.com/databank/27/1320/article14219.asp.

2556. Butler D. 2005. Bird flu vaccine not up to scratch: positive results of little practical use, experts warn. Nature News, August 10. bioedonline.org/news/news.cfm?art=1964.

2557. Butler D. 2005. Bird flu vaccine not up to scratch: positive results of little practical use, experts warn. Nature News, August 10. bioedonline.org/news/news.cfm?art=1964.

2558. Butler D. 2005. Bird flu vaccine not up to scratch: positive results of little practical use, experts warn. Nature News, August 10. bioedonline.org/news/news.cfm?art=1964.

2559. Butler D. 2005. Bird flu vaccine not up to scratch: positive results of little practical use, experts warn. Nature News, August 10. bioedonline.org/news/news.cfm?art=1964.

2560. McKie R. 2005. Vaccine failure could lead to flu pandemic. Observer, October 9. observer.guardian.co.uk/uk_news/story/0,6903,1588106,00.html.

2561. Branswell H. Bird flu vaccine requires huge doses; stretching strategies critical: experts. Canadian Press, August 9. www.freerepublic.com/focus/f-news/1459633/posts.

2562. 2005. "No one" ready for bird flu. CBS/AP, October 6. cbsnews.com/stories/2005/10/06/health/main918141.shtml.

2563. 2005. Vaccines, drugs offer little help in bird flu fight. Governments should instead focus on controlling pandemic, expert cautions. Reuters, October 10.

2564. 2005. Race against a lethal virus. Sydney Morning Herald. October 25. smh.com.au/news/world/race-against-a-lethal-virus/2005/10/24/1130006061717.html.

2565. Altman LK, Bradsher K. 2005. Vaccine for bird flu tests well, but making enough may be problem. New York Times, August 8. iht.com/articles/2005/08/07/news/vaccine.php.

2566. 2005. Some quotes about the state of the world's readiness to face a flu pandemic. Canadian Press NewsWire, May 25.

2567. Hawkes N. 2005. Flu pandemic "could kill 360 million worldwide." The Times, May 6.

2568. 2005. Race against a lethal virus. Sydney Morning Herald. October 25. smh.com.au/news/world/race-against-a-lethal-virus/2005/10/24/1130006061717.html.

2569. Barlett DL, Steele JB. About us. barlettandsteele.com/about.html.

2570. Barlett DL, Steele JB. 2004 The health of nations. New York Times, October 24. www.anabaptistethics.org/HAS/News/The%20Health%20of%20Nations.htm.

2571. Revill J. 2005. A tragic, wasted opportunity to avert disaster. Observer, October 16. observer.guardian.co.uk/focus/story/0,6903,1593220,00.html.

2572. Barlett DL, Steele JB. 2004 The health of nations. New York Times, October 24. www.anabaptistethics.org/HAS/News/The%20Health%20of%20Nations.htm.

2573. Berkley S. 2006. We're running out of time. Newsweek International, January 30. msnbc.msn.com/id/10965125/site/newsweek/.

2574. Pollack A. 2005. Talk of bird flu pandemic revives interest in passed-over drugs. New York Times, October 7.

2575. Drexler M. 2005. Bird flu blues. October 18. tompaine.com/print/bird_flu_blues.php.

2576. Japsen B. 2005. Bird-flu vaccine: we may be last in line. Chicago Tribune, October 19 seattletimes.nwsource.com/html./health/2002569783_flufactory19.html.

2577. Japsen B. 2005. Bird-flu vaccine: we may be last in line. Chicago Tribune, October 19 seattletimes.nwsource.com/html./health/2002569783_flufactory19.html.

2578. Osterholm MT. 2005. Preparing for the next pandemic. Foreign Affairs 84(4). www.foreignaffairs.org/20050701faessay84402/michael-t-osterholm/preparing-for-the-next-pandemic.html.

2579. McManus K. 2004. Asian avian influenza—a call to action. Australian Veterinary Journal 82:135.

2580. Weekly Epidemiological Record. 2005. H5N1 avian influenza: first steps towards development of a human vaccine. Weekly Epidemiological Record 80:277–8.

2581. Japsen B. 2005. Bird-flu vaccine: we may be last in line. Chicago Tribune, October 19 seattletimes.nwsource.com/html./health/2002569783_flufac tory19.html.

2582. Gibbs WW, Soares C. 2005. Preparing for a pandemic. Scientific American, October 24. www.sciam.com/print_version.cfm?articleID=000DCB5A -9CC7-134E-9CC783414B7F0000.

2583. Butler D. 2005. Avian flu special. The flu pandemic: were we ready? Nature 425:400. nature.com/nature/journal/v435/n7041/full/435400a.html.

2584. Mackenzie D, Choo K. 2005. Bird flu: kick-start vaccination or face the consequences. New Scientist, October 14. www.newscientist.com/channel/health /mg18825215.900.html.

2585. Bush RM. 2004. Influenza as a model system for studying the cross-species transfer and evolution of the SARS coronavirus. Philosophical Transactions of the Royal Society of London B 359:1067–73.

2586. Goodman J. 2005. Meeting the challenge of pandemic vaccine preparedness: an FDA perspective. In: Institute of Medicine of the National Academies, John R. La Montagne Memorial Symposium on Pandemic Influenza Research: Meeting Proceedings (Washington, DC: National Academies Press, pp. 19–28).

2587. United States Conference of Catholic Bishops Secretariat for Pro-Life Activities. Fact sheet: Embryonic stem cell research and vaccines using fetal tissue . usccb.org/prolife/issues/bioethic/vaccfac2.htm.

2588. Sanghavi D. 2003. Flu: a shot worth taking. Boston Globe, December 9. boston .com/news/globe/health_science/articles/2003/12/09/flu_a_shot_worth _taking?mode=PF.

2589. Gibbs WW, Soares C. 2005. Preparing for a pandemic. Scientific American, October 24.

2590. Centers for Disease Control and Prevention. [date unknown]. How flu vaccines are made. U.S. Department of Health and Human Services; [last reviewed 2019 Dec 12; accessed 2020 Apr 7]. https://www.cdc.gov/flu/prevent/how -fluvaccine-made.htm.

2591. Drexler M. 2005. Bird flu blues. October 18. tompaine.com/print/bird_flu _blues.php.

2592. Board on Health Promotion and Disease Prevention. Institute of Medicine. 2002. The Future of the Public's Health in the 21st Century (Washington, DC: National Academies Press, p. 96).

2593. Branswell H. 2005. Pandemic planning shouldn't overlook need to fix source agricultural. Canadian Press, October 24. www.cp.org/premium/ONLINE /member/National/051024/n1024135A.html.

2594. Lett D. 2005. Feds to stockpile antivirals as pandemic "speed bump." Canadian Medical Association Journal 172(9):1167. www.cmaj.ca/cgi/reprint/172/9/1167.

2595. Uhlman M. 2005. In a flu pandemic, hygiene is a lifesaver. Philadelphia Inquirer, October 11.

2596. Institute of Medicine Board on Health Promotion and Disease Prevention. 2002. The Future of the Public's Health in the 21st Century (Washington, DC: National Academies Press, p. 96).

2597. Legters LJ, Brink LH, Takafuji ET. 1993. Are we prepared for a viral epidemic emergency? In: Morse SS, editor. Emerging Viruses (New York, NY: Oxford University Press, p. 272).

2598. Institute of Medicine. 1988. The Future of Public Health (Washington, DC: National Academies Press, p. 19). fermat.nap.edu/books/0309038308/html ./19.html.

2599. Institute of Medicine Board on Health Promotion and Disease Prevention. 2002. The Future of the Public's Health in the 21st Century (Washington, DC: National Academies Press, p. 100).

2600. Cowen T. 2005. Avian flu: what should be done. Mercatus Center at George Mason University: Working Paper Series. November 11.

2601. VandHei J, Baker P. 2005. Critics say Bush undercut New Orleans flood control. Washington Post, September 2, p. A16. www.washingtonpost.com/wp -dyn/content/article/2005/09/01/AR2005090102261.html.

2602. Oritz P. 2005. Credentials questioned: another Bush crony is point man on avian flu. Diversity Inc. Magazine, November 1.

2603. Brewin B. 2005. Health directors say HHS flu cuts are for the birds. Government Health IT, October 18. www.govhealthit.com/article91152-10-18-05 -Web.

2604. Pelosi N. 2005. Statement on President's avian flu pandemic preparedness strategy. Press Release, November 1. democraticleader.house.gov/press/releases .cfm?pressReleaseID=1255.

2605. 2005. Proposed reductions in preparedness funds would leave USA vulnerable to public health emergencies warn public health officials. Medical News Today, July 16. medicalnewstoday.com/medicalnews.php?newsid=27505.

2606. Sandalow M. 2005. In Hurricane Katrina's wake, some question whether battle against terrorism is the right fight. San Francisco Chronicle, September 11. sfgate.com/cgi-bin/article.cgi?file=/c/a/2005/09/11/MNG40EM00T1 .DTL&type=printable.

2607. 2005. They knew what to expect. Reuters, September 2. wired.com/news/planet /0,2782,68738,00.html.

2608. Shute N, Querna E, Bainbridge B, Brink S, Ramachandran N. 2005. Of birds and men. U.S. News and World Report 138(12):40–9. tinyurl.com/jkacf.

2609. Palma B. 2020 Feb 26. Did Trump administration fire the US pandemic response team? Snopes; [updated 2020 Mar 13; accessed 2020 Apr 7]. https:// www.snopes.com/fact-check/trump-fire-pandemic-team/.

2610. Sun LH. 2018 May 10. Top White House official in charge of pandemic response exits abruptly. Washington Post [accessed 2020 Apr 7]. https://www .washingtonpost.com/news/to-your-health/wp/2018/05/10/top-white-house -official-in-charge-of-pandemic-response-exits-abruptly/.

2611. Transcript of President Bush's October 4, 2005. Press Conference. Courtesy of FDCH/e-Media, October 4.

2612. Harris G. 2005. Fear of flu outbreak rattles Washington. New York Times, October 7. query.nytimes.com/gst/fullpage.html.?sec=health&res=9B05EED A1130F936A35753C1A9639C8B63.

2613. Sternberg S. 2005. Imagine what would happen if a Category 5 viral storm hit every state. USA Today, November 10, p. 1A. www.usatoday.com/printedi tion/news/20051011/1a_cover11.art.htm.

2614. Knobler SL, Mack A, Mahmoud A, Lemon SL (eds.), 2005. The Threat of pandemic influenza: are we ready? Workshop Summary (Washington, DC: National Academies Press). p. 64.

2615. Harris G. 2005. Fear of flu outbreak rattles Washington. New York Times, October 7. query.nytimes.com/gst/fullpage.html.?sec=health&res=9B05EED A1130F936A35753C1A9639C8B63.

2616. Sternberg S. 2005. Officials race to head off a bird flu pandemic. USA Today, October 10. www.usatoday.com/news/health/2005-10-10-avian-flu-cover_x.htm.

2617. Rosenthal E. 2005. Nations redouble their efforts against bird flu. International Herald Tribune, September 17. /iht.com/bin/print_ipub.php?file=/articles /2005/09/16/news/flu.php.

2618. Sandman PM. Katrina: hurricanes, catastrophes, and risk communication. September 8. psandman.com/col/katrina.htm.

2619. 2005. U.S. lawmakers call for creation of "bird flu czar." Democrats say nation unprepared for outbreak of deadly avian influenza. Reuters, October 7.

2620. 2005. Thai newspaper: pandemic phase 4? Effect Measure, September 05. effect measure.blogspot.com/2005/09/thai-newspaper-pandemic-phase-4.html.

2621. Boyd RS. H5N1: a killer strain of flu. Knight Ridder Newspapers, October 16.

2622. Goldstein J. 2005. The next flu pandemic: are we ready? (You don't want to know). Miami Herald.com, September 20. tinyurl.com/efnl3.

2623. Rovera R. 2006. Prepare for pandemic, localities are warned. Washington Post, February 25, p. B04. washingtonpost.com/wp-dyn/content/article /2006/02/24/AR2006022401802.html.

2624. Democracy Now. 2005. Transcript—Mike Davis on The Monster at Our Door: The Global Threat of Avian Flu. Democracy Now. October 19. democ racynow.org/article.pl?sid=05/10/19/1332209.

2625. Wilson A. 2006. Officials discuss reaction to influenza. The Olympian, April 15. 159.54.227.3/apps/pbcs.dll/article?AID=/20060415/NEWS01/60415007.

2626. Heslam J. 2005. Can flu guru do the job? Critics question his credentials. The Boston Herald, October 7.

2627. Sternberg S. 2005. Imagine what would happen if a Category 5 viral storm hit every state. USA Today, November 10, p. 1A.

2628. Cowen T. 2005. Avian flu: what should be done. Mercatus Center at George Mason University: Working Paper Series, November 11.

2629. Osterholm MT. 2005. Preparing for the next pandemic. Foreign Affairs 84(4). www.foreignaffairs.org/20050701faessay84402/michael-t-osterholm/prepar ing-for-the-next-pandemic.html.

2630. Cowen T. 2005. Avian flu: what should be done. Mercatus Center at George Mason University: Working Paper Series, November 11.

2631. Heiberg M. 2005. Asian nations plan for pandemic flu, another treatment is suggested. Center for Infectious Disease Research and Policy News. August 12.

2632. Guarner J. 2020. Three emerging coronaviruses in two decades. Am J Clin Pathol. 153(4):420–421. https://doi.org/10.1093/ajcp/aqaa029.

2633. He J, Tao H, Yan Y, Huang S-Y, Xiao Y. 2020 Feb 21. Molecular mechanism of evolution and human infection with the novel coronavirus (2019-nCoV). bioRxiv .org. [accessed 2020 Mar 30]. https://doi.org/10.1101/2020.02.17.952903.

2634. Wölfel R, Corman VM, Guggemos W, Seilmaier M, Zange S, Müller MA, Niemeyer D, Jones TC, Vollmar P, Rothe C, et al. 2020. Virological assessment of hospitalized patients with COVID-2019. Nature. [Epub ahead of print 2020 Apr 1; accessed 2020 Apr 18]. https://doi.org/10.1038/s41586-020-2196-x.

2635. Liu Z, Magal P, Seydi O, Webb G. 2020. Understanding unreported cases in the COVID-19 epidemic outbreak in Wuhan, China, and the importance of major public health interventions. Biology. 9(3):50. https://doi.org/10.3390 /biology9030050.

2636. Marty AM, Jones MK. 2020. The novel Coronavirus (SARS-CoV-2) is a one health issue. One Health. 9:100123. https://doi.org/10.1016/j.onehlt.2020 .100123.

2637. Park M, Thwaites RS, Openshaw PJM. 2020. COVID-19: lessons from SARS and MERS. Eur J Immunol. 50(3):308–311. https://doi.org/10.1002/eji .202070035.

2638. Adalja AA, Watson M, Toner ES, Cicero A, Inglesby TV. 2019. Characteristics of microbes most likely to cause pandemics and global catastrophes. In: Inglesby TV, Adalja AA, editors. Global Catastrophic Biological Risks. Current Topics in Microbiology and Immunology, vol 424. Switzerland: Springer. p. 1–20. https://doi.org/10.1007/82_2019_176.

2639. Hui DSC, Zumla A. 2019. Severe acute respiratory syndrome: historical, epidemiologic, and clinical features. Infect Dis Clin North Am. 33(4):869–889. https://doi.org/10.1016/j.idc.2019.07.001.

2640. Hui DSC, Zumla A. 2019. Severe acute respiratory syndrome: historical, epidemiologic, and clinical features. Infect Dis Clin North Am. 33(4):869–889. https://doi.org/10.1016/j.idc.2019.07.001.

2641. Wilder-Smith A, Chiew CJ, Lee VJ. 2020 Mar 5. Can we contain the COVID-19 outbreak with the same measures as for SARS? Lancet Infect Dis. [accessed 2020 Mar 30]. https://doi.org/10.1016/s1473-3099(20)30129-8.

2642. Li J-Y, You Z, Wang Q, Zhou Z-J, Qiu Y, Luo R, Ge X-Y. 2020. The epidemic of 2019-novel-coronavirus (2019-nCoV) pneumonia and insights for emerging infectious diseases in the future. Microbes Infect. 22(2):80–85. https://doi.org /10.1016/j.micinf.2020.02.002.

2643. Hui DSC, Zumla A. 2019. Severe acute respiratory syndrome: historical, epidemiologic, and clinical features. Infect Dis Clin N Am. 33(4):869–889. https://doi.org/10.1016/j.idc.2019.07.001.

2644. Wilder-Smith A, Chiew CJ, Lee VJ. 2020 Mar 5. Can we contain the COVID-19 outbreak with the same measures as for SARS? Lancet Infect Dis. [accessed 2020 Mar 30]. https://doi.org/10.1016/s1473-3099(20)30129-8.

2645. Marty AM, Jones MK. 2020. The novel coronavirus (SARS-CoV-2) is a one health issue. One Health. 9:100123. https://doi.org/10.1016/j.onehlt.2020 .100123.

2646. Fraser C, Riley S, Anderson RM, Ferguson NM. 2004. Factors that make an infectious disease outbreak controllable. Proc Natl Acad Sci U S A. 101(16):6146–6151. https://doi.org/10.1073/pnas.0307506101.

2647. Lee N, Hui D, Wu A, Chan P, Cameron P, Joynt GM, Ahuja A, Yung MY, Leung CB, To KF, et al. 2003. A major outbreak of severe acute respiratory syndrome in Hong Kong. N Engl J Med. 348(20):1986–1994. https://doi.org /10.1056/NEJMoa030685.

2648. Assiri A, Al-Tawfiq JA, Al-Rabeeah AA, Al-Rabiah FA, Al-Hajjar S, Al-Barrak A, Flemban H, Al-Nassir WN, Balkhy HH, Al-Hakeem RF, et al. 2013. Epidemiological, demographic, and clinical characteristics of 47 cases of Middle East respiratory syndrome coronavirus disease from Saudi Arabia: a descriptive study. Lancet Infect Dis. 13(9):752–761. https://doi.org/10.1016/S1473 -3099(13)70204-4.

2649. Fang Z, Yi F, Wu K, Lai K, Sun X, Zhong N, Liu Z. 2020 Mar 12. Clinical characteristics of coronavirus pneumonia 2019 (COVID-19): an updated systematic review. medRxiv.org. [accessed 2020 Mar 30]. https://doi.org/10.1101 /2020.03.07.20032573.

2650. Zou L, Ruan F, Huang M, Liang L, Huang H, Hong Z, Yu J, Kang M, Song Y, Xia J, et al. 2020. SARS-CoV-2 viral load in upper respiratory specimens of infected patients. N Engl J Med. 382(12):1177–1179. https://doi.org/10.1056 /NEJMc2001737.

2651. He X, Lau EHY, Wu P, Deng X, Wang J, Hao X, Lau YC, Wong JY, Guan Y, Tan X, et al. 2020 Apr 15. Temporal dynamics in viral shedding and transmissibility of COVID-19. Nat Med. https://doi.org/10.1038/s41591-020-0869-5.

2652. Luo S-H, Liu W, Liu Z-J, Zheng X-Y, Hong C-X, Liu Z-R, Liu J, Weng J-P. 2020 Mar 6. A confirmed asymptomatic carrier of 2019 novel coronavirus (SARS-CoV-2). Chin Med J (Engl). [accessed 2020 Mar 30]. https://doi.org/10 .1097/cm9.0000000000000798.

2653. Cheng H-Y, Jian S-W, Liu D-P, Ng T-C, Huang W-T, Lin H-H. 2020 Mar 19. High transmissibility of COVID-19 near symptom onset. medRxiv.org. [accessed 2020 Mar 30]. https://doi.org/10.1101/2020.03.18.20034561.

2654. The Lancet. 2020. COVID-19: fighting panic with information. Lancet. 395(10224):537. [accessed 2020 Mar 30]. https://doi.org/10.1016/S0140 -6736(20)30379-2.

2655. Malta M, Rimoin AW, Strathdee SA. 2020. The coronavirus 2019-nCoV epidemic: is hindsight 20/20? EClinicalMedicine. 20:100289. https://doi.org/10 .1016/j.eclinm.2020.100289.

2656. Peckham R. 2020. COVID-19 and the anti-lessons of history. Lancet. 395(10227):850–852. [accessed 2020 Mar 30]. https://doi.org/10.1016/s0140 -6736(20)30468-2.

2657. Yang Y, Peng F, Wang R, Guan K, Jiang T, Xu G, Sun J, Chang C. 2020 Mar 3. The deadly coronaviruses: the 2003 SARS pandemic and the 2020 novel coronavirus epidemic in China. J Autoimmun. [accessed 2020 Mar 30]. https://doi.org/10.1016/j.jaut.2020.102434.

2658. Carbone M, Green JB, Bucci EM, Lednicky JA. 2020. Coronaviruses: facts, myths, and hypotheses. J Thorac Oncol. Article in press. [accessed 2020 Mar 30]. https://doi.org/10.1016/j.jtho.2020.02.024.

2659. Garrett L. 2020. COVID-19: the medium is the message. Lancet. 395(10228):942–943. [accessed 2020 Mar 30]. https://doi.org/10.1016/S0140 -6736(20)30600-0.

2660. Jones DS. 2020 Mar 12. History in a crisis—lessons for Covid-19. N Engl J Med. [accessed 2020 Mar 30]. https://doi.org/10.1056/NEJMp2004361.

2661. The Lancet. 2020. COVID-19: fighting panic with information. Lancet. 395(10224):537. [accessed 2020 Mar 30]. https://doi.org/10.1016/S0140 -6736(20)30379-2.

2662. Lee VJ, Chiew CJ, Khong WX. 2020 Mar 13. Interrupting transmission of COVID-19: lessons from containment efforts in Singapore. J Travel Med. [accessed 2020 Mar 30]. https://doi.org/10.1093/jtm/taaa039.

2663. The Lancet. 2020. COVID-19: fighting panic with information. Lancet. 395(10224):537. [accessed 2020 Mar 30]. https://doi.org/10.1016/S0140 -6736(20)30379-2.

2664. Lau H, Khosrawipour V, Kocbach P, Mikołajczyk A, Schubert J, Bania J, Khosrawipour T. 2020 Mar 27. The positive impact of lockdown in Wuhan on containing the COVID-19 outbreak in China. J Travel Med. [accessed 2020 Mar 30]. https://doi.org/10.1093/jtm/taaa037.

2665. Eve F. 2020 Feb 2. China's reaction to the coronavirus outbreak violates human rights. Guardian. [accessed 2020 Apr 18]; https://www.theguardian.com /world/2020/feb/02/chinas-reaction-to-the-coronavirus-outbreak-violates -human-rights.

2666. Chen X, Yu B. 2020 Mar 2. First two months of the 2019 Coronavirus Disease (COVID-19) epidemic in China: real-time surveillance and evaluation with a second derivative model. Glob Health Res Policy. 5:7. [accessed 2020 Mar 30]. https://doi.org/10.1186/s41256-020-00137-4.

2667. Kupferschmidt K, Cohen J. 2020 Mar 6. Can China's COVID-19 strategy work elsewhere? Science. 367(6482):1061–1062. https://doi.org/10.1126/science .367.6482.1061.

2668. Health Commission of Hubei Province. 2020 Mar 19. Epidemic situation of new crown pneumonia in Hubei province on March 18, 2020. [accessed 2020 Mar 31]. http://wjw.hubei.gov.cn/fbjd/dtyw/202003/t20200319_2185058 .shtml.

2669. Jasarevic T, Ryan M, van Kerkhove M, Ghebreyesus TA. 2020 Jan 29. Novel coronavirus press conference at United Nations of Geneva. World Health Organization. [accessed 2020 Mar 31]. https://www.who.int/docs/default-source /coronaviruse/transcripts/who-audio-script-ncov-rresser-unog-29jan2020.pdf.

2670. Tedros AG. 2020 Jan 30. WHO Director-General's statement on IHR Emergency Committee on Novel Coronavirus (2019-nCoV). World Health Organization. [accessed 2020 Mar 31]. https://www.who.int/dg/speeches/detail/who

-director-general-s-statement-on-ihr-emergency-committee-on-novel-corona
virus-(2019-ncov).

2671. World Health Organization. 2019 Mar 19. Coronavirus disease 2019 (COVID-19) situation report—59. Geneva: WHO; [accessed 2020 Apr 1]. https://www.who.int/docs/default-source/coronaviruse/situation-reports/20200319-sitrep-59-covid-19.pdf?sfvrsn=c3dcdef9_2.

2672. Cohen J, Kupferschmidt K. 2020 Feb 28. Strategies shift as coronavirus pandemic looms. Science. 367(6481):962–963. https://doi.org/10.1126/science.367.6481.962.

2673. Kupferschmidt K, Cohen J. 2020 Mar 6. Can China's COVID-19 strategy work elsewhere? Science. 367(6482):1061–1062. https://doi.org/10.1126/science.367.6482.1061.

2674. Cohen J, Kupferschmidt K. 2020 Mar 20. Countries test tactics in 'war' against COVID-19. Science. 367(6484):1287–1288. https://doi.org/10.1126/science.367.6484.1287.

2675. Normile D. 2020 Mar 17. Coronavirus cases have dropped sharply in South Korea. What's the secret to its success? Science. [accessed 2020 Mar 31]. https://doi.org/10.1126/science.abb7566.

2676. Tanne JH, Hayasaki E, Zastrow M, Pulla P, Smith P, Rada AG. 2020 Mar 18. Covid-19: how doctors and healthcare systems are tackling coronavirus worldwide. BMJ. 368:m1090. https://doi.org/10.1136/bmj.m1090.

2677. Tanne JH, Hayasaki E, Zastrow M, Pulla P, Smith P, Rada AG. 2020 Mar 18. Covid-19: how doctors and healthcare systems are tackling coronavirus worldwide. BMJ. 368:m1090. https://doi.org/10.1136/bmj.m1090.

2678. Tedros AG. 2020 Mar 16. WHO Director-General's opening remarks at the media briefing on COVID-19—16 March 2020. World Health Organization. [accessed 2020 Mar 31]. https://www.who.int/dg/speeches/detail/who-director-general-s-opening-remarks-at-the-media-briefing-on-covid-19—16-march-2020.

2679. Normile D. 2020 Mar 17. Coronavirus cases have dropped sharply in South Korea. What's the secret to its success? Science. [accessed 2020 Mar 31]. https://doi.org/10.1126/science.abb7566.

2680. Khazan O. 2020 Mar 13. The 4 key reasons the U.S. is so behind on coronavirus testing. The Atlantic. [accessed 2020 Mar 31]; https://www.theatlantic.com/health/archive/2020/03/why-coronavirus-testing-us-so-delayed/607954/.

2681. Meyer R, Madrigal AC. 2020 Mar 6. Exclusive: the strongest evidence yet that America is botching coronavirus testing. The Atlantic. [accessed 2020 Mar 31]; https://www.theatlantic.com/health/archive/2020/03/how-many-americans-have-been-tested-coronavirus/607597/.

2682. Branswell H. 2020 Mar 20. Understanding what works: how some countries are beating back the coronavirus. STAT. [accessed 2020 Mar 31]. https://www.statnews.com/2020/03/20/understanding-what-works-how-some-countries-are-beating-back-the-coronavirus/.

2683. Holshue ML, DeBolt C, Lindquist S, Lofy KH, Wiesman J, Bruce H, Spitters C, Ericson K, Wilkerson S, Tural A, et al. 2020. First case of 2019 novel

coronavirus in the United States. N Engl J Med. 382(10):929–936. https://doi
.org/10.1056/NEJMoa2001191.

2684. World Health Organization. 2020 Jan 21. Novel coronavirus (2019-nCoV)
situation report—1. Geneva: WHO; [accessed 2020 Apr 6]. https://www.who
.int/docs/default-source/coronaviruse/situation-reports/20200121-sitrep-1
-2019-ncov.pdf.

2685. New York Times. 2020 Mar 21. Pences test negative; states warn that supplies
are dwindling. NYT. [updated 2020 Mar 27; accessed 2020 Mar 31]; https://
www.nytimes.com/2020/03/21/world/coronavirus-updates-usa-world.html.

2686. Tanne JH, Hayasaki E, Zastrow M, Pulla P, Smith P, Rada AG. 2020 Mar 18.
Covid-19: how doctors and healthcare systems are tackling coronavirus worldwide. BMJ. 368:m1090. https://doi.org/10.1136/bmj.m1090.

2687. Anderson RM, Heesterbeek H, Klinkenberg D, Hollingsworth TD. 2020.
How will country-based mitigation measures influence the course of the
COVID-19 epidemic? Lancet. 395(10228):931–934. https://doi.org/10.1016
/S0140-6736(20)30567-5.

2688. Wilder-Smith A, Chiew CJ, Lee VJ. 2020 Mar 5. Can we contain the COVID-
19 outbreak with the same measures as for SARS? Lancet Infect Dis. [accessed
2020 Mar 30]. https://doi.org/10.1016/s1473-3099(20)30129-8.

2689. Anderson RM, Heesterbeek H, Klinkenberg D, Hollingsworth TD. 2020.
How will country-based mitigation measures influence the course of the
COVID-19 epidemic? Lancet. 395(10228):931–934. https://doi.org/10.1016
/S0140-6736(20)30567-5.

2690. Bayham J, Fenichel EP. 2020 Mar 17. The impact of school closure for COVID-
19 on the US healthcare workforce and the net mortality effects. medRxiv.org.
[accessed 2020 Mar 31]. https://doi.org/10.1101/2020.03.09.20033415.

2691. Kawano S, Kakehashi M. 2015. Substantial impact of school closure on the
transmission dynamics during the pandemic flu H1N1–2009 in Oita, Japan.
PLoS ONE. 10(12):e0144839. [accessed 2020 Mar 31]. https://doi.org/10
.1371/journal.pone.0144839.

2692. Petrie JG, Ohmit SE, Cowling BJ, Johnson E, Cross RT, Malosh RE, Thompson MG, Monto AS. 2013. Influenza transmission in a cohort of households
with children: 2010–2011. PLoS ONE. 8(9):e75339. https://doi.org/10.1371
/journal.pone.0075339.

2693. Zhu Y, Bloxham CJ, Hulme KD, Sinclair JE, Tong ZWM, Steele LE, Noye
EC, Lu J, Chew KY, Pickering J, et al. 2020 Mar 30. Children are unlikely to
have been the primary source of household SARS-CoV-2 infections. medRxiv
.org. [accessed 2020 Apr 6]. https://doi.org/10.1101/2020.03.26.20044826.

2694. Pang J, Wang MX, Ang IYH, Tan SHX, Lewis RF, Chen JI-P, Gutierrez RA,
Gwee SXW, Chua PEY, Yang Q, et al. 2020. Potential rapid diagnostics, vaccine and therapeutics for 2019 novel coronavirus (2019-nCoV): a systematic
review. J Clin Med. 9(3):623. http://doi.org/10.3390/jcm9030623.

2695. Kupferschmidt K, Cohen J. 2020. Can China's COVID-19 strategy work elsewhere? Science. 367(6482):1061–1062. https://doi.org/10.1126/science.367
.6482.1061.

2696. Hollingsworth TD, Klinkenberg D, Heesterbeek H, Anderson RM. 2011. Mitigation strategies for pandemic influenza A: balancing conflicting policy objectives. PLoS Comput Biol. 7(2):e1001076. http://doi.org/10.1371/journal.pcbi.1001076.

2697. Ferguson N, Laydon D, Nedjati Gilani G, Imai N, Ainslie K, Baguelin M, Bhatia S, Boonyasiri A, Cucunuba Perez Z, Cuomo-Dannenburg G, et al. 2020 Mar 16. Impact of non-pharmaceutical interventions (NPIs) to reduce COVID-19 mortality and healthcare demand. London: Imperial College COVID-19 Response Team. Report No.: 9. http://doi.org/10.25561/77482.

2698. Grasselli G, Pesenti A, Cecconi M. 2020 Mar 13. Critical care utilization for the COVID-19 outbreak in Lombardy, Italy: early experience and forecast during an emergency response. JAMA. [accessed 2020 Mar 31]. https://doi.org/10.1001/jama.2020.4031.

2699. Daugherty Biddison EL, Faden R, Gwon HS, Mareiniss DP, Regenberg AC, Schoch-Spana M, Schwartz J, Toner ES. 2019. Too many patients . . . a framework to guide statewide allocation of scarce mechanical ventilation during disasters. CHEST. 155(4)848–854. https://doi.org/10.1016/j.chest.2018.09.025.

2700. Emanuel EJ, Persad G, Upshur R, Thome B, Parker M, Glickman A, Zhang C, Boyle C, Smith M, Phillips JP. 2020 Mar 23. Fair allocation of scarce medical resources in the time of Covid-19. N Engl J Med. [accessed 2020 Apr 2]. https://doi.org/10.1056/NEJMsb2005114.

2701. Cowling BJ, Lim WW. 2020 Mar 13. They've contained the coronavirus. Here's how. New York Times. [accessed 2020 Mar 31]; https://www.nytimes.com/2020/03/13/opinion/coronavirus-best-response.html.

2702. Yang CH, Jung H. 2020. Topological dynamics of the 2015 South Korea MERS-CoV spread-on-contact networks. Sci Rep. 10:4327. https://doi.org/10.1038/s41598-020-61133-9.

2703. Wilder-Smith A, Chiew CJ, Lee VJ. 2020 Mar 5. Can we contain the COVID-19 outbreak with the same measures as for SARS? Lancet Infect Dis. [accessed 2020 Mar 30]. https://doi.org/10.1016/s1473-3099(20)30129-8.

2704. Lauer SA, Grantz KH, Bi Q, Jones FK, Zheng Q, Meredith HR, Azman AS, Reich NG, Lessler J. 2020. The incubation period of coronavirus disease 2019 (COVID-19) from publicly reported confirmed cases: estimation and application. Ann Intern Med. [Epub ahead of print 2020 Mar 10; accessed 2020 Mar 31]. https://doi.org/10.7326/M20-0504.

2705. Centers for Disease Control and Prevention. 2020. Coronavirus disease 2019 (COVID-19): travel-associated exposures. U.S. Department of Health and Human Services; [last reviewed 2020 Mar 30; accessed 2020 Mar 31]. https://www.cdc.gov/coronavirus/2019-ncov/php/risk-assessment.html.

2706. Tan L, Kang X, Zhang B, Zheng S, Liu B, Yu T, Yang F, Wang Q, Miao H. 2020 Mar 27. A special case of COVID-19 with long duration of viral shedding for 49 days. medRxiv.org. [accessed 2020 Mar 31]. https://doi.org/10.1101/2020.03.22.20040071.

2707. Zhou F, Yu T, Du R, Fan G, Liu Y, Liu Z, Xiang J, Wang Y, Song B, Gu X, et al. 2020. Clinical course and risk factors for mortality of adult inpatients with COVID-19 in Wuhan, China: a retrospective cohort study. Lancet.

395(10229):1054–1062. [corrected 2020 Mar 12; accessed 2020 Mar 31]. https://doi.org/10.1016/S0140-6736(20)30566-3.

2708. Sun P, Qie S, Liu Z, Ren J, Li K, Xi J. 2020 Feb 28. Clinical characteristics of hospitalized patients with SARS-CoV-2 infection: a single arm meta-analysis. J Med Virol. [corrected 2020 Mar 17; accessed 2020 Mar 31]. https://doi.org/10.1002/jmv.25735.

2709. Fang Z, Yi F, Wu K, Lai K, Sun X, Zhong N, Liu Z. 2020 Mar 12. Clinical characteristics of coronavirus pneumonia 2019 (COVID-19): an updated systematic review. medRxiv.org. [accessed 2020 Mar 30]. https://doi.org/10.1101/2020.03.07.20032573.

2710. Zou X, Chen K, Zou J, Han P, Hao J, Han Z. 2020 Mar 12. Single-cell RNA-seq data analysis on the receptor ACE2 expression reveals the potential risk of different human organs vulnerable to 2019-nCoV infection. Front Med. [accessed 2020 Mar 31]. https://doi.org/10.1007/s11684-020-0754-0.

2711. Sun K, Gu L, Ma L, Duan Y. 2020 Mar 31. Atlas of ACE2 gene expression in mammals reveals novel insights in transmission of SARS-Cov-2. bioRxiv.org. [accessed 2020 Apr 6]. https://doi.org/10.1101/2020.03.30.015644.

2712. Jain V, Yuan J-M. 2020 Mar 16. Systematic review and meta-analysis of predictive symptoms and comorbidities for severe COVID-19 infection. medRxiv.org. [accessed 2020 Mar 31]. https://doi.org/10.1101/2020.03.15.20035360.

2713. Zhang Y. 2020 Feb 17. The epidemiological characteristics of an outbreak of 2019 novel coronavirus diseases (COVID-19)—China, 2020. Chinese Center for Disease Control and Prevention. CCDC Weekly. [accessed 2020 Mar 31]. http://weekly.chinacdc.cn/en/article/id/e53946e2-c6c4-41e9-9a9b-fea8db1a8f51.

2714. Yang J, Zheng Y, Gou X, Pu K, Chen Z, Guo Q, Ji R, Wang H, Wang Y, Zhou Y. 2020. Prevalence of comorbidities in the novel Wuhan coronavirus (COVID-19) infection: a systematic review and meta-analysis. Int J Infect Dis. [Epub ahead of print 2020 Mar 12; accessed 2020 Mar 31]. https://doi.org/10.1016/j.ijid.2020.03.017.

2715. Jain V, Yuan J-M. 2020 Mar 16. Systematic review and meta-analysis of predictive symptoms and comorbidities for severe COVID-19 infection. medRxiv.org. [accessed 2020 Mar 31]. https://doi.org/10.1101/2020.03.15.20035360.

2716. Jain V, Yuan J-M. 2020 Mar 16. Systematic review and meta-analysis of predictive symptoms and comorbidities for severe COVID-19 infection. medRxiv.org. [accessed 2020 Mar 31]. https://doi.org/10.1101/2020.03.15.20035360.

2717. Ogen Y. 2020. Assessing nitrogen dioxide (NO2) levels as a contributing factor to coronavirus (COVID-19) fatality. Sci Total Environ. 726:138605. https://doi.org/10.1016/j.scitotenv.2020.138605.

2718. Chen K, Wang M, Huang C, Kinney PL, Anastas PT. 2020 Mar 27. Air pollution reduction and mortality benefit during the COVID-19 outbreak in China. medRxiv.org. [accessed 2020 Mar 31]. https://doi.org/10.1101/2020.03.23.20039842.

2719. He G, Pan Y, Tanaka T. 2020 Apr 1. COVID-19, city lockdown, and air pollution: evidence from China. medRxiv.org. [accessed 2020 Apr 6]. https://doi.org/10.1101/2020.03.29.20046649.

2720. Booth CM, Matukas LM, Tomlinson GA, Rachlis AR, Rose DB, Dwosh HA, Walmsley SL, Mazzulli T, Avendano M, Derkach P, et al. 2003. Clinical features and short-term outcomes of 144 patients with SARS in the greater Toronto area. JAMA. 289(21):2801–2809. https://doi.org/10.1001/jama.289.21.JOC30885.

2721. Garbati MA, Fagbo SF, Fang VJ, Skakni L, Joseph M, Wani TA, Cowling BJ, Peiris M, Hakawi A. 2016. A comparative study of clinical presentation and risk factors for adverse outcome in patients hospitalised with acute respiratory disease due to MERS coronavirus or other causes. PLoS ONE. 11(11):e0165978. https://doi.org/10.1371/journal.pone.0165978.

2722. Li B, Yang J, Zhao F, Zhi L, Wang X, Liu L, Bi Z, Zhao Y. 2020 Mar 11. Prevalence and impact of cardiovascular metabolic diseases on COVID-19 in China. Clin Res Cardiol. [accessed 2020 Mar 31]. https://doi.org/10.1007/s00392-020-01626-9.

2723. Yang JK, Feng Y, Yuan MY, Yuan SY, Fu HJ, Wu BY, Sun GZ, Yang GR, Zhang XL, Wang L, et al. 2006. Plasma glucose levels and diabetes are independent predictors for mortality and morbidity in patients with SARS. Diabet Med. 23(6):623–628. https://doi.org/10.1111/j.1464-5491.2006.01861.x.

2724. Huang R, Zhu L, Xue L, Liu L, Yan X, Wang J, Zhang B, Xu T, Ji F, Zhao Y, et al. 2020 Feb 28. Clinical findings of patients with coronavirus disease 2019 in Jiangsu province, China: a retrospective, multi-center study. SSRN: Preprints with The Lancet; [accessed 2020 Apr 6]. https://dx.doi.org/10.2139/ssrn.3548785.

2725. Simonnet A, Chetboun M, Poissy J, Raverdy V, Noulette J, Duhamel A, Labreuche J, Mathieu D, Pattou F, Jourdain M, et al. 2020. High prevalence of obesity in severe acute respiratory syndrome coronavirus-2 (SARS-CoV-2) requiring invasive mechanical ventilation. Obesity. Accepted articles. [accessed 2020 Apr 11]. https://doi.org/10.1002/oby.22831.

2726. Huang R, Zhu L, Xue L, Liu L, Yan X, Wang J, Zhang B, Xu T, Ji F, Zhao Y, et al. 2020 Feb 28. Clinical findings of patients with coronavirus disease 2019 in Jiangsu province, China: a retrospective, multi-center study. SSRN: Preprints with The Lancet; [accessed 2020 Apr 6]. https://dx.doi.org/10.2139/ssrn.3548785.

2727. Fryar CD, Kruszon-Moran D, Gu Q, Ogden CL. 2018 Dec 20. Mean body weight, height, waist circumference, and body mass index among adults: United States, 1999–2000 through 2015–2016. Natl Health Stat Report. 122:1–16.

2728. Muscogiuri G, Pugliese G, Barrea L, Savastano S, Colao A. 2020. Obesity: the "Achilles heel" for COVID-19? Metabolism. [Epub ahead of print 2020 Apr 27; accessed 2020 May 11]. https://dx.doi.org/10.1016/j.metabol.2020.154251.

2729. Zhao L. 2020. Obesity accompanying COVID-19: the role of epicardial fat. Obesity. Article in press. [accessed 2020 May 11]. https://doi.org/10.1002/oby.22867.

2730. Huang JF, Wang XB, Zheng KI, Liu WY, Chen JJ, George J, Zheng MH. 2020. Obesity hypoventilation syndrome and severe COVID-19. Metabolism. 108:154249. https://dx.doi.org/10.1016/j.metabol.2020.154249.

2731. Adams ML, Katz DL, Grandpre J. 2020 Apr 2. Population based estimates of comorbidities affecting risk for complications from COVID-19 in the US. medRxiv.org. [accessed 2020 Apr 6]. https://doi.org/10.1101/2020.03.30 .20043919.

2732. Liu W, Tao ZW, Lei W, Ming-Li Y, Kui L, Ling Z, Shuang W, Yan D, Jing L, Liu HG, et al. 2020. Analysis of factors associated with disease outcomes in hospitalized patients with 2019 novel coronavirus disease. Chin Med J (Engl). [Epub ahead of print 2020 Feb 28; accessed 2020 Mar 31]. https://doi.org/10 .1097/CM9.0000000000000775.

2733. Alqahtani JS, Oyelade T, Aldhahir AM, Alghamdi SM, Almehmadi M, Alqahtani AS, Quaderi S, Mandal S, Hurst J. 2020 Mar 27. Prevalence, severity and mortality associated with COPD and smoking in patients with COVID-19: a rapid systematic review and meta-analysis. medRxiv.org. [accessed 2020 Apr 6]. https://doi.org/10.1101/2020.03.25.20043745.

2734. Lippi G, Henry BM. 2020. Active smoking is not associated with severity of coronavirus disease 2019 (COVID-19). Eur J Intern Med. Article in press. [accessed 2020 Mar 31]. https://doi.org/10.1016/j.ejim.2020.03.014.

2735. Corrales-Medina VF, Musher DM, Wells GA, Chirinos JA, Chen L, Fine MJ. 2012. Cardiac complications in patients with community-acquired pneumonia: incidence, timing, risk factors, and association with short-term mortality. Circulation. 125(6):773–781. https://doi.org/10.1161/CIRCULATIONAHA .111.040766.

2736. Marrie TJ, Shariatzadeh MR. 2007. Community-acquired pneumonia requiring admission to an intensive care unit: a descriptive study. Medicine (Baltimore). 86(2):103–111. https://doi.org/10.1097/MD .0b013e3180421c16.

2737. Corrales-Medina VF, Alvarez KN, Weissfeld LA, Angus DC, Chirinos JA, Chang CC, Newman A, Loehr L, Folsom AR, Elkind MS, et al. 2015. Association between hospitalization for pneumonia and subsequent risk of cardiovascular disease. JAMA. 313(3):264–274. https://doi.org/10.1001/jama.2014 .18229.

2738. Cilli A, Erdem H, Karakurt Z, Turkan H, Yazicioglu-Mocin O, Adiguzel N, Gungor G, Bilge U, Tasci C, Yilmaz G, et al. 2013. Community-acquired pneumonia in patients with chronic obstructive pulmonary disease requiring admission to the intensive care unit: risk factors for mortality. J Crit Care. 28(6):975–979. https://doi.org/10.1016/j.jcrc.2013.08.004.

2739. Aitken M, Kleinrock M. 2018 Apr 19. Medicine use and spending in the U.S.: a review of 2017 and outlook to 2022. Parsippany (NJ): IQVIA Institute for Human Data Science; [accessed 2020 Mar 31]. https://www.iqvia.com/insights /the-iqvia-institute/reports/medicine-use-and-spending-in-the-us-review-of -2017-outlook-to-2022.

2740. Caldeira D, Alarcão J, Vaz-Carneiro A, Costa J. 2012. Risk of pneumonia associated with use of angiotensin converting enzyme inhibitors and angiotensin receptor blockers: systematic review and meta-analysis. BMJ. 345:e4260. https://doi.org/10.1136/bmj.e4260.

2741. Cure E, Cumhur Cure M. 2020. Angiotensin-converting enzyme inhibitors and angiotensin receptor blockers may be harmful in patients with diabetes during COVID-19 pandemic. Diabetes Metab Syndr. 14(4):349–350. https://doi.org/10.1016/j.dsx.2020.04.019.

2742. Pinto BGG, Oliveira AER, Singh Y, Jimenez L, Goncalves ANA, Ogava RLT, Creighton R, Peron JPS, Nakaya HI. 2020 Mar 27. ACE2 expression is increased in the lungs of patients with comorbidities associated with severe COVID-19. medRxiv.org. [accessed 2020 Mar 31]. https://doi.org/10.1101/2020.03.21.20040261.

2743. Kuster GM, Pfister O, Burkard T, Zhou Q, Twerenbold R, Haaf P, Widmer AF, Osswald S. 2020 Mar 20. SARS-CoV2: should inhibitors of the renin–angiotensin system be withdrawn in patients with COVID-19? Eur Heart J. [accessed 2020 Mar 31]. https://doi.org/10.1093/eurheartj/ehaa235.

2744. Aronson JK, Ferner RE. 2020 Apr 2. Drugs and the renin-angiotensin system in covid-19. BMJ. 369:m1313. [accessed 2020 Apr 6]. https://doi.org/10.1136/bmj.m1313.

2745. Ibuprofen pack with pull-quote [infographic]. 2020 Mar 17. NutritionFacts.org. [accessed 2020 Mar 31]. https://www.facebook.com/NutritionFacts.org/photos/a.505323302817517/3398378763511942/.

2746. Fang L, Karakiulakis G, Roth M. 2020 Mar 11. Are patients with hypertension and diabetes mellitus at increased risk for COVID-19 infection? Lancet. [accessed 2020 Mar 31]. https://doi.org/10.1016/S2213-2600(20)30116-8.

2747. Bhatt AP, Gunasekara DB, Speer J, Reed MI, Peña AN, Midkiff BR, Magness ST, Bultman SJ, Allbritton NL, Redinbo MR. 2018. Nonsteroidal anti-inflammatory drug-induced leaky gut modeled using polarized monolayers of primary human intestinal epithelial cells. ACS Infect Dis. 4(1):46–52. https://doi.org/10.1021/acsinfecdis.7b00139.

2748. Voiriot G, Philippot Q, Elabbadi A, Elbim C, Chalumeau M, Fartoukh M. 2019. Risks related to the use of non-steroidal anti-inflammatory drugs in community-acquired pneumonia in adult and pediatric patients. J Clin Med. 8(6):786. https://doi.org/10.3390/jcm8060786.

2749. Park S, Brassey J, Heneghan C, Mahtani K. 2020 Mar 19. Managing fever in adults with possible or confirmed COVID-19 in primary care. Oxford: Centre for Evidence-Based Medicine; [accessed 2020 Mar 31]. https://www.cebm.net/covid-19/managing-fever-in-adults-with-possible-or-confirmed-covid-19-in-primary-care/.

2750. Little P. 2020 Mar 27. Non-steroidal anti-inflammatory drugs and covid-19. BMJ. 368:m1185. [accessed 2020 Apr 6]. https://doi.org/10.1136/bmj.m1185.

2751. Oakes JM, Fuchs RM, Gardner JD, Lazartigues E, Yue X. 2018. Nicotine and the renin-angiotensin system. Am J Physiol Regul Integr Comp Physiol. 315(5):R895–R906. https://doi.org/10.1152/ajpregu.00099.2018.

2752. Lippi G, Henry BM. 2020. Active smoking is not associated with severity of coronavirus disease 2019 (COVID-19). Eur J Intern Med. Article in press. [accessed 2020 Mar 31]. https://doi.org/10.1016/j.ejim.2020.03.014.

2753. Liu W, Tao ZW, Wang L, Yuan M-L, Liu K, Zhou L, Wei S, Deng Y, Liu J,

Liu HG, et al. 2020. Analysis of factors associated with disease outcomes in hospitalized patients with 2019 novel coronavirus disease. Chin Med J (Engl). [Epub ahead of print 2020 Feb 28; accessed 2020 Mar 31]. https://doi.org/10.1097/CM9.0000000000000775.

2754. Fang Z, Yi F, Wu K, Lai K, Sun X, Zhong N, Liu Z. 2020 Mar 10. Clinical characteristics of coronavirus pneumonia 2019 (COVID-19): an updated systematic review. medRxiv.org. [accessed 2020 Mar 30]. https://doi.org/10.1101/2020.03.07.20032573.

2755. Jain V, Yuan J-M. 2020 Mar 16. Systematic review and meta-analysis of predictive symptoms and comorbidities for severe COVID-19 infection. medRxiv.org. [accessed 2020 Mar 31]. https://doi.org/10.1101/2020.03.15.20035360.

2756. Chow N, Fleming-Dutra K, Gierke R, Hall A, Hughes M, Pilishvili T, Ritchey M, Roguski K, Skoff T, Ussery E. 2020. Preliminary estimates of the prevalence of selected underlying health conditions among patients with coronavirus disease 2019—United States, February 12–March 28, 2020. Morb Mortal Wkly Rep. 69(13):382–386. http://dx.doi.org/10.15585/mmwr.mm6913e2.

2757. Ioannidis JPA, Axfors C, Contopoulos-Ioannidis DG. 2020 Apr 8. Population-level COVID-19 mortality risk for non-elderly individuals overall and for non-elderly individuals without underlying diseases in pandemic epicenters. medRxiv.org. [accessed 2020 Apr 11]. https://doi.org/10.1101/2020.04.05.20054361.

2758. Korea Centers for Disease Control and Prevention. 2020 Apr 10. 27 additional cases have been confirmed. Case distribution by gender and age group. Korea: KCDC; [accessed 2020 Apr 10]. https://www.cdc.go.kr/board/board.es?mid=a30402000000&bid=0030&act=view&list_no=366801&tag=&nPage=1.

2759. Bialek S, Boundy E, Bowen V, Chow N, Cohn A, Dowling N, Ellington S, Gierke R, Hall A, MacNeil J, et al. 2020. Severe outcomes among patients with coronavirus disease 2019 (COVID-19)—United States, February 12–March 16, 2020. Morb Mortal Wkly Rep. 69(12):343–346. [corrected 2020 Mar 18; accessed 2020 Apr 6]. http://dx.doi.org/10.15585/mmwr.mm6912e2.

2760. McMichael TM, Currie DW, Clark S, Pogosjans S, Kay M, Schwartz NG, Lewis J, Baer A, Kawakami V, Lukoff MD, et al. 2020. Epidemiology of Covid-19 in a long-term care facility in King County, Washington. N Engl J Med. [Epub ahead of print 2020 Mar 27; accessed 2020 Apr 6]. https://doi.org/10.1056/NEJMoa2005412.

2761. Carbone M, Green JB, Bucci EM, Lednicky JJ. 2020. Editorial: coronaviruses: facts, myths and hypotheses. J Thorac Oncol. Article in press. [accessed 2020 Mar 30]. https://doi.org/10.1016/j.jtho.2020.02.024.

2762. Sun P, Qie S, Liu Z, Ren J, Li K, Xi J. 2020 Feb 28. Clinical characteristics of hospitalized patients with SARS-CoV-2 infection: a single arm meta-analysis. J Med Virol. [accessed 2020 Mar 31]. https://doi.org/10.1002/jmv.25735.

2763. Hui DS, Joynt GM, Wong KT, Gomersall CD, Li TS, Antonio G, Ko FW, Chan MC, Chan DP, Tong MW, et al. 2005. Impact of severe acute respiratory syndrome (SARS) on pulmonary function, functional capacity and quality of life in a cohort of survivors. Thorax. 60(5):401–409. https://doi.org/10.1136/thx.2004.030205.

2764. Shi Y, Wang Y, Shao C, Huang J, Gan J, Huang X, Bucci E, Piacentini M, Ippolito G, Melino G. 2020 Mar 23. COVID-19 infection: the perspectives on immune responses. Cell Death Differ. [accessed 2020 Mar 31]. https://doi.org/10.1038/s41418-020-0530-3.

2765. Leng Z, Yin D, Zhao Z, Yan M, Yang Y, He X, Zhao RC, Liu H. 2020. A survey of 434 clinical trials about coronavirus disease 2019 in China. J Med Virol. [Epub ahead of print 2020 Mar 27; accessed 2020 Apr 6]. https://doi.org/10.1002/jmv.25779.

2766. Anderson RM, Heesterbeek H, Klinkenberg D, Hollingsworth TD. 2020. How will country-based mitigation measures influence the course of the COVID-19 epidemic? Lancet. 395(10228):931–934. https://doi.org/10.1016/S0140-6736(20)30567-5.

2767. Greger M. 2015. How not to die. New York: Flatiron Books.

2768. Greger M. 2020. Immune function. NutritionFacts.org; [updated 2020 Mar 4; accessed 2020 Mar 31]. https://nutritionfacts.org/topics/immune-function/.

2769. Noah TL, Zhang H, Zhou H, Glista-Baker E, Müller L, Bauer RN, Meyer M, Murphy PC, Jones S, Letang B, et al. 2014. Effect of broccoli sprouts on nasal response to live attenuated influenza virus in smokers: a randomized, double-blind study. PLoS ONE. 9(6):e98671. https://doi.org/10.1371/journal.pone.0098671.

2770. Müller L, Meyer M, Bauer RN, Zhou H, Zhang H, Jones S, Robinette C, Noah TL, Jaspers I. 2016. Effect of broccoli sprouts and live attenuated influenza virus on peripheral blood natural killer cells: a randomized, double-blind study. PLoS One. 11(1):e0147742. https://doi.org/10.1371/journal.pone.0147742.

2771. American College of Lifestyle Medicine. 2020 Mar 23. Lifestyle choices to boost immunity. Chesterfield (MO): ACLM; [accessed 2020 Mar 31]. https://files.constantcontact.com/abfbc81b001/4e7c0973-293d-4cd1-89c7-796d86808393.pdf.

2772. World Health Organization. 2020. Stay physically active during self-quarantine. Copenhagen: WHO Regional Office for Europe; [accessed 2020 Mar 31]. http://www.euro.who.int/en/health-topics/health-emergencies/coronavirus-covid-19/novel-coronavirus-2019-ncov-technical-guidance/stay-physically-active-during-self-quarantine.

2773. World Health Organization. 2018 Oct 23. Healthy diet. Geneva: WHO; [accessed 2020 Mar 31]. https://www.who.int/news-room/fact-sheets/detail/healthy-diet.

2774. Coates BM, Staricha KL, Wiese KM, Ridge KM. 2015. Influenza A virus infection, innate immunity, and childhood. JAMA Pediatr. 169(10):956–963. https://doi.org/10.1001/jamapediatrics.2015.1387.

2775. Zimmermann P, Curtis N. 2020. Coronavirus infections in children including COVID-19: an overview of the epidemiology, clinical features, diagnosis, treatment and prevention options in children. Pediatr Infect Dis J. [Epub ahead of print 2020 Mar 25; accessed 2020 Mar 31]. https://doi.org/10.1097/INF.0000000000002660.

2776. Spezzani V, Piunno A, Iselin HU. 2020. Benign COVID-19 in an immuno-compromised cancer patient—the case of a married couple. Swiss Med Wkly. 150:w20246. https://doi.org/10.4414/smw.2020.20246.

2777. D'Antiga L. 2020. Coronaviruses and immunosuppressed patients. The facts during the third epidemic. Liver Transpl. [Epub ahead of print 2020 Mar 20; accessed 2020 Apr 1]. https://doi.org/10.1002/lt.25756.

2778. Nickbakhsh S, Ho A, Marques DFP, McMenamin J, Gunson RR, Murcia P. 2020 Mar 20. Epidemiology of seasonal coronaviruses: establishing the context for COVID-19 emergence. medRxiv.org. [accessed 2020 Apr 1]. https://doi.org/10.1101/2020.03.18.20037101.

2779. Mizumoto K, Omori R, Nishiura H. 2020 Mar 13. Age specificity of cases and attack rate of novel coronavirus disease (COVID-19). medRxiv.org. [accessed 2020 Apr 1]. https://doi.org/10.1101/2020.03.09.20033142.

2780. Wang SF, Tseng SP, Yen CH, Yang JY, Tsao CH, Shen CW, Chen KH, Liu FT, Liu WT, Chen YMA, et al. 2014. Antibody-dependent SARS coronavirus infection is mediated by antibodies against spike proteins. Biochem Biophys Res Commun. 451(2):208–214. https://doi.org/10.1016/j.bbrc.2014.07.090.

2781. Fu Y, Cheng Y, Wu Y. 2020. Understanding SARS-CoV-2-mediated inflammatory responses: from mechanisms to potential therapeutic tools. Virol Sin. [Epub ahead of print 2020 Mar 3; accessed 2020 Apr 1]. https://doi.org/10.1007/s12250-020-00207-4.

2782. Wang YB, Wang LP, Li P. 2018. Perspectives on novel vaccine development. Pol J Vet Sci. 21(3):643–649. https://doi.org/10.24425/124302.

2783. Mizumoto K, Omori R, Nishiura H. 2020 Mar 13. Age specificity of cases and attack rate of novel coronavirus disease (COVID-19). medRxiv.org. [accessed 2020 Apr 1]. https://doi.org/10.1101/2020.03.09.20033142.

2784. Kasprak A. 2020 Mar 2. Did a noted pathologist write this viral coronavirus advice letter? Snopes.com; [updated 2020 Mar 13; accessed 2020 Apr 1]. https://www.snopes.com/fact-check/zinc-lozenges-coronavirus/.

2785. Monto AS. 1974. Medical reviews. Coronaviruses. Yale J Biol Med. 47(4):234–251.

2786. Valadbeigi S, Javadian S, Ebrahimi-Rad M, Khatami S, Saghiri R. 2019. Assessment of trace elements in serum of acute lymphoblastic and myeloid leukemia patients. Exp Oncol. 41(1):69–71.

2787. Eby GA, Davis DR, Halcomb WW. 1984. Reduction in duration of common colds by zinc gluconate lozenges in a double-blind study. Antimicrob Agents Chemother. 25(1):20–24. https://doi.org/10.1128/aac.25.1.20.

2788. Hemilä H. 2017. Zinc lozenges and the common cold: a meta-analysis comparing zinc acetate and zinc gluconate, and the role of zinc dosage. JRSM Open. 8(5):2054270417694291. https://doi.org/10.1177/2054270417694291.

2789. Singh M, Das RR. 2011. Zinc for the common cold. Cochrane Database Syst Rev. 2:CD001364. https://doi.org/10.1002/14651858.CD001364.pub3.

2790. Hemilä H, Petrus EJ, Fitzgerald JT, Prasad A. 2016. Zinc acetate lozenges for treating the common cold: an individual patient data meta-analysis. Br J Clin Pharmacol. 82(5):1393–1398. https://doi.org/10.1111/bcp.13057.

2791. Hemilä H, Chalker E. 2015. The effectiveness of high dose zinc acetate lozenges on various common cold symptoms: a meta-analysis. BMC Fam Pract. 16:24. https://doi.org/10.1186/s12875-015-0237-6.

2792. Hemilä H. 2017. Zinc lozenges and the common cold: a meta-analysis comparing zinc acetate and zinc gluconate, and the role of zinc dosage. JRSM Open. 8(5):2054270417694291. https://doi.org/10.1177/2054270417694291.

2793. Singh M, Das RR. 2011. Zinc for the common cold. Cochrane Database Syst Rev. 2:CD001364. https://doi.org/10.1002/14651858.CD001364.pub3.

2794. Hemilä H. 2017. Zinc lozenges and the common cold: a meta-analysis comparing zinc acetate and zinc gluconate, and the role of zinc dosage. JRSM Open. 8(5):2054270417694291. https://doi.org/10.1177/2054270417694291.

2795. Singh M, Das RR. 2011. Zinc for the common cold. Cochrane Database Syst Rev. 2:CD001364. https://doi.org/10.1002/14651858.CD001364.pub3.

2796. Novick SG, Godfrey JC, Godfrey NJ, Wilder HR. 1996. How does zinc modify the common cold? Clinical observations and implications regarding mechanisms of action. Med Hypotheses. 46(3):295–302. https://doi.org/10.1016/s0306-9877(96)90259-5.

2797. Korant BD, Kauer JC, Butterworth BE. 1974. Zinc ions inhibit replication of rhinoviruses. Nature. 248(449):588–590. https://doi.org/10.1038/248588a0.

2798. te Velthuis AJW, van den Worm SHE, Sims AC, Baric RS, Snijder EJ, van Hemert MJ. 2010. Zn(2+) inhibits coronavirus and arterivirus RNA polymerase activity in vitro and zinc ionophores block the replication of these viruses in cell culture. PLoS Pathog. 6(11):e1001176. https://doi.org/10.1371/journal.ppat.1001176.

2799. Dabbagh-Bazarbachi H, Clergeaud G, Quesada IM, Ortiz M, O'Sullivan CK, Fernández-Larrea JB. 2014. Zinc ionophore activity of quercetin and epigallocatechin-gallate: from Hepa 1–6 cells to a liposome model. J Agric Food Chem. 62(32):8085–8093. https://doi.org/10.1021/jf5014633.

2800. Zou X, Chen K, Zou J, Han P, Hao J, Han Z. 2020 Mar 12. Single-cell RNA-seq data analysis on the receptor ACE2 expression reveals the potential risk of different human organs vulnerable to 2019-nCoV infection. Front Med. [accessed 2020 Mar 31]. https://doi.org/10.1007/s11684-020-0754-0.

2801. Wang L, Song Y. 2018. Efficacy of zinc given as an adjunct to the treatment of severe pneumonia: a meta-analysis of randomized, double-blind and placebo-controlled trials. Clin Respir J. 12(3):857–864. https://doi.org/10.1111/crj.12646.

2802. Srinivasan MG, Ndeezi G, Mboijana CK, Kiguli S, Bimenya GS, Nankabirwa V, Tumwine JK. 2012. Zinc adjunct therapy reduces case fatality in severe childhood pneumonia: a randomized double blind placebo-controlled trial. BMC Med. 10:14. https://doi.org/10.1186/1741-7015-10-14.

2803. Wadhwa N, Chandran A, Aneja S, Lodha R, Kabra SK, Chaturvedi MK, Sodhi J, Fitzwater SP, Chandra J, Rath B, et al. 2013. Efficacy of zinc given as an adjunct in the treatment of severe and very severe pneumonia in hospitalized children 2-24 mo of age: a randomized, double-blind, placebo-controlled trial. Am J Clin Nutr. 97(6):1387–1394. https://doi.org/10.3945/ajcn.112.052951.

2804. Sempértegui F, Estrella B, Rodríguez O, Gómez D, Cabezas M, Salgado G, Sabin LL, Hamer DH. 2014. Zinc as an adjunct to the treatment of severe pneumonia in Ecuadorian children: a randomized controlled trial. Am J Clin Nutr. 99(3):497–505. https://doi.org/10.3945/ajcn.113.067892.

2805. Shah D, Sachdev HS, Gera T, De-Regil LM, Peña-Rosas JP. 2016. Fortification of staple foods with zinc for improving zinc status and other health outcomes in the general population. Cochrane Database Syst Rev. 6:CD010697. https://doi .org/10.1002/14651858.CD010697.pub2.

2806. Singh M, Das RR. 2011. Zinc for the common cold. Cochrane Database Syst Rev. 2:CD001364. https://doi.org/10.1002/14651858.CD001364.pub3.

2807. Davidson TM, Smith WM. 2010. The Bradford Hill criteria and zinc-induced anosmia: a causality analysis. Arch Otolaryngol Head Neck Surg. 136(7):673–676. https://doi.org/10.1001/archoto.2010.111.

2808. Eby GA. 2005. Treatment of acute lymphocytic leukemia using zinc adjuvant with chemotherapy and radiation—a case history and hypothesis. Med Hypotheses. 64(6):1124–1126. https://doi.org/10.1016/j.mehy.2004.12.019.

2809. Sugishita Y, Kurita J, Sugawara T, Ohkusa Y. 2020 Mar 16. Preliminary evaluation of voluntary event cancellation as a countermeasure against the COVID-19 outbreak in Japan as of 11 March, 2020. medRxiv.org. [accessed 2020 Apr 1]. https://doi.org/10.1101/2020.03.12.20035220.

2810. Anderson RM, Heesterbeek H, Klinkenberg D, Hollingsworth TD. 2020. How will country-based mitigation measures influence the course of the COVID-19 epidemic? Lancet. 395(10228):931–934. https://doi.org/10.1016 /S0140-6736(20)30567-5.

2811. Jombart T, van Zandvoort K, Russell TW, Jarvis CI, Gimma A, Abbott S, Clifford S, Funk S, Gibbs H, Liu Y, et al. 2020 Mar 13. Inferring the number of COVID-19 cases from recently reported deaths. medRxiv.org. [accessed 2020 Apr 1]. https://doi.org/10.1101/2020.03.10.20033761.

2812. Stein R. 2020. COVID-19 and rationally layered social distancing. Int J Clin Pract. 14:e13501. [Epub ahead of print 2020 Mar 14; accessed 2020 Apr 1]. https://doi.org/10.1111/ijcp.13501.

2813. Yang Y, Peng F, Wang R, Guan K, Jiang T, Xu G, Sun J, Chang C. 2020 Mar 3. The deadly coronaviruses: the 2003 SARS pandemic and the 2020 novel coronavirus epidemic in China. J Autoimmun. [accessed 2020 Mar 30]. https://doi.org/10.1016/j.jaut.2020.102434.

2814. Zou L, Ruan F, Huang M, Liang L, Huang H, Hong Z, Yu J, Kang M, Song Y, Xia J, et al. 2020. SARS-CoV-2 viral load in upper respiratory specimens of infected patients. N Engl J Med. 382(12):1177–1179.

2815. Yeo C, Kaushal S, Yeo D. 2020. Enteric involvement of coronaviruses: is faecal–oral transmission of SARS-CoV-2 possible? Lancet Gastroenterol Hepatol. 5(4):335–337. https://doi.org/10.1016/S2468-1253(20)30048-0.

2816. Johnson D, Lynch R, Marshall C, Mead K, Hirst D. 2013. Aerosol generation by modern flush toilets. Aerosol Sci Technol. 47(9):1047–1057. https://doi.org/10.1080/02786826.2013.814911.

2817. Knowlton SD, Boles CL, Perencevich EN, Diekema DJ, Nonnenmann MW, CDC Epicenters Program. 2018. Bioaerosol concentrations generated from toilet flushing in a hospital-based patient care setting. Antimicrob Resist Infect Control. 7:16. https://doi.org/10.1186/s13756-018-0301-9.

2818. Wallis C, Melnick JL, Rao VC, Sox TE. 1985. Method for detecting viruses in aerosols. Appl Environ Microbiol. 50(5):1181–1186.

2819. Booth TF, Kournikakis B, Bastien N, Ho J, Kobasa D, Stadnyk L, Li Y, Spence M, Paton S, Henry B, et al. 2005. Detection of airborne severe acute respiratory syndrome (SARS) coronavirus and environmental contamination in SARS outbreak units. J Infect Dis. 191(9):1472–1477. https://doi.org/10.1086/429634.

2820. Ong SWX, Tan YK, Chia PY, Lee TH, Ng OT, Wong MSY, Marimuthu K. 2020. Air, surface environmental, and personal protective equipment contamination by severe acute respiratory syndrome coronavirus 2 (SARS-CoV-2) from a symptomatic patient. JAMA. [Epub ahead of print 2020 Mar 4; accessed 2020 Apr 1]. https://doi.org/10.1001/jama.2020.3227.

2821. Santarpia JL, Rivera DN, Herrera V, Morwitzer MJ, Creager H, Santarpia GW, Crown KK, Brett-Major D, Schnaubelt E, Broadhurst MJ, et al. 2020 Mar 26. Transmission potential of SARS-CoV-2 in viral shedding observed at the University of Nebraska Medical Center. medRxiv.org. [accessed 2020 May 7]. https://doi.org/10.1101/2020.03.23.20039446.

2822. van Doremalen N, Bushmaker T, Morris DH, Holbrook MG, Gamble A, Williamson BN, Tamin A, Harcourt JL, Thornburg NJ, Gerber SI, et al. 2020. Aerosol and surface stability of SARS-CoV-2 as compared with SARS-CoV-1. N Engl J Med. [Epub ahead of print 2020 Mar 17; accessed 2020 Apr 1]. https://doi.org/10.1056/NEJMc2004973.

2823. Firquet S, Beaujard S, Lobert P-E, Sané F, Caloone D, Izard D, Hober D. 2015. Survival of enveloped and non-enveloped viruses on inanimate surfaces. Microbes Environ. 30(2):140–144. https://doi.org/10.1264/jsme2.ME14145.

2824. Geller C, Varbanov M, Duval RE. 2012. Human coronaviruses: insights into environmental resistance and its influence on the development of new antiseptic strategies. Viruses. 4(11):3044–3068. https://doi.org/10.3390/v4113044.

2825. Casanova LM, Jeon S, Rutala WA, Weber DJ, Sobsey MD. 2010. Effects of air temperature and relative humidity on coronavirus survival on surfaces. Appl Environ Microbiol. 76(9):2712–2717. https://doi.org/10.1128/AEM.02291-09.

2826. Kampf G, Todt D, Pfaender S, Steinmann E. 2020. Persistence of coronaviruses on inanimate surfaces and their inactivation with biocidal agents. J Hosp Infect. 104(3):246–251. https://doi.org/10.1016/j.jhin.2020.01.022.

2827. Warnes SL, Little ZR, Keevil CW. 2015. Human coronavirus 229E remains infectious on common touch surface materials. mBio. 6(6):e01697–15. https://doi.org/10.1128/mBio.01697-15.

2828. van Doremalen N, Bushmaker T, Morris DH, Holbrook MG, Gamble A, Williamson BN, Tamin A, Harcourt JL, Thornburg NJ, Gerber SI, et al. 2020.

Aerosol and surface stability of SARS-CoV-2 as compared with SARS-CoV-1. N Engl J Med. [Epub ahead of print 2020 Mar 17; accessed 2020 Apr 1]. https://doi.org/10.1056/NEJMc2004973.

2829. Otter JA, Donskey C, Yezli S, Douthwaite S, Goldenberg SD, Weber DJ. 2016. Transmission of SARS and MERS coronaviruses and influenza virus in healthcare settings: the possible role of dry surface contamination. J Hosp Infect. 92(3):235–250. https://doi.org/10.1016/j.jhin.2015.08.027.

2830. Duan SM, Zhao XS, Wen RF, Huang JJ, Pi GH, Zhang SX, Han J, Bi SL, Ruan L, Dong XP, et al. 2003. Stability of SARS coronavirus in human specimens and environment and its sensitivity to heating and UV irradiation. Biomed Environ Sci. 16(3):246–255.

2831. Lai MY, Cheng PK, Lim WW. 2005. Survival of severe acute respiratory syndrome coronavirus. Clin Infect Dis. 41(7):e67–71. https://doi.org/10.1086/433186.

2832. van Doremalen N, Bushmaker T, Morris DH, Holbrook MG, Gamble A, Williamson BN, Tamin A, Harcourt JL, Thornburg NJ, Gerber SI, et al. 2020. Aerosol and surface stability of SARS-CoV-2 as compared with SARS-CoV-1. N Engl J Med. [Epub ahead of print 2020 Mar 17; accessed 2020 Apr 1]. https://doi.org/10.1056/NEJMc2004973.

2833. Chin A, Chu J, Perera M, Hui K, Yen HL, Chan M, Peiris M, Poon L. 2020 Jan 1. Stability of SARS-CoV-2 in different environmental conditions. medRxiv.org. [accessed 2020 Apr 1]. https://doi.org/10.1101/2020.03.15.20036673.

2834. van Doremalen N, Bushmaker T, Morris DH, Holbrook MG, Gamble A, Williamson BN, Tamin A, Harcourt JL, Thornburg NJ, Gerber SI, et al. 2020. Aerosol and surface stability of SARS-CoV-2 as compared with SARS-CoV-1. N Engl J Med. [Epub ahead of print 2020 Mar 17; accessed 2020 Apr 1]. https://doi.org/10.1056/NEJMc2004973.

2835. Chin A, Chu J, Perera M, Hui K, Yen HL, Chan M, Peiris M, Poon L. 2020 Jan 1. Stability of SARS-CoV-2 in different environmental conditions. medRxiv .org. [accessed 2020 Apr 1]. https://doi.org/10.1101/2020.03.15.20036673.

2836. Winther B, Gwaltney JM, Mygind N, Turner RB, Hendley JO. 1986. Sites of rhinovirus recovery after point inoculation of the upper airway. JAMA. 256(13):1763–1767.

2837. Kwok YLA, Gralton J, McLaws M-L. 2015. Face touching: a frequent habit that has implications for hand hygiene. Am J Infect Control. 43(2):112–114. https://doi.org/10.1016/j.ajic.2014.10.015.

2838. Nicas M, Best D. 2008. A study quantifying the hand-to-face contact rate and its potential application to predicting respiratory tract infection. J Occup Environ Hyg. 5(6):347–352. https://doi.org/10.1080/15459620802003896.

2839. Hendley JO, Wenzel RP, Gwaltney JM. 1973. Transmission of rhinovirus colds by self-inoculation. N Engl J Med. 288(26):1361–1364. https://doi.org/10.1056/NEJM197306282882601.

2840. Elder NC, Sawyer W, Pallerla H, Khaja S, Blacker M. 2014. Hand hygiene and face touching in family medicine offices: a Cincinnati Area Research and Improvement Group (CARInG) network study. J Am Board Fam Med. 27(3):339–346.

2841. Erasmus V, Daha TJ, Brug H, Richardus JH, Behrendt MD, Vos MC, van Beeck EF. 2010. Systematic review of studies on compliance with hand hygiene guidelines in hospital care. Infect Control Hosp Epidemiol. 31(3):283–294. https://doi.org/10.1086/650451.

2842. Quraishi ZA, McGuckin M, Blals FX. 1984. Duration of handwashing in intensive care units: a descriptive study. Am J Infect Control. 12(2):83–87. https://doi.org/10.1016/0196-6553(84)90021-x.

2843. Centers for Disease Control and Prevention. 2020 Mar 18. How to protect yourself. U.S. Department of Health and Human Services; [accessed 2020 Apr 1]. https://www.cdc.gov/coronavirus/2019-ncov/prepare/prevention .html.

2844. Centers for Disease Control and Prevention. 2020 Mar 4. Show me the science—how to wash your hands. U.S. Department of Health and Human Services; [accessed 2020 Apr 1]. https://www.cdc.gov/handwashing/show-me -the-science-handwashing.html.

2845. Jensen DA, Danyluk MD, Harris LJ, Schaffner DW. 2015. Quantifying the effect of hand wash duration, soap use, ground beef debris, and drying methods on the removal of Enterobacter aerogenes on hands. J Food Prot. 78(4):685–690. https://doi.org/10.4315/0362-028X.JFP-14-245.

2846. Todd EC, Michaels BS, Smith D, Greig JD, Bartleson CA. 2010. Outbreaks where food workers have been implicated in the spread of foodborne disease. Part 9. Washing and drying of hands to reduce microbial contamination. J Food Prot. 73(10):1937–1955. https://doi.org/10.4315/0362-028x-73.10.1937.

2847. Wong JSW, Lee JKF. 2019. The common missed handwashing instances and areas after 15 years of hand-hygiene education. J Environ Public Health. 2019:5928924. https://doi.org/10.1155/2019/5928924.

2848. McNeil SA, Foster CL, Hedderwick SA, Kauffman CA. 2001. Effect of hand cleansing with antimicrobial soap or alcohol-based gel on microbial coloni- zation of artificial fingernails worn by health care workers. Clin Infect Dis. 32(3):367–372. https://doi.org/10.1086/318488.

2849. Carrico AR, Spoden M, Wallston KA, Vandenbergh MP. 2013. The environ- mental cost of misinformation: why the recommendation to use elevated tem- peratures for handwashing is problematic. Int J Consum Stud. 37(4):433–441. https://doi.org/10.1111/ijcs.12012.

2850. Price PB. 1938. The bacteriology of normal skin; a new quantitative test ap- plied to a study of the bacterial flora and the disinfectant action of mechanical cleansing. J Infect Dis. 63(3):301–318. https://doi.org/10.1093/infdis/63.3 .301.

2851. Michaels B, Gangar V, Schultz A, Arenas M, Curiale M, Ayers T, Paulson D. 2002. Water temperature as a factor in handwashing efficacy. Food Serv Tech- nol. 2(3):139–149. https://doi.org/10.1046/j.1471-5740.2002.00043.x.

2852. Carrico AR, Spoden M, Wallston KA, Vandenbergh MP. 2013. The environ- mental cost of misinformation: why the recommendation to use elevated temperatures for handwashing is problematic. Int J Consum Stud. 37(4):433–441. https://doi.org/10.1111/ijcs.12012.

2853. McCormick RD, Buchman TL, Maki DG. 2000. Double-blind, randomized trial of scheduled use of a novel barrier cream and an oil-containing lotion for protecting the hands of health care workers. Am J Infect Control. 28(4):302–310. https://doi.org/10.1067/mic.2000.107425.

2854. World Health Organization. 2009. WHO guidelines on hand hygiene in health care: a summary. Geneva: WHO. Report No.: WHO/IER/PSP/2009.07. https://www.who.int/gpsc/information_centre/hand-hygiene-summary/en/.

2855. Centers for Disease Control and Prevention. 2020 Mar 18. Frequently asked questions about hand hygiene for healthcare personnel responding to COVID-2019. U.S. Department of Health and Human Services; [accessed 2020 Apr 1]. https://www.cdc.gov/coronavirus/2019-ncov/infection-control/hcp-hand -hygiene-faq.html.

2856. Elder NC, Sawyer W, Pallerla H, Khaja S, Blacker M. 2014. Hand hygiene and face touching in family medicine offices: a Cincinnati Area Research and Improvement Group (CARInG) network study. J Am Board Fam Med. 27(3):339–346. https://doi.org/10.3122/jabfm.2014.03.130242.

2857. Siddharta A, Pfaender S, Vielle NJ, Dijkman R, Friesland M, Becker B, Yang J, Engelmann M, Todt D, Windisch MP, et al. Virucidal activity of World Health Organization-recommended formulations against enveloped viruses, including Zika, Ebola, and emerging coronaviruses. J Infect Dis. 215(6):902–906. https://doi.org/10.1093/infdis/jix046.

2858. Boyce JM, Pittet D. 2002. Guideline for hand hygiene in health-care settings. Recommendations of the Healthcare Infection Control Practices Advisory Committee and the HICPAC/SHEA/APIC/IDSA Hand Hygiene Task Force. MMWR Recomm Rep. 51(RR-16):1–45. https://www.cdc.gov/mmwr/preview /mmwrhtml/rr5116a1.htm.

2859. World Health Organization. [date unknown]. Guide to local production: WHO-recommended handrub formulations. Geneva: WHO; [revised 2010 Apr; accessed 2020 Apr 1]. https://www.who.int/gpsc/information_centre /handrub-formulations/en/.

2860. Evon D. 2020 Mar 5. Can a homemade Tito's Vodka hand sanitizer help stem coronavirus? Snopes.com; [accessed 2020 Apr 1]. https://www.snopes.com/fact -check/hand-sanitizer-titos-vodka/.

2861. Kratzel A, Todt D, V'kovski P, Steiner S, Gultom M, Thao TTN, Ebert N, Holwerda M, Steinmann J, Niemeyer D, et al. 2020. Inactivation of severe acute respiratory syndrome coronavirus 2 by WHO-recommended hand rub formulations and alcohols. Emerg Infect Dis. [Epub ahead of print 2020 Apr 13; accessed 2020 Apr 18]. https://doi.org/10.3201/eid260.

2862. World Health Organization. [date unknown]. Guide to local production: WHO-recommended handrub formulations. Geneva: WHO [revised 2010 Apr; accessed 2020 Apr 1]. https://www.who.int/gpsc/information_centre /handrub-formulations/en/.

2863. Food and Drug Administration. 2020. Policy for temporary compounding of certain alcohol-based hand sanitizer products during the public health emergency. FDA. Report No.: FDA-2020-D-1106. https://www.fda.gov/regulatory-information/search-fda-guidance-documents/policy-temporary-compounding-certain-alcohol-based-hand-sanitizer-products-during-public-health.

2864. U.S. Pharmacopeia. 2020. Compounding alcohol-based hand sanitizer during COVID-19 pandemic. USP; [updated 2020 Mar 25; accessed 2020 Apr 1]. https://www.usp.org/sites/default/files/usp/document/about/public-policy/usp-covid19-handrub.pdf.

2865. National Environmental Agency. 2020 Jan 25. Interim guidelines for environmental cleaning and disinfection of areas exposed to confirmed case(s) of COVID-19 non-healthcare premises. Singapore: NEA; [revised 2020 Mar 16; accessed 2020 Apr 1]. https://www.nea.gov.sg/our-services/public-cleanliness/environmental-cleaning-guidelines/guidelines-for-environmental-cleaning-and-disinfection.

2866. Kampf G, Todt D, Pfaender S, Steinmann E. 2020. Persistence of coronaviruses on inanimate surfaces and their inactivation with biocidal agents. J Hosp Infect. 104(3):246–251. https://doi.org/10.1016/j.jhin.2020.01.022.

2867. Patel P, Sanghvi S, Malik K, Khachemoune A. 2020. Back to the basics: diluted bleach for COVID-19. J Am Acad Dermatol. [Epub ahead of print 2020 Apr 10; accessed 2020 Apr 18]. https://doi.org/10.1016/j.jaad.2020.04.033.

2868. National Environmental Agency. 2020 Jan 25. Interim guidelines for environmental cleaning and disinfection of areas exposed to confirmed case(s) of COVID-19 non-healthcare premises. Singapore: NEA; [revised 2020 Mar 16; accessed 2020 Apr 1]. https://www.nea.gov.sg/our-services/public-cleanliness/environmental-cleaning-guidelines/guidelines-for-environmental-cleaning-and-disinfection.

2869. Chin AWH, Chu JTS, Perera MRA, Hui KPY, Yen HL, Chan MCW, Peiris M, Poon LLM. 2020 Mar 27. Stability of SARS-CoV-2 in different environmental conditions. medRxiv.org. [accessed 2020 Apr 1]. https://www.medrxiv.org/content/10.1101/2020.03.15.20036673v2.

2870. Wu YC, Chen CS, Chan YJ. 2020. The outbreak of COVID-19: an overview. J Chin Med Assoc. 83(3):217–220. https://doi.org/10.1097/JCMA.0000000000000270.

2871. Centers for Disease Control and Prevention. 1991. Epidemiologic notes and reports chlorine gas toxicity from mixture of bleach with other cleaning products—California. Morb Mortal Wkly Rep. 40(36):619–621,627–629. [last reviewed 2001 May 2; accessed 2020 Apr 6]. https://www.cdc.gov/mmwr/preview/mmwrhtml/00015111.htm.

2872. National Environmental Agency. 2020 Jan 25. Interim guidelines for environmental cleaning and disinfection of areas exposed to confirmed case(s) of COVID-19 non-healthcare premises. Singapore: NEA; [revised 2020 Mar 16; accessed 2020 Apr 1]. https://www.nea.gov.sg/our-services/public-cleanliness/environmental-cleaning-guidelines/guidelines-for-environmental-cleaning-and-disinfection.

2873. Chin AWH, Chu JTS, Perera MRA, Hui KPY, Yen HL, Chan MCW, Peiris M, Poon LLM. 2020 Mar 27. Stability of SARS-CoV-2 in different environmental conditions. medRxiv.org. [accessed 2020 Apr 1]. https://www.medrxiv.org/content/10.1101/2020.03.15.20036673v2.

2874. Lai MY, Cheng PK, Lim WW. 2005. Survival of severe acute respiratory syndrome coronavirus. Clin Infect Dis. 41(7):e67–71. https://doi.org/10.1086/433186.

2875. Dellanno C, Vega Q, Boesenberg D. 2009. The antiviral action of common household disinfectants and antiseptics against murine hepatitis virus, a potential surrogate for SARS coronavirus. Am J Infect Control. 37(8):649–652. https://doi.org/10.1016/j.ajic.2009.03.012.

2876. Rabenau HF, Cinatl J, Morgenstern B, Bauer G, Preiser W, Doerr HW. 2005. Stability and inactivation of SARS coronavirus. Med Microbiol Immunol. 194(1-2):1–6. https://doi.org/10.1007/s00430-004-0219-0.

2877. U.S. Environmental Protection Agency. [date unknown]. List N: disinfectants for use against SARS-CoV-2. U.S. EPA; [updated 2020 Mar 26; accessed 2020 Apr 1]. https://www.epa.gov/pesticide-registration/list-n-disinfectants-use-against-sars-cov-2.

2878. Sattar SA, Springthorpe VS, Karim Y, Loro P. 1989. Chemical disinfection of non-porous inanimate surfaces experimentally contaminated with four human pathogenic viruses. Epidemiol Infect. 102(3):493–505. https://doi.org/10.1017/s0950268800030211.

2879. Desai AN, Aronoff DM. 2020 Apr 9. Food safety and COVID-19. JAMA. [accessed 2020 Apr 11]. https://doi.org/10.1001/jama.2020.5877.

2880. Chin AWH, Chu JTS, Perera MRA, Hui KPY, Yen HL, Chan MCW, Peiris M, Poon LLM. 2020. Stability of SARS-CoV-2 in different environmental conditions. Lancet Microbe. [Epub ahead of print 2020 Apr 2; accessed 2020 Apr 11]. https://doi.org/10.1016/S2666-5247(20)30003-3.

2881. Desai AN, Aronoff DM. 2020 Apr 9. Food safety and COVID-19. JAMA. [accessed 2020 Apr 11]. https://doi.org/10.1001/jama.2020.5877.

2882. Wu YC, Chen CS, Chan YJ. 2020. The outbreak of COVID-19: an overview. J Chin Med Assoc. 83(3):217–220. https://doi.org/10.1097/JCMA.0000000000000270.

2883. Zhang J, Zhou L, Yang Y, Peng W, Wang W, Chen X. 2020. Therapeutic and triage strategies for 2019 novel coronavirus disease in fever clinics. Lancet Respir Med. 8(3):e11–e12. https://doi.org/10.1016/S2213-2600(20)30071-0.

2884. Centers for Disease Control and Prevention. 2020 Mar 25. What to do if you are sick: steps to help prevent the spread of COVID-19 if you are sick. U.S. Department of Health and Human Services; [last reviewed 2020 Mar 25; accessed 2020 Mar 31]. https://www.cdc.gov/coronavirus/2019-ncov/if-you-are-sick/steps-when-sick.html.

2885. Loeb J. 2020. Pet dog confirmed to have coronavirus. Vet Rec. 186(9):265. https://doi.org/10.1136/vr.m892.

2886. Cheng L. 2020 Mar 19. Coronavirus: Hong Kong confirms a second dog is infected. South China Morning Post. [accessed 2020 Apr 6]; https://www.scmp

.com/news/hong-kong/health-environment/article/3075993/coronavirus
-hong-kong-confirms-second-dog.

2887. Shi J, Wen Z, Zhong G, Yang H, Wang C, Liu R, He X, Shuai L, Sun Z, Zhao Y, et al. 2020 Mar 31. Susceptibility of ferrets, cats, dogs, and different domestic animals to SARS-coronavirus-2. bioRxiv.org. [accessed 2020 Apr 6]. https://doi.org/10.1101/2020.03.30.015347.

2888. Huang Q, Zhan X, Zeng XT. 2020. COVID-19 pandemic: stop panic abandonment of household pets. J Travel Med. [Epub ahead of print 2020 Apr 9; accessed 2020 Apr 11]. https://doi.org/10.1093/jtm/taaa046.

2889. Shi J, Wen Z, Zhong G, Yang H, Wang C, Liu R, He X, Shuai L, Sun Z, Zhao Y, et al. 2020 Mar 31. Susceptibility of ferrets, cats, dogs, and different domestic animals to SARS-coronavirus-2. bioRxiv.org. [accessed 2020 Apr 6]. https://doi.org/10.1101/2020.03.30.015347.

2890. Zhang Q, Zhang H, Huang K, Yang Y, Hui X, Gao J, He X, Li C, Gong W, Zhang Y, et al. 2020 Apr 3. SARS-CoV-2 neutralizing serum antibodies in cats: a serological investigation. bioRxiv.org. [accessed 2020 Apr 6]. https://doi.org/10.1101/2020.04.01.021196.

2891. U.S. Department of Agriculture. 2020 Apr 5. USDA statement on the confirmation of COVID-19 in a tiger in New York. USDA; [modified 2020 Apr 6; accessed 2020 Apr 6]. https://www.aphis.usda.gov/aphis/newsroom/news/sa _by_date/sa-2020/ny-zoo-covid-19.

2892. Centers for Disease Control and Prevention. 2020 Mar 25. What to do if you are sick: steps to help prevent the spread of COVID-19 if you are sick. U.S. Department of Health and Human Services; [last reviewed 2020 Mar 25; accessed 2020 Mar 31]. https://www.cdc.gov/coronavirus/2019-ncov/if-you-are -sick/steps-when-sick.html.

2893. Allen J, Lipsitch M. 2020 Mar 24. 6 things to know if you're living with someone who has coronavirus, or think you might be. USA Today (McLean, VA) [accessed 2020 Apr 1]; https://www.usatoday.com/story/opinion/2020 /03/24/coronavirus-testing-shortage-take-precautions-just-in-case-column /2899989001/.

2894. Zhao BB, Liu Y, Chen C. 2020. Air purifiers: a supplementary measure to remove airborne SARS-CoV-2. Build Environ. [Epub ahead of print 2020 Apr 24; accessed 2020 May 11]. https://doi.org/10.1016/j.buildenv.2020.106918.

2895. Qian H, Zheng X. 2018. Ventilation control for airborne transmission of human exhaled bio-aerosols in buildings. J Thorac Dis. 10(Suppl 19):S2295– S2304. https://dx.doi.org/10.21037/jtd.2018.01.24.

2896. Casanova LM, Jeon S, Rutala WA, Weber DJ, Sobsey MD. 2010. Effects of air temperature and relative humidity on coronavirus survival on surfaces. Appl Environ Microbiol. 76(9):2712–2717. https://dx.doi.org/10.1128/AEM.02291-09.

2897. Jiang S, Huang L, Chen X, Wang J, Wu W, Yin S, Chen W, Zhan J, Yan L, Ma L, et al. 2003. Ventilation of wards and nosocomial outbreak of severe acute respiratory syndrome among healthcare workers. Chin Med J. 116(9):1293–1297.

2898. Centers for Disease Control and Prevention. 2020 Mar 25. What to do if you are sick: steps to help prevent the spread of COVID-19 if you are sick. U.S.

Department of Health and Human Services [last reviewed 2020 Mar 25; accessed 2020 Mar 31]. https://www.cdc.gov/coronavirus/2019-ncov/if-you-are-sick/steps-when-sick.html.

2899. Chughtai AA, Seale H, Islam MS, Owais M, Macintyre CR. 2020. Policies on the use of respiratory protection for hospital health workers to protect from coronavirus disease (COVID-19). Int J Nurs Stud. [Epub ahead of print 2020 May; accessed 2020 Apr 1]. https://doi.org/10.1016/j.ijnurstu.2020.103567.

2900. Leung NHL, Chu DKW, Shiu EYC, Chan K-H, McDevitt JJ, Hau BJP, Yen H-L, Li Y, Ip DKM, Peiris JSM, et al. 2020 Apr 3. Respiratory virus shedding in exhaled breath and efficacy of face masks. Nat Med. [accessed 2020 Apr 6]. https://doi.org/10.1038/s41591-020-0843-2.

2901. National Research Council. 2020. Rapid expert consultation on the possibility of bioaerosol spread of SARS-CoV-2 for the COVID-19 pandemic (April 1, 2020). Washington(DC): National Academies Press. https://doi.org/10.17226/25769.

2902. Cohen J. 2020 Mar 27. Not wearing masks to protect against coronavirus is a 'big mistake,' top Chinese scientist says. Science. [accessed 2020 Apr 6]. https://doi.org/10.1126/science.abb9368.

2903. Centers for Disease Control and Prevention. 2020. Coronavirus disease 2019 (COVID-19): recommendations for cloth face covers. U.S. Department of Health and Human Services; [last reviewed 2020 Apr 3; accessed 2020 Apr 6]. https://www.cdc.gov/coronavirus/2019-ncov/prevent-getting-sick/cloth-face-cover.html.

2904. U.S. Surgeon General. 2020 Feb 29. Seriously people—STOP BUYING MASKS! Twitter.com; [accessed 2020 Apr 6]. https://twitter.com/surgeon_general/status/1233725785283932160.

2905. Centers for Disease Control and Prevention. 2020. Coronavirus disease 2019 (COVID-19): recommendations for cloth face covers. U.S. Department of Health and Human Services; [last reviewed 2020 Apr 3; accessed 2020 Apr 6]. https://www.cdc.gov/coronavirus/2019-ncov/prevent-getting-sick/cloth-face-cover.html.

2906. Centers for Disease Control and Prevention. 2009 Sep 24. Interim recommendations for facemask and respirator use to reduce 2009 influenza A (H1N1) virus transmission. Atlanta: CDC; [accessed 2020 Apr 1]. https://www.cdc.gov/h1n1flu/masks.htm.

2907. Jefferson T, Foxlee R, Del Mar C, Dooley L, Ferroni E, Hewak B, Prabhala A, Nair S, Rivetti A. 2008. Physical interventions to interrupt or reduce the spread of respiratory viruses: systematic review. BMJ. 336(7635):77–80. https://doi.org/10.1136/bmj.39393.510347.BE.

2908. Jung H, Kim J, Lee S, Lee J, Kim J, Tsai P, Yoon C. 2014. Comparison of filtration efficiency and pressure drop in anti-yellow sand masks, quarantine masks, medical masks, general masks, and handkerchiefs. Aerosol Air Qual Res. 14(3):991–1002. https://doi.org/10.4209/aaqr.2013.06.0201.

2909. Kellogg WH, MacMillan G. 1920. An experimental study of the efficacy of gauze face masks. Am J Public Health (N Y). 10(1):34–42. https://dx.doi.org/10.2105/ajph.10.1.34.

2910. World Health Organization. 2020. Advice on the use of masks in the community, during home care and in healthcare settings in the context of the novel coronavirus (2019-nCoV) outbreak: interim guidance, 6 April 2020. Geneva: WHO; [accessed 2020 May 7]. https://apps.who.int/iris/rest/bitstreams/1274280/retrieve.

2911. Leung CC, Lam TH, Cheng KK. 2020. Mass masking in the COVID-19 epidemic: people need guidance. Lancet. 395(10228):945. https://doi.org/10.1016/S0140-6736(20)30520-1.

2912. Feng S, Shen C, Xia N, Song W, Fan M, Cowling BJ. 2020. Rational use of face masks in the COVID-19 pandemic. Lancet Respir Med. [Epub ahead of print 2020 Mar 20; accessed 2020 Apr 1]. https://doi.org/10.1016/S2213-2600(20)30134-X.

2913. Centers for Disease Control and Prevention. 2020. Coronavirus disease 2019 (COVID-19): cloth face covers FAQs. U.S. Department of Health and Human Services; [last reviewed 2020 Apr 4; accessed 2020 Apr 6]. https://www.cdc.gov/coronavirus/2019-ncov/prevent-getting-sick/cloth-face-cover-faq.html.

2914. Livingston E, Desai A, Berkwits M. 2020. Sourcing personal protective equipment during the COVID-19 pandemic. JAMA. [Epub ahead of print 2020 Mar 28; accessed 2020 Apr 6]. https://doi.org/10.1001/jama.2020.5317.

2915. van der Sande M, Teunis P, Sabel R. 2008. Professional and home-made face masks reduce exposure to respiratory infections among the general population. PLoS ONE. 3(7):e2618. https://doi.org/10.1371/journal.pone.0002618.

2916. Davies A, Thompson KA, Giri K, Kafatos G, Walker J, Bennett A. 2013. Testing the efficacy of homemade masks: would they protect in an influenza pandemic? Disaster Med Public Health Prep. 7(4):413–418. https://doi.org/10.1017/dmp.2013.43.

2917. Rengasamy S, Eimer B, Shaffer RE. 2010. Simple respiratory protection—evaluation of the filtration performance of cloth masks and common fabric materials against 20–1000 nm size particles. Ann Occup Hyg. 54(7):789–798. https://doi.org/10.1093/annhyg/meq044.

2918. O'Kelly E, Pirog S, Ward J, Clarkson PJ. 2020 Apr 17. Informing homemade emergency facemask design: the ability of common fabrics to filter ultrafine particles. medRxiv.org. [accessed 2020 Apr 19]. https://doi.org/10.1101/2020.04.14.20065375.

2919. Centers for Disease Control and Prevention. 2020. Coronavirus disease 2019 (COVID-19): cloth face covers. U.S. Department of Health and Human Services; [last reviewed 2020 Apr 4; accessed 2020 Apr 6]. https://www.cdc.gov/coronavirus/2019-ncov/prevent-getting-sick/diy-cloth-face-coverings.html.

2920. National Environmental Agency. 2020 Jan 28. Interim guidelines for environmental cleaning and disinfection in residences that may be exposed to the COVID-19 virus. Singapore: NEA; [revised 2020 Feb 24; accessed 2020 Apr 1]. https://www.nea.gov.sg/our-services/public-cleanliness/environmental-cleaning-guidelines/guidelines/interim-guidelines-for-environmental-cleaning-and-disinfection-in-residences.

2921. Cheng CY. 2003. SARS and PPE (part 5). Singapore Med Assoc News. 35:17–22.

2922. Soucheray S. 2020 Feb 13. Unmasked: experts explain necessary respiratory protection for COVID-19. Minneapolis: Center for Infectious Disease Research and Policy; [accessed 2020 Apr 1]. http://www.cidrap.umn.edu/news-perspec tive/2020/02/unmasked-experts-explain-necessary-respiratory-protection -covid-19.

2923. U.S. Department of Health and Human Services. 2006 March. Draft pandemic influenza preparedness and response plan. Washington: HHS; http://www .dhhs.gov/nvpo/pandemicplan/.

2924. Chughtai AA, Seale H, Islam MS, Owais M, Macintyre CR. 2020. Policies on the use of respiratory protection for hospital health workers to protect from coronavirus disease (COVID-19). Int J Nurs Stud. [Epub ahead of print 2020 May; accessed 2020 Apr 1]. https://doi.org/10.1016/j.ijnurstu.2020.103567.

2925. Soucheray S. 2020 Feb 13. Unmasked: experts explain necessary respiratory protection for COVID-19. Minneapolis: Center for Infectious Disease Research and Policy; [accessed 2020 Apr 1]. http://www.cidrap.umn.edu/news-perspec tive/2020/02/unmasked-experts-explain-necessary-respiratory-protection -covid-19.

2926. Dick EC, Jennings LC, Mink KA, Wartgow CD, Inhorn SL. 1987. Aerosol transmission of rhinovirus colds. J Infect Dis. 156(3):442–448. https://doi.org /10.1093/infdis/156.3.442.

2927. Gwaltney JM, Hendley JO. 1982. Transmission of experimental rhinovirus infection by contaminated surfaces. Am J Epidemiol. 116(5):828–833. https://doi .org/10.1093/oxfordjournals.aje.a113473.

2928. Brankston G, Gitterman L, Hirji Z, Lemieux C, Gardam M. 2007. Transmission of influenza A in human beings. Lancet Infect Dis. 7(4):257–265. https://doi .org/10.1016/S1473-3099(07)70029-4.

2929. Ashour HM, Elkhatib WF, Rahman MM, Elshabrawy HA. 2020. Insights into the recent 2019 novel coronavirus (SARS-CoV-2) in light of past human coronavirus outbreaks. Pathogens. 9(3):186. https://doi.org/10.3390/pathogens 9030186.

2930. Sandaradura I, Goeman E, Pontivivo G, Fine E, Gray H, Kerr S, Marriott D, Harkness J, Andresen D. 2020. A close shave? Performance of P2/N95 respirators in healthcare workers with facial hair: results of the BEARDS (BEnchmarking Adequate Respiratory DefenceS) study. J Hosp Infect. Article in press [accessed 2020 Apr 1]. https://doi.org/10.1016/j.jhin.2020.01.006.

2931. Jefferson T, Del Mar CB, Dooley L, Ferroni E, Al-Ansary LA, Bawazeer GA, van Driel ML, Nair S, Jones MA, Thorning S, et al. 2011. Physical interventions to interrupt or reduce the spread of respiratory viruses. Cochrane Database Syst Rev. 7:CD006207. https://doi.org/10.1002/14651858.CD006207 .pub4.

2932. Han Q, Lin Q, Ni Z, You L. 2020. Letter to the editor: uncertainties about the transmission routes of 2019 novel coronavirus. Influenza Other Respir Viruses. [Epub ahead of print 2020 Mar 4; accessed 2020 Apr 1]. https://doi.org/10 .1111/irv.12735.

2933. Deng W, Bao L, Gao H, Xiang Z, Qu Y, Song Z, Gong S, Liu J, Liu J, Yu P, et al. 2020 Mar 14. Rhesus macaques can be effectively infected with SARS-CoV-2 via ocular conjunctival route. bioRxiv.org. https://doi.org/10.1101/2020.03.13.990036.

2934. Shaw K. 2006. The 2003 SARS outbreak and its impact on infection control practices. Public Health. 120(1):8–14. https://doi.org/10.1016/j.puhe.2005.10.002.

2935. Chughtai AA, Seale H, Islam MS, Owais M, Macintyre CR. 2020. Policies on the use of respiratory protection for hospital health workers to protect from coronavirus disease (COVID-19). Int J Nurs Stud. [Epub ahead of print 2020 May; accessed 2020 Apr 1]. https://doi.org/10.1016/j.ijnurstu.2020.103567.

2936. Centers for Disease Control and Prevention. 2020 Mar 18. 10 things you can do to manage your health at home. U.S. Department of Health and Human Services; [accessed 2020 Apr 1]. https://www.cdc.gov/coronavirus/2019-ncov/if-you-are-sick/caring-for-yourself-at-home.html.

2937. Centers for Disease Control and Prevention. 2020 Mar 25. What to do if you are sick: steps to help prevent the spread of COVID-19 if you are sick. U.S. Department of Health and Human Services [last reviewed 2020 Mar 25; accessed 2020 Mar 31]. https://www.cdc.gov/coronavirus/2019-ncov/if-you-are-sick/steps-when-sick.html?deliveryName=USCDC_2067-DM23796.

2938. World Health Organization. 2020 Mar 25. Coronavirus disease 2019 (COVID-19) situation report—65. Geneva: WHO; [accessed 2020 Mar 31]. https://www.who.int/docs/default-source/coronaviruse/situation-reports/20200325-sitrep-65-covid-19.pdf?sfvrsn=ce13061b_2.

2939. Neher RA, Dyrdak R, Druelle V, Hodcroft EB, Albert J. 2020. Potential impact of seasonal forcing on a SARS-CoV-2 pandemic. Swiss Med Wkly. 150(11-12):w20224. https://doi.org/10.4414/smw.2020.20224.

2940. Moriyama M, Hugentobler WJ, Iwasaki A. 2020. Seasonality of respiratory viral infections. Annu Rev Virol. [Epub ahead of print 2020 Mar 20; accessed 2020 Apr 1]. https://doi.org/10.1146/annurev-virology-012420-022445.

2941. Altamimi A, Ahmed AE. 2019. Climate factors and incidence of Middle East respiratory syndrome coronavirus. J Infect Public Health. [Epub ahead of print 2019 Dec 6; accessed 2020 Apr 1]. https://doi.org/10.1016/j.jiph.2019.11.011.

2942. Moriyama M, Hugentobler WJ, Iwasaki A. 2020. Seasonality of respiratory viral infections. Annu Rev Virol. [Epub ahead of print 2020 Mar 20; accessed 2020 Apr 1]. https://doi.org/10.1146/annurev-virology-012420-022445.

2943. Lipsitch M. 2020. Seasonality of SARS-CoV-2: will COVID-19 go away on its own in warmer weather? Boston: Center for Communicable Disease Dynamics; [accessed 2020 Apr 1]. https://ccdd.hsph.harvard.edu/will-covid-19-go-away-on-its-own-in-warmer-weather/.

2944. Fox SJ, Miller JC, Meyers LA. 2017. Seasonality in risk of pandemic influenza emergence. PLoS Comput Biol. 13(10):e1005749. https://doi.org/10.1371/journal.pcbi.1005749.

2945. Juzeniene A, Ma LW, Kwitniewski M, Polev GA, Lagunova Z, Dahlback A, Moan J. 2010. The seasonality of pandemic and non-pandemic influenzas: the roles of solar radiation and vitamin D. Int J Infect Dis. 14(12):e1099–1105. https://doi.org/10.1016/j.ijid.2010.09.002.

2946. Lipsitch M. 2020. Seasonality of SARS-CoV-2: will COVID-19 go away on its own in warmer weather? Boston: Center for Communicable Disease Dynamics; [accessed 2020 Apr 1]. https://ccdd.hsph.harvard.edu/will-covid-19-go-away-on-its-own-in-warmer-weather/.

2947. Kwok KO, Lai F, Wei WI, Wong SYS, Tang J. 2020. Herd immunity—estimating the level required to halt the COVID-19 epidemics in affected countries. J Infect. [Epub ahead of print 2020 Mar 21; accessed 2020 Apr 1]. https://doi.org/10.1016/j.jinf.2020.03.027.

2948. Sayburn A. 2020 Mar 25. Covid-19: experts question analysis suggesting half UK population has been infected. BMJ 368:m1216. [accessed 2020 Apr 1]. https://doi.org/10.1136/bmj.m1216.

2949. Kwok KO, Lai F, Wei WI, Wong SYS, Tang J. 2020. Herd immunity—estimating the level required to halt the COVID-19 epidemics in affected countries. J Infect. [Epub ahead of print 2020 Mar 21; accessed 2020 Apr 1]. https://doi.org/10.1016/j.jinf.2020.03.027.

2950. Bao L, Deng W, Gao H, Xiao C, Liu J, Xue J, Lv Q, Liu J, Yu P, Xu Y, et al. 2020 Mar 14. Reinfection could not occur in SARS-CoV-2 infected rhesus macaques. bioRxiv.org. [accessed 2020 Apr 1]. https://doi.org/10.1101/2020.03.13.990226.

2951. Duan K, Liu B, Li C, Zhang H, Yu T, Qu J, Zhou M, Chen L, Meng S, Hu Y, et al. 2020. Effectiveness of convalescent plasma therapy in severe COVID-19 patients. Proc Natl Acad Sci U S A. [Epub ahead of print 2020 Mar 5; accessed 2020 Apr 9]. https://doi.org/10.1073/pnas.2004168117.

2952. Tang F, Quan Y, Xin ZT, Wrammert J, Ma MJ, Lv H, Wang TB, Yang H, Richardus JH, Liu W, et al. 2011. Lack of peripheral memory B cell responses in recovered patients with severe acute respiratory syndrome: a six-year follow-up study. J Immunol. 186(12):7264–7268. https://doi.org/10.4049/jimmunol.0903490.

2953. Kissler SM, Tedijanto C, Goldstein E, Grad YH, Lipsitch M. 2020 Apr 14. Projecting the transmission dynamics of SARS-CoV-2 through the postpandemic period. Science [accessed 2020 Apr 18]. https://doi.org/10.1126/science.abb5793.

2954. Hunter P. 2020 Mar 17. The spread of the COVID-19 coronavirus: health agencies worldwide prepare for the seemingly inevitability of the COVID-19 coronavirus becoming endemic. EMBO Rep. e50334. [accessed 2020 Mar 30]. https://doi.org/10.15252/embr.202050334.

2955. Fung S-Y, Yuen K-S, Ye Z-W, Chan C-P, Jin D-Y. 2020. A tug-of-war between severe acute respiratory syndrome coronavirus 2 and host antiviral defence: lessons from other pathogenic viruses. Emerg Microbes Infect. 9(1):558–570. https://doi.org/10.1080/22221751.2020.1736644.

2956. Adalja AA, Watson M, Toner ES, Cicero A, Inglesby TV. 2019. Characteristics of microbes most likely to cause pandemics and global catastrophes. In: Inglesby TV, Adalja AA, editors. Global Catastrophic Biological Risks. Current Topics in Microbiology and Immunology, vol 424. Switzerland: Springer. p. 1–20. https://doi.org/10.1007/82_2019_176.

2957. Mandl JN, Schneider C, Schneider DS, Baker ML 2018. Going to bat(s) for studies of disease tolerance. Front Immunol. 9:2112. https://doi.org/10.3389/fimmu.2018.02112.

2958. Mandl JN, Schneider C, Schneider DS, Baker ML 2018. Going to bat(s) for studies of disease tolerance. Front Immunol. 9:2112. https://doi.org/10.3389/fimmu.2018.02112.

2959. Benvenuto D, Giovanetti M, Salemi M, Prosperi M, De Flora C, Alcantara LCJ, Angeletti S, Ciccozzi M. 2020 Feb 12. The global spread of 2019-nCoV: a molecular evolutionary analysis. Pathog Glob Health. [accessed 2020 Mar 30]. https://doi.org/10.1080/20477724.2020.1725339.

2960. Cui J, Li F, Shi Z-L. 2019. Origin and evolution of pathogenic coronaviruses. Nat Rev Microbiol. 17:181–192. https://doi.org/10.1038/s41579-018-0118-9.

2961. Grubaugh ND, Petrone ME, Holmes EC. 2020. We shouldn't worry when a virus mutates during disease outbreaks. Nat Microbiol. 5:529–530. https://doi.org/10.1038/s41564-020-0690-4.

2962. Zhang J, Jia W, Zhu J, Li B, Xing J, Liao M, Qi W. 2020. Letter to the editor: insights into the cross-species evolution of 2019 novel coronavirus. J Infect. Article in press. [accessed 2020 Mar 30]. https://doi.org/10.1016/j.jinf.2020.02.025.

2963. Weaver J. 2005. What can nervous Americans do about bird flu? MSNBC, October 18.

2964. Potter CW. 2001. A history of influenza. J Appl Microbiol. 91(4):572–579. https://doi.org/10.1046/j.1365-2672.2001.01492.x.

2965. Nebehay S. 2005. WHO's Chan aims to prepare world for bird flu outbreak. Reuters, September 13.

2966. Abbott A. 2005. Avian flu special: what's in the medicine cabinet? Nature 435:407–9. nature.com/news/2005/050523/full/435407a.html.

2967. Gostin L. 2004. Influenza pandemic preparedness: legal and ethical dimensions. Hastings Center Report 35:10–11.

2968. Public Broadcasting System. American Experience Transcript. 1918 Influenza Timeline. pbs.org/wgbh/amex/influenza/timeline/index.html.

2969. Lezzoni L. 1999. Influenza 1918: The Worst Epidemic in American History (New York, NY: TV Books).

2970. Evans WA, Armstrong DB, Davis WH, Kopf EW, Woodward WC. 1918. Influenza: report of a special committee of the American Public Health Association. Journal of the American Medical Association 71:2068–73.

2971. Hudson C. 1999. Something in the air. Daily Mail, August 21, pp. 30–31.

2972. Lezzoni L. 1999. Influenza 1918: The Worst Epidemic in American History (New York, NY: TV Books).

2973. Traxel D. 1998. Outbreak: the 1918 flu epidemic killed 13,000 Philadelphians in eight weeks. Scientists still don't know what made it so deadly. Philadelphia Inquirer, October 4.

2974. Barry JM. 2004. The Great Influenza: The Epic Story of the Deadliest Plague in History (New York, NY: Penguin Books).

2975. Collier R. 1974. The Plague of the Spanish Lady: The Influenza Pandemic of 1918–1919 (New York, NY: Atheneum).

2976. Crosby AW. 2003. America's Forgotten Pandemic: The Influenza of 1918 (Cambridge, UK: Cambridge University Press).

2977. Torrey EF, Yolken RH. 2005. Beasts of the Earth: Animals, Humans, and Disease (New Brunswick, NJ: Rutgers University Press).

2978. Scanlon B. 2005. Recalling 1918's perilous plague. Rocky Mountain News, November 26.

2979. Evans WA, Armstrong DB, Davis WH, Kopf EW, Woodward WC. 1918. Influenza: report of a special committee of the American Public Health Association. Journal of the American Medical Association 71:2068–73.

2980. 1918. British Medical Journal, December 21 as cited in Billings M. The influenza pandemic of 1918: the public health response. June 1997. virus.stanford.edu/uda/fluresponse.html.

2981. Correia S, Luck S, Verner E. 2020 Mar 30. Pandemics depress the economy, public health interventions do not: evidence from the 1918 flu. SSRN [revised 2020 Apr 13; accessed 2020 Apr 18]. https://dx.doi.org/10.2139/ssrn.3561560.

2982. Cowen T. 2005. Avian flu: what should be done. Mercatus Center at George Mason University: Working Paper Series, November 11.

2983. Kelvin AA, Halperin S. 2020. COVID-19 in children: the link in the transmission chain. Lancet Infect Dis. [Epub ahead of print 2020 Mar 25; accessed 2020 Apr 8]. https://doi.org/10.1016/S1473-3099(20)30236-X.

2984. World Health Organization. 2005. Avian influenza: assessing the pandemic threat, January 1. www.who.int/csr/disease/influenza/H5N1-9reduit.pdf.

2985. Jones L. 2005. America under attack. Men's Health, November, pp. 154–9.

2986. Neergaard L. 2005. Is it time to vaccinate more kids to stop flu's spread? Associated Press, October 5. www.oanow.com/servlet/Satellite?pagename=OAN%2FMGArticle%2FOAN_BasicArticle&c=MGArticle&cid=1031785427827&path=%21features%21.

2987. Massie MK. 2004. Precautions can help prevent flu or ease pain. Pittsburgh Post-Gazette, October 13, p. A6.

2988. Lee PJ, Krilov LR. 2005. When animal viruses attack: SARS and avian influenza. Pediatric Annals 34(1):43–52.

2989. Oxford JS, Bossuyt S, Balasingam S, Mann A, Novelli P, Lambkin R. 2003. Treatment of epidemic and pandemic influenza with neuraminidase and M2 proton channel inhibitors. Clinical Microbiology and Infection 9:1–14.

2990. Massie MK. 2004. Precautions can help prevent flu or ease pain. Pittsburgh Post-Gazette, October 13, p. A6.

2991. Drexler M. 2002. Secret Agents: The Menace of Emerging Infections (Washington, DC: Joseph Henry Press).

2992. Phillips H, Killingray D. 2003. Introduction. In: Phillips H, Killingray D (eds.), The Spanish Influenza Pandemic of 1918–19: New Perspectives (London, UK: Routledge, pp. 1–26).

2993. Zwillich T. 2005. Warnings grow dire on bird flu threat. WebMD Medical News, June 16. www.webmd.com/content/article/107/108562?src=RSS_PUBLIC.

2994. Specter M. 2005. Nature's bioterrorist. New Yorker, February 28, pp. 52–61.

2995. Brown D. 1992. It all started in Kansas. Washington Post Weekly Edition 9(21). March 23–30.

2996. American Samoa Government. Historical calendar. November. www.asg-gov .net/026HISTORICALCAL_NOVEMBER.htm.

2997. American Samoa Government. Historical calendar. November. www.asg-gov .net/026HISTORICALCAL_NOVEMBER.htm.

2998. American Samoa Government. Historical calendar. November. www.asg-gov .net/026HISTORICALCAL_NOVEMBER.htm.

2999. Herda PS. 1995. The 1918 influenza pandemic in Fiji, Tonga, and the Samoas. In: Bryder L, Dow DA (eds.), New Countries and Old Medicine: Proceedings of an International Conference on the History of Medicine and Health (Auckland, New Zealand: Pyramid Press, pp. 46–53).

3000. American Samoa Government. Historical calendar. November. www.asg-gov .net/026HISTORICALCAL_NOVEMBER.htm.

3001. Herda PS. 1995. The 1918 influenza pandemic in Fiji, Tonga, and the Samoas. In: Bryder L, Dow DA (eds.), New Countries and Old Medicine: Proceedings of an International Conference on the History of Medicine and Health (Auckland, New Zealand: Pyramid Press, pp. 46–53).

3002. American Samoa Government. Historical calendar. November. www.asg-gov .net/026HISTORICALCAL_NOVEMBER.htm.

3003. Ravenholt RT, Foege WH. 1982. 1918 Influenza, encephalitis lethargica, parkinsonism. Lancet 320(8303):860–4.

3004. Phillips H, Killingray D. 2003. Introduction. In: Phillips H, Killingray D (eds.), The Spanish Influenza Pandemic of 1918–19: New Perspectives (London, UK: Routledge, pp. 1–26).

3005. Collier R. 1974. The Plague of the Spanish Lady: The Influenza Pandemic of 1918–1919 (New York, NY: Atheneum).

3006. Brown D. 1992. It all started in Kansas. Washington Post Weekly Edition 9(21). March 23–30.

3007. Knobler SL, Mack A, Mahmoud A, Lemon SL (eds.), 2005. The Threat of Pandemic Influenza: Are We Ready? Workshop Summary (Washington, DC: National Academies Press).

3008. Collier R. 1974. The Plague of the Spanish Lady: The Influenza Pandemic of 1918–1919 (New York, NY: Atheneum).

3009. Knobler SL, Mack A, Mahmoud A, Lemon SL (eds.), 2005. The Threat of Pandemic Influenza: Are We Ready? Workshop Summary (Washington, DC: National Academies Press).

3010. Gulliford A (ed.), 2003. Living in the San Juan Mountains: prospectus on traditional cultural properties on the San Juan National Forest and adjacent public lands. Fort Lewis College Foundation, Center of Southwest Studies. swcenter .fortlewis.edu/inventory/UsfSanJuanTCP.htm.

3011. Porter KA. 1990. Pale Horse, Pale Rider (Orlando, Florida: Harcourt Brace and Company).

3012. Barry JM. 2004. The Great Influenza: The Epic Story of the Deadliest Plague in History (New York, NY: Penguin Books).

3013. Scanlon B. 2005. Recalling 1918's perilous plague. Rocky Mountain News, November 26

3014. Soper GA. 1918. Influenza pneumonia pandemic in the American army camps during September and October, 1918. Science 48:451–6.

3015. Bleakley L. 2005. Bird flu may see NZ close borders. The Press (New Zealand). September 23. stuff.co.nz/stuff/0,2106,3419499a11,00.html.

3016. Louv R. 2005. We are not prepared for a pandemic. San Diego Union-Tribune, October 11. www.signonsandiego.com/news/metro/louv/20051011-9999 -lz1e11louv.html.

3017. GlobalSecurity.org. 2005. Flu pandemic mitigation-social distancing. www .globalsecurity.org/security/ops/hsc-scen-3_flu-pandemic-distancing.htm.

3018. Monroe JA. 2005. Pandemic influenza plan. Indiana State Department of Health. www.in.gov/isdh/pdf.s/PandemicInfluenzaPlan.pdf.

3019. Connolly C. 2006. U.S. plan for flu pandemic revealed. Washington Post, April 16, p. A01. washingtonpost.com/wp-dyn/content/article/2006/04/15 /AR2006041500901.html.

3020. Kennedy M. 2005. No way of knowing effectiveness of pandemic plan until outbreak hits. Vancouver Sun, March 11, p. A4.

3021. Lenehan GP. 2004. Universal respiratory etiquette: a modest proposal. Journal of Emergency Nursing 30(1):3.

3022. Tierno, PM Jr. 2001. The Secret Life of Germs (New York, NY: Atria Books).

3023. Barker J, Stevens D, Bloomfield SF. 2001. Spread and prevention of some common viral infections in community facilities and domestic homes. Journal of Applied Microbiology 91(1):7–21.

3024. Boone SA, Gerba CP. 2005. The occurrence of influenza A virus on household and day care center fomites. Journal of Infection 51(2):103–9.

3025. Couch RB. 1995. Medical Microbiology (Galveston, Texas: University of Texas Medical Branch, p. 1–22).

3026. De Castro AB, Peterson C. 2005. Preventing exposure to influenza: steps health care workers can take. American Journal of Nursing 105(1):112.

3027. Tierno, PM Jr. 2001. The Secret Life of Germs (New York, NY: Atria Books).

3028. Tierno, PM Jr. 2001. The Secret Life of Germs (New York, NY: Atria Books).

3029. Bean B, Moore BM, Sterner B, Petersen RN, Gerding DN, Balfour HH. 1982. Survival of influenza viruses in environmental surfaces. Journal of Infectious Diseases 146(1):47–51.

3030. Boone SA, Gerba CP. 2005. The occurrence of influenza A virus on household and day care center fomites. Journal of Infection 51(2):103–9.

3031. England B. 1982. Detection of viruses on fomites. In: Gerba CP, Goyal SM (eds.), Methods in Environmental Virology: Microbiology Series, vol. 7 (New York, NY: Marcel Dekker Inc, pp. 179–91).

3032. De Castro AB, Peterson C. 2005. Preventing exposure to influenza: steps health care workers can take. American Journal of Nursing 105(1):112.

3033. Cairncross S. 2003. Handwashing with soap—a new way to prevent ARIs? Tropical Medicine and International Health 8(8):677–9.

3034. Morens DM, Rash VM. 1995. Lessons from a nursing home outbreak of influenza A. Infection Control and Hospital Epidemiology 16(5):275–80.

3035. Larson E. 2001. Hygiene of the skin: when is clean too clean? Emerging Infectious Diseases 7:225–30.

3036. Tierno PM Jr. 2001. The Secret Life of Germs (New York, NY: Atria Books).

3037. Teleman MD, Boudville IC, Heng BH, Zhu D, Leo YS. 2004. Factors associated with transmission of severe acute respiratory syndrome among health-care workers in Singapore. Epidemiology and Infection 132:797–803.

3038. Bren L. 2001. Fighting the flu. FDA Consumer 35(1):12–3.

3039. Bakalar N. 2003. Where the Germs Are: A Scientific Safari (New York, NY: Wiley).

3040. Klevens RM, Edwards JR, Richards CL, Horan TC, Gaynes RP, Pollock DA, Cardo DM. 2007. Estimating health care-associated infections and deaths in U.S. hospitals, 2002. Public Health Rep. 122(2):160–166. https://dx.doi.org/10.1177/003335490712200205.

3041. Albert RK, Condie F. 1981. Hand-washing patterns in medical intensive-care units. New England Journal of Medicine 304(24):1465–6.

3042. Tibballs J. 1996. Teaching medical staff to handwash. Medical Journal of Australia 164:395–8.

3043. Pritchard RC, Raper RF. 1996. Doctors and hand washing. Medical Journal of Australia 164:389–390.

3044. Boyce JM. 1999. It is time for action: Improving hand hygiene in hospitals. Annals of Internal Medicine 130(2):153–5.

3045. Boyce JM. 1999. It is time for action: Improving hand hygiene in hospitals. Annals of Internal Medicine 130(2):153–5.

3046. Tierno PM Jr. 2001. The Secret Life of Germs (New York, NY: Atria Books).

3047. Centers for Disease Control and Prevention. [date unknown]. When & how to wash your hands. U.S. Department of Health and Human Services [last reviewed 2020 Apr 2; accessed 2020 Apr 9]. https://www.cdc.gov/handwashing/when-how-handwashing.html.

3048. Tierno PM Jr. 2001. The Secret Life of Germs (New York, NY: Atria Books).

3049. Laestadius JG, Dimberg L. 2005. Hot water for handwashing—where is the proof? Journal of Occupational and Environmental Medicine 47(4):434–5.

3050. Meadows M. 2001. Beat the winter bugs: how to hold your own against colds and flu. FDA Consumer 35(6):11–7. www.fda.gov/fdac/features/2001/601_flu.html.

3051. Tierno PM Jr. 2001. The Secret Life of Germs (New York, NY: Atria Books).

3052. World Health Organization Consultation on Hand Hygiene in Health Care. 2005. WHO Guidelines on Hand Hygiene in Health Care (Advanced Draft). Global Patient Safety Challenge, 2005–2006. who.int/entity/patientsafety/events/05/HH_en.pdf.

3053. Macias AE, Ponce-de-Leon S. 2005. Infection control: old problems and new challenges. Archives of Medical Research 36(6):637–45.

3054. World Health Organization Consultation on Hand Hygiene in Health Care.

2005. WHO Guidelines on Hand Hygiene in Health Care (Advanced Draft). Global Patient Safety Challenge, 2005–2006. who.int/entity/patientsafety/events /05/HH_en.pdf.

3055. World Health Organization Consultation on Hand Hygiene in Health Care. 2005. WHO Guidelines on Hand Hygiene in Health Care (Advanced Draft). Global Patient Safety Challenge, 2005–2006. who.int/entity/patientsafety/events /05/HH_en.pdf.

3056. Starkman D. 2000. Y2K related buying distorts some companies results; concerns about foul ups lead to stock-piling. Wall Street Journal, January 31.

3057. Centers for Disease Control and Prevention. [date unknown]. When & how to use hand sanitizer. U.S. Department of Health and Human Services; [last reviewed 2020 Mar 3; accessed 2020 Apr 7]. https://www.cdc.gov/handwash ing/show-me-the-science-hand-sanitizer.html.

3058. Travers AH, Sosnowski T. 2002. St. Patrick, the organic chemist and Sherlock Holmes meet in the emergency department: a case report. Canadian Journal of Emergency Medicine 4(4). www.caep.ca/004.cjem-jcmu/004-00.cjem/vol-4 .2002/v44-289.htm.

3059. World Health Organization Consultation on Hand Hygiene in Health Care. 2005. WHO Guidelines on Hand Hygiene in Health Care (Advanced Draft). Global Patient Safety Challenge, 2005–2006. who.int/entity/patientsafety/events /05/HH_en.pdf.

3060. Laurance J. 2005. Washing hands defense against bird flu. New Zealand Herald, October 14. www.nzherald.co.nz/author/story.cfm?a_id=93&objec tid=10350158.

3061. Kuchment A. 2003. A matter of hygiene. Newsweek, April 14, p. 49.

3062. Uhlman M. 2005. In a flu pandemic, hygiene is a lifesaver. Philadelphia Inquirer, October 11.

3063. Collier R. 1974. The Plague of the Spanish Lady: The Influenza Pandemic of 1918–1919 (New York, NY: Atheneum).

3064. Kleffman S. 2006. As flu pandemic swept world, locals sought isolation. Contra Costa Times, March 26. contracostatimes.com/mld/cctimes/news/local/states /california/14191058.htm.

3065. Chow CB. 2004. Post-SARS infection control in the hospital and clinic. Paediatric Respiratory Reviews 5:289–95.

3066. Teleman MD, Boudville IC, Heng BH, Zhu D, Leo YS. 2004. Factors associated with transmission of severe acute respiratory syndrome among health-care workers in Singapore. Epidemiology and Infection 132:797–803.

3067. Department of Health and Human Services. 2006. Draft pandemic influenza preparedness and response plan. March. dhhs.gov/nvpo/pandemicplan/.

3068. Hong Kong University Task Force on SARS. 2004. Guidelines on the Use of Facemasks. August 10. hku.hk/uhs/he/flu/facemask.htm.

3069. Chow CB. 2004. Post-SARS infection control in the hospital and clinic. Paediatric Respiratory Reviews 5:289–95.

3070. Chow CB. 2004. Post-SARS infection control in the hospital and clinic. Paediatric Respiratory Reviews 5:289–95.

3071. U.S. Institute of Medicine Board on Health Sciences Policy. 2006. Reusability of Facemasks During an Influenza Pandemic: Facing the Flu (Washington, DC: National Academies Press). darwin.nap.edu/books/0309101824/html.

3072. Teleman MD, Boudville IC, Heng BH, Zhu D, Leo YS. 2004. Factors associated with transmission of severe acute respiratory syndrome among health-care workers in Singapore. Epidemiology and Infection 132:797–803.

3073. Department of Health and Human Services. 2006. Draft pandemic influenza preparedness and response plan. March. dhhs.gov/nvpo/pandemicplan/.

3074. Abbott A. 2005. Avian flu special: what's in the medicine cabinet? Nature 435:407–9. nature.com/news/2005/050523/full/435407a.html.

3075. Goldmann DA. 2001. Epidemiology and prevention of pediatric viral respiratory infections in health-care institutions. Emerging Infectious Diseases 7:249–53.

3076. Bridges CB, Kuehnert MJ, Hall CB. Transmission of influenza: implications for control in health care settings. Clinical Infectious Diseases 37:1094–101.

3077. Cheng CY. 2003. SARS and PPE (part 5). Singapore Medical Association News 35:17–22.

3078. Piotrowski J. 2003. Respiratory etiquette. Modern Healthcare 33(43):13.

3079. Cheng CY. 2003. SARS and PPE (part 5). Singapore Medical Association News 35:17–22.

3080. Cheng CY. 2003. SARS and PPE (part 5). Singapore Medical Association News 35:17–22.

3081. Oldenburg D. 2003. N95 masks flying off shelves, but they offer scant protection. Washington Post, February 15. www.ph.ucla.edu/EPI/bioter/n95masks.html.

3082. Cheng CY. 2003. SARS and PPE (part 5). Singapore Medical Association News 35:17–22.

3083. U.S. Institute of Medicine Board on Health Sciences Policy. 2006. Reusability of Facemasks During an Influenza Pandemic: Facing the Flu (Washington, DC: National Academies Press). darwin.nap.edu/books/0309101824/html.

3084. Abbott A. 2005. Avian flu special: what's in the medicine cabinet? Nature 435:407–9. nature.com/news/2005/050523/full/435407a.html.

3085. Cheng CY. 2003. SARS and PPE (part 5). Singapore Medical Association News 35:17–22.

3086. Cheng CY. 2003. SARS and PPE (part 5). Singapore Medical Association News 35:17–22.

3087. Bridges CB, Kuehnert MJ, Hall CB. Transmission of influenza: implications for control in health care settings. Clinical Infectious Diseases 37:1094–101.

3088. Cheng CY. 2003. SARS and PPE (part 5). Singapore Medical Association News 35:17–22.

3089. Bosman A, Mulder YM, de Leeuw JRJ, et al. 2004. Executive summary: avian flu epidemic 2003: public health consequences. RIVM (Research for Man and Environment) Report 630940004 (Bilthoven, The Netherlands: National Institute for Public Health and the Environment)

3090. World Health Organization. 2005. WHO global influenza preparedness plan. The role of WHO and recommendations for national measures before and during pandemics. www.who.int/csr/resources/publications/influenza/GIP_2005 _5Eweb.pdf.

3091. World Health Organization. 2020. Coronavirus disease (COVID-19) advice for the public: when and how to use masks. Geneva: WHO; [accessed 2020 Apr 7]. https://www.who.int/emergencies/diseases/novel-coronavirus-2019 /advice-for-public/when-and-how-to-use-masks.

3092. Cheng CY. 2003. SARS and PPE (part 5). Singapore Medical Association News 35:17–22.

3093. Uhlman M. 2005. Bird flu threat spurs run on masks: experts say it's hard to tell what's needed to protect against a pandemic. Knight-Ridder Tribune News, October 29. www.bird-flu-symptom.info/news/face-mask/.

3094. Cheng CY. 2003. SARS and PPE (part 5). Singapore Medical Association News 35:17–22.

3095. Cheng CY. 2003. SARS and PPE (part 5). Singapore Medical Association News 35:17–22.

3096. Cheng CY. 2003. SARS and PPE (part 5). Singapore Medical Association News 35:17–22.

3097. Nickerson C. 2005. Europe bracing to battle bird flu: fears heighten of global outbreak. Boston Globe, October 10. www.boston.com/news/world/europe /articles/2005/10/10/europe_bracing_to_battle_bird_flu/.

3098. Cooper S. 2005. Don't fear fear or panic panic: an economist's view of pandemic flu. BMO Nesbitt Burns Inc. bmonesbittburns.com/economics/reports /20051011/dont_fear_fear.pdf.

3099. Branswell H. 2003. Vomiting? The trots? You don't have flu. Toronto Star, January 20, p. E06. www.ctv.ca/servlet/ArticleNews/story/CTVNews /20030114/flu_not030114/Health?s_name=&no_ads=.

3100. Bouchard GA. Watch out for holiday leftovers. University of Alberta Faculty News. www.afhe.ualberta.ca/Index.asp?page=News&news=463.

3101. Cunha BA. 2004. Influenza: historical aspects of epidemics and pandemics. Infectious Disease Clinics of North America 18:141–55.

3102. Bren L. 2001. Fighting the flu. FDA Consumer 35(1):12–3. fda.gov/FDAC /features/2001/101_flu.html.

3103. Bender BS. 2000. Barbara, what's a nice girl like you doing writing an article like this? The scientific basis of folk remedies for colds and flu. Chest 118:887–8. chestjournal.org/cgi/content/full/118/4/887.

3104. Phillips H, Killingray D. 2003. Introduction. In: Phillips H, Killingray D (eds.), The Spanish Influenza Pandemic of 1918–19: New Perspectives (London, UK: Routledge, pp. 1–26).

3105. Bender BS. 2000. Barbara, what's a nice girl like you doing writing an article like this? The scientific basis of folk remedies for colds and flu. Chest 118:887–8. chestjournal.org/cgi/content/full/118/4/887.

3106. Meadows M. 2001. Beat the winter bugs: how to hold your own against colds and flu. FDA Consumer 35(6):11–7. www.fda.gov/fdac/features/2001/601 _flu.html.

3107. Egland AG. 2006. March 23. Pediatrics, dehydration. emedicine.com/emerg /topic372.htm. emedicine.com/emerg/topic372.htm.

3108. Woodson G. 2005. Preparing for the Coming Influenza Pandemic. crofsblogs .typepad.com/h5n1/files/ComingPandemic.pdf.

3109. Bender BS. 2000. Barbara, what's a nice girl like you doing writing an article like this? The scientific basis of folk remedies for colds and flu. Chest 118:887–8. chestjournal.org/cgi/content/full/118/4/887.

3110. Kamienski MC. 2003. Reye syndrome. American Journal of Nursing. 103(7):54–7.

3111. Acha PN. 2003. Influenza. In: Zoonoses and Communicable Diseases Common to Man and Animals, Volume II, Chlamydioses, Rickettsioses, and Viroses (Washington, DC: Pan American Health Organization, pp. 155–71).

3112. Herskovits B. 2005. Popeyes, KFC forge plans in case of bird flu outbreak. PR Week, November 11. prweek.com/us/thisissue/article/527525/popeyes-kfc-forge-plans-case-bird-flu-outbreak.

3113. Palamara AT, Nencioni L, Aquilano K, et al. 2005. Inhibition of influenza A virus replication by Resveratrol. Journal of Infectious Diseases 191(10):1719–29.

3114. Walle T, Hsieh F, DeLegge MH, Oatis JE Jr, Walle UK. 2004. High absorption but very low bioavailability of oral resveratrol in humans. Drug Metabolism and Disposition 32(12):1377–82. dmd.aspetjournals.org/cgi/content/full/32/12/1377.

3115. Roy H, Lundy S. 2005. Resveratrol. Pennington Nutrition Series: Number 7. www.pbrc.edu/education/pdf./PNS_resveratrol.pdf.

3116. Grammaticas D. 2005. Bird flu. Is it the new BSE? Independent, August 28. findarticles.com/p/articles/mi_qn4159/is_20050828/ai_n14899800/print.

3117. Lee PJ, Krilov LR. 2005. When animal viruses attack: SARS and avian influenza. Pediatric Annals, January 2005:43–51.

3118. Karesh W, Cook RA. 2005. The human-animal link. Foreign Affairs 84(4): 38–50. foreignaffairs.org/20050701faessay84403/william-b-karesh-robert -a-cook/the-human-animal-link.html.?mode=print.

3119. Osterholm MT. 2005. Preparing for the next pandemic. Foreign Affairs 84(4). foreignaffairs.org/20050701faessay84402/michael-t-osterholm/preparing-for-the-next-pandemic.html.?mode=print.

3120. Powell J. 2004. Bird flu seen as the next pandemic. Minneapolis Star Tribune, November 16. www.all-hands.net/Article1467.html.

3121. Appleby J. 2005. Economists say avian flu could have huge impact. USA Today, October 6. www.usatoday.com/money/economy/2005-10-06-bird-flu-usat_x .htm.

3122. Osterholm MT. 2005. Preparing for the next pandemic. Foreign Affairs 84(4). www.foreignaffairs.org/20050701faessay84402/michael-t-osterholm/preparing-for-the-next-pandemic.html.

3123. Cooper S, Coxe D. 2005. An investor's guide to avian flu. BMO Nesbit Burns Research, August. bmonesbittburns.com/economics/reports/20050812/avian _flu.pdf.

3124. Branswell H. 2005. Flu pandemic could trigger second Great Depression, brokerage warns clients. Canadian Press, August 17.

3125. Council on Foreign Relations. 2005. Q&A with Laurie Garrett. Foreign Affairs, May 25. www.foreignaffairs.org/background/pandemic/Garrett2.

3126. International Monetary Fund. 2020 Apr. World economic outlook. Chapter 1. The great lockdown. Washington(DC): IMF [accessed 2020 Apr 18]. https://www.imf.org/en/Publications/WEO/Issues/2020/04/14/World-Economic-Outlook-April-2020-The-Great-Lockdown-49306.

3127. Osterholm MT. 2005. Preparing for the next pandemic. New England Journal of Medicine 352(18):1839–42. content.nejm.org/cgi/content/full/352/18/1839.

3128. Branswell H. 2005. Flu pandemic could wreak economic havoc. Canadian Press, October 18.

3129. Reynolds G. 2004. The flu hunters. New York Times, November 7. www.nytimes.com/2004/11/07/magazine/07FLU.html.?ex=1257570000&en=03e105e1ce5a804e&ei=5090&partner=rssuserland.

3130. Osterholm M, Colwell R, Garrett L, Fauci AS. 2005. The Council on Foreign Relations meeting: the threat of global pandemics. Federal News Service, June 16. www.cfr.org/publication/8198/threat_of_global_pandemics.html.

3131. Schwartz R, Bicks M, Chapman S, et al. 2005. Avian flu: is the government ready for an epidemic? ABC News. www.wirednewyork.com/forum/archive/index.php/t-7324.html.

3132. Garrett L. 2005. The next pandemic? Probable cause. Foreign Affairs 84(4). www.foreignaffairs.org/20050701faessay84401/laurie-Garrett/the-next-pandemic.html.

3133. Osterholm MT. 2005. Preparing for the next pandemic. Foreign Affairs 84(4). www.foreignaffairs.org/20050701faessay84402/michael-t-osterholm/preparing-for-the-next-pandemic.html.

3134. Sandman PM. 2005. The flu pandemic preparedness snowball. Peter Sandman Column, October 10. www.psandman.com/col/panflu3.htm.

3135. Walsh B. 2005. A wing and a prayer. Time Asia, September 19. www.time.com/time/asia/magazine/printout/0,13675,501050926-1106457,00.html.

3136. Weintraub A. 2005. The "horrific" economics of avian flu. Business Week, September 19. www.businessweek.com/magazine/content/05_38/b3951011.htm.

3137. Wysocki Jr B, Lueck S. 2006. Just-in-time inventories leave U.S. vulnerable. Wall Street Journal, January 6, p. 1. calnurses.org/media-center/in-the-news/2006/january/page.jsp?itemID=27523122.

3138. 2005. The threat of global pandemics. Council on Foreign Relations Meeting. Federal News Service, June 16. cfr.org/publication/8198/threat_of_global_pandemics.html.

3139. Branswell H. 2005. Pandemic could create serious and sustained food shortages, expert warns. Canadian Press, June 20. mediresource.sympatico.ca/health_news_detail_pf.asp?news_id=7069.

3140. Huff AG, Beyeler WE, Kelley NS, McNitt JA. 2015. How resilient is the United States' food system to pandemics? J Environ Stud Sci. 5(3):337–347. https://doi.org/10.1007/s13412-015-0275-3.

3141. Booz Allen Hamilton. 2006. Influenza pandemic simulation: implications for

the public and private sectors. boozallen.com/media/file/Influenza_Pandemic
_Simulation.pdf.

3142. 2006. Bird flu: the untold story. Oprah Winfrey Show, January 24.

3143. Milbank D. 2005. Capitol Hill flu briefing was no trick, and no treat. Washington Post, October 13, p. A02. www.washingtonpost.com/wp-dyn/content
/article/2005/10/12/AR2005101202250.html.

3144. Homeland Security Council. 2006. National Strategy for Pandemic Influenza
Implementation Plan. May. www.whitehouse.gov/homeland/nspi_implemen
tation.pdf.

3145. Robins B. 2005. If the chickens come home to roost . . . Sydney Morning Herald, September 12. www.smh.com.au/news/business/if-the-chickens-come
-home-to-roost-133/2005/09/11/1126377202189.html.

3146. Atkins T. 2006. U.N. may use "flu-casters" if pandemic hits. Reuters, January
28. www.alertnet.org/thenews/newsdesk/L28274955.htm.

3147. Weintraub A. 2005. The "horrific" economics of avian flu. Business Week,
September 19. www.businessweek.com/magazine/content/05_38/b3951011
.htm.

3148. Schwartz R, Bicks M, Chapman S, et al. 2005. Avian flu: is the government
ready for an epidemic? ABC News. www.wirednewyork.com/forum/archive
/index.php/t-7324.html.

3149. Osterholm M, Branswell H. 2005. Emerging pandemic: costs and consequences of an avian influenza outbreak (webcast). Woodrow Wilson International Center for Scholars, September 19. www.wilsoncenter.org/index.cfm
?topic_id=116811&fuseaction=topics.event_summary&event_id=142787.

3150. Verity R, Okell LC, Dorigatti I, Winskill P, Whittaker C, Imai N, Cuomo-
Dannenburg G, Thompson H, Walker PGT, Fu H, et al. 2020. Estimates of the
severity of coronavirus disease 2019: a model-based analysis. Lancet Infect Dis.
[Epub ahead of print 2020 Mar 30; accessed 2020 Apr 7]. https://doi.org/10
.1016/S1473-3099(20)30243-7.

3151. Osterholm M, Branswell H. 2005. Emerging pandemic: costs and consequences of an avian influenza outbreak (webcast). Woodrow Wilson
International Center for Scholars, September 19. www.wilsoncenter.org
/index.cfm?topic_id=116811&fuseaction=topics.event_summary&event
_id=142787.

3152. Stern A. 2006. Preparing for pandemic: know how to bury your dead. The
Star (Malaysia), February 16. jphpk.gov.my/English/Feb06%2016h.htm.

3153. Osterholm M, Branswell H. 2005. Emerging pandemic: costs and consequences of an avian influenza outbreak (webcast). Woodrow Wilson International Center for Scholars, September 19. www.wilsoncenter.org/index.cfm
?topic_id=116811&fuseaction=topics.event_summary&event_id=142787.

3154. Osterholm M, Branswell H. 2005. Emerging pandemic: costs and consequences of an avian influenza outbreak (webcast). Woodrow Wilson International Center for Scholars, September 19. www.wilsoncenter.org/index.cfm
?topic_id=116811&fuseaction=topics.event_summary&event_id=142787.

3155. Public Health Agency of Canada. 2005. Canadian Pandemic Influenza Plan.

Guidelines for the Management of Mass Fatalities During an Influenza Pandemic. phac-aspc.gc.ca/cpip-pclcpi/pdf.-cpip-03/cpip-appendix-i.pdf.

3156. Jones L. 2005. America under attack. Men's Health, November, pp. 154–9.

3157. Jones L. 2005. America under attack. Men's Health, November, pp. 154–9.

3158. Agence France Press. 2020 Mar 23. Madrid ice rink turned into morgue due to coronavirus. CTV News. [updated 2020 Mar 23; accessed 2020 Apr 7]; https://www.ctvnews.ca/world/madrid-ice-rink-turned-into-morgue-due-to-coronavirus-1.4864644.

3159. Durkin E. 2020 Mar 30. FEMA sends refrigerated trucks to New York City to hold bodies. Politico. [accessed 2020 Apr 7]; https://www.politico.com/states/new-york/albany/story/2020/03/30/fema-sends-refrigerated-trucks-to-new-york-city-to-hold-bodies-1269600.

3160. Armus T. 2020 Apr 3. 'Every day it's getting worse': bodies of coronavirus victims are left on the streets in Ecuador's largest city. Washington Post. [accessed 2020 Apr 7]; https://www.washingtonpost.com/nation/2020/04/03/ecuador-coronavirus-bodies/.

3161. Kilgannon C. 2020 Apr 10. As morgues fill, N.Y.C. to bury some virus victims in Potter's Field. New York Times. [accessed 2020 Apr 12]; https://www.nytimes.com/2020/04/10/nyregion/coronavirus-deaths-hart-island-burial.html.

3162. Davis M. 2005. The coming avian flu pandemic. Tomdispatch.com www.tomdispatch.com/indexprint.mhtml.?pid=13470.

3163. Wilson B. 2005. Grim flu theory: millions could die. Advertiser, January 29, p. 70. theglobeandmail.com/servlet/ArticleNews/TPStory/LAC/20051025/HEALTHPOLL25/TPNational/TopStories.

3164. Pyne C. 2005. Mass graves for bird flu. Sunday Mail, October 30, p. 93.

3165. Priest L. 2005. Pandemic fears moderate, poll says. Globe and Mail, October 25, p. A11.

3166. Cooper S. 2005. Don't fear fear or panic panic: an economist's view of pandemic flu. BMO Nesbitt Burns Inc. bmonesbittburns.com/economics/reports/20051011/dont_fear_fear.pdf.

3167. Olivari N. 2005. Some currency investors debate bird flu mutation. Reuters, October 17.

3168. Cooper S, Coxe D. 2005. An investor's guide to avian flu. BMO Nesbit Burns Research, August. bmonesbittburns.com/economics/reports/20050812/avian_flu.pdf.

3169. Citigroup. 2006. Global portfolio strategist: avian flu. March 9. smithbarney.com/pdf./global_port_strat.pdf.

3170. Quisenberry D. 2005. Remembering the 1918 flu pandemic. Grand Rapids Press, October 30.

3171. Folley A. 2020 Mar 11. Alex Jones promotes toothpaste he claims 'kills' coronavirus; FDA warns it's fraudulent. The Hill. [updated 2020 Mar 12; accessed 2020 Apr 7]. https://thehill.com/blogs/blog-briefing-room/news/487149-alex-jones-promotes-toothpaste-he-claims-kills-coronavirus-as.

3172. Davies P. 2000. The Devil's Flu (New York, NY: Henry Holt and Company).

3173. Levenson M. 2020 Mar 27. Price gouging complaints surge amid coronavirus pandemic. New York Times. [accessed 2020 Apr 7]; https://www.nytimes .com/2020/03/27/us/coronavirus-price-gouging-hand-sanitizer-masks-wipes .html.

3174. Davis B. In Washington, tiny think tank wields big stick on regulation. Wall Street Journal, July 16. mercatus.org/pdf./materials/806.pdf.

3175. Cowen T. 2005. Avian flu: what should be done. Mercatus Center at George Mason University: Working Paper Series, November 11. mercatus.org/article. php?id=1435&print=1.

3176. Osterholm M, Branswell H. 2005. Emerging pandemic: costs and consequences of an avian influenza outbreak (webcast). Woodrow Wilson International Center for Scholars, September 19. www.wilsoncenter.org/index.cfm ?topic_id=116811&fuseaction=topics.event_summary&event_id=142787.

3177. Branswell H. 2005. Businesses need to do continuity planning for flu pandemic, report suggests. Canadian Press, October 11. cbc.ca/cp/business /051011/b1011108.html.

3178. Cooper S, Coxe D. 2005. An investor's guide to avian flu. BMO Nesbit Burns Research, August. bmonesbittburns.com/economics/reports/20050812/avian _flu.pdf.

3179. Cooper S, Coxe D. 2005. An investor's guide to avian flu. BMO Nesbit Burns Research, August. bmonesbittburns.com/economics/reports/20050812/avian _flu.pdf.

3180. Brainerd E, Siegler MV. 2002. The economic effects of the 1918 influenza epidemic. National Bureau of Economic Research, Inc. (Washington, DC: Summer Institute). williams.edu/Economics/wp/brainerdDP3791.pdf.

3181. Council on Foreign Relations. 2005. Conference on the Global Threat of Pandemic Influenza, Session 5: What would the world look like after a pandemic? November 16. cfr.org/publication/9246/council_on_foreign_ relations_conference_on_the_global_threat_of_pandemic_influenza_ses sion_5.html.

3182. Hamilton G. 2005. Surviving the influenza pandemic. Vancouver Sun, August 25.

3183. Berkrot B. 2005. Flu-resistant investments? Try vaccines, gold. Reuters, October 24.

3184. Cooper S, Coxe D. 2005. An investor's guide to avian flu. BMO Nesbit Burns Research, August. bmonesbittburns.com/economics/reports/20050812/avian _flu.pdf.

3185. Cowen T. 2005. Avian flu: what should be done. Mercatus Center at George Mason University: Working Paper Series, November 11. mercatus.org/pdf ./materials/1435.pdf.

3186. Kirby A. 2004. Bird flu's "huge potential risk." BBC News, April 21. www .news.bbc.co.uk/2/hi/science/nature/3643643.stm.

3187. Berkrot B. 2005. Flu-resistant investments? Try vaccines, gold. Reuters, October 24.

3188. Tilney FC. 1916. Commentary during a symposium on poliomyelitis. Long Island Medical Journal 10:469. medscape.com/viewarticle/472896?src=mp.

3189. Sandman PM. 2005. The flu pandemic preparedness snowball. Peter Sandman Column, October 10. www.psandman.com/col/panflu3.htm.

3190. Mackay N. 2005. Warning: this bird could kill. Sunday Herald, August 28. www.sundayherald.com/51482.

3191. Farago A. 2005. History's actors catch a cold. Orlando Sentinel, September 13.

3192. 2005. Relief workers confront "urban warfare." CNN, September 1. www.cnn .com/2005/WEATHER/09/01/katrina.impact/.

3193. 2005. Pandemic project needed, expert says. The Vancouver Sun, May 5, p. A2.

3194. Osterholm MT. 2005. Preparing for the next pandemic. Foreign Affairs 84(4). www.foreignaffairs.org/20050701faessay84402/michael-t-osterholm/prepar ing-for-the-next-pandemic.html.

3195. An Account of the Influenza Epidemic in Perry County, Kentucky. 1919. 8/14/19, NA, RG 200, Box 689 as cited in Institute of Medicine Board of Health. The Threat of Pandemic Influenza: Are We Ready? (Washington, DC: National Academies Press).

3196. Barry JM. 2004. The Great Influenza: The Epic Story of the Deadliest Plague in History (New York, NY: Penguin Books).

3197. Barry JM. 2004. The Great Influenza: The Epic Story of the Deadliest Plague in History (New York, NY: Penguin Books).

3198. Jordan E. 1927. Epidemic Influenza, 1st Edition (Chicago, Illinois: American Medical Association).

3199. Crosby A. 1999. Influenza 1918. PBS American Experience. pbs.org/wgbh/amex /influenza/filmmore/transcript/transcript1.html.

3200. Garrett L. 2005. The next pandemic? Probable cause. Foreign Affairs 84(4). www.foreignaffairs.org/20050701faessay84401/laurie-Garrett/the-next-pan demic.html.

3201. Rodies KE. 1998. That great call: the pandemic of 1918. Nursing and Health Care Perspectives 19(5):204–5.

3202. Crosby A. 1999. Influenza 1918. PBS American Experience. pbs.org/wgbh/amex /influenza/filmmore/transcript/transcript1.html.

3203. Harris G. 2005. Bush plan shows U.S. not ready for deadly flu. New York Times, October 8. query.nytimes.com/gst/fullpage.html.?res=9E07E7DB1F3 0F93BA35753C1A9639C8B63&sec=health&pagewanted=print.

3204. Harbrecht L. 2005. Doctoral student's research brings lessons, insight to a looming pandemic. AScribe Newswire, October 25. newswire.ascribe .org/cgi-bin/behold.pl?ascribeid=20051025.095424&time=10%2023%20 PDT&year=2005&public=0.

3205. Beech H. 2003. The quarantine blues: with suspected SARS patients getting dumped in their backyards, China's villagers rebel. Time Asia, May 19. time .com/time/asia/magazine/article/0,13673,501030519-451009,00.html.

3206. O'Toole T, Mair M, Inglesby TV. 2002. Shining light on "Dark Winter." Clinical Infectious Diseases 34(7):972–83. www.journals.uchicago.edu/CID /journal/issues/v34n7/020165/020165.web.pdf.

3207. Wright D. 2004. Bioterrorism: the new threat of infectious diseases. Science and Technology, October. brynmawr.edu/sandt/2004_october/index.html.

3208. Enserink M. 2004. Influenza: girding for disaster. Looking the pandemic in the eye. Science 306(5695)392–4.

3209. Nordqvist C. 2006. Who should get pandemic vaccine first? The strong, the weak, the young or the elderly? Medical News Today, May 12. medicalnewstoday .com/healthnews.php?newsid=43348.

3210. Branswell H. 2006. Priority urged for youth in pandemic: Top ethicist suggests "life-cycle" principle approach for vaccines. Canadian Press, May 12. hamil tonspectator.com/NASApp/cs/ContentServer?pagename=hamilton/Layout /Article_Type1&c=Article&cid=1147384212873&call_pageid=102042066503 6&col=1112101662670.

3211. Emanuel EJ, Wertheimer A. 2006. Public health. Who should get influenza vaccine when not all can? Science 312(5775):854–5.

3212. Enserink M. 2004. Influenza: girding for disaster. Looking the pandemic in the eye. Science 306(5695)392–4.

3213. Cosic M. 2003. Panic attack. Australian Magazine, May 10, p. 26.

3214. Bollet AJ. 2004. Plagues and Poxes: The Impact of Human History on Epidemic Disease (New York, NY: Demos).

3215. Souter CR. 2005. "Psychology of looting" explained. New England Psychologist, November. masspsy.com/leading/0511_ne_qa.html.

3216. 2002. In the wake of the plague: the Black Death and the world it made. New England Journal of Medicine 247(4):297–8.

3217. Phua K, Lee LK. 2005. Meeting the challenges of epidemic infectious disease outbreaks: an agenda for research. Journal of Public Health Policy 26:122–32. palgrave-journals.com/jphp/journal/v26/n1/pdf./3200001a .pdf.

3218. Kelley A. 2020 Mar 31. Attacks on Asian Americans skyrocket to 100 per day during coronavirus pandemic. The Hill. [accessed 2020 Apr 7]; https://thehill .com/changing-america/respect/equality/490373-attacks-on-asian-americans -at-about-100-per-day-due-to.

3219. Porter R. 1997. The Greatest Benefit to Mankind (New York, NY: W.W. Norton and Company, Inc).

3220. Collier R. 1974. The Plague of the Spanish Lady: The Influenza Pandemic of 1918–1919 (New York, NY: Atheneum).

3221. Crosby A. Alfred Crosby on: influenza's very democratic. Influenza 1918. Public Broadcasting System American Experience transcript. pbs.org/wgbh/amex /influenza/filmmore/reference/interview/drcrosby4.html.

3222. Schoch-Spana M. 2000. Implications of pandemic influenza for bioter-rorism response. Clinical Infectious Diseases 31:1409–13. www.journals .uchicago.edu/CID/journal/issues/v31n6/000949/000949.text.html. ?erFrom=113277705876320080Guest.

3223. Collier R. 1974. The Plague of the Spanish Lady: The Influenza Pandemic of 1918–1919 (New York, NY: Atheneum).

3224. 2002. In the wake of the plague: the Black Death and the world it made. New England Journal of Medicine 247(4):297–8.

3225. Knobler S, Mahmoud A, Lemon S, Mack A, Sivitz L, Oberholtzer K (eds.), Learning from SARS, Preparing for the Next Disease Outbreak, Workshop Summary (Washington, DC: National Academies Press, pp. 116–36). darwin. nap.edu/html./SARS/0309091543.pdf.

3226. Risse GB. 1988. Epidemics and history: ecological perspectives and social responses. In: Fee E, Fox DM (eds.), AIDS: The Burdens of History (Berkeley, CA: University of California Press, pp. 33–66).

3227. Phillips H, Killingray D. 2003. Introduction. In: Phillips H, Killingray D (eds.), The Spanish Influenza Pandemic of 1918–19: New Perspectives (London, UK: Routledge, pp. 1–26).

3228. 2005. Religious conservatives claim Katrina was God's omen, punishment for the United States. Media Matters for America. September 13. mediamatters .org/items/200509130004.

3229. 2005. Hurricane is God's work: Christian extremists. Sydney Morning Herald, September 3. www.smh.com.au/news/world/hurricane-is-gods-work-chris tian-extremists/2005/09/03/1125302770141.html.

3230. Brown J, Martin A. 2005. New Orleans residents: God's mercy evident in Katrina's wake. Agape Press, September 2. www.headlines.agapepress.org/archive /9/22005b.asp.

3231. Collier R. 1974. The Plague of the Spanish Lady: The Influenza Pandemic of 1918–1919 (New York, NY: Atheneum).

3232. Homeland Security Council. 2006. National Strategy for Pandemic Influenza Implementation Plan. May. www.whitehouse.gov/homeland/nspi_implemen tation.pdf.

3233. Collier R. 1974. The Plague of the Spanish Lady: The Influenza Pandemic of 1918–1919 (New York, NY: Atheneum).

3234. Citigroup. 2006. Global Portfolio Strategist: Avian Flu. March 9. smithbarney .com/pdf./global_port_strat.pdf.

3235. Osterholm M, Branswell H. 2005. Emerging pandemic: costs and consequences of an avian influenza outbreak (webcast). Woodrow Wilson International Center for Scholars, September 19. www.wilsoncenter.org/index.cfm ?topic_id=116811&fuseaction=topics.event_summary&event_id=142787.

3236. Osterholm MT. 2005. Preparing for the next pandemic. Foreign Affairs 84(4). www.foreignaffairs.org/20050701faessay84402/michael-t-osterholm/prepar ing-for-the-next-pandemic.html.

3237. Solomon C. 2005. Sims warns of flu pandemic. Seattle Times, October 4. seattle times.nwsource.com/cgi-bin/PrintStory.pl?document_id=2002538085&zsection _id=2002120005&slug=fluforum04m&date=20051004.

3238. Rosenthal E, Bradsher K. 2006. Is business ready for a flu pandemic? New York Times, March 16.

3239. Neergaard L. 2005. Few U.S. companies ready for flu pandemic. Associated Press, December 2.

3240. Sandman PM. 2005. The flu pandemic preparedness snowball. Peter Sandman Column, October 10. www.psandman.com/col/panflu3.htm.

3241. Harris S. 2005. Federal government's role in bird-flu response limited. National Journal, October 21. govexec.com/story_page.cfm?articleid=32616&printerfriendlyVers=1&.

3242. Johnston M. 2005. Bird flu victims may be forced to fend for themselves. New Zealand Herald, October 13. www.nzherald.co.nz/author/story.cfm?a_id=110&ObjectID=10349987.

3243. New Zealand Ministry of Health. 2005. Influenza, avian influenza, pandemic influenza FAQ. Scoop Independent News, September 15. www.scoop.co.nz/stories/GE0509/S00077.htm.

3244. Sandman PM. 2005. The flu pandemic preparedness snowball. Peter Sandman Column, October 10. www.psandman.com/col/panflu3.htm.

3245. Mason M. 2005. Official: preventing pandemic impossible. ABC News, October 15. abcnews.go.com/Health/wireStory?id=1216962&CMP=OTC-RSS Feeds0312.

3246. Sandman PM. 2005. The flu pandemic preparedness snowball. Peter Sandman Column, October 10. www.psandman.com/col/panflu3.htm.

3247. Hawaleshka D. 2005. Bracing for bird flu. Maclean's, March, p.46. www.macleans.ca/topstories/health/article.jsp?content=20050321_102364_102364.

3248. Bialik C. 2005 Jan 13. Just how deadly is bird flu? It depends on whom you ask. Wall Street Journal. [accessed 2020 Apr 12]; https://www.wsj.com/articles/SB110512998255120225.

3249. Gorman C. 2005. How scared should we be? Scared enough to take action. Time, October 17. www.time.com/time/archive/preview/0,10987,1115685,00.html.

3250. De Gennaro N. 2005. Avian flu pandemic real threat, says national expert. Daily News Journal, October 8.

3251. Sandman PM. 2005. The flu pandemic preparedness snowball. Peter Sandman Column, October 10. www.psandman.com/col/panflu3.htm.

3252. New Zealand Ministry of Health. 2005. Ministry of Health flu fact sheet. October 21. xtramsn.co.nz/news/0,11964-4925488,00.html.

3253. Vasquez J. 2006. U.S. govt. bird flu advice: stockpile tuna, milk. CBS 5, March 13. cbs5.com/topstories/local_story_073011212.html.

3254. Leno J. 2006. Late-night political jokes. March 12–18. politicalhumor.about.com/library/bldailyfeed3.htm.

3255. Leno J. 2006. Late-night political jokes. March 12–18. politicalhumor.about.com/library/bldailyfeed3.htm.

3256. U.S. Department of Health and Humane Services. 2006. Pandemic flu planning checklist for individuals and families. January. pandemicflu.gov/plan/pdf./Individuals.pdf.

3257. Robertson J, Robertson R. 2005. Apocalypse Chow: How to Eat Well When the Power Goes Out (New York, NY: Simon Spotlight Entertainment).

3258. 2006. Bird flu: things to know, not fear. USA Today, April 12. usatoday.com/news/opinion/editorials/2006-04-11-bird-flu_x.htm.

3259. 2006. Bird flu: the untold story. Oprah Winfrey Show, January 24.

3260. Avila J, Ramsey M. 2006. Renowned bird flu expert warns: be prepared. March 14. abcnews.go.com/WNT/AvianFlu/story?id=1724801&page=1.

3261. Screenshot of google cache archived at http://ryanschultz.vox.com/library /post/us-consulate-in-hong-kong-backtracks-on-bird-flu-warning-why.html

3262. U.S. Department of Health and Human Services. 2006 Jan. Pandemic flu planning checklist for individuals and families. HHS; http://www.pandemicflu.gov /plan/pdf/individuals.pdf,

3263. Baum D. 2006 Nov 11. State Department simply offers good advice. Greenhammer. http://www.greenhammer.net/2006/week45.htm.

3264. Dreifus C. 2006. Bird flu and you. AARP.34–35.

3265. Smallheer S. 2006. Towns told: no federal help if bird flu strikes. Rutland Herald, May 12.

3266. Woodson G. 2005. Preparing for the Coming Influenza Pandemic (Decatur, GA: The Druid Oak Health Center). crofsblogs.typepad.com/h5n1/files/Coming Pandemic.pdf.

3267. Deutsche Presse-Agentur. 2006 Nov 7. Stockpiling suggested for possible bird flu. Bangkok Post Breaking News. http://www.bangkokpost.net/breaking _news/breakingnews.php?id=114048

3268. Federal Emergency Management Agency. 2004. Are you ready? An in-depth guide to citizen preparedness. August. fema.gov/pdf./areyouready/arey oready_full.pdf.

3269. Dreifus C. 2006. Bird flu and you. AARP. 34–35.

3270. U.S. Environmental Protection Agency. 2005. Emergency disinfection of drinking water. September. epa.gov/safewater/faq/emerg.html.

3271. Owens SR. 2001. Being prepared: preparations for a pandemic of influenza. European molecular Biology Organization Reports 2(12):1061–3.

3272. Kennedy M. 2005. Turning fear into action. Ottawa Citizen, March 9, p. A6.

3273. Association of Avian Pathologists American College of Poultry Veterinarians fact sheet. 2005. Asian bird flu.

3274. Pluimers F (Chairman). 2003. Workshop 4: Control measures and legislation. In: Schrijver RS, Koch G (eds.), Proceedings of the Frontis Workshop on Avian Influenza: Prevention and Control (Wageningen, The Netherlands, at library. wur.nl/frontis/avian_influenza/workshop4.pdf.).

3275. U.S. Department of Agriculture National Agricultural Statistics Service. 2006. Poultry slaughter-2005 annual summary. February. usda.mannlib.cornell .edu/reports/nassr/poultry/ppy-bban/pslaan06.pdf.

3276. 2003. Workshop 4. Control measures and legislation. In: Schrijver RS, Koch G (eds.), Avian Influenza: Prevention and Control. Proceedings of the Frontis Workshop on Avian Influenza: Prevention and Control. The Netherlands 13–15 October. library.wur.nl/frontis/avian_influenza/workshop4.pdf.

3277. Campitelli L, Fabiani C, Puzelli S, et al. 2002. H3N2 influenza viruses from domestic chickens in Italy: an increasing role for chickens in the ecology of influenza? Journal of General Virology 83:413–20.

3278. World Health Organization. 2004. Avian influenza A(H5) in rural areas in Asia: food safety considerations. February 12. who.int/foodsafety/micro/avian2 /en/index.html.

3279. Capua I, Mutinelli F, Marangon S, Alexander DJ. 2000. H7N1 avian influenza in Italy (1999 to 2000) in intensively reared chickens and turkeys. Avian Pathology 29:537–43.

3280. Editorial. 2005. Avian influenza virus: are we prepared? Canadian Medical Association Journal 172:965. cmaj.ca/cgi/content/full/172/8/965.

3281. Food and Agriculture Organization of the United Nations 2005. Animal health special report. avian influenza—questions and answers. www.fao.org/ag/againfo /subjects/en/health/diseases-cards/avian_qa.html.#1.

3282. Dierauf L. Avian influenza in wild birds. U.S. Department of the Interior U.S. Geological Survey. Wildlife Health Bulletin 04-01. www.nwhc.usgs.gov/publi cations/wildlife_health_bulletins/WHB_04_01.jsp.

3283. Marangon S, Capua SI, Rossi E, Ferre N Dalla Pozza M, Bonfanti L, Manelli A. 2003. The control of avian influenza in areas at risk: the Italian experience 1997. In: Schrijver RS, Koch G (eds), Proceedings of the Frontis Workshop on Avian Influenza: Prevention and Control. The Netherlands 13–15 October. library.wur.nl/frontis/avian_influenza/05_marangon.pdf.

3284. Enserink M. 2004. Bird flu infected 1,000, Dutch researchers say. Science 306:590.

3285. World Health Organization, Department of Communicable Disease Surveillance and Response, Global Influenza Programme. 2004. Vaccines for pandemic influenza: informal meeting of WHO, influenza vaccine manufacturers,

3286. McNeil DG. 2004. Experts call wild birds victims, not vectors. New York Times, October 12, p. 6.

3287. Ruef C. 2004. A new influenza pandemic—unprepared for a big threat? Infection 32:313–4.

3288. Sturm-Ramirez KM, Ellis T, Bousfield B, et al. 2004. Reemerging H5N1 influenza viruses in Hong Kong in 2002 are highly pathogenic to ducks. Journal of Virology 78:4892–901. jvi.asm.org/cgi/content/full/78/9/4892?view=long& pmid=15078970.

3289. BirdLife International. 2006. BirdLife statement on avian influenza. April 11. birdlife.org/action/science/species/avian_flu/index.html.

3290. 2004. Flu pandemic could wreck ecosystem. Australia Seven News, December 11 as cited in Davis M. 2005. The Monster at Our Door: The Global Threat of Avian Flu (New York, NY: The New Press, p. 123).

3291. Hulse-Post DJ, Sturm-Ramirez KM, Humberd J, et al. 2005. Role of domestic ducks in the propagation and biological evolution of highly pathogenic H5N1 influenza viruses in Asia. Proceedings of the National Academy of Sciences of the United States of America 102(30):10682–87.

3292. Hulse-Post DJ, Sturm-Ramirez KM, Humberd J, et al. 2005. Role of domestic ducks in the propagation and biological evolution of highly pathogenic H5N1 influenza viruses in Asia. Proceedings of the National Academy of Sciences of the United States of America 102(30):10682–87.

3293. Adler J. 2005. The fight against the flu. Newsweek, October 31.

3294. Sturm-Ramirez KM, Hulse-Post DJ, Govorkova EA, et al. 2005. Are ducks contributing to the endemicity of highly pathogenic H5N1 influenza virus in Asia? Journal of Virology 79(17):11269–79.

3295. Chong J. 2006. Bird flu defies control efforts. Los Angeles Times, March 27.

3296. University of Georgia Southeastern Cooperative Wildlife Disease Study. 2002. Low pathogenicity AI in Virginia. SCWDS Briefs, July.

3297. 2006. Farmers protest against free-range duck ban. World Poultry 22(3):6.

3298. Piller C. 2005. Vietnam officials ban duck, goose farming to staunch bird flu. Los Angeles Times, February 5.

3299. Brown D. 2005. Scientists race to head off lethal potential of avian flu. Washington Post, August 23.

3300. Nstate, LLC. 2005. Minnesota. Netstate.com June 2. netstate.com/states/intro/mn_intro.htm.

3301. Halvorson DA. 1995. Avian influenza control in Minnesota. Poultry Digest, September, pp. 12–19.

3302. Stegeman A (Chairman). 2003. Workshop 1: Introduction and spread of avian influenza. In: Schrijver RS, Koch G (eds.), Proceedings of the Frontis Workshop on Avian Influenza: Prevention and Control. library.wur.nl/frontis/avian_influenza/workshop1.pdf.

3303. Minnesota Agricultural Statistics Service. 2005. Turkeys raised. Minnesota Ag News, January 7. www.nass.usda.gov/mn/tkrsd05.pdf.

3304. Stegeman A (Chairman). 2003. Workshop 1: Introduction and spread of avian influenza. In: Schrijver RS, Koch G (eds.), Proceedings of the Frontis Workshop on Avian Influenza: Prevention and Control. library.wur.nl/frontis/avian_influenza/workshop1.pdf.

3305. Suarez DL. 2000. Evolution of avian influenza viruses. Veterinary Microbiology 74:15–27.

3306. Suarez DL. 2000. Evolution of avian influenza viruses. Veterinary Microbiology 74:15–27.

3307. Easterday BC. 1975. Animal influenza. In: Kilbourne ED (ed.), The Influenza Viruses and Influenza (New York, NY: Academic Press, pp. 449–81).

3308. Minnesota Department of Agriculture. 2005. Poultry Your Way: A Guide to Management Alternatives for the Upper Midwest (University of Minnesota, St. Paul Minnesota Institute for Sustainable Agriculture). www.cias.wisc.edu/pdf/poultryway.pdf.

3309. Bureau of Natural Resources—Wildlife Division. 2000. Wild turkey (meleagris gallopavo). Wildlife in Connecticut Informational Series. January. dep.state.ct.us/burnatr/wildlife/factshts/wldtrky.htm.

3310. Bureau of Natural Resources—Wildlife Division. 2000. Wild turkey (meleagris gallopavo). Wildlife in Connecticut Informational Series. January. dep.state.ct.us/burnatr/wildlife/factshts/wldtrky.htm.

3311. Minnesota Department of Agriculture. 2005. Poultry Your Way: A Guide to Management Alternatives for the Upper Midwest (University of Minnesota, St. Paul Minnesota Institute for Sustainable Agriculture). cias.wisc.edu/pdf./poultryway.pdf.

3312. Halvorson DA, Kelleher CJ, Senne DA. 1985. Epizootiology of avian influenza: effect of seasonal incidence in sentinel ducks and domestic turkey in Minnesota. Applied and Environmental Microbiology 49:914–9.

3313. Swayne DE, Akey BL. 2003. Avian influenza control strategies in the United States of America. In: Schrijver RS, Koch G (eds.), Proceedings of the Frontis Workshop on Avian Influenza: Prevention and Control (Wageningen, The Netherlands, pp. 113–30).

3314. Stegeman A (Chairman). 2003. Workshop 1: Introduction and spread of avian influenza. In: Schrijver RS, Koch G (eds.), Proceedings of the Frontis Workshop on Avian Influenza: Prevention and Control. library.wur.nl/frontis/avian _influenza/workshop1.pdf.

3315. Furtman M. 2006. Waterfowling's tug of war. Minnesota Department of Natural Resources. www.dnr.state.mn.us/volunteer/novdec99/flyway.html.

3316. Alexander DJ. 1993. Orthomyxovirus infection. In: McFerran JB, McNulty MS (eds.), Virus Infections of Birds (Amsterdam, The Netherlands: Elsevier Science Publishers, pp. 287–316).

3317. Alexander DJ. 1993. Orthomyxovirus infection. In: McFerran JB, McNulty MS (eds.), Virus Infections of Birds (Amsterdam, The Netherlands: Elsevier Science Publishers, pp. 287–316).

3318. Hall C. 2004. Impact of avian influenza on U.S. poultry trade relations-2002: H5 or H7 low pathogenic avian influenza. Annals of the New York Academy of Science 1026:47–53. www.blackwell-synergy.com/doi/abs/10.1196/annals .1307.006.

3319. Halvorson DA. 1995. Avian influenza control in Minnesota. Poultry Digest, September, pp. 12–19.

3320. Davis M. 2005. The Monster at Our Door: The Global Threat of Avian Flu (New York, NY: The New Press).

3321. Shortridge KF, Peiris JSM, Guan Y. 2003. The next influenza pandemic: lessons from Hong Kong. Journal of Applied Microbiology 94:70–9.

3322. Stegeman A (Chairman). 2003. Workshop 1: Introduction and spread of avian influenza. In: Schrijver RS, Koch G (eds.), Proceedings of the Frontis Workshop on Avian Influenza: Prevention and Control. library.wur.nl/frontis/avian _influenza/workshop1.pdf.

3323. Swayne DE, Akey BL. 2003. Avian influenza control strategies in the United States of America. In: Schrijver RS, Koch G (eds.), Proceedings of the Frontis Workshop on Avian Influenza: Prevention and Control (Wageningen, The Netherlands, pp. 113–30).

3324. Flesher J. 2005. Low-grade case of H5N1 bird flu found in Michigan three years ago. Associated Press, October 26. curevents.com/vb/archive/index .php/t-26103.html.

3325. 2005. Web focus—avian flu timeline. Nature Web. www.nature.com/nature /focus/avianflu/timeline.html.

3326. Swayne DE. 2003.Transcript of the question and answer sessions from the Fifth International Symposium on Avian Influenza. Avian Diseases 47:1219–55.

3327. FAOSTAT. 2019. Livestock primary. Food and Agriculture Organization of the United Nations; [updated 2020 Mar 4; accessed 2020 Apr 7]. http://www.fao .org/faostat/en/#data/QL.

3328. Whiting D. 2004. Herculean task to clean up Asia's family farms. The Star Online, January 29. forests.org/articles/reader.asp?linkid=28841.

3329. Food and Agriculture Organization of the United Nations. 2004. FAO Recommendations on the prevention, control and eradication of highly pathogenic avian influenza (HPAI) in Asia. www.fao.org/ag/againfo/subjects/en/health /diseases-cards/27septrecomm.pdf.

3330. Food and Agriculture Organization of the United Nations. 2004. Questions and answers on avian influenza; briefing paper prepared by AI Task Force, Internal FAO Document, January 30. animal-health-online.de/drms/faoinflu enza.pdf.

3331. Gilbert M, Wint W, Slingenbergh J. 2004. The ecology of highly pathogenic avian influenza in East and South-east Asia: outbreaks distribution, risk factors and policy implications. Consultancy report for the Animal Health Service of the Animal Production and Health Division of the Food and Agriculture Organization of the United Nations, Rome, Italy, August.

3332. Pitt D. 2020 Apr 10. Industry scrambles to stop fatal bird flu in South Carolina. Associated Press. [accessed 2020 Apr 18]. https://apnews.com /7e284ee45dae602841d246f933fae6ec.

3333. Branswell H. 2005. Penning poultry indoors doesn't eliminate risk of bird flu spread: officials. Canadian Press, August 24. avianflu.futurehs.com /?m=20050824.

3334. MacKenzie D. 2005. Bird flu may have reached Europe. New Scientist, October 10.

3335. 2005. Europe puts poultry indoors as bird flu cases multipy. Agence France Presse, February 7. breitbart.com/news/2006/02/17/060217125003.zx 1q7vqk.html.

3336. Soil Association. 2001. Organic farming, food quality and human health. A review of the evidence. August. soilassociation.org/Web/SA/saweb.nsf/9f78 8a2d1160a9e580256a71002a3d2b/de88ae6e5aa94aed80256abd00378489/$F ILE/foodqualityreport.pdf.

3337. Gilbert M, Chaitaweesub P, Parakamawongsa T, et al. 2006. Free-grazing ducks and highly pathogenic avian influenza, Thailand. Emerging Infectious Diseases 12(2):227–34.

3338. Order of British Columbia. Perry Robert William Kendall. www.protocol.gov .bc.ca/protocol/prgs/obc/2005/2005_Kendall.htm.

3339. Branswell H. 2005. Penning poultry indoors doesn't eliminate risk of bird flu spread: Officials. Canadian Press, August 24. promedmail.org/pls/promed /f?p=2400:1001:::NO::F2400_P1001_BACK_PAGE,F2400_P1001_PUB _MAIL_ID:1000%2C30173.

3340. Centers for Disease Control and Prevention. 2004. Update on avian influenza A (H5N1). April 12. www.cdc.gov/flu/avian/professional/han081304 .htm.

3341. Richmond JY. 1998. The 1, 2, 3's of Biosafety Levels. Centers for Disease Control and Prevention Office of Health and Safety, February 6. www.cdc.gov/od /ohs/symp5/jyrtext.htm.

3342. Centers for Disease Control and Prevention. 2004. Update on avian influenza A (H5N1). April 12. www.cdc.gov/flu/avian/professional/han081304.htm.

3343. Environment, Health and Safety Division: Ernes Orlando Lawrence Berkeley National Laboratory. Biosafety program. lbl.gov/ehs/biosafety/Biosafety_Manual /html./bio__level_3.shtml.

3344. Richmond JY. 1998. The 1, 2, 3's of Biosafety Levels. Centers for Disease Control and Prevention Office of Health and Safety, February 6. www.cdc.gov/od /ohs/symp5/jyrtext.htm.

3345. Environment, Health and Safety Division: Ernes Orlando Lawrence Berkeley National Laboratory. Biosafety program. lbl.gov/ehs/biosafety/Biosafety_Manual /html./bio__level_3.shtml.

3346. Richmond JY. 1998. The 1, 2, 3's of Biosafety Levels. Centers for Disease Control and Prevention Office of Health and Safety, February 6. www.cdc.gov/od /ohs/symp5/jyrtext.htm.

3347. Environment, Health and Safety Division: Ernes Orlando Lawrence Berkeley National Laboratory. Biosafety program. lbl.gov/ehs/biosafety/Biosafety_Manual /html./bio__level_3.shtml.

3348. Stegeman A (Chairman). 2003. Workshop 1: Introduction and spread of avian influenza. In: Schrijver RS, Koch G (eds.), Proceedings of the Frontis Workshop on Avian Influenza: Prevention and Control. library.wur.nl/frontis/avian _influenza/workshop1.pdf.

3349. Cutler GJ. 1986. The nature and impact of layer industry changes. Proceedings of the Second International Symposium on Avian Influenza (University of Wisconsin: U.S. Animal Health Association, pp. 423–6).

3350. Osterholm M, Colwell R, Garrett L, Fauci AS. 2005. The threat of global pandemics. Presentation for the Council on Foreign Relations, June 16. cfr.org /publication.html.?id=8198.

3351. Delgado CL, Narrod CA, Tiongco MM. 2003. Policy, technical, and environmental determinants and implications of the scaling-up of livestock production in four fast-growing developing countries: a synthesis. Submitted to the Food and Agricultural Organization of the United Nations by the International Food Policy Research Institute. July 24. www.fao.org/WAIRDOCS/LEAD/x6170e /x6170e00.htm.

3352. Garrett L. 2005. The next pandemic? Probable cause. Foreign Affairs 84(4). www.foreignaffairs.org/20050701faessay84401/laurie-Garrett/the-next-pandemic.html.

3353. Webster R, Plotkin S, Dodet B. 2005. Emergence and control of viral respiratory diseases. Emerging Infectious Disease. www.cdc.gov/ncidod/EID/vol11 no04/05-0076.htm.

3354. Gilbert M, Wint W, Slingenbergh J. 2004. The ecology of highly pathogenic avian influenza in East and South-east Asia: outbreaks distribution, risk factors and policy implications. Consultancy report for the Animal Health Service of the Animal Production and Health Division of the Food and Agriculture Organization of the United Nations, Rome, Italy, August.

3355. Council on Foreign Relations. 2005. Session 1: Avian flu—where do we stand?

Conference on the Global Threat of Pandemic Influenza, November 16. cfr
.org/publication/9230/council_on_foreign_relations_conference_on_the
_global_threat_of_pandemic_influenza_session_1.html.

3356. Council on Foreign Relations. 2005. Session 1: Avian flu—where do we stand?
Conference on the Global Threat of Pandemic Influenza, November 16. cfr
.org/publication/9230/council_on_foreign_relations_conference_on_the
_global_threat_of_pandemic_influenza_session_1.html.

3357. Shortridge K. 2006. H5N1 "bird flu"—some insight. New Zealand Pharmacy,
April, pp. 23–7.

3358. Woods M. 2001. How to brew flu: put ducks, people, and pigs together. Pittsburgh Post-Gazette, April 29, p. A18.

3359. Rudd K. 1995. Poultry reality check needed. Poultry Digest, December 1995,
pp. 12–20. www.ansci.cornell.edu/poultry/ppapril99.pdf.

3360. Berry W. 1999. Nation's destructive farm policy is everyone's concern. Herald-
Leader, July 11. agrenv.mcgill.ca/agrecon/ecoagr/doc/berry.htm.

3361. Tyson Foods, Inc. 2006. History: timeline. www.tysonfoodsinc.com/About
Tyson/History/Timeline.aspx.

3362. Perdue ML, Swayne DE. 2005. Public health risk from avian influenza viruses.
Avian Diseases 49:317–27.

3363. Zanella A. 2002. Avian influenza attributable to Serovar H7N1 in light layers
in Italy. Avian Diseases 47:1177–80.

3364. Food and Agriculture Organization of the United Nations. 2004. Emergency
Prevention System Transboundary Animal Diseases, Bulletin No. 25 January-
June. fao.org/documents/show_cdr.asp?url_file=/docrep/007/y5537e/y5537
e09.htm.

3365. Linares JA, Gayle L, Sneed L, Wigle W. 2004. H5N2 avian influenza outbreak
in Texas. In: 76th Northeastern Conference on Avian Diseases: June 9–11
(State College, Pennsylvania: Department of Veterinary Science, College of
Agricultural Sciences, Pennsylvania State University, p. 14). www.vetsci.psu
.edu/NECAD/NECADProceedings.pdf.

3366. Van Kerkhove MD, Vong S, Guitian J, Holl D, Mangtani P, San S, Ghani AC.
2009. Poultry movement networks in Cambodia: implications for surveillance
and control of highly pathogenic avian influenza (HPAI/H5N1). Vaccine. 2009
Oct 23;27(45):6345–6352. https://doi.org/10.1016/j.vaccine.2009.05.004.

3367. Alexander DJ. 2007. An overview of the epidemiology of avian influenza. Vaccine. 25:5637–5644.

3368. Veterinary Services; Surveillance, Preparedness, and Response Services;
Animal and Plant Health Inspection Service. 2016. Final report for the
2014–2015 outbreak of highly pathogenic avian influenza (HPAI) in the
United States. U.S. Department of Agriculture [revised 2016 Aug 11;
accessed 2020 Apr 7].

3369. U.S. Department of Agriculture. 2020 Apr 9. USDA confirms highly pathogenic H7N3 avian influenza in a commercial flock in Chesterfield County,
South Carolina. USDA. [accessed 2020 Apr 18]. https://www.aphis.usda.gov
/aphis/newsroom/stakeholder-info/sa_by_date/sa-2020/sa-04/hpai-sc.

3370. Enserink M. 2005. Veterinary scientists shore up defenses against bird flu. Science 308(5720):341.

3371. Capua I, Alexander DJ. 2004. Avian influenza: recent developments. Avian Pathology 33:393–404.

3372. Webby RJ, Webster RG. 2001. Emergence of influenza A viruses. Philosophical Transactions of the Royal Society of London 356:1817–28.

3373. World Health Organization. 2005. Avian influenza: assessing the pandemic threat, January 1. www.who.int/csr/disease/influenza/H5N1-9reduit.pdf.

3374. Enserink M. 2005. Veterinary scientists shore up defenses against bird flu. Science 308(5720):341.

3375. Capua I, Alexander DJ. 2004. Avian influenza: recent developments. Avian Pathology 33:393–404.

3376. Davis M. 2005. The Monster at Our Door: The Global Threat of Avian Flu (New York, NY: The New Press).

3377. U.S. Government Accountability Office. 2017 Apr 13. Avian influenza: USDA has taken actions to reduce risks but needs a plan to evaluate its efforts. Washington: GAO. Report No.: GAO-17-360. [accessed 2020 Apr 7]. https://www.gao.gov/assets/690/684086.pdf.

3378. Zanella A. 2002. Avian influenza attributable to Serovar H7N1 in light layers in Italy. Avian Diseases 47:1177–80.

3379. Swayne DE. 2003. Transcript of the question and answer session from the Fifth International Symposium on Avian Influenza. Avian Diseases 47:1219–55.

3380. Normile D. 2004. Stopping Asia's avian flu: a worrisome third outbreak. Science 303:447.

3381. Ross E. 2004. Asia is the traditional cradle of influenza, although disease can originate anywhere. Biotech Week, February 25, p. 628.

3382. Abbot A. 2004. Canadian bird flu prompts mass cull. Nature News, April 6.

3383. Food and Agriculture Organization of the United Nations. FAOSTAT database. faostat.fao.org/faostat/collections?subset=agriculture.

3384. Osterholm MT. 2005. Preparing for the next pandemic. New England Journal of Medicine 352(18):1839–42. content.nejm.org/cgi/content/full/352/18/1839.

3385. Food and Agriculture Organization of the United Nations. FAOSTAT database. faostat.fao.org/faostat/collections?subset=agriculture.

3386. Sipress A. 2005. As SE Asian farms boom, stage set for a pandemic; conditions ripe for spread of bird flu. Washington Post, February 5, p. A01.

3387. Osterholm MT. 2005. Preparing for the next pandemic. New England Journal of Medicine 352(18):1839–42. content.nejm.org/cgi/content/full/352/18/1839.

3388. Delgado CL, Narrod CA 2002. Impact of the changing market forces and policies on structural change in the livestock industries of selected fast-growing developing countries. Final Research Report of Phase I, International Food Policy Research Institute.

3389. Wallace RG, Bergmann L, Hogerwerf L, Gilbert M. 2010. Are influenzas in southern China byproducts of the region's globalising historical present? In:

Giles-Vernick T, Craddock S, Gun JL, editors. Influenza and public health: learning from past pandemics. London: Earthscan. p. 101–144.

3390. Orent W. 2006. Big chicken farms gave birds the flu. Pittsburgh Post-Gazette, March 19. post-gazette.com/pg/06078/672413-109.stm.

3391. ZhichuuYan J, et al. 2003. Inside China. Pig Progress 19(1).

3392. 2004. Current quotations. Associated Press, February 2.

3393. Shortridge KF. 1982. Avian influenza A viruses of southern China and Hong Kong: ecological aspects and implications for man. Bulletin of the World Health Organization 60:129–35.

3394. Ross E. 2004. Asia is the traditional cradle of influenza, although disease can originate anywhere. Biotech Week, February 25, p. 628.

3395. 2005. Poultry is fastest-growing sector of meat industry: UN expert. Agence France Presse, February 24.

3396. Bellaver C, Bellaver IH. 1999. Livestock production and quality of societies' life in transition economies. Livestock Production Science 59:125–35.

3397. FAOSTAT. 2019. Food and agriculture data. Rome: Food and Agriculture Organization of the United Nations; http://faostat.fao.org/faostat/collections?subset=agriculture.

3398. Delgado CL, Narrod CA. 2002. Impact of the changing market forces and policies on structural change in the livestock industries of selected fast-growing developing countries. Final Research Report of Phase I, International Food Policy Research Institute.

3399. Food and Agriculture Organization of the United Nations (FAO). 1998. Industrial livestock production, concentrate feed demand and natural resource requirements in China Ke Bingsheng. Beijing, China: China Agricultural University.

3400. Food and Agriculture Organization of the United Nations (FAO). 2007b. FAOSTAT. Rome, Italy.

3401. Food and Agriculture Organization of the United Nations (FAO). 1998. Industrial livestock production, concentrate feed demand and natural resource requirements in China Ke Bingsheng. Beijing, China: China Agricultural University.

3402. Simpson JR, Shi Y, Li O, Chen W, Liu S. 1999. Pig, broiler and laying hen farm structure in China, 1996. Proposal to International Agrohydrology Research and Training Center (IARTC) International Symposium, June 25–26.

3403. Osterholm M, Colwell R, Garrett L, Fauci AS. 2005. The Council on Foreign Relations meeting: the threat of global pandemics. Federal News Service, June 16. www.cfr.org/publication/8198/threat_of_global_pandemics.html.

3404. Oshitani H. Communicable diseases in the Western Pacific region. Inaugural Ceremony of the Scientific Advisory Structure of the Centre for Health Protection, Department of Health, Hong Kong. www.info.gov.hk/gia/general/200406/23/ppt2.pdf.

3405. Motavalli J. 2005. Laurie Garrett: are we prepared for avian flu? Interviewed by Jim Motavalli. E Magazine, July–August 2005, www.emagazine.com/view/??2826.

3406. De Haan C, Steinfeld H, Blackburn H. 1997. Livestock and the Environment: Finding a Balance (Brussels, Belgium: European Commission Directorate-General for Development). fao.org/docrep/x5303e/x5303e00.htm.

3407. United National Environment Programme Global Environment Facility. 2003. Protecting the Environment from the Impact of the Growing Industrialization of Livestock Production in East Asia. Working paper. Thailand as cited in Davis M. 2005. The Monster at Our Door: The Global Threat of Avian Flu (New York, NY: The New Press, p. 83).

3408. Tao B. 2003. A stitch in time: addressing the environmental, health, and animal welfare effects of China's expanding meat industry. Georgetown International Environmental Law Review, Winter. findarticles.com/p/articles/mi_qa3970/is_200301/ai_n9187183/print.

3409. Taylor M. 2005. Is there a plague on the way? Farm Journal, March 10.

3410. U.S. Department of Agriculture. Center for Emerging Issues 2000. Overseas investments by U.S. meat corporations what's the future for U.S. exports? Changing Times in Animal Agriculture, July.

3411. Powell J. 2004. A global game of chicken: with lives and billions of dollars at stake, a Cargill processing plant in Thailand has become an industry model in the war against avian influenza. Star Tribune (Minneapolis, MN), November 1, p. 1D.

3412. Powell J. 2004. A global game of chicken: with lives and billions of dollars at stake, a Cargill processing plant in Thailand has become an industry model in the war against avian influenza. Star Tribune (Minneapolis, MN), November 1, p. 1D.

3413. Dominguez A. 2005. Antiviral use on Chinese poultry makes bird flu fight tougher. Associated Press, June 20.

3414. Uyeki TM, Peiris M. 2019. Novel avian influenza A virus infections of humans. Infect Dis Clin North Am. 33(4):907–932. https://doi.org/10.1016/j.idc.2019.07.003.

3415. Philippon DAM, Wu P, Cowling BJ, Lau EHY. 2020 Mar 10. Avian influenza human infections at the human-animal interface. J Infect Dis. [Epub ahead of print 2020 Mar 10; accessed 2020 Apr 6]. https://doi.org/10.1093/infdis/jiaa105.

3416. Centers for Disease Control and Prevention. 2005. Avian influenza infections in humans, May 24. www.cdc.gov/flu/avian/gen-info/avian-flu-humans.htm.

3417. Poirot E, Levine MZ, Russell K, Stewart RJ, Pompey JM, Chiu S, Fry AM, Gross L, Havers FP, Li ZN, et al. 2019. Detection of avian influenza A(H7N2) virus infection among animal shelter workers using a novel serological approach—New York City, 2016–2017. J Infect Dis. 219(11):1688–1696. https://doi.org/10.1093/infdis/jiy595.

3418. Centers for Disease Control and Prevention. 2005. Avian influenza infections in humans, May 24. www.cdc.gov/flu/avian/gen-info/avian-flu-humans.htm.

3419. Lopez-Martinez I, Balish A, Barrera-Badillo G, Jones J, Nuñez-García TE, Jang Y, Aparicio-Antonio R, Azziz-Baumgartner E, Belser JA, Ramirez-Gonzalez JE, et al. 2013. Highly pathogenic avian influenza A(H7N3) virus in poultry workers, Mexico, 2012. Emerg Infect Dis. 19(9):1531–1534. https://doi.org/10.3201/eid1909.130087.

3420. Puzelli S, Rossini G, Facchini M, Vaccari G, Di Trani L, Di Martino A, Gaibani P, Vocale C, Cattoli G, Bennett M, et al. 2014. Human infection with highly pathogenic A(H7N7) avian influenza virus, Italy, 2013. Emerg Infect Dis. 20(10):1745–1749. https://doi.org/10.3201/eid2010.140512.

3421. Uyeki TM, Peiris M. 2019. Novel avian influenza A virus infections of humans. Infect Dis Clin North Am. 33(4):907–932. https://doi.org/10.1016/j.idc.2019.07.003.

3422. Philippon DAM, Wu P, Cowling BJ, Lau EHY. 2020 Mar 10. Avian influenza human infections at the human-animal interface. J Infect Dis. [Epub ahead of print 2020 Mar 10; accessed 2020 Apr 6]. https://doi.org/10.1093/infdis/jiaa105.

3423. Mudeva A. 2005. Bird flu fears haunt Netherlands again. Reuters, September 15. www.jphpk.gov.my/English/Sept05%2016.htm.

3424. The World Factbook. 2006. Netherlands. January 10. www.cia.gov/cia/publications/factbook/geos/nl.html.

3425. Capua I, Alexander DJ. 2004. Avian influenza: recent developments. Avian Pathology 33:393–404.

3426. Enserink M. 2004. Bird flu infected 1,000, Dutch researchers say. Science 306:590.

3427. Enserink M. 2004. Bird flu infected 1,000, Dutch researchers say. Science 306:590.

3428. World Health Organization. 2003. Avian influenza in the Netherlands: disease outbreak reported. Epidemic and Pandemic Alert and Response. April 24. www.who.int/csr/don/2003_04_24/en/.

3429. Koopmans M, Wilbrink B, Conyn M, et al. 2004. Transmission of H7N7 avian influenza A virus to human beings during a large outbreak in commercial poultry farms in the Netherlands. Lancet 363(9409):587–93.

3430. Shortridge KF. 2003. Avian influenza viruses in Hong Kong: zoonotic considerations. In: Schrijver RS, Koch G (eds.), Proceedings of the Frontis Workshop on Avian Influenza: Prevention and Control (Wageningen, The Netherlands. pp. 9–18).

3431. Democracy Now. 2005. Transcript—Mike Davis on The Monster at Our Door: The Global Threat of Avian Flu. Democracy Now. October 19. democracynow.org/article.pl?sid=05/10/19/1332209.

3432. Perry S. 2006. Bird flu: "This thing just continues to march." City Pages, March 22. citypages.com/databank/27/1320/article14219.asp.

3433. Alexander DJ, Capua I, Brown IH. 2003. Avian influenza viruses and influenza in humans. In: Schrijver RS, Koch G (eds.), Proceedings of the Frontis Workshop on Avian Influenza: Prevention and Control (Wageningen, The Netherlands, pp. 1–12).

3434. Daily G, Ehrlich PR. 1996. Global change and human susceptibility to disease. Annual Review of Energy and the Environment 21:125–44.

3435. New Harvest. new-harvest.org.

3436. Webster RG, Wright SM, Castrucci MR, Bean WJ, Kawaoka Y. 1993. Influenza—a model of an emerging virus disease. Intervirology 35:16–25.

3437. Goetz T. 2006. The battle to stop bird flu. Wired, January, p. 111–5.

3438. Macmahon E. 2005. Preface. Journal of Antimicrobial Chemotherapy 55:i1.

3439. Thomas G, Morgan-Witts M. 1982. Anatomy of an Epidemic (Garden City, New York, NY: Doubleday)

3440. MacKenzie D. 2006. Genes of deadly bird flu reveal Chinese origin. New Scientist, February 6. www.newscientist.com/article.ns?id=dn8686.

3441. U.S. Department of the Interior, U.S. Geological Survey. 2005. The avian influenza H5N1 threat. August. www.nwhc.usgs.gov/publications/fact_sheets /pdf.s/ai/HPAI082005.pdf.

3442. Gambaryan A, Tuzikov A, Pazynina G, Bovin N, Balish A, Klimov A. 2005. Evolution of the receptor binding phenotype of influenza A (H5) viruses. Virology 344(2):432–8.

3443. Davis M. 2005. The Monster at Our Door: The Global Threat of Avian Flu (New York, NY: The New Press).

3444. Myers KP, Olsen CW, Setterquist SF, et al. 2006. Are swine workers in the United States at increased risk of infection with zoonotic influenza virus? Clinical Infectious Diseases 42(1):14–20.

3445. Beare AS, Webster RG. 1991. Replication of avian influenza viruses in humans. Archives of Virology 119:37–42.

3446. Ison MG, Mills J, Openshaw P, Zambon M, Osterhaus A, Hayden F. 2002. Current research on respiratory viral infections: Fourth International Symposium. Antiviral Research 55:227–8.

3447. Gray R. 2005. Scientists aim for clone cure to bird flu. Scotland on Sunday, October 23.

3448. Truyen U, Parrish CR, Harder TC, Kaaden O. 1995. There is nothing permanent except change. The emergence of new virus diseases. Veterinary Microbiology 43:103–22.

3449. Perez DR, Nazarian SH, McFadden G, Gilmore MS. 2005. Miscellaneous threats: highly pathogenic avian influenza, and novel bio-engineered organisms. In: Bronze MS, Greenfield RA (eds.), Biodefense: Principles and Pathogens (Norfolk, UK: Horizon Bioscience).

3450. Food and Agriculture Organization of the United Nations. 2004. FAO workshop on social and economic impacts of avian influenza control, Bangkok, Thailand. www.fao.org/ag/againfo/subjects/documents/execsumm_avian .pdf.

3451. Shortridge KF. 2003. Severe acute respiratory syndrome and influenza. American Journal of Respiratory and Critical Care Medicine 168:1416–20.

3452. Christensen K. 2003. Population genetics. kursus.kvl.dk/shares/vetgen/_Pop gen/genetics/8/2.htm.

3453. University of Waikato. Human evolution. sci.waikato.ac.nz/evolution/Human Evolution.shtml.

3454. Food and Agriculture Organization of the United Nations. 2004. FAO workshop on social and economic impacts of avian influenza control, Bankok, Thailand. www.fao.org/ag/againfo/subjects/documents/execsumm_avian.pdf.

3455. Center for Infectious Disease Research and Policy. 2005. WHO: flu pandemic

threat may be growing. CIDRAP News, May 18. www.cidrap.umn.edu/cidrap
/content/influenza/avianflu/news/may1805who.html.

3456. Bevins SN, Dusek RJ, White CL, Gidlewski T, Bodenstein B, Mansfield KG, DeBruyn P, Kraege D, Rowan E, Gillin C, et al. 2016. Widespread detection of highly pathogenic H5 influenza viruses in wild birds from the Pacific Flyway of the United States. Sci Rep. 6(1):1–9. https://dx.doi.org/10.1038/srep28980.

3457. Schuettler D. 2005. Asia's bird flu here to stay, FAO says. Reuters, February 23.

3458. Henig RM. 1992. The flu pandemic. New York Times, November 29, p. 28.

3459. Gadsby P. 1999. Fear of flu—pandemic influenza outbreaks. Discover, January.

3460. BirdLife International. 2004. Avian flu and wild birds. July.

3461. Davies P. 2000. The Devil's Flu (New York, NY: Henry Holt and Company).

3462. Young E. 2002. Hong Kong chicken flu slaughter "failed." New Scientist, April 19.

3463. Piller C. 2005. Vietnam moves to curb bird flu. Los Angeles Times, February 3. www.biotech.wisc.edu/seebiotech/seemail/020705.html.#485.

3464. Osterholm M, Colwell R, Garrett L, Fauci AS. 2005. The Council on Foreign Relations meeting: the threat of global pandemics. Federal News Service, June 16. www.cfr.org/publication/8198/threat_of_global_pandemics.html.

3465. Tangwisutijit N. 2005. Virus shock: bird-flu mutates, adapts to humans. The Nation (Thailand), May 20.

3466. American Association for the Advancement of Science, Atlas of Population and Environment. Meat and fish. atlas.aaas.org/index.php?part=2&sec=natres&sub =meatfish.

3467. Xianglin L. 2004. The livestock revolution and feed demand in China. www .eseap.cipotato.org/MF-ESEAP/Publications/PH-China-2004/03-Chapter-3 .pdf.

3468. Willett W. 2001. Eat, Drink, and Be Healthy: The Harvard Medical School Guide to Healthy Eating (New York, NY: Simon & Schuster).

3469. Webster RG, Bean WJ, Gorman OT, Chambers TM, Kawaoka Y. 1992. Evolution and ecology of influenza A viruses. Microbiological Reviews 56(1):152–79.

3470. Shortridge KF. 1992. Pandemic influenza: a zoonosis? Seminars in Respiratory Infections 7:11–25.

3471. Motavalli J. 2005. Laurie Garrett: are we prepared for avian flu? Interviewed by Jim Motavalli. E Magazine, July/August 2005, www.emagazine.com/view /?2826.

3472. McKenna MAJ. 2004. Animal diseases threaten humans. Cox News Service, March 2.

3473. Webster RG, Bean WJ, Gorman OT, Chambers TM, Kawaoka Y. 1992. Evolution and ecology of influenza A viruses. Microbiological Reviews 56(1):152–79.

3474. Webster RG, Bean WJ, Gorman OT, Chambers TM, Kawaoka Y. 1992. Evolution and ecology of influenza A viruses. Microbiological Reviews 56(1):152–79.

3475. Sompayrac L. 2002. How Pathogenic Viruses Work (Sudbury, Massachusetts: Jones and Bartlett Publishers).

3476. Centers for Disease Control and Prevention. 2006. Epidemiology and Prevention of Vaccine-Preventable Diseases: The Pink Book. www.cdc.gov/nip/publi cations/pink/flu.pdf.

3477. Zambon M. 2006. Influenza, respiratory syncytial virus and SARS. Medical Progress, January. www.medicalprogress.com/dispdf.cfm?fname=Influenza.pdf.

3478. Webster RG, Bean WJ, Gorman OT, Chambers TM, Kawaoka Y. 1992. Evolution and ecology of influenza A viruses. Microbiological Reviews 56(1):152–79.

3479. Ferguson L, Luo K, Olivier AK, Cunningham FL, Blackmon S, Hanson-Dorr K, Sun H, Baroch J, Lutman MW, Quade B, et al. 2018. Influenza D virus infection in feral swine populations, United States. Emerg Infect Dis. 24(6):1020–1028. https://doi.org/10.3201/eid2406.172102.

3480. Silveira S, Falkenberg SM, Kaplan BS, Crossley B, Ridpath JF, Bauermann FB, Fossler CP, Dargatz DA, Dassanayake RP, Vincent AL, et al. 2019. Serosurvey for influenza D virus exposure in cattle, United States, 2014–2015. Emerg Infect Dis. 25(11):2074–2080. https://doi.org/10.3201/eid2511.190253.

3481. White SK, Ma W, McDaniel CJ, Gray GC, Lednicky JA. 2016. Serologic evidence of exposure to influenza D virus among persons with occupational contact with cattle. J Clin Virol. 81:31–33. https://doi.org/10.1016/j.jcv.2016.05.017.

3482. Asha K, Kumar B. 2019. Emerging influenza D virus threat: what we know so far! J Clin Med. 8(2):192. https://doi.org/10.3390/jcm8020192.

3483. Capua I, Mutinelli F, Marangon S, Alexander DJ. 2000. H7N1 avian influenza in Italy (1999 to 2000) in intensively reared chickens and turkeys. Avian Pathology 29:537–43.

3484. Yousaf M. 2004. Avian influenza outbreak hits the industry again. World Poultry, Volume 20, No. 3, pp. 22–5.

3485. Lee S, Kasif S. 2006. The complete genome sequence of a dog: a perspective. BioEssays. 28(6):569–573. https://doi.org/10.1002/bies.20421.

3486. Iwami S, Takeuchi Y, Liu X. 2009. Avian flu pandemic: can we prevent it? J Theor Biol. 257(1):181–190. https://doi.org/10.1016/j.jtbi.2008.11.011.

3487. Lopez-Martinez I, Balish A, Barrera-Badillo G, Jones J, Nuñez-García TE, Jang Y, Aparicio-Antonio R, Azziz-Baumgartner E, Belser JA, Ramirez-Gonzalez JE, et al. 2013. Highly pathogenic avian influenza A(H7N3) virus in poultry workers, Mexico, 2012. Emerg Infect Dis. 19(9):1531–1534. https://doi.org/10.3201/eid1909.130087.

3488. Iwami S, Takeuchi Y, Liu X. 2009. Avian flu pandemic: can we prevent it? J Theor Biol. 257(1):181–190. https://doi.org/10.1016/j.jtbi.2008.11.011.

3489. New Zealand Press Association. 2005. Bird flu expert says virus entering critical phase. Stuff, November 24. stuff.co.nz/stuff/0,2106,3488861a7144,00.html.

3490. Axford RFE, Bishop SC, Nicholas FW, Owen JB (eds.), Breeding for disease resistance in its evolutionary context. In: Breeding for Disease Resistance in Farm Animals (Wallingford, UK: CABI Publishing, pp. ix–xiv).

3491. Olsen CW, Carey S, Hinshaw L, Karasin AI. 2000. Virologic and serologic surveillance for human, swine and avian influenza virus infections among pigs in the north-central United States. Arch Virol. 145(7):1399–1419. https://doi.org/10.1007/s007050070098.

3492. Lee JH, Gramer MR, Joo HS. 2007. Efficacy of swine influenza A virus vaccines against an H3N2 virus variant. Can J Vet Res. 71(3):207–212.

3493. Karasin AI, Schutten MM, Cooper LA, Smith CB, Subbarao K, Anderson GA, Carman S, Olsen CW. 2000. Genetic characterization of H3N2 influenza viruses isolated from pigs in North America, 1977–1999: evidence for wholly human and reassortant virus genotypes. Virus Res. 68(1):71–85. https://doi.org/10.1016/s0168-1702(00)00154-4.

3494. Olsen CW, Carey S, Hinshaw L, Karasin AI. 2000. Virologic and serologic surveillance for human, swine and avian influenza virus infections among pigs in the north-central United States. Arch Virol. 145(7):1399–1419. https://doi.org/10.1007/s007050070098.

3495. Fraser L. 2002. Doctors fear deadly flu virus will lead to new pandemic. Daily Telegraph, September 22.

3496. Slingenbergh J, Gilbert M, de Balogh K, Wint W. 2004. Ecological sources of zoonotic diseases. Revue Scientifique et Technique Office International des Epizooties 23:467–84.

3497. U.S. Department of Agriculture, Animal Plant Health Inspection Service, Veterinary Services, National Animal Health Monitoring System. 2005. Poultry '04 part II: Reference of health and management of gamefowl breeder flocks in the United States, 2004. www.aphis.usda.gov/vs/ceah/ncahs/nahms/poultry/poultry04/poultry04_report_gamefowl.pdf.

3498. Brooymans H. 2004. Organic farms called potential avian flu portal. Edmonton Journal (Alberta), April 4, p. A6.

3499. Frabotta D. 2005. Bird flu's U.S. flyby? DVM Newsmagazine, December 1. www.dvmnewsmagazine.com/dvm/article/articleDetail.jsp?id=274373.

3500. McNeil DG. 2004. Experts call wild birds victims, not vectors. New York Times, October 12, p. 6.

3501. Food and Agriculture Organization of the United Nations Avian Influenza Technical Task Force. 2004. Update on the avian influenza situation. Avian Influenza Disease Emergency News, issue 16. fao.org/AG/AGAInfo/subjects/documents/ai/AVIbull016.pdf.

3502. Blokhuis HJ, de Jong IC, Koolhaas JM, Korte SM, Lambooij E, Prelle IT, van de Burgwal JA. 2000. Effects of environmental enrichment on behavioural responses to novelty, learning, and memory, and the circadian rhythm in cortisol in growing pigs. Physiology and Behaviour 68(4), 571–578.

3503. Ritchie BW. 1995. Avian Viruses: Function and Control (Lake Worth, FL: Wingers Publishing).

3504. Avens JS. Colorado State University. 1987. Overview: Salmonella—what's the problem? Third Poultry symposium Proceedings: Managing for Profit.

3505. Soil Association. 2002. Animal health—the prevention of infectious livestock diseases. Written evidence from the Soil Association to the Royal Society, for the inquiry into infectious livestock diseases. www.soilassociation.org/web/sa/saweb.nsf/librarytitles/1AE72.Html./$file/Animal%20Health%20-.pdf.

3506. Peste des petits ruminants—an emerging plague? New Agriculturist. www.new-agri.co.uk/00-6/focuson/focuson9.html.

3507. Food and Agriculture Organization of the United Nations. 2003. No evidence that SARS stems from farm animals. Interview with Peter Roeder. FAO news release, May 5.

3508. Pesticide Action Network (PAN) Asia and the Pacific. 2004. Avian Flu: One more indictment of unsafe industrial food production. February 20. lists.iatp .org/listarchive/archive.cfm?id=89067.

3509. Pesticide Action Network (PAN) Asia and the Pacific. 2004. Avian Flu: One more indictment of unsafe industrial food production. February 20. lists.iatp .org/listarchive/archive.cfm?id=89067.

3510. Young E. 2002. Hong Kong chicken flu slaughter "failed." New Scientist, April 19.

3511. Food and Agriculture Organization of the United Nations 2004. FAO workshop on social and economic impacts of avian influenza control. Siam City Hotel, Bangkok, Thailand, December 8–9. fao.org/ag/againfo/subjects/docu ments/AIReport.pdf.

3512. National Live Stock and Meat Board. 1991. Facts from the Meat Board: The animal welfare/rights challenge.

3513. Wisconsin Agri-Business Foundation. 1989. Our Farmers Care, p. 15.

3514. Cheeke P. 1999 Contemporary Issues in Animal Agriculture, 2nd ed (Danville, IL: Interstate Publishers).

3515. Cheeke P. 1999 Contemporary Issues in Animal Agriculture, 2nd ed (Danville, IL: Interstate Publishers).

3516. Knobler SL, Mack A, Mahmoud A, Lemon SL (eds.), 2005. The Threat of Pandemic Influenza: Are We Ready? Workshop Summary (Washington, DC: National Academies Press). p. 29.

3517. Knobler SL, Mack A, Mahmoud A, Lemon SL (eds.), 2005. The Threat of Pandemic Influenza: Are We Ready? Workshop Summary (Washington, DC: National Academies Press). p. 29.

3518. Davis M. 2005. The Monster at Our Door: The Global Threat of Avian Flu (New York, NY: The New Press, p. 92).

3519. Environmental Defense. 2000. Factory hog farming: the big picture. Hogwatch, November. www.environmentaldefense.org/documents/2563_Factory HogFarmingBigPicture.pdf.

3520. U.S. Animal Health Association. 2004. Report of the committee on transmissible diseases of poultry and other avian species. www.usaha.org/committees /reports/2004/report-pad-2004.pdf.

3521. Marano N (Moderator). 2004. Avian Influenza Symposium transcript. Centers for Disease Control and Prevention. November 3, p.1.

3522. Byrne D. 2004. Combating emerging zoonoses: Challenges and prospects at community level. Conference on Infectious Disease: European Response to Public Health Risks from Emerging Zoonotic Diseases, The Hague, September 17. medicalnewstoday.com/medicalnews.php?newsid=13681.

3523. Madec F and Rose N. 2003. How husbandry practices may contribute to the course of infectious diseases in pigs. In: 4th International Symposium on Emerging and Re-emerging Pig Diseases (Rome, Italy June 29–July 2, pp. 9–18).

3524. Network for the Prevention and Control of Zoonoses. 2005. How zoonoses are transmitted. www.medvetnet.org/cms/templates/doc.php?id=21

3525. Heasman M, Mellentin J. 2006. Will Europe's BSE crisis bring about a new relationship between food and health? The Centre for Food and Health Studies, March 1. www.euractiv.com/Article?tcmuri=tcm:29-117667-16& type=Analysis

3526. Piper E. 2000. Stop factory farming and end BSE, UK scientists say. Reuters, December 4.

3527. Heasman M, Mellentin J. 2006. Will Europe's BSE crisis bring about a new relationship between food and health? The Centre for Food and Health Studies, March 1. www.euractiv.com/Article?tcmuri=tcm:29-117667-16& type=Analysis

3528. Cornelius de Haan et al. 2001. Directions in Development, Livestock Development, Implications for Rural Poverty, the Environment, and Global Food Security (Washington, DC: World Bank, pp. xii-xiii).

3529. Waltner-Toews D, Lang T. 2000. A new conceptual base for food and agricultural policy: the emerging model of links between agriculture, food, health, environment and society. Global Change and Human Health 1:116–30.

3530. American Public Health Association. 2003. Precautionary moratorium on new concentrated animal feed operations. Association News: 2003 Policy Statements. www.apha.org/legislative/policy/2003/2003-007.pdf.

3531. Duncan IJH. 2005. Science-based assessment of animal welfare: farm animals. Revue Scientifique et Technique 24(2):483–92.

3532. Gruhn P, Goletti F, Yudelman M. 2000. Integrated nutrient management, soil fertility, and sustainable agriculture: current issues and future challenges. Food, Agriculture, and the Environment: Discussion Paper 32 (Washington, DC: International Food Policy Research Institute). www.ifpri.org/2020/dp/2020dp32.pdf.

3533. Brown LR, Flavin C, French H, et al. 2000. The State of the World 2000 (New York, NY: W. W. Norton and Co, pp. 24–26).

3534. McMichael AJ, Haines A, Sloof R, Kovats S (eds.), 1996. Climate change and human health. World Health Organization, World Metereological Organization, UN Environment Programme.

3535. United Nations Development Programme. 2000. Human Development Report 2000 (New York, NY: Oxford University Press).

3536. Gardner G, Halweil B. 2000. Underfed and overfed: the global epidemic of malnutrition. Worldwatch Paper 150, Worldwatch Institute. www.worldwatch.org/pubs/paper/150.html.

3537. Epstein PR. 2000 The WTO, globalization and a new world order. Global Change and Human Health 1:41–43.

3538. Citizens' Environmental Coalition and Sierra Club. 2005. The wasting of rural New York State. newyork.sierraclub.org/conservation/agriculture/Wasting _NYS_Report.pdf.

3539. 2004. The American Heritage Dictionary of the English Language, 4th Edition (Boston, MA: Houghton Mifflin).

3540. American Public Health Association. 2003. Precautionary moratorium on new concentrated animal feed operations. Association News: 2003 Policy Statements. www.apha.org/legislative/policy/2003/2003-007.pdf.

3541. American Public Health Association. 2019 Nov 5. Precautionary morato-rium on new and expanding concentrated animal feeding operations. Wash-ington: APHA; [accessed 2020 Apr 7]. https://www.apha.org/policies-and -advocacy/public-health-policy-statements/policy-database/2020/01/13/ precautionary-moratorium-on-new-and-expanding-concentrated-animal -feeding-operations.

3542. Metheringham J, Hubrecht R. 1996. Poultry in transit—a cause for concern? British Veterinary Journal 152:247–9.

3543. Specter M, Greenman B. Fighting the flu. New Yorker Online. 21 February 2005.

3544. The Humane Society of the United States. 2006. An HSUS report: the eco nomic consequences of adopting alternative production practices to genetic selection for rapid growth in poultry. hsus.org/farm/resources/research/eco nomics/fast_growth_econ.html.

3545. Salvador RJ, Zdorkowski GA. Cheap food that isn't. www.public.iastate.edu /~rjsalvad/cheapfood.htm.

3546. Waltner-Toews D, Lang T. 2000. A new conceptual base for food and agricul-tural policy: the emerging model of links between agriculture, food, health, environment and society. Global Change and Human Health 1:116–30.

3547. Tilman D, Cassman KG, Matson PA, Naylor R, Polasky S. 2002. Agricultural sustainability and intensive production practices. Nature 418:671–7.

3548. Michigan State University. 2004. MSU veterinary college dean named to Institute of Medicine. News release, October 18. newsroom.msu.edu/site /indexer/2177/content.htm.

3549. O'Rourke K. 2004. O.I.E. takes action at annual meeting. Journal of the American Veterinary Medical Association 225:486–7.

3550. National Agricultural Research, Extension, Education, and Economics Advisory Board Meeting and Focus Session. 2004. Protecting our food system from current and emerging animal and plant diseases and pathogens: implications for research, education, extension, and economics. Washington Court Hotel, 525 New Jersey Ave., N.W., Washington, DC. October 27–29.

3551. National Agricultural Research, Extension, Education, and Economics Advisory Board Meeting and Focus Session. 2004. Protecting our food system from current and emerging animal and plant diseases and pathogens: implications for research, education, extension, and economics. Washington Court Hotel, 525 New Jersey Ave., N.W., Washington, DC. October 27–29.

3552. National Agricultural Research, Extension, Education, and Economics Advisory Board Meeting and Focus Session. 2004. Protecting our food system from current and emerging animal and plant diseases and pathogens: implications for research, education, extension, and economics. Washington Court Hotel, 525 New Jersey Ave., N.W., Washington, DC. October 27–29.

3553. Torres-Vélez F, Brown C. 2004. Emerging infections in animals—potential new zoonoses. Clinics in Laboratory Medicine 24:825–38.

3554. Garrett L. 1994. The Coming Plague (New York, NY: Penguin Books).

3555. Cullington BJ. 1990. Emerging viruses, emerging threat. Science 247:279–80.

3556. Lythgoe KA, Read AF. 1998. Catching the Red Queen? The advice of the rose. Trends Ecology and Evolution 13:473–474.

3557. Carrol L. 1872. Through the Looking Glass and What Alice Found There (London, UK: Macmillan).

3558. Cullington BJ. 1990. Emerging viruses, emerging threat. Science 247:279–80.

3559. Mitchison A. 1993. Will we survive? As host and pathogen evolve together, will the immune system retain the upper hand? Scientific American, September, pp. 136–44.

3560. Torrey EF, Yolken RH. 2005. Beasts of the Earth: Animals, Humans, and Disease (New Brunswick, NJ: Rutgers University Press).

3561. Drexler M. 2002. Secret Agents: The Menace of Emerging Infections (Washington, DC: Joseph Henry Press).

3562. Mitchison A. 1993. Will we survive? As host and pathogen evolve together, will the immune system retain the upper hand? Scientific American, September, pp. 136–44.

3563. Shortridge K. 2006 April. H5N1 "bird flu"—some insight. New Zealand Pharm. p. 23–27.

3564. Branswell H. 2006 April 15. Decade after H5N1 virus emerged, experts ponder best-before-date question. Canadian Press. cnews.canoe.ca/CNEWS /Canada/2006/04/15/1535656-cp.html.

3565. Perdue ML, Swayne DE. 2005. Public health risk from avian influenza viruses. Avian Dis. 49(3):317–327.

3566. Oxford J. 2006. The next pandemic? Nature. 444:1007–1008.

3567. Redlener I. 2006. Americans at risk: why we are not prepared for megadisasters and what we can do. New York: Alfred A Knopf.

3568. Wallace R. 2016. Big farms make big flu: dispatches on infectious disease, agribusiness, and the nature of science. New York: Monthly Review Press.

3569. Goneau LW, Mehta K, Wong J, L'Huillier AG, Gubbay JB. 2018. Zoonotic influenza and human health—part 1: virology and epidemiology of zoonotic influenzas. Curr Infect Dis Rep. 20(10):37. https://doi.org/10.1007/s11908 -018-0642-9.

3570. Philippon DAM, Wu P, Cowling BJ, Lau EHY. 2020 Mar 10. Avian influenza human infections at the human-animal interface. J Infect Dis. [Epub ahead of print 2020 Mar 10; accessed 2020 Apr 6]. https://doi.org/10.1093/infdis /jiaa105.

3571. Li YT, Linster M, Mendenhall IH, Su YCF, Smith GJD. 2019. Avian influenza viruses in humans: lessons from past outbreaks. Br Med Bull. 132(1):81–95. https://doi.org/10.1093/bmb/ldz036.

3572. Liu B, Havers FP, Zhou L, Zhong H, Wang X, Mao S, Li H, Ren R, Xiang N, Shu Y, et al. 2017. Clusters of human infections with avian influenza A(H7N9) virus in China, March 2013 to June 2015. J Infect Dis. 216(suppl_4):S548–554. https://doi.org/10.1093/infdis/jix098.

3573. Zhang ZH, Meng LS, Kong DH, Liu J, Li SZ, Zhou C, Sun J, Song RJ, Wu JJ. 2017. A suspected person-to-person transmission of avian influenza A (H7N9) case in ward. Chin Med J (Engl). 130(10):1255–1256. https://dx.doi.org/10.4103/0366-6999.205849.

3574. Centers for Disease Control and Prevention. [date unknown]. Influenza risk assessment results. U.S. Department of Health and Human Services; [last reviewed 2019 Oct 9; accessed 2020 Apr 7]. https://www.cdc.gov/flu/pandemic-resources/monitoring/irat-virus-summaries.htm.

3575. Silva W, Das TK, Izurieta R. 2017. Estimating disease burden of a potential A(H7N9) pandemic influenza outbreak in the United States. BMC Public Health. 17(1):898. https://doi.org/10.1186/s12889-017-4884-5.

3576. Smith R. 2005. Poultry has two central issues. Feedstuffs, November 14, p. 26.

3577. Mabbett T. 2005. People, poultry and avian influenza. Poultry International 44(9):34–9.

3578. Suarez DL, Perdue ML, Cox N, et al. 1998. Comparisons of highly virulent H5N1 influenza A viruses isolated from humans and chickens from Hong Kong. Journal of Virology 72:6678–88.

3579. Capua I, Alexander DJ. 2004. Avian influenza: recent developments. Avian Pathology 33:393–404.

3580. Shane SM. 2003. Disease continues to impact the world's poultry industries. World Poultry 19(7):22–7.

3581. Raju M. 2005. Inside EPA 26(42).

3582. Thaxton YV. 2005. Are you prepared for AI? Poultry, April–May, p. 5.

3583. Benatar D. 2006. The chickens come home to roost. Am J Public Health. 97(9):1545–1546.

3584. Rockeman O, Mulvany L. 2020 Jan 10. Milk processors are going bankrupt as Americans ditch dairy. Bloomberg. [accessed 2020 Apr 7]; https://www.bloomberg.com/news/articles/2020-01-10/distaste-for-dairy-sends-milk-processors-to-bankruptcy-court.

3585. U.S. Government Publishing Office. 2009. Senate hearing 110–693. Hallmark/Westland meat recall. Washington: GPO; [accessed 2020 Apr 7]. https://www.govinfo.gov/content/pkg/CHRG-110shrg44333/html/CHRG-110shrg44333.htm.

3586. Willett W, Rockström J, Loken B, Springmann M, Lang T, Vermeulen S, Garnett T, Tilman D, DeClerck F, Wood A, et al. 2019. Food in the Anthropocene: the EAT-Lancet Commission on healthy diets from sustainable food systems. Lancet. 393(10170):447–492. https://doi.org/10.1016/S0140-6736(18)31788-4.

3587. Chinese Nutrition Society. 2016 May 18. Statement about the official version of the Chinese Resident Balanced Pagoda. Beijing: Chinese Nutrition Society; [accessed 2020 Apr 11]. http://dg.cnsoc.org/article/04/8a2389f-d54b964c80154c1d781d90197.html.

3588. Springmann M, Godfray HC, Rayner M, Scarborough P. 2016. Analysis and valuation of the health and climate change cobenefits of dietary change. Proc Natl Acad Sci U S A. 113(15):4146–4151. https://doi.org/10.1073/pnas.1523119113.

3589. Akhtar A. 2013. The need to include animal protection in public health poli-

cies. J Public Health Policy. 34(4):549–559. https://dx.doi.org/10.1057/jphp
.2013.29.

3590. Dodek P. 2004. Diabetes and other comorbid conditions were associated with
a poor outcome in SARS. ACP J Club. 140(1):19. https://doi.org/10.7326/ACPJC
-2004-140-1-019.

3591. Rivers CM, Majumder MS, Lofgren ET. 2016. Risks of death and severe
disease in patients with Middle East respiratory syndrome coronavirus,
2012–2015. Am J Epidemiol. 184(6):460–464. https://doi.org/10.1093/aje
/kww013.

3592. Simonnet A, Chetboun M, Poissy J, Raverdy V, Noulette J, Duhamel A,
Labreuche J, Mathieu D, Pattou F, Jourdain M, et al. 2020. High prevalence
of obesity in severe acute respiratory syndrome coronavirus-2 (SARS-CoV-2)
requiring invasive mechanical ventilation. Obesity. [Epub ahead of print 2020
Apr 9; accessed 2020 Apr 18]. https://doi.org/10.1002/oby.22831.

3593. Yang J, Zheng Y, Gou X, Pu K, Chen Z, Guo Q, Ji R, Wang H, Wang Y,
Zhou Y. 2020. Prevalence of comorbidities in the novel Wuhan coronavirus
(COVID-19) infection: a systematic review and meta-analysis. Int J Infect Dis.
[Epub ahead of print 2020 Mar 12; accessed 2020 Mar 31]. https://doi.org/10
.1016/j.ijid.2020.03.017.

3594. Greger M. 2015. How not to die. New York: Flatiron Books.

3595. Walla K. 2019 June. Meat in the middle: blended options join eaters in sustainability. Washington(DC): Foodtank; [accessed 2020 Apr 7]. https://foodtank
.com/news/2019/06/meat-in-the-middle-blended-options-join-eaters-in
-sustainability/.

3596. Shanker D, Mulvany L. 2019 Aug 12. Pork giant Smithfield pushes into the
market for plant protein. Bloomberg. [accessed 2020 Apr 7]; https://www
.bloomberg.com/news/articles/2019-08-12/pork-giant-smithfield-pushes-into
-the-market-for-plant-protein.

3597. Dunkin'. 2019 Oct 21. The story behind our Beyond Sausage® sandwich. DD
IP Holder LLC and BR IP Holder LLC; [accessed 2020 Apr 7]. https://news
.dunkindonuts.com/blog/dunkin-beyond-meat-sausage-breakfast.

3598. The Good Food Institute. 2020. Plant-based market overview. Washington: GFI [accessed 2020 Apr 7]. https://www.gfi.org/marketresearch?utm
_source=blog&utm_medium=website&utm_campaign=marketresearch.

3599. Quorn Foods. 2018 Nov 15. The world's biggest meat alternative production facility opens in the heart of the North East. Stokesly(United Kingdom):
Quorn; [accessed 2020 Apr 7]. https://www.quorn.co.uk/company/press/world's
-biggest-meat-alternative-production-facility-opens.

3600. Duewer LA, Krause KR, Nelson KE. 1993 Oct. U.S. poultry and red meat
consumption, prices, spreads, and margins. U.S. Department of Agriculture.
Report No.: 684.

3601. Churchill W. 1932. Fifty years hence. Popular Mechanics. [accessed 2020 Apr 7].
http://rolandanderson.se/Winston_Churchill/Fifty_Years_Hence.php.

3602. Tuomisto HL, de Mattos MJT. 2011. Environmental impacts of cultured meat production. Environ Sci Technol. 45(14):6117–46123. https://doi.org/10.1021/es200130u.

3603. Bhat ZF, Kumar S, Bhat HF. 2017. In vitro meat: a future animal-free harvest. Crit Rev Food Sci Nutr. 57(4):782–789. https://doi.org/10.1080/10408398.2014.924899.

3604. Shapiro P. 2018. Clean meat: how growing meat without animals will revolutionize dinner and the world. New York: Simon & Schuster.

3605. U.S. Food and Drug Administration. NARMS integrated report: 2012–2013. The National Antimicrobial Resistance Monitoring System: enteric bacteria. FDA; [accessed 2020 Apr 7]. https://www.fda.gov/media/92769/download.

3606. Benatar D. 2006. The chickens come home to roost. Am J Public Health. 97(9):1545–1546.

3607. Torrey EF, Yolken RH. 2005. Beasts of the Earth: Animals, Humans, and Disease (New Brunswick, NJ: Rutgers University Press).

3608. 1997. Mad cow outbreak may have been caused by animal rendering plants. New York Times News Service, March 11.

3609. Center for Food Safety. History of rendering: cattle cannibalism in the USA. centerforfoodsafety.org/page267.cfm.

3610. Frist B. 2005. The threat of avian flu. Washington Times, September 29. www.washtimes.com/op-ed/20050928-084420-7052r.htm.

3611. 2005. Bird flu may be more deadly than tsunami. Associated Press, October 24.

3612. Kennedy M. 2005. Bird flu could kill millions: global pandemic warning from WHO. "We're not crying wolf. There is a wolf. We just don't know when it's coming." Gazette (Montreal), March 9, p. A1.

3613. Center for Infectious Disease Research and Policy. 2005. Foreign Affairs focuses on pandemic threat. CIDRAP News, June 10.

3614. Kennedy M. 2005. Bird flu could kill millions: global pandemic warning from WHO. "We're not crying wolf. There is a wolf. We just don't know when it's coming." Gazette (Montreal), March 9, p. A1.

About the Author

A founding member and Fellow of the American College of Lifestyle Medicine, Michael Greger, MD, is a physician, *New York Times* bestselling author, and internationally recognized speaker on nutrition, food safety, and public health issues. He has lectured at the Conference on World Affairs, testified before Congress and was invited as an expert witness in the defense of Oprah Winfrey in the infamous "meat defamation" trial. In 2017, Dr Greger was honored with the ACLM Lifestyle Medicine Trailblazer Award. He is a graduate of Cornell University School of Agriculture and Tufts University School of Medicine. His first book *How Not to Die* became an instant *New York Times* bestseller. He has videos on more than 2,000 health topics freely available at NutritionFacts.org, with new videos and articles uploaded every day.